DERMATOPATHOLOGY IN SYSTEMIC DISEASE

DERMATOPATHOLOGY IN SYSTEMIC DISEASE

Bruce R. Smoller, M.D.

Professor of Pathology and Dermatology
Director, Dermatopathology Division
University of Arkansas for Medical Sciences
Little Rock, Arkansas

Thomas D. Horn, M.D.

Professor and Chair of Dermatology
Professor of Pathology
University of Arkansas for Medical Sciences
Little Rock, Arkansas

OXFORD
UNIVERSITY PRESS
2001

OXFORD
UNIVERSITY PRESS

Oxford   New York
Athens   Auckland   Bangkok   Bogotá   Buenos Aires   Calcutta
Cape Town   Chennai   Dar es Salaam   Delhi   Florence   Hong Kong   Istanbul
Karachi   Kuala Lumpur   Madrid   Melbourne   Mexico City   Mumbai
Nairobi   Paris   São Paulo   Shanghai   Singapore   Taipei   Tokyo   Toronto   Warsaw

and associated companies in
Berlin   Ibadan

Library of Congress Cataloging-in-Publication Data
Smoller, Bruce R.
Dermatopathology in systemic disease /
Bruce R. Smoller, Thomas D. Horn.
p. ; cm.   Includes bibliographical references and index.
ISBN 0-19-513038-3 (cloth)
1. Cutaneous manifestations of general diseases.
I. Horn, Thomas D. II.
Title.
[DNLM: 1. Skin Manifestations.
2. Skin—pathology.
WR 143 S666d 2001]
RL100.S565 2001   616.5'07—dc21   00-044610

The science of medicine is a rapidly changing field. As new research and clinical experience broaden our knowledge, changes in treatment and drug therapy do occur. The author and the publisher of this work have checked with sources believed to be reliable in their efforts to provide information that is accurate and complete, and in accordance with the standards accepted at the time of publication. However, in light of the possibility of human error or changes in the practice of medicine, neither the author, nor the publisher, nor any other party who has been involved in the preparation or publication of this work warrants that the information contained herein is in every respect accurate or complete. Readers are encouraged to confirm the information contained herein with other reliable sources, and are strongly advised to check the product information sheet provided by the pharmaceutical company for each drug they plan to administer.

1 3 5 7 9 8 6 4 2
Printed in Hong Kong
on acid-free paper

PREFACE

Dermatopathology is a subspecialty within the fields of dermatology and pathology that often confounds the general practitioner. This is, at least in part, due to the complicated and nonintuitive nomenclature. Most textbooks in the field are arranged by one of two organizational schemes. Some books categorize diseases by histologic patterns, which is very helpful for pathologists who can access diseases by simple observation. These schemes do not offer any understanding of disease processes within the context of a patient's medical problems, but allow diagnosticians to compare histologic patterns in order to arrive at a diagnosis. Other texts are arranged in schemes based on clinical grouping of diseases. These books are often helpful for clinicians who have a firm knowledge of dermatology, but may fall short for the pathologist who is not trained specifically in the field.

This textbook is organized by systemic disease processes, presenting the cutaneous manifestations associated with different systemic diseases and conditions. It is the authors' hope that this textbook will serve as an ancillary volume that will supplement other, more comprehensive dermatopathology textbooks by providing a focus on the clinical content in which biopsy results must be interpreted. Pathologists confronted with a patient who has a certain underlying systemic disease and has undergone a skin biopsy will be able to find cutaneous diseases that have been associated with that underlying condition. Diseases limited to the skin are not addressed in this volume. Diagnosticians should be able to cross-reference information regarding the patient's overall medical condition with histologic changes found on skin biopsy specimens.

Little Rock, Arkansas

B.R.S.
T.D.H.

CONTENTS

For my wife, Laura, my two wonderful sons, Jason and Gabey, and my parents, Bobby and Mark, without whom none of this would be worth doing.

B.R.S.

To Richard Rosen and Margarete Horn, with gratitude.

T.D.H.

The authors thank their mentors, Drs. N. Scott McNutt, Antoinette Hood, and Evan Farmer for all they have done for us, professionally and personally, over the years.

Systemic Diseases Involving the Skin and Multiple Internal Organ Systems

Lupus Erythematosus

Discoid Lupus Erythematosus

Epidemiology. Discoid lesions may occur as an isolated condition in patients with discoid lupus erythematosus (DLE) or as a cutaneous manifestation in some patients with systemic lupus erythematosus (SLE). In total, approximately 15%–25% of patients with SLE will have discoid lesions [1, 2]. Approximately 5% of patients with DLE will ultimately progress to systemic involvement and be reclassified as having SLE [3, 4].

Cutaneous Features. Discoid lupus erythematosus has been divided into localized and diffuse disease based on involvement of the head and neck alone or in addition to disease below the neck [2, 5]. Discoid lesions are present in approximately 15%–25% of patients with SLE [1, 2].

The classic discoid lesion seen in lupus erythematosus is a discrete, erythematous, round plaque with an adherent thick, hyperkeratotic scale. The epidermis underlying the scale is atrophic. Follicular plugging, scarring, and mottled pigmentation are often present [6]. The face, ears, and scalp are the most commonly affected sites. Scalp involvement may result in scarring alopecia. The lips, tongue, and oral mucosa can also be involved. Most eruptions are asymptomatic. Koebnerization is reported [7].

Rare variants of DLE include verrucous or hypertrophic lupus erythematosus, which is more commonly seen on the forearms, an acral variant, and tumid lupus erythematosus, which appears as indurated, edematous plaques lacking surface changes on the face or trunk [7].

Associated Disorders. Patients classified as having DLE, by definition, do not demonstrate any systemic signs and symptoms of lupus erythematosus.

Histologic Features. It is virtually impossible to differentiate the type of lupus erythematosus based solely on histologic criteria. Although there are studies that have attempted to make such distinctions, most investigators find that the overlap in changes is too great to allow accurate discrimination [6]. Histologic changes of DLE include hyperkeratosis and follicular plugging. The epidermis is initially of normal thickness, but as the lesions progress epidermal atrophy may become prominent (Fig. 1–1). Thickening of the basement membrane zone of the epidermis and hair follicles may be apparent in well-developed lesions (Fig. 1–2). An interface dermatitis is present, with lymphocytes present within the epidermis, often in proximity to dying keratinocytes. Basal vacuolization is often extensive (Fig. 1–3). There is a superficial and deep perivascular lymphohistiocytic inflammatory infiltrate within the dermis. A similar infiltrate is seen within and around cutaneous appendages (Fig. 1–4). Plasma cells may be present, but eosinophils are extremely uncommon. Vessels within the superficial dermis are often dilated, and slight extravasation of erythrocytes may be present [6]. Mucin is present in small amounts within the reticular dermis. It has been suggested that the presence of basement membrane thickening, dermal colloid bodies, atrophy of pilosebaceous units, and periappendageal inflammation are all more commonly seen in DLE than in subacute cutaneous lupus erythematosus (SCLE) [8].

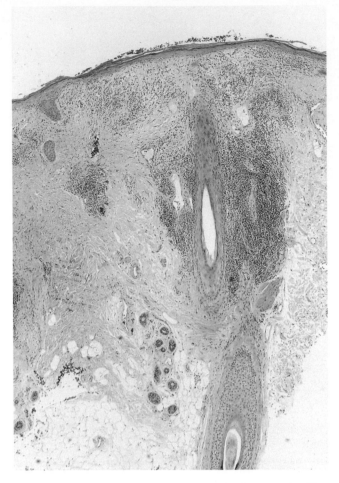

Fig. 1–1. Discoid lupus erythematosus is characterized by an interface dermatitis, follicular plugging, and superficial and deep perivascular and perifollicular inflammatory infiltrates.

The following entities must be considered in the histologic differential diagnosis of DLE:

- Dermatomyositis
- Graft-versus-host disease
- Lichen planus
- Lymphocytic infiltrate of Jessner
- Mixed connective tissue disease
- Polymorphous light eruption
- Subacute cutaneous lupus erythematosus
- Systemic lupus erythematosus

Tumid lupus erythematosus is characterized primarily by mucin deposition in the reticular dermis. Interface changes are minimal to absent, and inflammation is generally less conspicuous than in samples of DLE.

Verrucous lupus erythematosus demonstrates extensive epidermal hyperplasia and acanthosis with in-

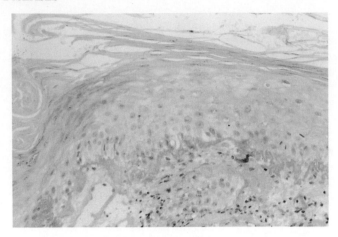

Fig. 1–2. After diastase digestion stain reveals thickening of the basement membrane zone in a well-established plaque of discoid lupus erythematosus.

terface changes, often resembling pseudoepitheliomatous hyperplasia, keratoacanthoma, or squamous cell carcinoma. Basement membrane thickening and mucin deposition are often less pronounced than in classic DLE [7]. It may be difficult to distinguish some cases of verrucous lupus erythematosus from hypertrophic lichen planus. In most cases, however, the dermal inflammatory infiltrate is more confluent in lichen planus.

Special Studies. For DLE, direct immunofluorescence demonstrates stippled, or thready, granular deposits of IgG, IgM, and/or IgA and, in more than 90% of skin from lesional biopsies, complement along the dermal–epidermal junction. Sun-exposed, clinically normal skin and non-sun-exposed, clinically normal skin do not demonstrate immunoglobulin deposition [9]. Antibodies directed against the membrane attack com-

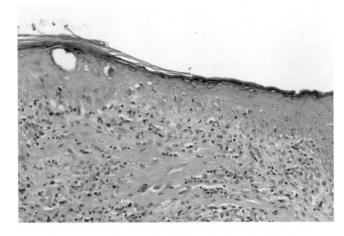

Fig. 1–3. An interface inflammatory reaction leads to epidermal atrophy and basal vacuolization in discoid lupus erythematosus.

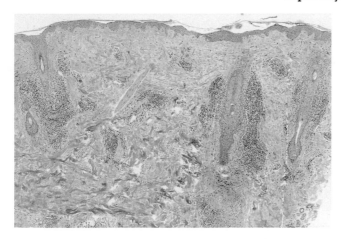

Fig. 1–4. The inflammatory reaction in lupus erythematosus is localized around dermal vessels and cutaneous appendages in the superficial and deep portions of the dermis.

plex (C5–C9) are also found along the dermal–epidermal junction in affected skin from patients with DLE. They are seen in up to 76% of affected skin [10, 11]. The deposition of immunoglobulins has been shown to be associated with disruption of collagen IV and collagen VII in affected skin [12]. A periodic acid–Schiff stain may be helpful in highlighting the thickening of the basement membrane in some cases.

Pathogenesis. Epidermal keratinocytes demonstrate upregulation of intracellular adhesion molecule 1, and lymphocytes in the dermis express leukocyte function-associated antigen 2. The interaction of these two molecules may play a role in target/effector recognition in cutaneous lupus erythematosus. Increased epidermal expression of D-related human leukocyte antigen (HLA-DR) may play a role in antigen presentation [13]. Cytotoxic T cells are thought to be important in the pathogenesis, as well [14]. The photosensitivity experienced by patients with lupus erythematosus may be related, in part, to ultraviolet radiation–induced cytokine release [15].

Lupus Profundus

Epidemiology. Less than 10% of patients with lupus profundus fulfill the criteria for having SLE [16]. Lupus profundus occurs most frequently in adult women [17]. Lupus profundus has also been reported to occur in association with neonatal lupus erythematosus [18] and DLE [19].

Cutaneous Features. Subcutaneous, asymptomatic to slightly tender, well-defined nodules on the extremities are the most common initial signs of lupus profundus

[20]. These may ulcerate, but more commonly there is no overlying epidermal change. Occasionally, epidermal and periappendageal changes suggesting DLE are seen overlying the panniculitis [19]. In one study, changes suggestive of DLE were present in 21% of patients with lupus profundus [21]. Lupus profundus rarely appears on the face [22]. Morphea-like changes have been described in patients with lupus profundus [23]. The cutaneous manifestations of lupus profundus lasted for a mean duration of 6 years in one study [17]. Rare cases of lupus profundus have appeared in a linear distribution [24].

Associated Disorders. Most patients with lupus profundus have a mild clinical course. Most never develop systemic abnormalities or laboratory anomalies [16]; however, in a minority of patients, signs and symptoms of SLE, as described earlier, may be present.

Histologic Features. Lupus profundus is a lobular panniculitis that is characterized by an infiltrate composed of lymphocytes, histiocytes, and plasma cells (Fig. 1–5). The lymphocytes form nodules, often with germinal centers [25]. Lymphocytic nuclear dust has been described in some cases [19]. The lymphocytes are a mixture of T helper and cytotoxic/suppressor cells. B lymphocytes are not part of the inflammatory reaction [26]. Eosinophils are present in small numbers in about 25% of cases [21, 27]. Amorphous, eosinophilic (hyaline) necrosis of the fat within the lobules is a common feature [25] (Fig. 1–6). Lipomembranous, or membranocystic, changes have also been reported in some patients with lupus profundus [28]. In a few cases, histologic changes more typical of DLE are found in the upper portions of the biopsy specimen.

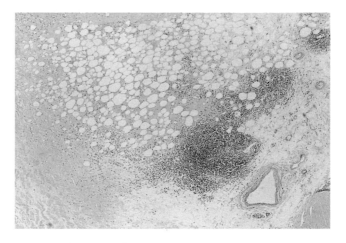

Fig. 1–5. Lupus profundus is characterized by nodules of inflammatory cells at the periphery of the fatty lobules in the subcutaneous fat.

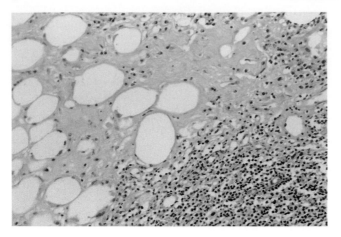

Fig. 1–6. Amorphous, eosinophilic degeneration of the surrounding fat is a common finding in lupus profundus.

Special Studies. Granular deposits of IgG and C3 may be present along the dermal–epidermal junction, but they are not found in all cases [23]. A similar pattern is often seen within the vessel walls of deep dermal blood vessels [26].

Pathogenesis. The pathogenesis of lupus profundus remains unknown.

Systemic Lupus Erythematosus

Epidemiology. Systemic lupus erythematosus is an autoimmune disease that demonstrates a 9:1 female predominance. It affects people of all races, although nonwhite are slightly more likely to be affected. Prevalence rates range from 4 to 250 per 100,000 people, depending on the population base studied [29]. Onset in women is most frequent during childbearing years. There is some genetic basis for the development of SLE as demonstrated by the concordance rate of 24% in monozygotic twins as compared with 2% in dizygotic twins [30]. An increased incidence of HLA-DR2 and HLA-DR3 is seen in patients with SLE [31]. There is some evidence for linkage of the chromosome 1q41–42 region in patients with SLE [32].

Cutaneous Features. Patients with SLE may present with cutaneous changes identical to those seen in DLE or SCLE, but also have signs of systemic involvement. Some 80%–90% of patients with SLE will have cutaneous manifestations at some point during the course of their disease [33].

The butterfly pattern, malar erythema, is the most common cutaneous manifestation, affecting up to 67% of patients with SLE [34]. In most cases, the erythema is part of an indurated, confluent plaque with distinct borders. Papules and vesicles are present less com-

monly. In many cases, the nasolabial folds are spared. Photosensitivity that presents as a severe sunburn after low ultraviolet light exposure is present in approximately 50% of patients with SLE.

Periungual and palmar erythema and dilation in nail fold capillary beds are common in patients with SLE. Livedo reticularis, a net-like pattern of erythema, occurs in 10%–15% of patients with SLE [35]. This manifestation may be exacerbated by exposure to cold.

The oral mucosa is involved in approximately 25% of patients with SLE. This can take the form of petechia, gingivitis, cheilitis, and ulcers [7]. Alopecia occurs in up to 30% of patients with SLE. In contrast to patients with DLE, the alopecia is often nonscarring and may be caused by a telogen effluvium.

Associated Disorders. Systemic lupus erythematosus involves many organ systems, as is summarized in Table 1–1. Joints are affected in up to 90% of patients with SLE [36]. Joint involvement manifests as arthralgia, most commonly in the small joints of the hands, wrists, and ankles. Actual arthritis, defined as inflammation of the joint space with visible clinical changes, is less commonly found. Avascular necrosis of the femoral heads is seen in patients with SLE, especially in those who have taken systemic corticosteroids.

Kidneys are affected in approximately 50% of patients [36], and this complication is associated with a worse prognosis. There is a wide range of renal pathology that is seen in these patients, and biopsy is often required to determine the nature and the extent of the renal compromise.

The respiratory system is involved in 40% of patients with SLE [36] and most often takes the form of pleuritic chest pain. Interstitial pneumonia and diaphragmatic myopathy have also been reported [37]. The central nervous system is affected in 30% of SLE patients [36]. Symptoms may be nonspecific, including depression, headaches, and inability to concentrate, or may include seizures, psychoses, and strokes. Lupoid hepatitis is described in rare patients with SLE [38].

Table 1–1. Organ Systems Involved in Systemic Lupus Erythematosus (Percentage of Patients Displaying Signs and Symptoms)	
Organ System	*Patients with Signs and Symptoms (%)*
Musculoskeletal	90
Renal	50
Pulmonary	40
Central nervous system	30
Cardiovascular	20–40
Hepatic	Rare

From references 36–39 and 41–43.

The heart may be affected by abnormalities in the conduction system, myocardium, valves, and coronary arteries in patients with SLE [39]. Raynaud's phenomenon is present in 18% [40] to 44% [41] of SLE patients. Perniosis has been reported to occur in patients with SLE [42]. Rheumatoid nodules occur in 5%–10% of patients with SLE [43]. SLE may coexist with a wide range of other diseases, including porphyria cutanea tarda [44] and psoriasis.

Histologic Features. The histologic features of the malar erythema seen in SLE are quite similar to the changes described in discoid lesions. The primary pathologic alteration is that of an interface dermatitis. Lymphocytes are present along the dermal–epidermal junction, extending into the overlying epidermis. Dying keratinocytes are present in variable numbers, and vacuolar degeneration of the basal layer is extensive. Hyperkeratosis and follicular plugging may be present, but are often less pronounced than what is seen in biopsy specimens from patients with DLE. Over time, the epidermis becomes progressively more atrophic, and the basement membrane appears thickened. Within the dermis, there is a moderately intense lymphocytic infiltrate surrounding vessels in the superficial and deep dermis, as well as cutaneous appendages. Plasma cells are often present in small numbers, but eosinophils are rarely seen. Vascular ectasia is often present, and slight amounts of acid mucopolysaccharides may be present within the superficial reticular dermis.

Special Studies. Direct immunofluorescence tests can be useful in determining the systemic nature of the disease in patients with SLE. Similar to the situation with DLE, direct immunofluorescence examination of affected, sun-exposed skin will reveal deposits of IgG, IgM, and/or IgA, along with C3 along the dermal–epidermal junction in a granular pattern. Unlike DLE, however, the same immunoreactant staining pattern will be present in up to 75% of sun-exposed, nonlesional skin and in up to 50% of non-sun-exposed, nonlesional skin of patients with SLE (lupus band test) [9].

Serologic studies have largely supplanted direct immunofluorescence studies for determining the systemic nature of the disease. Antinuclear antibodies are present in 98% of patients with SLE. Antihistone antibodies are present in 70% of these patients, and anti-double-stranded DNA antibodies are present in about 50%.

Pathogenesis. The pathogenesis of this autoimmune disease is not known. Genetic factors are thought to play some role, as are hormonal factors and environmental factors [45]. Infectious diseases, including parvovirus B19 [46], are believed to trigger the onset of SLE in some cases. Cytokine production related to genetic polymorphisms, often induced by ultraviolet light, in combination with selectin and adhesion molecule expression contribute to the inflammatory response seen in lupus erythematosus [47]. Serum interferon levels are also known to correlate with disease activity [48]. Increased dermal mucin present in cutaneous lesions of SLE is due to increased production of glycosaminoglycans by affected cutaneous fibroblasts [49].

Subacute Cutaneous Lupus Erythematosus

Epidemiology. Subacute cutaneous lupus erythematosus is present in 5%–10% of all patients with lupus erythematosus [50–52]. The disease is most frequent in young to middle-aged white women. It is much less common in black or Hispanic populations, and only about 30% of cases occur in men [53]. Approximately 50% of patients with SCLE fulfill the criteria for having SLE [53]. Increased frequencies of HLA-B8 and HLA-DR3 are reported in patients with SCLE [54].

Cutaneous Features. The cutaneous manifestations of SCLE include polycyclic or annular patches, or psoriasiform patches that occur predominantly on photodistributed areas. Extension of the rash to sun-protected sites occurs. The upper back, chest, arms, and lateral neck are the most common sites of involvement, with the face, scalp, and lower extremities affected less frequently [54]. Most patients have either annular lesions or psoriasiform lesions, but do not have lesions with both morphologies simultaneously [53]. Approximately equal numbers of patients display each type of lesion. About 15% of patients with SCLE will have discoid lesions of lupus erythematosus at some point during the course of their disease [51]. The primary lesions of SCLE are nonscarring.

Less commonly, a more generalized eruption consisting of patches with a pityriasiform appearance may be present [55]. Erythema multiforme–like lesions have also been described [56]. Vesicles and bullae are infrequently seen and have been associated with the HLA-DR3 phenotype [57]. Erythroderma has also been reported [58].

Photosensitivity is seen in 90% [59] to 100% [55] of patients with SCLE. Involvement of mucous membranes is relatively uncommon. Raynaud's phenomenon is present in about 25% of patients with SCLE. Periungual telangiectasias and livedo reticularis are also seen in only a minority of cases, and vasculitis is uncommon in these patients [53]. Alopecia [60] and livedo reticularis [51] have also been reported in patients with SCLE.

Upon resolution, hypopigmentation of affected areas is frequently noted. These changes may resemble vitiligo [53].

Associated Disorders. Systemic involvement is present in most patients with SCLE. Arthritis and arthralgias are present in 42% [59] to 80% [61] of patients. Myalgias are reported in about 20% of cases [51]. Renal disease and central nervous system disease are less common, affecting approximately 10% of patients with SCLE [51, 59, 61].

Subacute cutaneous lupus erythematosus has been reported in association with breast [62], lung [63], and gastric [64] carcinomas and may represent a paraneoplastic syndrome; however, it should be noted that this co-occurrence is quite rare. Subacute cutaneous lupus erythematosus has been reported to occur with greater than expected frequency in patients with Sjögren's syndrome and rheumatoid arthritis [54]. It has also been reported in association with deficiencies in complement components C2 [65], C3 [66], and C4 [66].

Drug-induced SCLE has also been reported [67]. This uncommon association occurs most frequently with hydrochlorothiazide ingestion. It has also been reported in patients taking piroxicam [68], penicillamine [53], glyburide [53], aldactone [69], and griseofulvin [70] and in patients receiving gold therapy [71].

Histologic Features. The histologic changes seen in biopsy specimens of the annular and the psoriasiform patches in SCLE are indistinguishable. Subacute cutaneous lupus erythematosus has been reported to demonstrate less hyperkeratosis, follicular plugging, and deep lymphocytic infiltrate than is the case with DLE [50]. It has also been reported that epidermal necrosis and colloid bodies are more prominent in SCLE than in DLE [57]. These changes are subtle, however, and definitive subclassification of lupus erythematosus is not usually possible based solely on interpretation of skin biopsy results [6].

Special Studies. Most, but not all patients with SCLE have anti-Ro (SS-A) antibodies [53]. Anti-La (SS-B) antibodies may also be found, although in a much lower percentage of patients. The presence of these antibodies is not, however, specific for SCLE. Anti-Ro antibodies are also reported in patients with other subtypes of lupus erythematosus and Sjögren syndrome. It has been suggested that anti-Ro antibodies may be a marker for a group of patients at higher risk for multiorgan vasculopathy, myositis, or progressive pulmonary disease [72]. The presence of these antibodies also correlates with photosensitivity.

Direct immunofluorescence examination of lesional skin reveals granular deposits of IgG and C3 along the dermal–epidermal junction in approximately 60% of cases. Nonlesional, sun-protected skin demonstrates a positive immunofluorescence pattern in 26%–46% of cases [51]. A unique immunostaining pattern has also been described in approximately 30% of patients with SCLE. These patients demonstrate dust-like particles of IgG in the epidermis and superficial dermis and within the dermal cellular infiltrates [73].

Pathogenesis. The pathogenesis of SCLE is not known. It has been suggested that antibody-dependent cellular cytotoxicity may play a role in the pathogenesis of cutaneous damage, especially in the presence of anti-Ro antibodies [4, 14].

Neonatal Lupus Erythematosus

Epidemiology. Neonatal lupus erythematosus (NLE) is quite uncommon. It presents within the first 6 months of life [74]. Although the exact incidence of the condition is not known, it has been estimated to be at least 1 in 20,000 live births [75]. In most cases, the cutaneous eruption resolves by 6 months of age. Ro antibody–positive mothers with HLA subtypes A1, B8, and DR3 may be at increased risk for having infants with NLE [76].

Cutaneous Features. The cutaneous features of neonatal lupus erythematosus are analogous to those of SCLE in adults [75]. About half of patients with NLE will demonstrate a cutaneous eruption. The face and scalp are the most commonly affected locations. Annular or psoriasiform patches typically heal without scarring. Follicular plugging and atrophy are not normally present. Sun exposure may induce or exacerbate the eruption [75].

Associated Disorders. Congenital complete heart block is the major extracutaneous manifestation in patients with NLE and is found in about 50% of patients [75]. The heart block may be detected as early as the second trimester of pregnancy [77] and is often irreversible [74].

Less common systemic manifestations include liver disease and thrombocytopenia. Noninfectious hepatitis that resolves without sequelae has been reported [78]. Liver disease has been reported in up to 10% of patients with NLE [79]. Splenomegaly and decreased complement levels may also be present [80]. Aplastic anemia has been described in a single infant with NLE [81].

Histologic Features. The histologic features of NLE include a sparse interface dermatitis, with necrosis of basal keratinocytes. There is a scant infiltrate of lymphocytes around vessels of the superficial vascular plexus. Histologic changes are often more subtle than those found in DLE or SCLE [82].

Special Studies. Direct immunofluorescence examination demonstrates granular deposits of IgG and C3 along the dermal–epidermal junction in most cases.

Pathogenesis. Mothers of babies with NLE usually have IgG anti-Ro/SS-A antibodies, which cross the placenta and presumably give rise to the signs and symptoms of lupus erythematosus [75].

Antiphospholipid Syndrome

Epidemiology. Antiphospholipid antibodies are responsible for the lupus anticoagulant and anticardiolipin antibodies. Antiphospholipid syndrome is present in 20%–50% of patients with SLE [83], but can occur in other settings. An autosomal dominant inheritance pattern has been suggested in some cases [84].

Cutaneous Features. Antiphospholipid syndrome often presents with a livedo reticularis pattern on the thighs, shins, and forearms. The trunk is less frequently involved [85].

Atrophie blanche, or livedoid vasculitis, is also seen in some patients with antiphospholipid syndrome [86]. Atrophic, hypopigmented scar-like depressions occur on the lower extremities, especially around the ankles. Patients with the antiphospholipid syndrome and thrombophlebitis may demonstrate edema and tenderness of the lower extremity [87]. Vascular occlusion may lead to ischemia, ulceration, and digital gangrene [87, 88].

Associated Disorders. Patients with the antiphospholipid syndrome are prone to the development of repeated venous and/or arterial thromboses, thrombocytopenia, and repeated fetal loss [89]. Deep venous thrombosis is the most common vascular occlusive phenomenon seen in this syndrome. Strokes are also encountered commonly. Depression, cognitive dysfunction, and psychoses have also been associated with the antiphospholipid syndrome [90].

The syndrome has also been reported in patients with other connective tissue diseases and in patients with malignant tumors and infectious diseases. Drug etiology is reported (Table 1–2).

Histologic Features. Histologic features of affected skin from patients with the antiphospholipid syndrome demonstrate vascular occlusion. In early lesions, vessels throughout the dermis are occluded by eosinophilic, amorphous material (Fig. 1–7). Affected vessels may be venous or arterial and at any level in the dermis or subcutaneous fat. As lesions progress, an inflammatory infiltrate appears around the vessels and in the surrounding dermis. Well-developed lesions demonstrate areas of necrosis within the dermis and epidermis deprived of normal blood flow along with a secondary inflammatory response. The following entities must be

Table 1–2. Diseases Associated with Antiphospholipid Syndrome

Autoimmune diseases
  Systemic lupus erythematosus
  Rheumatoid arthritis
  Scleroderma
  Dermatomyositis
  Sjögren's syndrome
  Behçet's syndrome
  Hashimoto's thyroiditis
  Myasthenia gravis
  Diabetes mellitus
  Multiple sclerosis
Drug induced
  Chlorpromazide
  Procainamide
  Hydralazine
  Quinidine
  Phenytoin
  Sulfonamides
Infectious diseases
  Bacterial
    Tuberculosis
    Leprosy
    Syphilis
    Lyme disease
    Klebsiella
    Mycoplasma penetrans
  Protozoal
    Pneumocystis carinii
    Plasmodium
  Viral
    Acquired immunodeficiency syndrome
    Mononucleosis
    Hepatitis C
    Rubella
    Parvovirus
Hematoproliferative disorders
  Thrombotic thrombocytopenic purpura
  Sickle cell disease
  Polycythemia vera
  Myelofibrosis
  Monoclonal gammopathies
  Von Willebrand's disease
Malignant neoplasms
  Hairy cell leukemia
  Lymphoma
  Waldenström's macroglobulinemia
  Carcinoma
    Lung
    Prostate
    Head and neck
    Esophagus
    Cervix
    Renal
  Thymoma
Miscellaneous
  Chronic renal failure
  Nodular hyperplasia of the liver
  Celiac disease

From references 83 and 114–118.

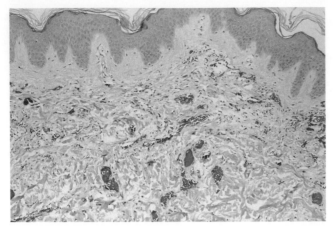

A

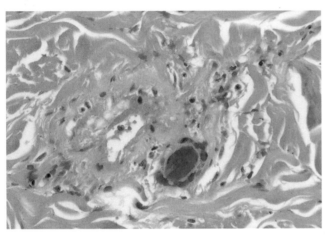

B

Fig. 1–7. *A, B,* In the antiphospholipid syndrome, dermal blood vessels are occluded by eosinophilic material.

considered in the histologic differential diagnosis of antiphospholipid syndrome:

- Cryoglobulinemia
- Disseminated intravascular coagulation
- Protein C or S deficiency
- Purpura fulminans
- Septic vasculitis
- Waldenström's macroglobulinemia

Special Studies. Coagulation studies provide the most exact information regarding the disease process. A Russell viper venom test and a search for anticardiolipin antibodies are helpful in making a specific diagnosis. Special studies performed on histologic sections do not enhance the diagnostic specificity.

Pathogenesis. Apoptosis occurring as part of the autoimmune disease process may provide antigenic stimulus for the production of antiphospholipid antibodies

[91]. Patients demonstrate antibodies to epitopes on β_2-glycoprotein I and prothrombin, as well as antiendothelial cell antibodies [92].

Bullous Lupus Erythematosus

Epidemiology. Bullous lupus erythematosus (BLE) is relatively uncommon and usually occurs as part of SLE. The diagnosis is most often made in patients who fulfill the American Rheumatism Association (ARA) criteria for SLE and who have vesicles and bullae arising on, but not limited to, sun-exposed skin and direct immunofluorescence findings consistent with lupus erythematosus [93]. It should be noted that BLE has been reported in patients who do not fulfill the ARA criteria for SLE [94]. Black women are most commonly affected [95].

Cutaneous Features. The clinical appearance of BLE is similar to that of dermatitis herpetiformis. Small vesicles and bullae are present, more commonly on the trunk and extremities. The face can also be affected. The blisters tend to be tense and to arise on previously uninvolved skin. They heal without scarring. Mucosal surfaces may be involved. Cutaneous blisters have not been reported as the presenting manifestation of lupus erythematosus.

Associated Disorders. In most cases, BLE is associated with systemic involvement, especially of the kidneys, joints, and brain [93].

Histologic Features. The specific features of BLE include a subepidermal blister with aggregates of neutrophils present in small microabscesses within the papillary dermis (Figs. 1–8 and 1–9). Intraepidermal neutrophilic abscesses have also been reported [96]. Lymphocytes and eosinophils may also be present. Papillary dermal edema is usually present [95]. In some cases, leukocytoclastic vasculitis is present [96]. The histologic changes may rarely include changes characteristic of other types of lupus erythematosus such as interface dermatitis and liquefactive degeneration of the basal layer of the epidermis, but in most cases these changes are absent. The following entities must be considered in the histologic differential diagnosis of BLE:

- Bullous drug eruption
- Dermatitis herpetiformis
- Epidermolysis bullosa acquisita
- Linear IgA bullous dermatosis

Special Studies. Direct immunofluorescence examination reveals granular deposits of IgG, IgM, and C3 along the dermal–epidermal junction in most cases. IgA

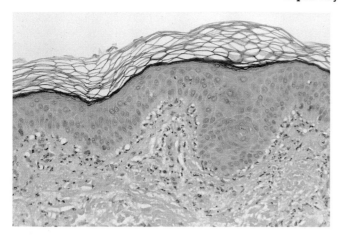

Fig. 1–8. Early lesions of bullous lupus erythematosus are characterized by neutrophils along the dermal–epidermal junction.

deposits are also present in a similar distribution in up to 76% of patients, a much higher percentage than is found in other subtypes of lupus erythematosus [97]. Circulating autoantibodies to type VII collagen have been reported in most cases of BLE [98, 99]. In these cases, the immunoglobulin deposition along the dermal–epidermal junction may be linear in appearance and will localize to the floor of the blister on salt-split skin preparations.

Pathogenesis. The relationship between BLE and epidermolysis bullosa acquisita is presently unclear. It is not yet known if the circulating anti-type VII antibodies found in most patients with SLE are pathogenetic. Some authors believe that these antibodies play a central role in the inflammatory destruction of the base-

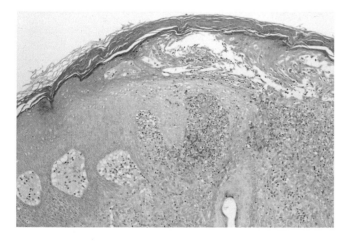

Fig. 1–9. In well-established lesions of bullous lupus erythematosus, the neutrophils form microabscesses within the papillary dermal tips.

ment membrane zone [95]. It has been suggested that there are two types of patients with BLE, those with antibodies directed against type VII collagen and those without [95].

Livedoid Vasculitis (Atrophie Blanche)

Epidemiology. Livedoid vasculitis is also known as *segmental hyalinizing vasculitis.* The clinical correlate is known as *atrophie blanche.* In many, but not all cases, affected patients also have lupus erythematosus. Atrophie blanche occurs predominantly in young to middle-aged women. The mean age of onset is approximately 32 years of age [100]. Rare cases have been reported in children [101]. The term *atrophie blanche* has also been applied to the sequela of ulcers in the setting of stasis dermatitis. Upon healing, these ulcers leave a depressed, white scar.

Cutaneous Features. Livedoid vasculitis almost always involves the lower extremities. Petechiae are often the initial presentation. Hemorrhagic bullae and purpuric papules are other early lesions [102]. The disease progresses to irregularly shaped, angulated ulcerations that heal with depressed scarring and porcelain white hypopigmentation [103]. The ulcerations tend to exacerbate in the summer months and may be quite painful [100].

Associated Disorders. Livedoid vasculitis and cerebral thromboses or progressive dementia occur simultaneously in some patients and together are known as Sneddon's syndrome [104]. Kidney involvement has also been described [105]. Some of these patients have SLE, and anticardiolipin antibodies are present in most of them [106, 107]. It has been demonstrated that 91% of patients with SLE and livedoid vasculitis developed lupus involving the central nervous system. Lupus nephritis was present in 11% of these patients [108].

Pigmented purpuric eruption has been associated with livedoid vasculitis [100]. Raynaud's phenomenon is present in many of these patients [102].

Histologic Features. Histologic changes in livedoid vasculitis include deposition of fibrin within the walls of affected dermal vessels (Figs. 1–10 and 1–11). Older lesions demonstrate occlusion of the vascular lumen with fibrin. There is minimal inflammation surrounding the vessels, and leukocytoclasis is not seen in most cases [109]. In these cases, the epidermis may be ulcerated or atrophic, and increased dermal fibrosis and scarring are common [103].

Special Studies. Direct immunofluorescence studies may demonstrate immunoglobulins and complement

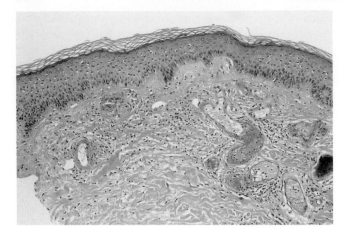

Fig. 1–10. Livedoid vasculitis is characterized by fibrin at the periphery of affected vessels, with minimal inflammation.

within the vessel walls in some cases [110]. In most cases, this is not helpful in making the diagnosis.

Elevated fibrinopeptide A levels are present in patients with livedoid vasculitis and suggest a thrombotic disorder as opposed to an inflammatory process [111].

Pathogenesis. Most investigators believe that livedoid vasculitis is a vasculopathy and not a true vasculitis [109, 112]. Atrophie blanche has been attributed to the defective release of tissue plasminogen-activating factor from blood vessel walls [113]. Considering the finding of anticardiolipin antibodies in some patients with livedoid vasculitis, it has been suggested that livedoid vasculitis may be related to antiphospholipid syndrome [103].

Miscellaneous

Leukocytoclastic vasculitis may be encountered in patients with lupus erythematosus. The clinical and his-

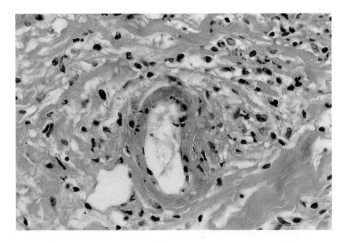

Fig. 1–11. Higher power demonstrates the peripheral deposition of fibrin in the vessel walls in a lesion of livedoid vasculitis.

tologic presentations are identical to other forms of leukocytoclastic vasculitis and are discussed in Chapter 4.

Drug-induced lupus erythematosus is discussed in Chapter 23.

References

1. Pistiner, M., Wallace, D. J., Nessim, S., Metzger, A. L., and Klinenberg, J. R., *Lupus erythematosus in the 1980's: A survey of 570 patients.* Semin Arthritis Rheum, 1991. 21:55–64.
2. Callen, J. P., Tuffanelli, D. L., and Provost, T. T., *Collagen vascular disease: An update.* J Am Acad Dermatol, 1993. 28:477–484.
3. Sontheimer, R. D., *Clinical manifestations of cutaneous lupus erythematosus.* In *Dubois' Lupus Erythematosus*, D. J. Wallace and B. H. Hahn, Eds. 1993, Lea & Febiger: Philadelphia, pp. 290–295.
4. Hymes, S. R., and Jordan, R. E., *Chronic cutaneous lupus erythematosus.* Med Clin North Am, 1989. 73: 1055–1071.
5. Beutner, E. H., Jablonska, S., White, D. B., Blaszczyk, M., Chorzelski, T. P., Cunningham, R. K., and Davis, B. M., *Dermatologic criteria for classifying the major forms of cutaneous lupus erythematosus: Methods for systematic discriminant analysis and questions on the interpretation of findings.* Clin Dermatol, 1993. 10: 443–456.
6. Jerdan, M. S., Hood, A. F., Moore, G. W., and Callen, J. P., *Histopathologic comparison of the subsets of lupus erythematosus.* Arch Dermatol, 1990. 126:52–55.
7. Connolly, K., *Lupus erythematosus,* in *Cutaneous Medicine and Surgery*, K. A. Arndt, et al., Eds. 1996, W. B. Saunders Company: Philadelphia, pp. 260–278.
8. Bielsam, I., Herrero, C., Collado, A., Cobos, A., Palou, J., and Mascaro, J. M., *Histopathologic findings in cutaneous lupus erythematosus.* Arch Dermatol, 1994. 130:54–58.
9. Harrist, T. J., and Mihm, M. C., Jr., *The specificity and clinical usefulness of the lupus band test.* Arthritis Rheum, 1980. 23:479–490.
10. Biesecker, G., Lavin, L., Ziskind, M., and Koffler, D., *Cutaneous localization of the membrane attack complex in discoid and systemic lupus erythematosus.* N Engl J Med, 1982. 306:264–270.
11. Helm, K. F., Peters, M. S., *Deposition of membrane attack complex in cutaneous lesions of lupus erythematosus.* J Am Acad Dermatol, 1993. 28:687–691.
12. Mooney, E., Gammon, W. R., and Jennette, J. C., *Characterization of the changes in matrix molecules at the dermal epidermal junciton in lupus erythematosus.* J Cutan Pathol, 1991. 18:417–422.
13. Tebbe, B., Mazur, L., Stadler, R., and Orfanos, C. E., *Immunohistochemical analysis of chronic discoid and subacute cutaneous lupus erythematosus—relation to immunopathologic mechanisms.* Br J Dermatol, 1995. 132:25–31.

14. Provost, T. T., and Reichlin, M., *Immunopathologic studies of cutaneous lupus erythematosus.* J Clin Immunol, 1988. 8:223–233.

15. Norris, D. A., *Pathomechanisms of photosensitive lupus erythematosus.* J Invest Dermatol, 1993. 1993:100.

16. Watanabe, T., and Tsuchida, T., *Lupus erythematosus profundus: A cutaneous marker for a distinct clinical entity.* Br J Dermatol, 1996. 134:123–125.

17. Martens, P. B., Moder, K. G., and Ahmed, I., *Lupus panniculitis: Clinical perspectives from a case series.* J Rheumatol, 1999. 26:68–72.

18. Nitta, Y., *Lupus erythematosus profundus associated wtih neonatal lupus erytehmatosus.* Br J Dermatol, 1997. 136:112–114.

19. Caproni, M., Palleschi, G. M., Papi, C., and Fabbri, P., *Discoid lupus erythematosus lesions developed on lupus erythematosus profundus nodules.* Int J Dermatol, 1995. 34:357–359.

20. Chung, H. S., and Hann, S. K., *Lupus panniculitis treated by a combination therapy of hydroxychloroquine and quinacrine.* J Dermatol, 1997. 24:569–572.

21. Sanchez, N. P., Peters, M. S., and Winkelmann, R. K., *The histopathology of lupus erythematosus panniculitis.* J Am Acad Dermatol, 1981. 5:673–680.

22. Muncaster, A., Stewart, G., Moss, C., and Southwood, T., *Facial lupus erythematosus profundus in a 9-year-old boy.* J R Soc Med, 1998. 91:207–208.

23. Stork, J., and Vosmik, F., *Lupus erythematosus panniculitis with morphea-like lesions.* Clin Exp Dermatol, 1994. 19:79–82.

24. Heid, E., *A 17-year old Italian boy with a linear lupus erythematosus profundus.* Eur J Dermatol, 1998. 8:69.

25. Peters, M. S., and Su, W. P. D., *Lupus erythematosus panniculitis.* Med Clin North Am, 1989. 73:1113–1126.

26. Riccieri, V., Sili Scavalli, A., Spadaro, A., Taccari, E., and Zoppini, A., *Lupus erythematosus panniculitis: An immunohistochemical study.* Clin Rheumatol, 1994. 13:641–644.

27. Peters, M. S., and Su, W. P. D., *Eosinophils in lupus panniculitis and morphea profunda.* J Cutan Pathol, 1991. 18:189–192.

28. Snow, J. L., and Su, W. P. D., *Lipomembranous (membranocystic) fat necrosis. Clinicopathologic correlation of 38 cases.* Am J Dermatopathol, 1996. 18:151–155.

29. Lawrence, R. C., Hochberg, M. C., Kelsey, J. L., McDuffie, F. C., Medsger, T. A., Jr., Felts, W. R., and Sulman, L. E., *Estimates of the prevalence of selective arthritis and musculoskeletal diseases in the United States.* J Rheumatol, 1989. 16:427–441.

30. Deapen, D., Escalante, A., Weinrib, L., Horwitz, D., Bachman, B., Roy-Burman, P., Walker, A., and Mack, T. M., *A revised estimate of twin concordance in systemic lupus erythematosus.* Arthritis Rheum, 1992. 35:311–318.

31. Woods, V. L., *Pathogenesis of systemic lupus erythematosus,* in *Textbook of Rheumatology,* W. M. Kelley et al., Eds. 1993, W. B. Saunders Company: Philadelphia, pp. 999–1016.

32. Tsao, B. P., Cantor, R. M., Kalunian, K. C., Wallace, D. J., Hahn, B. H., and Rotter, J. I., *The genetic basis of systemic lupus erythematosus.* Proc Assoc Am Phys, 1998. 110:113–117.

33. Hochberg, M. C., and Petri, M., *Clinical features of systemic lupus erythematosus.* Curr Opin Rheumatol, 1993. 5:575–586.

34. Wallace, D. J., *Cutaneous manifestations of SLE,* in *Dubois' Lupus Erythematosus,* D. J. Wallace and B. H. Hahn, Eds. 1993, Lea & Febiger: Philadelphia, pp. 356–369.

35. Cervera, R., Khamashta, M. A., Font, J., Sebastiani, G. D., Gil, A., Lavilla, P., Domenech, I., and Aydintug, A. O., et al., *Systemic Lupus Erythematosus: Clinical and immunologic patterns of disease expression in a cohort of 1,000 patients.* Medicine (Baltimore), 1993. 72: 113–124.

36. Wallace, D. J., *The clinical presentation of SLE,* in *Dubois' Lupus Erythematosus,* D.J. Wallace, Ed. 1993, Lea & Febiger: Philadelphia, pp. 317–321.

37. Purice, S., Tudor, A., Gheorghiu, M., Matei, I., Balta, M., Cojocaru, M., and Pecec, C., *Pulmonary involvement in systemic lupus erythematosus.* Med Interne, 1987. 25:227–232.

38. Tanasescu, C., and Purice, S., *Liver disease in systemic lupus erythematosus.* Rom J Intern Med, 1992. 30:169–174.

39. Moder, K. G., Miller, T. D., and Tazelaar, H. D., *Cardiac involvement in systemic lupus erythematosus.* Mayo Clin Proc, 1999. 74:275–284.

40. Dubois, E. L., and Tuffanelli, D. L., *Clinical manifestations of systemic lupus erythematosus: Computer analysis of 520 cases.* JAMA, 1964. 190:104–111.

41. Hochberg, M. C., Boyd, R. E., Ahearn, J. M., Arnett, F. C., Bias, W. R., Provost, T. T., and Stevens, M. B., *Systemic lupus erythematosus: A review of clinico-laboratory features and immunogenetic markers in 150 patients with emphasis on demographic subsets.* Medicine (Baltimore), 1985. 64:285–295.

42. Millard, L. G., and Rowell, N. R., *Chilblains lupus erythematosus (Hutchinson's): A clinical and laboratory study of 17 patients.* Br J Dermatol, 1978. 98:497–506.

43. Hahn, B. H., Yardly, J. H., and Stevens, M. B., *Rheumatoid nodules in systemic lupus erythematosus.* Ann Intern Med, 1970. 72:49–58.

44. Gibson, G. E., and MeEvoy, M. T., *Coexistence of lupus erythematosus and porphyria cutanea tarda in fifteen patients.* J Am Acad Dermatol, 1998. 38:569–573.

45. Cooper, G. S., Dooley, M. A., Treadwill, E. L., St. Clair, E. W., Parks, C. G., and Gilkeson, G. S., *Hormonal, environmental, and infectious risk factors for developing systemic lupus erythematosus.* Arthritis Rheum, 1998. 41:1714–1724.

46. Roblot, P., Roblot, F., Ramassamy, A., and Becq-Giraudon, B., *Lupus syndrome after parvovirus B19 infection.* Rev Rhum Engl Ed, 1997. 64:849–851.

47. Werth, V. P., Dutz, J. P., and Sontheimer, R. D., *Pathogenetic mechanisms and treatment of cutaneous lupus erythematosus.* Curr Opin Rheumatol, 1997. 9:400–409.

48. Matei, I., Ghyka, G., Savi, I., and Tudor, A., *Correlation of serum interferon with some clinical and humoral*

signs of systemic lupus erythematosus. Med Interne, 1990. 28:289–294.

49. Pandya, A. G., Sontheimer, R. D., Cockerell, C. J., Takashima, A., and Piepkorn, M., *Papulonodular mucinosis associated with systemic lupus erythematosus: Possible mechanisms of increased glycosoaminoglycan accumulation.* J Am Acad Dermatol, 1995. 32:199–205.

50. Bangert, J., Freeman, R., Sontheimer, R. D., and Gilliam, J. N., *Subacute cutaneous lupus erythematosus and discoid lupus erythematosus. Comparative histologic findings.* Arch Dermatol, 1984. 120:332–337.

51. Sontheimer, R. D., Thomas, J. R., and Gilliam, J. N., *Subacute cutaneous lupus erythematosus: A cutaneous marker for a distinct lupus erythematosus subset.* Arch Dermatol, 1979. 115:1409–1415.

52. Mooney, E., and Wade, T. R., *Subacute cutaneous lupus erythematosus in Iceland.* Int J Dermatol, 1989. 28:104–106.

53. Sontheimer, R. D., *Subacute cutaneous lupus erythematosus: A decade's perspective.* Med Clin North Am 1989. 73:1073–1091.

54. David-Bajar, K. M., *Subacute cutaneous lupus erythematosus.* J Invest Dermatol, 1993. 100:2S–8S.

55. Hymes, S. R., Russell, T. J., and Jordan, R. E., *The anti-Ro antibody system.* Int J Dermatol, 1986. 25:1–7.

56. Sontheimer, R. D., and Gilliam, J. N., *Subacute cutaneous lupus erythematosus.* Curr Concepts Skin Disord, 1983. 4:11–17.

57. Herrero, C., Bies, I., Font, J., Lozano, F., Ercilla, G., Lecha, M., Ingelmo, M., and Mascaro, J. M., *Subacute cutaneous lupus erythematosus: Clinical pathologic findings in 13 cases.* J Am Acad Dermatol, 1988. 19: 1057–1062.

58. DeSpain, J. D., and Clark, D. P., *Subacute cutaneous lupus erythematosus presenting as erythroderma.* J Am Acad Dermatol, 1988. 19:388–392.

59. Callen, J. P., and Klein, J., *Subacute cutaneous lupus erythematosus. Clinical, serologic, immunogenetic, and therapeutic considerations in 72 patients.* Arthritis Rheum, 1988. 31:1007–1013.

60. Molad, Y., Weinberger, A., David, M., Garty, B., Wysenbeek, A. J., and Pinkhas, J., *Clinical manifestations and laboratory data of subacute cutaneous lupus erythematosus (abstr).* Isr J Med Sci, 1987. 23:278–280.

61. Sontheimer, R. D., *Subacute cutaneous lupus erythematosus.* Clin Dermatol, 1985. 3:58–68.

62. Neumann, R., Schmidt, J. B., and Niebauer, G., *Subacute lupus erythematosus-like gyrate erythema. Report of a case with a breast cancer.* Dermatologica, 1986. 173:146–149.

63. Blane, D., and Kienzler, J. L., *Lupus erythematosus gyratus repens. Report of a case associated with lung carcinoma.* Clin Exp Dermatol, 1982. 7:129–134.

64. Kuhn, A., and Kaufmann, I., *Subakuter kutaner lupus erythematodes als paraneoplastisches syndrom.* Z Hutkr, 1986. 61:581–583.

65. Provost, T. T., Arnett, F. C., and Reichlin, M., *Homozygous C_2 deficiency, lupus erythematosus and anti-Ro (SSA) antibodies.* Arthritis Rheum, 1983. 26:1279–1283.

66. Boom, B. W., and Daha, M. R., *Inherited deficiency of the third component of complement, associated with cutaneous lupus erythematosus.* Br J Dermatol, 1989. 121:809–812.

67. Reed, B. R., Huff, J. C., Jones, S. K., Orton, P. W., Lee, L. A., and Norris, D. A., *Subacute cutaneous lupus erythematosus associated with hydrochlorothiazide therapy.* Ann Intern Med, 1985. 103:49–51.

68. Roura, M., Lopez-Gil, F., and Umbert, P., *Systemic lupus erythematosus exacerbated by piroxicam.* Dermatologica, 1991. 182:56–58.

69. Leroy, D., Dompmartin, A., Le Jean, S., Guillemain, J. L., Mandard, J. C., and Deschamps, P., *Dermatitis caused by aldactone of a lupic annular erythema type.* Ann Dermatol Venereol, 1987. 114:1237–1240.

70. Miyagawa, S., Okuchi, T., Shiomi, Y., and Sakamoto, K., *Subacute cutaneous lupus erythematosus lesions precipitated by griseofulvin.* J Am Acad Dermatol, 1989. 21:343–346.

71. Balsa, A., Bernad, M., De Miguel, E., and Crespo, M., *Subacute cutaneous lupus erythematosus caused by chrysotherapy in rheumatoid arthritis (letter).* Rev Clin Esp, 1988. 182:505–506.

72. Magro, C. M., and Crowson, A. N., *The cutaneous pathology associated with seropositivity for antibodies to SSA (Ro). A clinicopathologic study of 23 adult patients without subacute lupus erythematosus.* J Cutan Pathol, 1999. 21:129–137.

73. Nieboer, C., Tak-Daimond, Z., and VanLeeuwen-Wallau, A. G., *Dust-like particles: A specific direct immunofluorescence pattern in sub-acute cutaneous lupus erythematosus.* Br J Dermatol, 1988. 118:725–734.

74. Olson, N. Y., and Lindsley, C. B., *Neonatal lupus erythematosus.* Am J Dis Child, 1987. 141:908–910.

75. Lee, L. A., *Neonatal lupus erythematosus.* J Invest Dermatol, 1993. 100:9S–13S.

76. Watson, R. M., Lane, A. T., Barnett, N. K., Bias, W. B., Arnett, F. C., and Provost, T. T., *Neonatal lupus erythematosus. A clincal, serological and immunogenetic study with review of the literature.* Medicine (Baltimore), 1984. 63:362–378.

77. Buyon, J. P., Swersky, S. H., Fox, H. E., Bierman, F. Z., and Winchester, R. J., *Intrauterine therapy for presumptive fetal myocarditis with acquired heart block due to systemic lupus erythematosus.* Arthritis Rheum, 1987. 30:44–49.

78. Laxer, R. M., Roberts, E. A., Gross, K. R., Britton, J. R., Cutz, F., Dimmick, J., Petty, R. E., and Silverman, E. D., *Liver disease in neonatal lupus erythematosus.* J Pediatr, 1990. 116:238–242.

79. Lee, L. A., Reichlin, M., Ruyle, S. Z., and Weston, W. L., *Neonatal lupus liver disease.* Lupus, 1993. 2:333–338.

80. Draznin, T. H., Esterly, N. B., Furey, N. L., and DeBofsky, H., *Neonatal lupus erythematosus.* J Am Acad Dermatol, 1979. 1:437–442.

81. Wolach, B., Choc, L., Pomeranz, A., Ben Ari, Y., Douer, D., and Metzker, A., *Aplastic anemia in neonatal lupus erythematosus.* Am J Dis Child, 1993. 147:941–944.

82. Maynard, B., Leiferman, K. M., and Peters, M. S.,

Neonatal lupus erythematosus syndrome. J Cutan Pahtol, 1991. 18:333–338.

83. Asheron, R. A., and Cervera, R., *Antiphospholipid syndrome.* J Invest Dermatol, 1993. 100:21S–27S.

84. Goel, N., Ortel, T. L., Bali, D., Anderson, J. P., Gourley, I. S., Smith, H., Morris, C. A., DeSimone, M., et al., *Familial antiphospholipid antibody syndrome: Criteria for disease and evidence for autosomal dominant inheritance.* Arthritis Rheum, 1999. 42:318–327.

85. Hughes, G. R. V., *Connective tissue disease and the skin. The Prosser-White Oration 1983.* Clin Exp Dermatol, 1984. 9:535–544.

86. Bard, J. W., and Winkelmann, R. K., *Livedo vasculitis–segmental hyalinizing vasculitis of the dermis.* Arch Dermatol, 1967. 96:489–499.

87. Alegre, V. A., Gastineau, D. A., and Winkelmann, R. K., *Skin lesions associated with circulating lupus anticoagulant.* Br J Dermatol, 1989. 120:419–429.

88. Dubois, E. L., and Arterberry, J. D., *Gangrene as a manifestation of systemic lupus erythematosus.* J Am Med Assoc, 1962. 181:366–374.

89. Love, P. E., and Santoro, S. A., *Antiphospholipid antibodies: Anticardiolipin and the lupus anticoagulant in systemic lupus erythematosus and in non-SLE disorders.* Ann Intern Med, 1990. 112:682–698.

90. Brey, R. L., and Escalante, A., *Neurological manifestations of antiphospholipid antibody syndrome.* Lupus, 1998. 7(suppl 2):S67–S74.

91. Pittoni, V., and Isenberg, D., *Apoptosis and antiphospholipid antibodies.* Semin Arthritis Rheum, 1998. 28:163–178.

92. Hill, M. B., Phipps, J. L., Hughes, P., and Greaves, M., *Anti-endothelial cell antibodies in primary antiphospholipid syndrome and SLE: Patterns of reactivity with membrane antigens on microvascular and umbilical venous cell membranes.* Br J Haematol, 1998. 103:416–421.

93. Camisa, C., *Vesiculobullous systemic lupus erythematosus.* J Am Acad Dermatol, 1988. 18:93–100.

94. Hall, R. P., Lawley, T. J., Smith, H. R., and Katz, S. I., *Bullous eruption of systemic lupus erythematosus. Dramatic response to dapsone therapy.* Ann Intern Med, 1982. 97:165–170.

95. Gammon, W. R., and Briggaman, R. A., *Bullous SLE: A phenotypically distinctive but immunologically heterogeneous bullous disorder.* J Invest Dermatol, 1993. 100:28S–34S.

96. Burrows, N. P., Bhogal, B. S., Black, M. M., Rustin, M. H. A., Ishida-Yamamoto, A., Kirtschig, G., and Russell Jones, R., *Bullous eruption of systemic lupus erythematosus: A clinicopathologic study of four cases.* Br J Dermatol, 1993. 128:332–338.

97. Camisa, C., and Sharma, H. M., *Vesiculobullous systemic lupus erythematosus.* J Am Acad Dermatol, 1983. 9:924–933.

98. Gammon, W. R., Woodley, D. T., Dole, K. C., and Briggaman, R. A., *Evidence that antibasement membrane zone antibodies in bullous eruption of systemic lupus erythematosus recognize epidermolysis bullosa acquisita autoantigen.* J Invest Deramtol, 1985. 84:472–476.

99. Barton, D. D., Fine, J.-D., Gammon, W. R., and Sams, W. M., Jr., *Bullous systemic lupus erythematosus: An unusual clinical course and detectable circulating autoantibodies to the epidermolysis bullosa acquisita antigen.* J Am Acad Dermatol, 1986. 15:369–373.

100. Yang, L. J., Chan, H. L., Chen, S. Y., Kuan, Y. Z., Chen, M. J., Wang, C. N., Chen, W. J., and Kuo, T. T., *Atrophie blanche. A clinicopathological study of 27 patients.* Chang Keng I Hsueh, 1991. 14:237–245.

101. Suarez, S. M., and Paller, A. S., *Atrophie blanche with onset in childhood.* J Pediatr, 1993. 123:753–755.

102. Elisaf, M., Nikou-Stefanski, S., Drosos, A. A., and Moutsopoulos, H. M., *Atrophie blanche. Clinical diagnosis and treatment.* Ann Med Interne (Paris), 1991. 142:415–418.

103. Acland, K. M., Darvay, A., Wakelin, S. H., and Russell-Jones, R., *Livedoid vasculitis: a manifestation of the antiphospholipid syndrome?* Br J Dermatol, 1999. 140:131–135.

104. Wright, R. A., and Kokmen, E., *Gradually proressive dementia without discrete cerebrovascular events in a patient with Sneddon's syndrome.* Mayo Clin Proc, 1999. 74:57–61.

105. Ohtani, H., Imai, H., Yasuda, T., Wakui, H., Komatsuda, A., Hamai, K., and Miura, A. B., *A combination of livedo racemosa, occlusion of cerebral blood vessels, and nephropathy: Kidney involvement in Sneddon's syndrome.* Am J Kidney Dis, 1995. 26:511–515.

106. Grattan, C. E., Burton, J. L., and Boon, A. P., *Sneddon's syndrome (livedo reticularis and cerebral thrombosis) with livedo vasculitis and anticardiolipin antibodies.* Br J Dermatol, 1989. 120:441–447.

107. Otoyama, K., Katayama, I., Suzuki, Y., Tone, T., Nishioka, K., and Nishiyama, S., *A case of Sneddon's syndrome with positive ANA and anti-cardiolipin antibodies: Primary anti-phospholipid syndrome?* J Dermatol, 1990. 17:489–492.

108. Yasue, T., *Livedoid vasculitis and central nervous system involvement in systemic lupus erythematosus.* Arch Dermatol, 1986. 122:66–70.

109. Shornick, J. K., Nicholes, B. K., Bergstresser, P. R., and Gilliam, J. N., *Idiopathic atrophie blanche.* J Am Acad Dermatol, 1983. 8:792–798.

110. Schroeter, A. L., Diaz-Perez, J. L., Winkelmann, R. K., and Jordan, R. E., *Livedo vasculitis (the vasculitis of atrophie blanche). Immunohistopathologic study.* Arch Dermatol, 1975. 111:188–193.

111. McCalmont, C. S., McCalmont, T. H., Jorizzo, J. L., White, W. L., Leshin, B., and Rothberger, H., *Livedo vasculitis: Vasculitis or thrombotic vasculopathy?* Clin Exp Dermatol, 1992. 17:4–8.

112. Papi, M., Didona, B., De Pita, O., Frezzolini, A., Di Giulio, S., De Matteis, W., Del Principe, D., and Cavalieri, R., *Livedo vasculopathy vs. small vessel cutaneous vasculitis: Cytokine and platelet P-selectin studies.* Arch Dermatol, 1998. 134:447–452.

113. Pizzo, S. V., Murray, J. C., and Gonias, S. L., *Atrophie blanche. A disorder associated wtih defective release of tissue plasminogen activator.* Arch Pathol Lab Med, 1986. 110:517–519.

114. Turcu, A., Bonnotte, B., Fein, F., Martin, F., Chauffert, B., and Lorcerie, B., *Association of celiac disease and antiphosphopholipid syndrome.* Presse Med, 1998. 14:1789.

115. Calvo Romero, J. M., and Diaz Rodriguez, E., *Chronic hepatitis C virus positive hepatitis and antiphospholipid syndrome.* Gastroenterol Hepatol, 1998. 21:437–438.

116. Yanez, A., Cedillo, L., Neyrolles, O., Alonzo, E., Prevost, M. C., Rojas, J., Watson, H. L., Blanchard, A., et al., *Mycoplasma penetrans bacteremia and primary antiphospholipid syndrome.* Emerg Infect Dis, 1999. 5:164–171.

117. Hughes, G. R., *The antiphospholipid syndrome and 'multiple sclerosis.'* Lupus, 1999. 8:89.

118. Marla, R. M., Ramos-Casals, M., Garcia-Carrasco, M., Cervera, R., Font, J., Bruguera, M., Rojas-Rodriguez, J., and Ingelmo, M., *Nodular regenerative hyperplasia of the liver and antiphospholipid antibodies: Report of two cases and review of the literature.* Lupus, 1999. 8:160–163.

Connective Tissue, Joint Diseases, and the Skin

Dermatomyositis

Epidemiology. Dermatomyositis and polymyositis are generally classified together as a connective tissue disorder. *Polymyositis* is a connective tissue disorder in which muscle weakness is the only sign; *dermatomyositis* includes both muscle weakness and cutaneous manifestations. The incidence of the disease ranges from 1 to 10 people per million per year, with a prevalence of 10–60 per million [1]. The incidence in children ranges from 1 to 3.2 per million [2]. Dermatomyositis is about twice as common in women as in men. The average age of disease onset is approximately 40 years, and the onset of dermatomyositis associated with cancer (see later) occurs at about age 55 years [1]. Dermatomyositis has been associated with human leukocyte antigen (HLA) types B8, B14, DR3, DRw52, and DQA1 [1]. Juvenile dermatomyositis has been associated with HLA-DR3 and HLA-B8 [3].

The 1 year survival rate has been estimated at 83%, with 74% 2 year survival and 55% overall survival at 9 years. In this study, cancer and cardiopulmonary complications were the most frequent causes of death [4].

Cutaneous Features. Cutaneous manifestations may appear 3–6 months before the development of muscle weakness [5]. The two most specific cutaneous manifestations of dermatomyositis are a heliotrope erythema and Gottron's papules. Heliotrope erythema consists of periorbital macules with marked edema that involves the eyelids. It is seen in 30%–60% of patients with dermatomyositis [6]. Gottron's papules are violaceous atrophic papules overlying the dorsal surfaces of the interphalangeal or metaphalangeal joints or, less commonly, the elbows or knees. They are seen in 70% of patients with dermatomyositis. Other changes include periungual telangiectasias, poikiloderma in a shawl-like distribution over the shoulders, overgrowth of nail cuticles and nail infarcts, and a scaly, erythematous, eruption on the scalp. Photosensitivity is usually prominent [7]. Less common manifestations include acquired ichthyosis [8], vasculitis [9], panniculitis [10], erythroderma [11], and bullae formation [12]. Juvenile dermatomyositis is complicated by calcinosis cutis in from 30% [13] to 70% [14] of cases.

Associated Disorders. Muscle weakness is present in most patients with dermatomyositis, although a form lacking muscle involvement, dermatomyositis sine myositis, has been described [5]. As many as 11% of patients with cutaneous findings of dermatomyositis will never develop muscle weakness [5]. Weakness is symmetric, involves proximal muscles, and is progressive.

Dermatomyositis has been associated with underlying cancer [15]. In one large study, 15% of adults with dermatomyositis had cancer, with a relative risk of 2.4 for men and 3.4 for women [16]. Other investigators believe that the cancer may be found in as many as 25% of adults with dermatomyositis [7]. In some series, ovarian carcinoma [17] and nasopharyngeal carcinomas [7] are related with disproportionate frequencies, but these observations are not replicated by all investigators. In men, a significant association between dermatomyositis and lymphoma has been reported [17]. Polymyositis is also associated with increased risk of internal cancer, albeit at a much lower rate. It has been suggested that the association with internal cancer may not be present for patients with dermatomyositis sine myositis [5].

A significant minority of patients with dermatomyositis/polymyositis (10%–40%) suffer from a second connective tissue disease such as scleroderma, systemic lupus erythematosus, rheumatoid arthritis, Sjögren's syndrome, or polyarteritis nodosa [18]. This relationship is more pronounced among affected women and is more likely to occur in patients with polymyositis than those with dermatomyositis [1]. Dermatomyositis has been described in a patient with bronchiolitis obliterans organizing pneumonia [19].

Juvenile dermatomyositis is associated with symmetric arthritis of large and small joints [1]. Decreased gastrointestinal absorption and occasional ulcerations and perforations of the gastrointestinal tract occur in these patients and may be related, in part, to treatment with corticosteroids [2]. About half of patients with juvenile dermatomyositis have electrocardiogram anomalies, including conduction abnormalities or bundle branch blocks [20]. Juvenile dermatomyositis is not associated with cancer [1]. Calcinosis cutis is a typical accompanying problem in juveniles with dermatomyositis.

Histologic Features. Histologic findings in dermatomyositis are characterized by an interface dermatitis that is relatively slight. Epidermal atrophy is present in later lesions, but the epidermis is of normal thickness in earlier lesions. Basal vacuolization is extensive, and lymphocytes are present within the epidermis. Within the dermis, there is a sparse to moderate infiltrate of lymphocytes and histiocytes surrounding the superficial vascular plexus. Occasional plasma cells may be seen. Eosinophils are not common. Cutaneous appendages are only minimally inflamed (Fig. 2–1). Abundant acid mucopolysaccharides can be seen in the papillary and superficial reticular dermis. A colloidal iron stain performed at pH 4.5 is helpful in highlighting the mucin deposition (Fig. 2–2). Compared with lupus erythematosus, the inflammatory infiltrate is sparse. The following entities must be considered in the histologic differential diagnosis of dermatomyositis:

- Erythema dyschromicum perstans
- Erythema multiforme
- Graft-versus-host disease
- Lupus erythematosus
- Mixed connective tissue disease

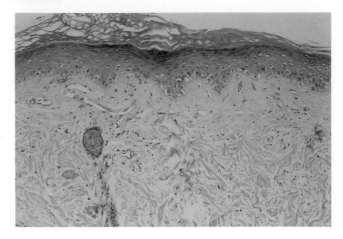

Fig. 2–1. Dermatomyositis is characterized by a vacuolar interface dermatitis with sparse inflammatory infiltrate.

- Pityriasis lichenoides chronica
- Poikiloderma atrophicans vasculare

Special Studies. Direct immunofluorescence examination may be helpful in making a diagnosis of dermatomyositis. Routine studies with IgG, IgA, IgM, and C3 are uniformly negative, unlike those for the histologically similar lupus erythematosus in which granular deposits of immunoreactants are usually present. Membrane attack complexes (C5b–9) have been demonstrated along the dermal–epidermal junction in 86% of biopsy specimems from affected skin of patients with dermatomyositis. Similar deposits are present in scattered dermal blood vessels in 77% of cases [21]. Some authors have found similar deposits of membrane attack complexes in skin affected by cutaneous lupus erythematosus [21]. In another study, investigators found that the presence of membrane attack com-

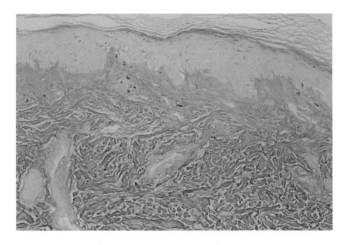

Fig. 2–2. A colloidal iron stain (pH 4.5) demonstrates abundant acid mucopolysaccharides in the reticular dermis in dermatomyositis.

plex along the dermal–epidermal junction and a negative lupus band test was 78.3% sensitive and 93.5% specific for the diagnosis of dermatomyositis [22].

Electromyogram and enzyme studies such as aldolase and creatine kinase levels are helpful in determining muscle involvement [7]. Direct immunofluorescence studies performed on muscle often demonstrate immunoglobulins, including IgA in one case [23].

Autoantibodies are present in most patients with dermatomyositis. Higher titers are present in those with associated connective tissue diseases. Anti-RNP is seen in patients with overlap syndromes, including dermatomyositis and lupus erythematosus or mixed connective tissue disease [24], and anti-Pm-Scl is found in patients with coexisting scleroderma and dermatomyositis [25]. Muscle-specific autoantibodies are present in only one-third of patients with dermatomyositis [1]. Low titer autoantibodies are present in a minority of patients with juvenile dermatomyositis and do not correlate with disease activity [1].

Pathogenesis. The cause of dermatomyositis is unknown. Autoantibodies directed specifically against muscle are found in only a few patients and thus cannot be implicated in most cases. Soluble interleukin-2 receptors have been demonstrated in patients with dermatomyositis [26], but the significance of this finding remains unknown. Although many viruses have been implicated in the pathogenesis, there is little evidence supporting these contentions [27]. *Toxoplasma gondii* has also been implicated by some researchers [28]. There does not appear to be a significant relationship between silicone implants and increased risk for dermatomyositis [29].

Scleroderma.
Patients with scleroderma (systemic sclerosis) have been divided into three groups based on clinical features [30]. About 50% of patients have limited disease and are described later (see Morphea). Patients with progressive systemic sclerosis have more aggressive disease and comprise the second largest group of patients with systemic sclerosis. A rare third group (acral sclerosis) has been described in which patients have sclerosis and disseminated telangiectasias, along with antibodies directed against RNA-associated protein fibrillarin [31].

Progressive Systemic Sclerosis
Epidemiology. The overall incidence of progressive systemic sclerosis (PSS) ranges from 2 to 20 people per 1 million per year. About half of these patients suffer from diffuse cutaneous sclerosis. There is a marked female predominance that ranges from 3:1 to 9:1. The peak age of onset is between the third and fifth decades

[30]. Patients with truncal scleroderma at the onset of disease have a 50% 5 year survival rate and a 25% 10 year survival rate [32]. Involvement of the kidneys, lungs, and heart are frequent causes of death in these patients.

Cutaneous features. The widespread thickening of the skin often begins in the the fingers and moves proximally to the trunk [33]. In patients with PSS, the skin changes quickly progress through three stages, including edema, induration, and, finally, atrophy, to involve the entire skin surface. In its late stages, the skin appears bound down to underlying structures. Many patients have "beaked" facial features.

Raynaud's phenomenon, or episodic digital ischemia, is present in 90%–98% of patients with PSS [34]. Pterygium inversum unguim-like changes of the nails in which the hyponychium adheres to the distal nail and obliterates the normal space have been reported in some patients with scleroderma [35]. Tapered fingers are frequently encountered, and digital ulcerations may be seen. Dilated tortuous capillary loops are seen, as well.

Associated disorders. Onset of PSS is often acute, with diffuse arthritis, carpal tunnel syndrome, and marked swelling of the extremities and Raynaud's phenomenon [33].

Gastrointestinal fibrosis is the most common visceral feature of PSS [36]. This manifests as esophageal reflux, delayed gastric emptying, and pseudo-obstruction of the small and large intestines. Pulmonary fibrosis is also common, occurring in 40%–90% of patients [37]. Pulmonary hypertension is seen in 5%–10% of patients with PSS. About 45% of patients with PSS have renal disease [34]. Malignant hypertension and renal failure are common causes of death [33]. Although cardiac involvement is present in up to one-third of patients with systemic sclerosis, it is only rarely clinically significant. Progressive systemic sclerosis has been reported in patients following exposure to environmental factors such as aromatic hydrocarbons, formaldehyde, and some drugs [30].

Sjögren's syndrome is present in 17% of patients with scleroderma, but may be seen more frequently in association with the limited form of the disease [38]. The relationship between PSS and mixed connective tissue disease is still unclear. Mixed connective tissue disease is discussed later.

Histologic features. The histologic features in PSS and morphea are indistinguishable. Early lesions demonstrate an infiltrate of lymphocytes and histiocytes around vessels in the superficial vascular plexus, as well as at the interface between the reticular dermis and subcutaneous fat. The epidermis is initially unremarkable, and there is no interface dermatitis. Plasma cells are often present, and perieccrine inflammation is

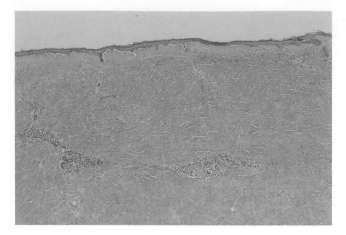

Fig. 2–3. A well-developed case of progressive systemic sclerosis demonstrating thickened collagen bundles in the presence of a dense perivascular inflammatory infiltrate.

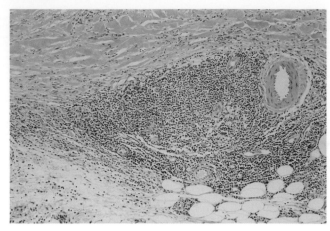

Fig. 2–5. A marked lymphocytic and plasmacellular infiltrate with lymphoid nodules is present in the deep reticular dermis in early lesions of morphea/progressive systemic sclerosis.

common (Fig. 2–3 and Fig. 2–4). Lymphocytic nodules are seen in the deep reticular dermis in some cases (Fig. 2–5). Occasional eosinophils are also seen in biopsy specimens from acute inflammatory lesions. Biopsy specimens from early lesions may also demonstrate intradermal edema separating collagen bundles in the reticular dermis (Fig. 2–6). As lesions become more fully developed and clinically indurated, the dermal collagen bundles appear thickened and more eosinophilic and have less space between bundles. The dermis becomes markedly thickened and leads to progressive thinning of the overlying epidermis. Rete ridges are ultimately lost or markedly decreased. The inflammatory infiltrate gradually becomes less pronounced. Eventually, eccrine coils are tightly enveloped by dense collagen bundles. Hair follicles are often lost due to the same

process, and arrector pili muscles are seen in the dermis without adjacent follicular epithelium (Fig. 2–7). The following entities must be considered in the histologic differential diagnosis of morphea/PSS:

- Connective tissue nevus (collagenoma)
- Lichen sclerosis et atrophicus
- Radiation dermatitis
- Scar
- Scleredema
- Sclerodermoid graft-versus-host disease

Special studies. Anti-Scl-70 is found in up to 75% of patients with PSS [39]. It is directed against topoisomerase I.

Pathogenesis. The cause of scleroderma remains

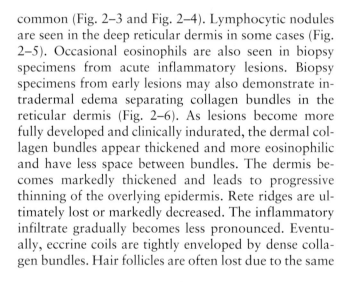

Fig. 2–4. Dense aggregates of plasma cells and lymphocytes are present around eccrine ducts in early lesions of progressive systemic sclerosis/morphea.

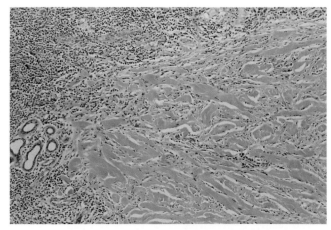

Fig. 2–6. Early lesions of progressive systemic sclerosis/morphea demonstrate a dense, diffuse dermal infiltrate and abundant interstitial edema.

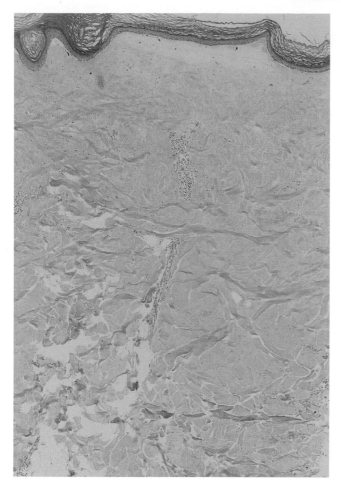

Fig. 2–7. Late in the course, lesions of morphea/progressive systemic sclerosis are characterized by markedly increased collagen bundles, loss of cutaneous appendages, and thinning of the epidermis.

unknown. Excessive collagen is deposited in the dermis and in the connective tissue matrices of other organs. T lymphocytes and monocytes are thought to initiate the disease process by targeting fibroblasts, platelets, mast cells, and endothelial cells to overproduce type I collagen [30, 40]. Abnormal endothelial cell function leading to microvascular injury has also been implicated in the pathogenesis [41–43].

Morphea. Morphea can be either localized or diffuse, but in both situations disease is limited to cutaneous changes, and there is no visceral involvement. Localized disease is characterized by several well-defined, indurated plaques. At the periphery of the plaques, there is a faint rim of violaceous erythema. The diffuse form of the disease is characterized by many similar-appearing lesions generally distributed. As mentioned earlier, it is not possible to differentiate morphea from PSS in a biopsy specimen.

Acral Scleroderma

Epidemiology. CREST is an acronym that describes patients with the constellation of calcinosis cutis, Raynaud's phenomenon, esophageal dysfunction, sclerodactyly, and telangiectasia and has been renamed *limited cutaneous scleroderma* [33]. In the United States, HLA-DR3 is associated with limited scleroderma, although this relationship does not appear to occur in Europeans with the disease [44]. Slightly more than one-half of all patients with scleroderma suffer from the limited cutaneous form [30].

Cutaneous features. Patients with limited cutaneous or localized scleroderma often have long-standing Raynaud's phenomenon before the onset of other cutaneous manifestations [33]. Changes are usually limited to thickening of the skin on the hands and digital ulceration [33]. Telangiectasias are often present and may be prominent, leading to bleeding diatheses in rare cases [45]. When matched with patients with PSS, patients with localized scleroderma have less muscle and skin involvement [46]. Calcinosis cutis manifests as eroded papules or nodules from which a chalky substance may extrude. In rare patients with localized scleroderma, ulcerations and mononeuritis, indicative of vasculitis, may be present [47].

Associated disorders. Localized scleroderma has been associated with primary biliary cirrhosis in about 16% of cases [48]. These patients often have an anticentromere antibody [49]. The relationship with primary biliary cirrhosis is stronger in patients with localized cutaneous scleroderma than in those with diffuse systemic sclerosis [50]. Nodular regenerative hyperplasia of the liver has also been reported in patients with localized cutaneous scleroderma and primary biliary cirrhosis [51].

Localized scleroderma has been associated with Sjögren's syndrome [49]. Esophageal dysmotility may be present in many of these patients [33]. Pulmonary hypertension and small intestinal hypomotility have also been reported, but are much less common than in systemic scleroderma [33]. Autoimmune hemolytic anemia has been reported in a patient with CREST syndrome [52].

Histologic features. Biopsy specimens from patients with localized scleroderma have changes identical to those in specimens from patients with systemic sclerosis (see above). In rare patients with localized scleroderma, leukocytoclastic vasculitis may be found in biopsy specimens. This corresponds to clinical ulcerations [47].

Special studies. Anticentromere antibodies are found in 70%–80% of patients with limited scleroderma and may be a marker for patients with the less severe form of the disease [53, 54].

Pathogenesis. The pathogenesis of localized scleroderma is currently unknown.

Eosinophilic Fasciitis

Epidemiology. Eosinophilic fasciitis, also known as *Shulman's syndrome,* was initially described as a syndrome of diffuse fasciitis, hypergammaglobulinemia, and peripheral eosinophilia [55]. It often presents shortly after intense physical exertion or trauma. It is more common in men and rarely occurs in children. Most patients present during their second to fifth decades.

Cutaneous Features. The skin of patients with eosinophilic fasciitis is firm and tightly bound [56]. The earliest changes may be marked pain and swelling of the extremities. The forearms are often diffusely involved, and the lower extremities may also be affected. Affected skin may give rise to a peau d'orange appearance. Fingers and toes are usually spared [57]. There is often a striking symmetry to the presentation.

Associated Disorders. Eosinophilic fasciitis has been associated with carpal tunnel syndrome and synovitis. Rare reports of restrictive pulmonary disease exist, but in most patients viscera are not affected. Eosinophilic fasciitis has been reported to occur as a paraneoplastic syndrome in conjunction with T-cell lymphomas [58], aplastic anemia [59], myelomonocytic leukemia, [60] and Hodgkin's disease [61].

Eosinophilic fasciitis, in conjunction with severe myalgias, arthralgias, fever, and weakness, has been reported in patients who ingested L-tryptophan [62]. Contaminants in the tryptophan preparations were implicated in the cause of the disease [63]. There are differences in the clinical, as well as laboratory, findings in these patients compared with patients with Shulman's syndrome [56].

Histologic features. The histologic findings of eosinophilic fasciitis include an unremarkable epidermis. Any inflammatory infiltrate within the dermis is sparse. Plasma cells and eosinophils are seen in a few cases. Inflammation is present within the subcutaneous fat and consists of lymphocytes, histiocytes, plasma cells, and eosinophils in most cases [56]. This most likely represents extension from the underlying inflamed fascia. Thickening may be present within the fibrous septa of the panniculus. Mucin is often abundant [56]. The fascia is markedly thickened (Fig. 2–8). A mixed inflammatory infiltrate, including plasma cells and eosinophils, is present and mucin deposition is pronounced (Fig. 2–9). The underlying muscle may demonstrate similar changes. It is important to note that, despite the name, eosinophils are not always present in biopsy tissue from patients with eosinophilic fasciitis.

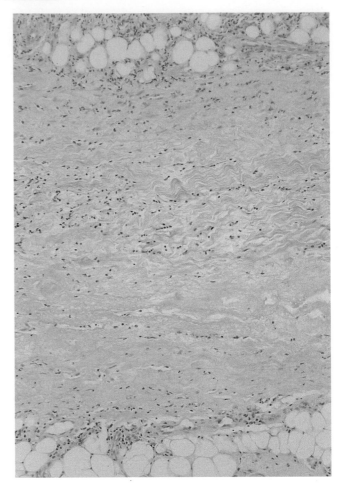

Fig. 2–8. Eosinophilic fasciitis is characterized by marked thickening of the fibrous septa within the panniculus and of the underlying fascia.

Special Studies. Rheumatoid factor and antinuclear antibodies are usually not observed in affected persons [64].

Pathogenesis. The pathogenesis of eosinophilic fasciitis remains unknown. Some authors have proposed a humoral immune mechanism based on the hypergammaglobulinemia frequently seen in these patients [55] and on immune deposits in affected fascia [65]. The presence of abundant factor XIIIa–positive cells within the inflamed panniculus and fascia may play a role in the fibroplasia that develops in these patients [56]. Cultured fibroblasts from affected skin of patients with eosinophilic fasciitis exhibit a marked increase in collagen production compared with unaffected skin [57].

Mixed Connective Tissue Disease

Epidemiology. Mixed connective tissue disease (MCTD) is a poorly defined entity that represents an overlap of clinical features in patients with systemic lu-

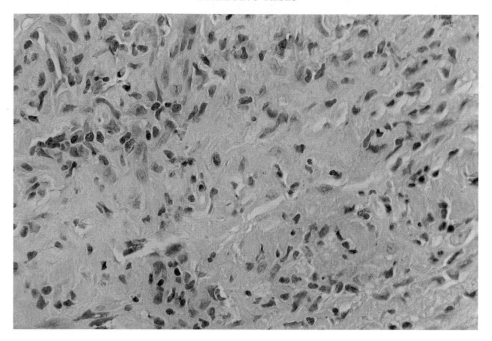

Fig. 2–9. A mixed inflammatory infiltrate with abundant lymphocytes and plasma cells and only scattered eosinophils, is characteristic of eosinophilic fasciitis.

pus erythematosus, scleroderma, and polymyositis [66]. Many authors do not believe that MCTD represents a discrete disease and classify it as a subtype of scleroderma [67]. Others believe that clinical, immunologic, and genetic data are sufficiently distinctive to warrant its designation as a separate entity [68]. Mixed connective tissue disease is associated with HLA-DR4 [69]. Given the lack of consensus regarding diagnostic criteria for this entity, it is difficult to arrive at exact morbidity and mortality statistics. As many as 38% of patients continued to have active disease or died of the disease with up to 29 years of follow-up [70]. In another study, 67% of patients studied for at least 5 years ultimately developed American Rheumatism Association criteria for systemic lupus erythematosus [71]. The mortality rate among children with MCTD is approximately 8%, with most deaths due to sepsis, cerebral complications, heart failure, renal failure, and pulmonary hypertension [72].

Cutaneous Features. The cutaneous eruption in MCTD is characterized by photodistributed, annular, erythematous macules and papules that may clinically resemble subacute lupus erythematosus. Less commonly, bullae on the dorsum of the hands, purpuric papules, and telangiectasias have been described [73].

Associated Disorders. Patients with MCTD often have Raynaud's phenomenon, polyarthralgias and arthritis, and edematous hands. Respiratory complications, including interstitial pneumonitis and fibrosis, pleural effusions and pleurisy, and pulmonary hypertension, occur

in 20%–80% of patients. Less commonly, pulmonary vasculitis, cysts, hemorrhage, and respiratory failure may be seen [74]. Patients with MCTD may suffer from esophageal hypomotility and myositis. Pneumatosis cystoides intestinalis has been reported in rare patients with MCTD [75]. Up to half of patients will have involvement of the central nervous system. Membranous glomerulonephritis [76] and sclerodermatous renal crises may also be seen [77]. Splenic vasculitis has been reported [78]. Second-trimester fetal loss may be more common than expected in patients with MCTD [79]. Rare patients with MCTD have presented with necrotizing histiocytic lymphadenitis (Kikuchi's disease) [80].

In children with MCTD, kidneys are involved in about half of cases and esophageal dysmotility in about 30% of cases. Myocarditis and cardiomyopathy may occur. Up to 86% of affected children experience Raynaud's phenomenon and scleroderma-like changes in their skin [72].

Histologic Features. Histologic features of cutaneous eruptions of MCTD include a paucicellular lichenoid infiltrate composed of lymphocytes, with exocytosis and scattered dying keratinocytes. Vascular ectasia may be prominent, and thrombosis may be present. There is no deep component to the inflammatory infiltrate, and follicular plugging is not as pronounced as in lupus erythematosus [73].

Special Studies. Direct immunofluorescence may be helpful in making a diagnosis of MCTD. In one study, keratinocyte nuclei were labeled with IgG and the C5b–9 membrane attack complex in all cases [73]. In about one-fourth of cases, granular deposits of IgG, IgM, and C3 may be present along the dermal–epidermal junction. The membrane attack complex is also present in dermal blood vessels, helping to distinguish MCTD from lupus erythematosus. The diagnosis is confirmed by presence of antibodies in the serum directed against U1 small nuclear ribonucleoprotein [74, 81].

Pathogenesis. The pathogenesis of MCTD is currently not known.

Sjögren's Syndrome

Epidemiology. Sjögren's syndrome may occur alone or in the presence of another connective tissue disease such as rheumatoid arthritis, PSS, or systemic lupus erythematosus. It is also known as *sicca syndrome* and is defined as the presence of a dry mouth (xerostomia) and dry eyes (xerophthalmia) [82]. Some authors believe Sjögren's syndrome to be as common as rheumatoid arthritis. It occurs most often in patients in their fifth decade [82]. Up to 90% of patients with Sjögren's syndrome have the HLA-DRw52 phenotype [82]. HLA-DR2 and HLA-DR3 are also present in 85%–90% of affected patients [83]. Sicca complex, but not true Sjögren's syndrome, occurs as part of chronic graft-versus-host disease.

Cutaneous Features. Vasculitis may occur in up to 25% of patients with Sjögren's syndrome and is most common in those with high titers of anti-Ro antibodies. The lower legs are most frequently involved, and the most common presentation is that of palpable purpura. Urticarial lesions are also present [84].

Rare patients with Sjögren's syndrome have been reported with panniculitis characterized by tender, indurated plaques on the lower extremities [85]. Other uncommon cutaneous manifestations include annular erythematous patches [86] and anhidrosis [87].

Associated Disorders. Patients with Sjögren's syndrome may suffer inflammatory reactions in many organs, giving rise to respiratory problems such as interstitial pneumonitis with fibrosis [84] and necrotizing bronchiolitis [88]. The gastrointestinal system can be affected by pancreatic dysfunction, chronic active hepatitis, or primary biliary cirrhosis [89]. The kidneys can be affected by interstitial nephritis and glomerulonephritis. Neurologic symptoms, including necrotizing arteritis, subarachnoid hemorrhages [90], and aseptic meningoencephalitis [91] have been reported. Myositis, pernicious anemia, and autoimmune thyroid diseases have also been reported in patients with Sjögren's syndrome [82]. Vasculitis involving peripheral nerves has been documented [84].

Rare cases of lymphoma, usually B-cell lymphoma, have been reported in patients with Sjögren's syndrome. Most are mucosa-associated lymphoid tissue lymphomas. They can appear within the salivary gland or in other organs throughout the body. The most significant predictors for the development of lymphoma in these patients are the presence of swollen salivary glands, lymphadenopathy, and leg ulcers [92]. Rare T-cell neoplasms have also been reported [93].

Histologic Features. The histologic features of vasculitis are identical to those of leukocytoclastic vasculitis due to other causes. There is a neutrophilic infiltrate surrounding vessels of the superficial vascular plexus, with transmural migration, vascular wall destruction, fibrin deposition, and extravasation of erythrocytes. About as commonly, a lymphocytic vasculitis has been reported. In these cases, there is also destruction of vessel walls, fibrin deposition, and extravasation of erythrocytes [94]. It has been suggested that the leukocytoclastic vasculitis pattern is seen more commonly in patients with Sjögren's syndrome and high titers of Ro (SS-A) and La (SS-B), hypergammaglobulinemia, and positive rheumatoid factors. The lymphocytic vasculitic pattern is more common in patients with Sjögren's syndrome with low titers of these antibodies [82].

The panniculitic plaques demonstrate a dense lobular panniculitis composed of plasma cells and lymphocytes. The infiltrate is predominantly perivascular and extends upward to surround eccrine structures in the deep reticular dermis. Mild fat necrosis may be seen [85].

Histologic examination of cutaneous erythematous patches reveal perivascular and periadnexal lymphocytic infiltrates. Atrophy of eccrine glands may be present. Myoepithelial islands have been described in biopsy specimens taken from cutaneous nodules. These islands are similar in appearance to those in salivary gland biopsy specimens.

Histologic examination of the lymphomas reveals lymphoid neoplasms that are indistinguishable from the sporadically occurring processes. Rare cases of pleomorphic T-cell lymphoma have been described in this population [93].

Microscopic examination of the salivary glands reveals a lymphoid infiltrate with destruction of glandular structures (Fig. 2–10). The lymphoid nodules can be extremely large (Fig. 2–11). Myoepithelial islands are frequently present and are believed to represent collapsed acini before their complete involution [95].

Special Studies. Special studies are not necessary to make a tissue diagnosis of Sjögren's syndrome. Serologic studies looking for circulating antibodies are essential.

Pathogenesis. Sjögren's syndrome is an autoimmune disease; however, the exact pathogenesis of the disease

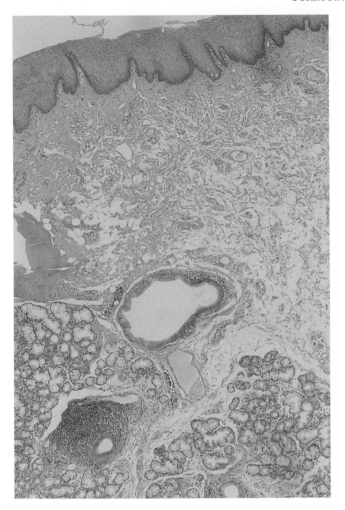

Fig. 2–10. Sjögren's syndrome is characterized by inflammatory cells within salivary glands.

remains largely elusive. Ro and La autoantibody-producing cells in salivary gland biopsy tissue have been detected in patients with Sjögren's syndrome. This raises the potential that these cells are directly involved in causing the inflammatory processes seen in this disease [96].

Psoriasis and Arthritis

Epidemiology. Psoriasis affects 1%–2% of the U.S. population [97]. It is a multifactorial disease, but genetics appear to play some role in the predisposition for the development of psoriasis. Patients with HLA-Cw6 have a relative risk of 24 for developing psoriasis. Up to one-half of patients with psoriasis report a family history of the disease [98]. There is a high rate of concordance of psoriasis in monozygotic twins [99]. Psoriasis is much more common in whites than in Asian, North and South American natives, and native North American blacks [100]. There is a high prevalence of psoriasis in Scandinavian countries. A potential psoriasis gene has been located on chromosome 17q [101]. Men and women are affected equally, and the usual age of onset is young adulthood [102].

The average age of onset of pustular psoriasis is 50 years, which is older than the average age of onset for plaque psoriasis. Men and women are equally at risk. Infections may be a triggering event in precipitating exacerbations [103].

Cutaneous Features. There are many classification systems for various clinical subtypes of psoriasis, and many names have been given to clinical variants of the disease. Classic plaque psoriasis is characterized by well-

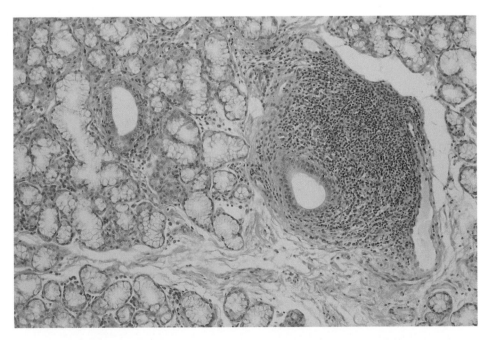

Fig. 2–11. Lymphoid aggregates may be quite large in some cases of Sjögren's syndrome.

demarcated, erythematous plaques with overlying thick scale distributed symmetrically on the extensor surfaces of the extremities. It is the most common form of psoriasis. Psoriatic plaques are symmetrically distributed on the knees and elbows, intergluteal cleft, and scalp. The trunk is also frequently affected. Gentle removal of the thick, adherent scale gives rise to characteristic punctate bleeding points, a sign known as the *Auspitz sign.* Some patients with localized forms of the disease may have plaques limited to the palms and soles.

Guttate psoriasis presents with the abrupt onset of oval patches ranging from several to 1–2 cm in diameter, with overlying scale, usually on the trunk and extremities. It is most commonly found in children.

Pustules may be a major cutaneous feature in some patients with psoriasis. The eruption may be localized to the extremities, or only the palms and soles, or it can be generalized. There are as many as five subtypes of generalized pustular psoriasis [103]. Pustular psoriasis has been associated with decreased levels of serum calcium.

Erythrodermic psoriasis occurs in about 2% of patients with psoriasis [104]. It can be seen as a result of an exacerbation of classic plaque psoriasis, or it can appear as a de novo condition. Erythrodermic psoriasis is more common in men.

Koebner's phenomenon, which is defined as the induction of a new psoriatic lesion on clinically uninvolved skin at the site of localized trauma, is a well-known feature of psoriasis. It is found in about one-third of patients with psoriasis.

Associated Disorders. Psoriasis can be precipitated by drugs such as β-blockers and lithium. Nonsteroidal antiinflammatory drugs may exacerbate psoriasis. Pustular psoriasis is often associated with the withdrawal of systemic corticosteroids in patients with plaque psoriasis. Pregnancy can also trigger a flare of pustular psoriasis. Guttate psoriasis has been shown to be closely associated with streptococcal infection in many patients [105]. Other potential triggering factors include stress [106], malignancy [107], climate, and hormonal factors [108].

Arthritis occurs in 4% [97] to 34% [109] of patients with psoriasis. Psoriatic arthritis is classified as a seronegative spondyloarthropathy. It affects men and women with equal likelihood, and most commonly presents after the skin disease. Although arthritis is more commonly seen in patients with more severe cutaneous psoriasis, the severity of the arthritis does not correlate completely with the severity of the skin disease [109]. When only one joint is involved, it is most commonly the knee, ankle, or metatarsophalangeal joint; however, several joints can be affected. Spondylitis and sacroiliitis may also be present. An increased incidence of HLA-B27 is seen in patients with psoriatic arthritis, and this association is even stronger for those with spondylitis. Increased frequencies of HLA types B16, B17, B38, B39, Cw6, DR4, and DR7 are also reported in patients with psoriatic arthritis [100]. Radiographic findings have been described as "pencil and cup" deformities in affected joints.

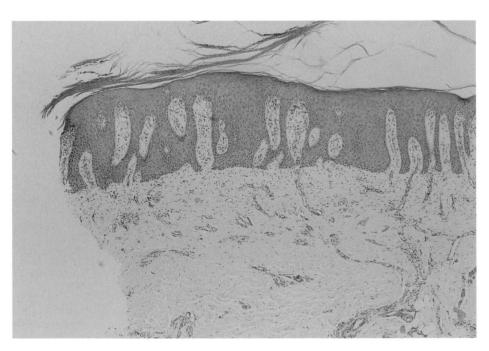

Fig. 2–12. Classic plaque psoriasis demonstrates regular elongation of the rete ridges with a characteristic bulbous pattern.

Erythrodermic and pustular psoriasis are associated with constitutional symptoms such as fever and malaise. Hypoalbuminemia is seen in some patients with erythrodermic psoriasis, and this in addition to increased cutaneous blood flow can result in "high output" cardiac failure. Psoriasis and psoriatic arthritis are seen with increased frequency in patients with human immunodeficiency virus infection [110].

Histologic Features. The many different clinical forms of psoriasis result in different histologic appearances. Classic psoriasis is characterized by diffuse, thick parakeratotic scale overlying an epidermis that demonstrates acanthosis and regular elongation of the bulbous-shaped rete ridges (Fig. 2–12). There is suprapapillary thinning of the epidermis between the rete ridges. The granular layer is lost or markedly diminished in thickness (Fig. 2–13). Neutrophils may be present in abscesses within the stratum corneum (Munro's microabscesses) (Fig. 2–14) or in the upper portion of the epidermis (Kogoj's spongiform pustule) (Fig. 2–15). Dilated capillaries are present within the tips of the dermal papillae (giving rise to the clinical Auspitz sign). This is one of the earliest histologic changes seen in psoriasis. A mild to moderately intense perivascular lymphocytic infiltrate is present, and scattered lymphocytes may be present within the epidermis. Scattered neutrophils may also be present within the dermis. Eosinophils and plasma cells are not generally present; however, plasma cells have been described in the psoriasiform eruption seen in patients with acquired immunodeficiency syndrome [111]. The following common entities must be considered in the histologic differential diagnosis of psoriasis:

- Acrodermatitis enteropathica
- Chronic spongiotic dermatitis/nummular eczema

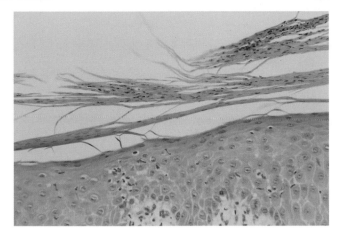

Fig. 2–14. Neutrophilic abscesses within the stratum corneum, known as Munro's microabscesses, are common in psoriasis.

- Dermatophytosis
- Lichen simplex chronicus
- Necrolytic migratory erythema
- Pityriasis rubra pilaris
- Seborrheic dermatitis

The histologic changes in guttate psoriasis are less prominent. The parakeratotic scale is often less thick and occurs in mounds as opposed to confluently over the epidermis (Fig. 2–16). The granular layer, while often focally diminished, is rarely completely absent. The epidermis is slightly acanthotic, but rarely demonstrates the regular elongation of the rete ridges that characterizes classic plaques of psoriasis. Slight spongiosis may be seen. Neutrophils may be present within the stratum corneum or epidermis. Dilated capillaries within the papillary dermal tips are often present and may serve as a

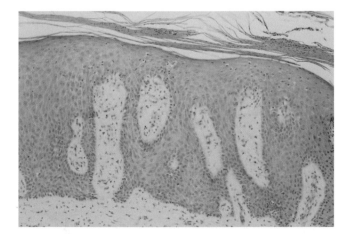

Fig. 2–13. Psoriasis is characterized by loss of the granular layer, parakeratosis with neutrophils within the stratum corneum, and suprapapillary thinning.

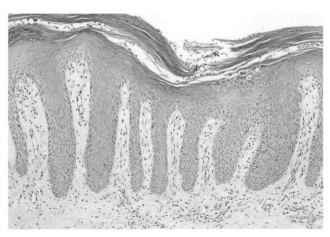

Fig. 2–15. Intraepidermal neutrophils (spongiform pustules of Kogoj) are also seen in psoriasis.

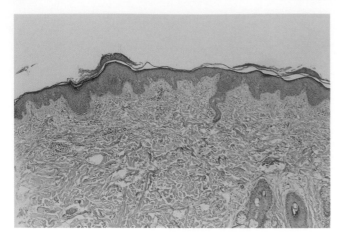

Fig. 2–16. The changes in guttate psoriasis include slight acanthosis and mounds of parakeratosis.

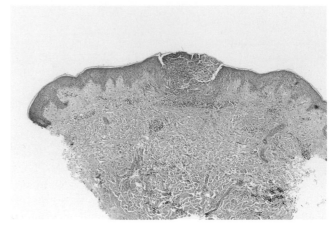

Fig. 2–18. Pustular psoriasis is characterized by large intraepidermal pustules often in the absence of other changes characteristic of psoriasis.

useful clue to the diagnosis (Fig. 2–17). A mild lymphohistiocytic infiltrate is present in the superficial dermis. The following entities must be considered in the histologic differential diagnosis of guttate psoriasis:

- Dermatophytosis
- Pityriasis rosea
- Pityriasis rubra pilaris
- Small plaque parapsoriasis/digitate dermatosis

Pustular psoriasis demonstrates yet another pattern of histologic changes. Parakeratosis may not be present but, when it is, is often limited to the area overlying the large pustules. The epidermis is minimally acanthotic, and no regular elongation of rete ridges is ordinarily seen. Within the epidermis, large neutrophilic abscesses are present (Fig. 2–18). The dermal changes are similar to those found

in other forms of psoriasis, although the dilated capillaries are often less prominent and may be surrounded by neutrophils instead of lymphocytes (Fig. 2–19) [112]. The following entities must be considered in the histologic differential diagnosis of pustular psoriasis:

- Acute generalized exanthematous pustulosis
- Candidiasis
- Dermatophytosis
- Dyshidrotic eczema
- Impetigo
- Pemphigus foliaceus/erythematosus
- Subcorneal pustular dermatosis of Sneddon and Wilkinson

Erythrodermic psoriasis paradoxically often has the least diagnostic changes in biopsy specimens. Paraker-

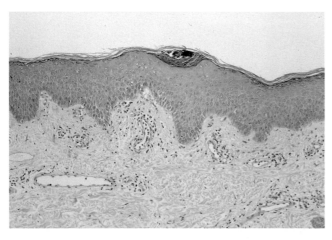

Fig. 2–17. Ectasia of vessels high in the papillary dermis may be one of the earliest changes seen in guttate psoriasis.

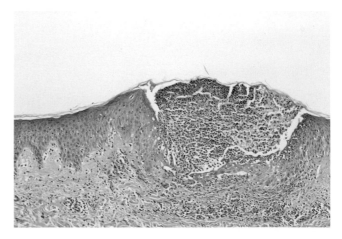

Fig. 2–19. Neutrophilic abscesses are large in many cases of pustular psoriasis and are often surrounded by slight degrees of spongiosis.

atosis is present, but not confluent or thick. The granular layer is diminished in thickness, but usually still present. Neutrophilic abscesses are rarely seen. The epidermis is mildly acanthotic, but does not usually demonstrate the classic regular elongation of rete ridges seen in patch/plaque psoriasis. The dermal inflammatory infiltrate is minimal. The following entities must be considered in the histologic differential diagnosis of erythrodermic psoriasis:

- Drug eruption
- Pityriasis rubra pilaris
- Subacute/chronic spongiotic dermatitis
- Sezary's syndrome

Special Studies. Special studies are not necessary to make a diagnosis of psoriasis. Often, however, it is helpful to evaluate a slide stained with periodic acid–Schiff to eliminate the possibility of a dermatophyte infection.

Pathogenesis. Psoriasis is a multifactorial disease. Approximately one-third of affected patients have a positive family history of psoriasis [113]. Epidermal hyperproliferation is marked. Increased cytokines such as interleukins-1, -6, and -8, which are proinflammatory and may stimulate keratinocyte proliferation, are present in psoriatic skin [114], as is leukotriene B_4, a neutrophilic chemoattractant [115]. A role for the immune system in the pathogenesis of psoriasis is suggested by the presence of activated T lymphocytes in affected skin and upregulation of intercellular adhesion molecule 1 and HLA-DR [116], as well as the beneficial effect of cyclosporine.

Rheumatoid Arthritis

Epidemiology. Rheumatoid arthritis affects patients of all ages, but is more common in older patients [117]. In one study, an incidence rate of 37 per 100,000 women and 14 per 100,000 men was calculated. The incidence increases with age, being approximately 8 per 100,000 for people aged 20–29 years and 61 per 100,000 for people aged 70–79 years [118]. Other studies give similar incidence figures [119]. Approximately 80% of those afflicted are women. About 10% of patients with rheumatoid arthritis have a positive family history for the disease and a history of other autoimmune diseases in 2% of family members [120]. Rheumatoid arthritis is more common in patients with HLA-Dw4 [121].

Cutaneous Features. Rheumatoid nodules are present in up to 20% of patients with rheumatoid arthritis and are more common in those with more severe disease [122]. The nodules present as nontender, subcutaneous masses on the extensor surfaces of forearms and el-

bows. Overlying surface changes are usually absent. Sites of trauma are especially prone to developing rheumatoid nodules. A rare, linear distribution of rheumatoid nodules has been described and attributed to possible trauma [123].

Rheumatoid papules, or palisaded neutrophilic and granulomatous dermatitis appear as symmetrically distributed erythematous papules with smooth or umbilicated surfaces over joints or on the extensor surfaces of extremities [124]. Less commonly, plaques and rarely vesicles may be present. Rheumatoid papules are associated with severe rheumatoid arthritis [125]. Although less common than rheumatoid nodules, rheumatoid papules are probably not as rare as reports suggest [125].

Rheumatoid vasculitis has been described in patients with long-standing, severe rheumatoid vasculitis. These lesions present as persistent cutaneous ulcerations that are almost always on the lower extremities [126]. In some cases, gangrene and digital infarcts may result.

Associated Disorders. Many cutaneous eruptions have been associated with rheumatoid arthritis. A partial list of these entities is provided in Table 2–1. Rheumatoid nodules have been described in extracuta-

Table 2–1. Cutaneous Eruptions Associated with Rheumatoid Arthritis

Blistering Diseases

Bullous pemphigoid
Cicatricial pemphigoid
Dermatitis herpetiformis
Epidermolysis bullosa acquisita
Erythema multiforme
Pemphigus vulgaris
Subcorneal pustular dermatosis

Vascular Disorders

Erythema elevatum diutinum
Erythermalgia
Mondor's disease
Noninflammatory purpura
Segmental hyalinizing vasculitis

Miscellaneous Conditions

Alopecia areata
Bronchiectasis
Erythema nodosum
Localized hyperhidrosis
Palmar erythema
Pyoderma gangrenosum
Urticaria
Vitiligo
Yellow nail syndrome
Yellow skin

From references 132 and 146–148.

neous sites, including heart, larynx, lungs, splenic capsule, peritoneum, eyes, and Achilles tendons [127].

The association of rheumatoid arthritis, granulocytopenia, and splenomegaly is known as Felty's syndrome. This syndrome is seen in less than 1% of patients with rheumatoid arthritis. These patients have more severe joint disease than others with rheumatoid arthritis and are susceptible to increased infections [128].

Histologic Features. Rheumatoid arthritis is associated with several types of cutaneous lesions, each with its own characteristic histologic changes. Rheumatoid nodules are usually located in the deep portion of the reticular dermis. They may extend upward into the papillary dermis and may even perforate through the epidermis. In addition, they often extend into the underlying subcutaneous fat. Central areas of fibrinoid necrosis are surrounded by palisades of histiocytes, some of which may be multinucleated (Fig. 2–20). A peripheral collarette of lymphocytes and plasma cells is often present, along with increased vascularity. Some authors have described leukocytoclastic vasculitis in the earliest nodules [129], but this finding is seldom present in well-formed nodules. The following entities must be considered in the differential diagnosis of a rheumatoid nodule:

- Epithelioid sarcoma
- Granuloma annulare
- Necrobiosis lipoidica
- Necrobiotic xanthogranuloma

Rheumatoid neutrophilic dermatitis [125, 130] is also termed *rheumatoid papules* [131] and *palisaded neutrophilic and granulomatous dermatitis* [124] in the literature. The epidermis is uninvolved in most cases. In a few cases, spongiotic intraepidermal blisters and subepidermal bullae may be present [125]. Within the dermis, there is a dense inflammatory infiltrate of neutrophils (Fig. 2–21). Some clusters of neutrophils may form microabscesses at the dermal–epidermal junction. Palisades of histiocytes form granulomas around karyorrhectic debris within the reticular dermis (Fig. 2–22). Fibrin is present in early papules, and fibrosis is more prominent in later lesions. Mucin is often present within the central foci of degeneration, especially in earlier lesions. Some authors believe that leukocytoclastic vasculitis is an invariable finding in the earliest papules and is the pathogenesis of this entity [124, 131], while others specifically deny the presence of true vasculitis in this condition [125]. The following entities must be considered in the histologic differential diagnosis of rheumatoid neutrophilic dermatitis:

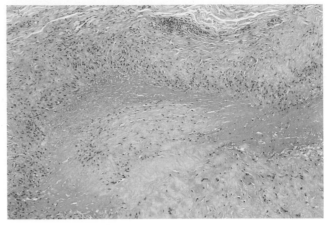

A

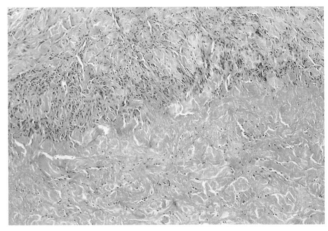

B

Fig. 2–20A. *A*, Rheumatoid nodules are located in the deep dermis and demonstrate central areas with abundant fibrin deposited on collagen. *B*, Multinucleated giant cells and other inflammatory cells are seen palisading around the central areas of altered collagen in rheumatoid nodules.

- Acute febrile neutrophilic dermatosis (Sweet's)
- Cutaneous Crohn s disease
- Erythema elevatum diutinum
- Granuloma annulare
- Leukocytoclastic vasculitis

Some authors have described rheumatoid vasculitis in patients with severe, long-standing rheumatoid arthritis [126]. In these cases, the histologic changes are indistinguishable from those of leukocytoclastic vasculitis as described elsewhere (see Chapter 4). A spectrum ranging from mild disease to severe vasculitis has been described [132].

Special Studies. Direct immunofluorescence of rheumatoid papules reveals massive deposits of fibrin, im-

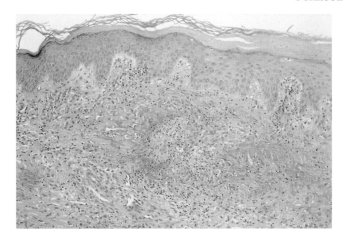

Fig. 2–21. A dense mixed inflammatory infiltrate with abundant neutrophils and giant cells is present within the dermis in rheumatoid papules.

munoglobulins, and complement in the foci of degenerated collagen [131]. The presence of immune complexes within vessel walls and along the dermal–epidermal junction appears to be variable and is somewhat controversial. Thus, direct immunofluorescence is rarely performed for these cases and is not deemed necessary to make a diagnosis.

Pathogenesis. It has been suggested that immune complex–mediated leukocytoclastic vasculitis is the inciting event in the formation of rheumatoid nodules [129]. Others refute this and argue that the primary process is one of enzymatic digestion [133]. It has been proposed that rheumatoid papules, or palisaded neutrophilic and granulomatous dermatitis associated with

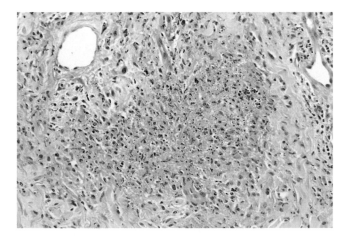

Fig. 2–22. Granulatomata with associated neutrophils are seen within the reticular dermis in well-developed rheumatoid papules.

rheumatoid arthritis, is an immune complex–mediated process [124].

Gout

Epidemiology. Gout is a disease that primarily affects older people and is more common in men than in women. In one study, the ratio of men to women was 3.3:1. Most affected women are postmenopausal [134]. A familial incidence of gout may be related to genetic factors involved in the renal clearance of uric acid [135]. There is a higher incidence in black than in white patients [136]. Additional risk factors for the development of gout include obesity [134], alcohol use [134], lead exposure [137], hypertension [134], diuretic treatment, and renal insufficiency [138]. It has been suggested that there is a seasonal variation in the incidence of acute gouty attacks, with these being most frequent in the spring [139].

Cutaneous Features. More than half of patients with gout present with acute inflammation of the first metatarsophalangeal joint. Ankles and knees are also affected in some cases. Presentation is with rapid onset of throbbing pain in the affected joint, with tenderness and erythema of the overlying skin. Initial attacks are reported to be polyarticular in up to 39% of cases [140]. Attacks recur at varying intervals of 6 months to 2 years and increase in frequency and severity if the condition is left untreated. Each attack lasts from several days to several weeks and resolves spontaneously. Tophi do not usually appear until at least 10 years after the initial attacks. Tophi are currently seen in less than 10% of patients with gout due to increased early medical intervention [141]. Tophi occur most commonly on the helix of the ear as firm, tender papules with variable erythema.

Associated Disorders. Gout is occasionally associated with conditions that lead to the overproduction of urates such as myeloproliferative disorders [142] and psoriasis. Gout is also associated with conditions that interfere with urate excretion, including treatment with thiazide diuretics and renal failure. Gout has been associated with hemolytic anemia and hypothyroidism [143].

Histologic Features. Histologic features of a gouty tophus are characterized by an unremarkable epidermis overlying a dermal or subcutaneous deposition of amorphous material (Fig. 2–23). Within the eosinophilic or amphophilic material, needle-like clefts can be seen in most cases (Fig. 2–24). The needle-like spaces represent urate crystals that have been dissolved with formalin fixation. A palisade of histiocytes, multi-

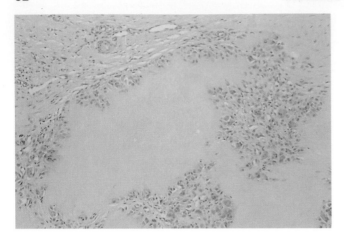

Fig. 2–23. Gout is characterized by palisades of histiocytes surrounding amorphous, acellular material.

nucleated giant cells, lymphocytes, and plasma cells surround the deposited material. Secondary calcification and ossification are commonly seen.

Special Studies. Polarization is very helpful in making a diagnosis of gout; however, in order to preserve the urate crystals within the biopsy specimen, alcohol fixation (such as Carnoy's fluid) is required. Polarizing microscopy reveals yellow crystals when they are parallel to the direction of a red compensator and blue crystals when they are perpendicular [144].

Serum hyperuricemia is helpful in making the diagnosis of gout. Leukocytosis and elevated erythrocyte sedimentation rates are also frequently present.

Pathogenesis. Gouty tophi are caused by the precipitation and deposition of urate crystals from supersat-

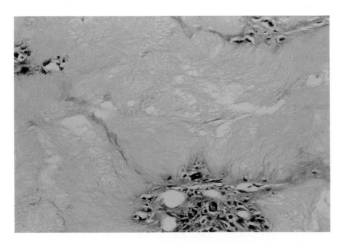

Fig. 2–24. Needle-like spaces representing dissolved urate crystals are present within the amorphous dermal material in gout.

urated body fluids into joint spaces. Deposited crystals elicit an immunologic response mediated by cytokines and monocytes that leads to the signs and symptoms experienced by affected patients [145].

References

1. Kovacs, S. O., and Kovacs, S. C., *Dermatomyositis.* J Am Acad Dermatol, 1998. 39:899–920.
2. Paller, A. S., *Juvenile dermatomyositis and overlap syndromes.* Adv Dermatol, 1995. 10:309–326.
3. Pachman, L. M., Jonasson, O., Cannon, R. A., and Friedman, J. M., *HLA-B8 in juvenile dermatomyositis.* Lancet, 1977. 2:567–568.
4. Love, L. A., Leff, R. L., Fraser, D. D., Targoff, I. N., Dalakas, M., Plotz, P. H., and Miller, F. W., *A new approach to the classification of idiopathic inflammatory myopathy: Myositis-specific autoantibodies define useful homogeneous patient groups.* Medicine (Baltimore), 1991. 70:360–364.
5. Euwer, R. L., and Sontheimer, R. D., *Amyopathic dermatomyositis (dermatomyositis sine myositis).* J Am Acad Dermatol, 1991. 24:959–966.
6. Callen, J. P., *Dermatomyositis.* Dermatol Clin, 1983. 1:461–473.
7. Callen, J. P., *Dermatomyositis and malignancy.* Clin Dermatol, 1993. 11:61–65.
8. Urrutia, S., Vazquez, F., Requena, L., and Sanchez Yus, E., *Acquired ichthyosis associated with dermatomyositis.* J Am Acad Dermatol, 1987. 16:627–629.
9. Feldman, D., Hochberg, M. C., Zizic, T. M., and Stevens, M. B., *Cutaneous vasculitis in adult polymyositis/dermatomyositis.* J Rheumatol, 1983. 10:85–89.
10. Neidenbach, P. J., Sahn, E. E., and Helton, J., *Panniculitis in juvenile dermatomyositis.* J Am Acad Dermatol, 1995. 33:305–307.
11. Pierson, J. C., and Taylor, J. S., *Erythrodermic dermatomyositis.* J Am Acad Dermatol, 1993. 28:136.
12. Glover, M., and Leigh, I., *Dermatomyositis pemphigoides: A case with coexistent dermatomyositis and bullous pemphigoid.* J Am Acad Dermatol, 1992. 27:849–852.
13. Pachman, L. M., Friedman, J. M., Maryjowski-Sweeney, M. L., Jonnason, O., Radvany, R. M., Sharp, G. C., Cobb, M. A., Battles, N. D., et al., *Immunogenetic studies of juvenile dermatomyositis. III. Study of antibody to organ-specific and nuclear antigens.* Arthritis Rheum, 1985. 28:151–157.
14. Bowyer, S. L., Clark, R. A., Ragsdale, C. G., Hollister, J. R., and Sullivan, D. B., *Juvenile dermatomyositis: Histologic findings and pathogenetic hypothesis for the associated skin changes.* J Rheumatol, 1986. 13:753–759.
15. Callen, J. P., *Malignancy in polymyositis/dermatomyositis.* Clin Dermatol, 1988. 6:55–63.
16. Sigurgeirsson, B., Lindelof, B., Edhag, O., and Allander, E., *Risk of cancer in patients with dermatomyositis and polymyositis.* N Engl J Med, 1992. 326:363–367.

17. Barnes, B. E., *Dermatomyositis and malignancy: A review of the literature.* Ann Intern Med, 1976. 84:68–76.
18. Tymms, D. E., and Webb, J., *Dermatomyositis and other connective tissue disease: A review of 105 cases.* J Rheumatol, 1985. 12:1140–1148.
19. Knoell, K. A., Hook, M., Grice, D. P., and Hendrix, J. D., Jr., *Dermatomyositis associated with bronchiolitis obliterans organizing pneumonia (BOOP).* J Am Acad Dermatol, 1999. 40:328–330.
20. Pachman, L. M., *Polymyositis and dermatomyositis in children.* In *Oxford Textbook of Rheumatology,* P.J. Maddison, et al., Eds. 1993, Oxford University Press, Oxford (UK), pp. 821–828.
21. Mascaro, J. M., Jr., Hausmann, G., Herrero, C., Grau, J. M., Cid, M. C., Palou, J., and Mascaro, J. M., *Membrane attack complex deposits in cutaneous lesions of dermatomyositis.* Arch Dermatol, 1995. 131:1386–1392.
22. Magro, C. M., and Crowson, A. N., *The immunofluorescent profile of dermatomyositis: A comparative study with lupus erythematosus.* J Cutan Pathol, 1997. 24:543–552.
23. Alexander, C. B., Croker, B. P., and Bossen, E. H., *Dermatomyositis associated with IgA deposition.* Arch Pathol Lab Med, 1982. 106:449–451.
24. Oddis, C. V., Okano, Y., Rudert, W. A., Trucco, M., Duquesnoy, R. J., and Medsger, T. A., Jr., *Serum autoantibody to the nucleolar antigen PM=Scl. Clinical and immunogenetic associations.* Arthritis Rheum, 1992. 35:1211–1217.
25. Genth, E., Mierau, R., Genetzy, P., von Muhlen, C. A., Kaufmann, S., von Wilmowsky, H., Meurer, M., Krieg, T., et al., *Immunogenetic associations of scleroderma-related antinuclear antibodies.* Arthritis Rheum, 1990. 33:657–665.
26. Tokano, Y., Kanai, Y., Hashimoto, H., Okumura, K., and Hirose, S., *Soluble interleukin-2 receptors in patients with polymyositis/dermatomyositis.* Ann Rheum Dis, 1992. 51:781–782.
27. Schiraldi, O., and Iandolo, E., *Polymyositis accompanying coxsackie B2 infection.* Infection, 1978. 6:32–34.
28. Magid, S. K., and Kagen, I. J., *Serologic evidence for acute toxoplasmosis in polymyositis-dermatomyositis.* Am J Med, 1983. 75:313–320.
29. Nyren, O., Yin, L., Josefsson, S., McLaughlin, J. K., Blot, W. J., Engqvist, M., Hakelius, L., Boice, J. D., Jr., et al., *Risk of connective tissue disease and related disorders among women with breast implants: A nationwide retrospective cohort study in Sweden.* BMJ, 1998. 316:417–422.
30. Perez, M. I., and Koh, S. R., *Systemic sclerosis.* J Am Acad Dermatol, 1993. 28:525–547.
31. Kurzhals, G., Meurer, M., Krieg, T., and Reimer, G., *Clinical association of autoantibodies to fibrillarin with diffuse scleroderma and disseminated telangiectasia.* J Am Acad Dermatol, 1990. 23:832–836.
32. Barnett, A. J., Miller, M. H., and Littlejohn, G. O., *A survival study of patients with scleroderma diagnosed over 30 years (1953–1983): The value of a simple cutaneous classification in the early stages of the disease.* J Rheumatol, 1988. 15:276–283.
33. Steen, V. D., *Clinical manifestations of systemic sclerosis.* Semin Cutan Med Surg, 1998. 17:48–54.
34. Tuffanelli, D. L., and Winkelmann, R. K., *Systemic scleroderma: A clinical study of 727 cases.* Arch Dermatol, 1961. 84:359–367.
35. Patterson, J. W., *Pterygium inversum unguis-like changes in scleroderma: Report of four cases.* Arch Dermatol, 1977. 113:1429–1430.
36. Silver, R. M., *Clinical aspects of systemic sclerosis (scleroderma).* Ann Rheum Dis, 1991. 50:846–853.
37. Steen, V. D., Owens, G. R., Fino, G. J., Rodnan, G. P., and Medsger, T. A., Jr., *Pulmonary involvement in systemic sclerosis (scleroderma).* Arthritis Rheum, 1985. 28:759–767.
38. Cipoletti, J. F., Buckingham, R. B., Barnes, E. L., Peel, R. L., Mahmood, K., Cignetti, F. E., Pierce, J. M., Rabin, B. S., et al., *Sjögren's syndrome in progressive systemic sclerosis.* Ann Intern Med, 1977. 87:535–541.
39. Tan, E. M., Rodnan, G. P., Garcia, I., Moroi, Y., Fritzler, M. J., and Peebles, C., *Diversity of anti-nuclear antibodies in progresive systemic sclerosis: Anti-centromere antibody and its relationship to CREST syndrome.* Arthritis Rheum, 1980. 23:617–625.
40. Denton, C. P., Shi-Wen, X., Sutton, A., Abraham, D. J., Black, C. M., and Pearson, J. D., *Scleroderma fibroblasts promote migration of mononuclear leucocytes across endothelial cell monolayers.* Clin Exp Immunol, 1998. 114:293–300.
41. Pignone, A., Scaletti, C., Matucci-Cerinic, M., Vazquez-Abad, D., Meroni, P. L., Del Papa, N., Falcini, F., Generini, S., et al., *Anti-endothelial cell antibodies in systemic sclerosis: significant association with vascular involvement and alveolo-capillary impairment.* Clin Exp Rheumatol, 1998. 16:527–532.
42. Furst, D. E., and Clements, P. J., *Hypothesis for the pathogenesis of systemic sclerosis.* J Rheumatol Suppl, 1997. 48:53–57.
43. Stratton, R. J., Coghlan, J. G., Pearson, J. D., Burns, A., Sweny, P., Abraham, D. J., and Black, C. M., *Different patterns of endothelial cell activation in renal and pulmonary vascular disease in scleroderma.* Q J Med, 1998. 91:561–566.
44. Livingston, J. Z., Scott, T. E., Wigley, F. M., Anhalt, G. J., Bias, W. B., McLean, R. H., and Hochberg, M. C., *Systemic sclerosis (scleroderma): clinical, genetic, and serological subsets.* J Rheumatol, 1987. 14:512–518.
45. Ueda, M., Abe, Y., Fujiwara, H., Fujimoto, W., Arakawa, K., Arata, J., Yoshioka, T., Tosmoda, J., et al., *Prominent telangiectasia associated with marked bleeding in CREST syndrome.* J Dermatol, 1993. 20:180–184.
46. Furst, D. E., Clements, P. J., Saab, M., Sterz, M. G., and Paulus, H. E., *Clinical and serological comparison of 17 chronic progressive systemic sclerosis (PSS) and 17 CREST syndrome patients matched for sex, age, and disease duration.* Ann Rheum Dis, 1984. 43:794–801.
47. Oddis, C. V., Eisenbeis, C. H., Jr., Reidbord, H. E., Steen, V. D., and Medsger, T. A., Jr., *Vasculitis in systemic sclerosis: Association with Sjögren's syndrome*

and the CREST syndrome variant. J Rheumatol, 1987. 14:942–948.

48. Clarke, A. K., Galbraith, R. M., Hamilton, E. B., and Williams, R., *Rheumatic disorders in primary biliary cirrhosis.* Ann Rheum Dis, 1978. 37:42–47.

49. Powell, F. C., Schroeter, A. L., and Dickson, E. R., *Primary biliary cirrhosis and the CREST syndrome: A report of 22 cases.* Q J Med, 1987. 62:75–82.

50. Goring, H. D., Panzer, M., Lakotta, W., and Ziemer, A., *Coincidence of scleroderma and primary biliary cirrhosis. Results of a systematic study of a dermatologic patient sample.* Hautarzt, 1998. 49:361–366.

51. McMahon, R. F., Babbs, C., and Warnes, T. W., *Nodular regenerative hyperplasia of the liver, CREST syndrome and primary biliary cirrhosis: An overlap syndrome?* Gut, 1989. 30:1430–1433.

52. Jordana, R., Tolosa, C., Selva, A., and Ordi, J., *Autoimmune hemolytic anemia and CREST syndrome.* Med Clin (Barc), 1990. 19:740–741.

53. Maricq, H. R., Harper, F. E., Khan, M. M., tan, E. M., and LeRoy, E. C., *Microvascular abnormalities as possible predictors of disease subsets in Raynaud's phenomenon and early connective tissue disease.* Clin Exp Rheumatol, 1983. 1:195–205.

54. Weiner, E. S., Earnshaw, W. C., Senecal, J. L., Bordwell, B., Johnson, P., and Rothfield, N. F., *Clinical associations of anticentromere antibodies and antibodies to topoisomerase I. A study of 355 patients.* Arthritis Rheum, 1988. 31:378–385.

55. Shulman, L. E., *Diffuse fasciitis with hypergammaglobulinemia and eosinophilia: A new syndrome?* J Rheumatol, 1974. 1:46A.

56. Feldman, S. R., Silver, R. M., and Maize, J. C., *A histopathologic comparison of Shulman's syndrome (diffuse fasciitis with eosinophilia) and the fasciitis associated with the eosinophilia-myalgia syndrome.* J Am Acad Dermatol, 1992. 26:95–100.

57. Kahari, V.-M., Heino, J., Niskanen, L., Fraki, J., and Uitto, J., *Eosinophilic fasciitis.* Arch Dermatol, 1990. 126:613–617.

58. Chan, L. S., Hanson, C. A., and Cooper, K. D., *Concurrent eosinophilic fasciitis and cutaneous T-cell lymphoma. Eosinophilic fasciitis as a paraneoplastic syndrome of T-cell malignant neoplasms?* Arch Dermatol, 1991. 127:862–865.

59. Hoffman, R., Dainiak, N., Sibrack, L., Pober, J. S., and Waldron, J. A., *Antibody-mediated aplastic anemia and diffuse fasciitis.* N Engl J Med, 1979. 300:718–721.

60. Michet, C. J., Doyle, J. A., and Ginsburg, W. W., *Eosinophilic fasciitis: Report of 15 cases.* May Clin Proc, 1981. 56:27–34.

61. Michaels, R. M., *Eosinophilic fasciitis complicated by Hodgkin's disease.* J Rheumatol, 1982. 9:473–476.

62. Silver, R. M., Heyes, M. P., Maize, J. C., Quearry, B., Vionnet-Fuasset, M., and Sternberg, E. M., *Scleroderma, fasciitis, and eosinophilia associated with the ingestion of tryptophan.* N Engl J Med, 1990. 322:874–881.

63. Carr, L., Ruther, E., Berg, P. A., and Lehnert, H., *Eosinophilia-myalgia syndrome in Germany: An epidemiologic review.* May Clin Proc, 1994. 69:620–625.

64. Doyle, J. A., *Eosinophilic fasciitis: Extracutaneous manifestations.* Cutis, 1984. 34:259–261.

65. Barnes, L., Rodnan, G. P., Medsger, T. A., and Short, D., *Eosinophilic fasciitis: A pathologic study of twenty cases.* Am J Pathol, 1979. 96:493–518.

66. Black, C., and Isenberg, D. A., *Mixed connective tissue disease—goodbye to all that.* Br J Rheumatol, 1992. 31:695–700.

67. Ostezan, L. B., and Callen, J. P., *Cutaneous manifestations of selected rheumatologic diseases.* Am Fam Phys 1996. 53:1625–1636.

68. Smolen, J. S., and Steiner, G., *Mixed connective tissue disease. To be or not to be?* Arthritis Rheum, 1998. 41:768–777.

69. Gendi, N. S. T., Welsh, K. I., van Venrooij, W. J., Vancheeswaran, R., Gilroy, J., and Black, C. M., *HLA type as a predictor of mixed connective tissue disease differentiation: ten-year clinical and immunogenetic followup of 46 patients.* Arthritis Rheum, 1995. 38:259–266.

70. Burdt, M. A., Hoffman, R. W., Deutscher, S. L., Wang, G. S., Johnson, J. C., and Sharp, G. C., *Long-term outcome in mixed connective tissue disease: Longitudinal clinical and serologic findings.* Arthritis Rheum, 1999. 42:899–909.

71. van den Hoogen, F. H., Spronk, P. E., Boerbooms, A. M., Bootsma, H., de Rooij, D. J., Kallenberg, C. G., and van de Putte, L. B., *Long-term follow-up of 46 patients with anti-(U1) snRNP antibodies.* Br J Rheumatol, 1994. 33:1117–1120.

72. Michels, H., *Course of mixed connective tissue disease in children.* Ann Med, 1997. 29:359–364.

73. Magro, C. M., Crowson, A. N., and Regauer, S., *Mixed connective tissue disease. A clinical, histologic, and immunofluorescence study of eight cases.* Am J Dermatopathol, 1997. 19:206–213.

74. Prakash, U. B., *Respiratory complications in mixed connective tissue disease.* Clin Chest Med, 1998. 19:733–746.

75. Wakamatsu, M., Inada, K., and Tsutsumi, Y., *Mixed connective tissue disease complicated by pneumatosis cystoides intestinalis and malabsorption syndrome: Case report and literature review.* Pathol Int, 1995. 45:875–878.

76. Kohler, P. F., and Vaughan, J., *The autoimmune diseases.* JAMA, 1982. 248:2646–2657.

77. Satoh, K., Imai, H., Yasuda, T., Wakui, H., Miura, A. B., and Nakamoto, Y., *Sclerodermatous renal crisis in a patient with mixed connective tissue disease.* Am J Kidney Dis, 1994. 24:215–218.

78. Akin, E., Tucker, L. B., Miller, L. C., and Schaller, J. G., *Splenic vasculitis in juvenile onset mixed connective tissue disease.* J Rheumatol, 1998. 25:1444–1445.

79. Ackerman, J., Gonzalez, E. F., and Gilbert-Barness, E., *Immunological studies of the placenta in maternal connective tissue disease.* Pediatr Dev Pathol, 1999. 2:19–24.

80. Gourley, I., Bell, A. L., and Biggart, D., *Kikuchi's disease as a presenting feature of mixed connective tissue disease.* Clin Rheumatol, 1995. 14:104–107.

81. Sharp, G. C., Irwin, W. S., May, C. M., Holman, H. R., McDuffie, F. C., Hess, E. V., and Schmid, F. R.,

Association of antibodies to ribonucleoprotein and Sm antigens with mixed connective tissue disease, systemic lupus erythematosus and other rheumatic diseases. N Engl J Med, 1976. 295:1149–1154.

82. Alexander, E., and Provost, T. T., *Sjögren's syndrome. Association of cutaneous vasculitis with central nervous system disease.* Arch Dermatol, 1987. 123:801–810.

83. Wilson, R. W., Provost, T. T., Bias, W. B., Alexander, E. L., Edlow, D. W., Hochberg, M. C., Stevens, M. B., and Arnett, F. C., *Sjögren's syndrome: influence of multiple HLA-D region alloantigens on clinical and serological expression.* Arthritis Rheum, 1984. 27:1245–1253.

84. Alexander, E. L., and Provost, T. T., *Cutaneous manifestations of primary Sjögren's syndrome: a reflection of vasculitis and association with anti-Ro(SS-A) antibodies.* J Invest Dermatol, 1983. 80:386–391.

85. McGovern, T. W., Erickson, A. R., and Fitzpatrick, J. E., *Sjögren's syndrome plasma cell panniculitis and hidradenitis.* J Cutan Pathol, 1996. 23:170–174.

86. Usuda, T., *Annular erythema as cutaneous manifestations of Sjögren's sydnrome.* Nippon Hifuka Gakkai Zasshi, 1982. 92:489–501.

87. Mitchell, J. M., Greenspan, J., Daniels, T., Whitcher, J. P., and Maibach, H. I., *Anhidrosis (hypohidrosis) in Sjögren's syndrome.* J Am Acad Dermatol, 1987. 16:233–235.

88. Newball, H. H., and Brahim, S. A., *Chronic obstructive airway disease in patients with Sjögren's syndrome.* Am Rev Respir Dis, 1977. 115:295–304.

89. Penner, E., and Reichlin, M., *Primary biliary cirrhosis associated with Sjögren's syndrome: Evidence for circulating and tissue deposited Ro/anti Ro immune complexes.* Arthritis Rheum, 1982. 25:1250–1253.

90. Alexander, E. L., Craft, C., Dorsch, C., Moser, R. L., Provost, T. T., and Alexander, G. E., *Necrotizing arteritis and spinal subarachnoid hemorrhage in Sjögren's syndrome.* Ann Neurol, 1982. 11:632–635.

91. Alexander, E. L., and Alexander, G. E., *Aseptic meningoencephalitis in primary Sjögren's syndrome.* Neurology, 1983. 33:593–598.

92. Sutcliffe, N., Inanc, M., Speight, P., and Isenberg, D., *Predictors of lymphoma development in primary Sjögren's syndrome.* Semin Arthritis Rheum, 1998. 28:80–87.

93. van der Valk, P. G. M., Hollema, H., van Voorst Vander, P. C., Brinker, M. G. L., and Poppema, S., *Sjögren's syndrome with specific cutaneous manifestations and multifocal clonal T-cell populations progressing to a cutaneous pleomorphic T-cell lymphoma.* Am J Clin Pathol, 1989. 92:357–361.

94. Molina, R., Provost, T. T., and Alexander, E. L., *Two types of inflammatory vascular disease in Sjögren's syndrome: Differential association with seroreactivity to rheumatoid factor in antibodies to Ro (SS-A) and with hypocomplementemia.* Arthritis Rheum, 1985. 28: 1251–1258.

95. Chaudhry, A. P., Cutler, L. S., Yamane, G. M., Satchidanand, S., Labay, G., and Sunderraj, M., *Light and ultrastructual features of lymphoepithelial lesions of the salivary glands in Mikulicz's disease.* J Pathol, 1986. 148:239–250.

96. Tenger, P., Halse, A. K., Haga, H. J., Jonsson, R., and Wahren-Herlenius, M., *Detection of anti-Ro/SSA and anti-La/SSB autoantibody-producing cells in salivary glands from patients with Sjögren's syndrome.* Arthritis Rheum, 1998. 41:2238–2248.

97. Phillips, T. J., and Dover, J. S., *Recent advances in dermatology.* N Engl J Med, 1992. 326:167–178.

98. Hellgren, L., *Psoriasis: A statistical, clinical and laboratory investigation of 255 psoriasis patients and matched healthy controls.* Acta Derm Venereol, 1964. 44:191–207.

99. Wuepper, K. D., Coulter, S. N., and Haberman, A., *Psoriasis vulgaris: A genetic approach.* J Invest Dermatol, 1990. 95:2S–4S.

100. Stern, R. S., and Wu, J., *Psoriasis. In Cutaneous Medicine and Surgery*, K. A. Arndt et al., Eds, 1996, W. B. Saunders Co., Philadelphia, pp. 295–321.

101. Stern, R. S., *Epidemiology of psoraisis.* Dermatol Clin, 1995. 13:717–722.

102. Farber, E. M., and Nall, L., *Epidemiology: Natural history and genetics. In Psoriasis*, H. H. Roenigk and H. I. Maibach, Eds. 1985, Marcel Dekker, New York, pp. 141–186.

103. Zelickson, B. D., and Muller, S. A., *Generalized pustular psoriasis. A review of 63 cases.* Arch Dermatol, 1991. 127:1339–1345.

104. Boyd, A. S., and Menter, A., *Erythrodermic psoriasis.* J Am Acad Dermatol, 1989. 21:1985–1991.

105. Telfer, N. R., Chalmers, R. J. G., Whale, K., and Colman, G., *The role of streptococcal infection in the intiation of guttate psoriasis.* Arch Dermatol, 1992. 128:39–42.

106. Farber, E. M., Rein, G., and Lanigan, S. W., *Stress and psoriasis: Psychoimmunologic mechanisms.* Int J Dermatol, 1991. 30:8–10.

107. Bhate, S. M., Sharpe, G. R., Marks, J. M., Shuster, S., and Ross, W. M., *Prevalence of skin and other cancers in patients with psoriasis.* Clin Exp Dermatol, 1993. 18:401–404.

108. Funk, J., Langeland, T., Schrumpf, E., and Hanssen, L. E., *Psoriasis induced by interferon-α.* Br J Dermatol, 1991. 125:463–465.

109. Stern, R. S., *The epidemiology of joint complaints in patients with psoriasis.* J Rheumatol, 1985. 12:315–320.

110. Duvic, M., Johnson, T. M., Rapini, R. P., Freese, T., Brewton, G., and Rios, A., *Acquired immunodeficiency syndrome-associated psoriasis and Reiter's syndrome.* Arch Dermatol, 1987. 123:1622–1632.

111. Horn, T. D., Herzberg, G. Z., and Hood, A. F., *Characterization of the dermal infiltrate in human immunodeficiency virus–infected patients with psoriasis.* Arch Dermatol, 1990. 126:1462–1465.

112. Heng, M. C. Y., Heng, J. A., and Allen, S. G., *Electron microscopic features in generalized pustular psoriasis.* J Invest Dermatol, 1987. 89:187–191.

113. Fry, L., *Psoriasis.* Br J Dermatol, 1988. 119:445–461.

114. Sauder, D. N., *The role of epidermal cytokines in inflammatory skin diseases.* J Invest Dermatol, 1990. 95:27S–28S.

115. Camp, R., Jones, R. R., Brain, S., Woollard, P., and

Greaves, M., *Production of microabscesses by topical application of leukotriene B₄.* J Invest Dermatol, 1984. 82:202–204.

116. Baadsgard, O., Fisher, G., Voorhees, J. J., and Cooper, K. D., *The role of immune system in the pathogenesis of psoriasis.* J Invest Dermatol, 1990. 95:32S–34S.

117. Masi, A. T., and Medsger, T. A., *Epidemiology of the rheumatic diseases.* In *Arthritis and Allied Conditions,* D. J. McCarty, Ed. 1979, Lea & Fabiger, Philadelphia. pp. 11–16.

118. Uhlig, T., Kvien, T. K., Glennas, A., Smedstad, L. M., and Forre, O., *The incidence and severity of rheumatoid arthritis, results from a county register in Oslo, Norway.* J Rheumatol, 1998. 25:1078–1084.

119. Aho, K., Kaipiainen-Seppanen, O., Heliovaara, M., and Klaukka, T., *Epidemiology of rheumatoid arthritis in Finland.* Semin Arthritis Rheum, 1998. 27:325–334.

120. Sany, J., Dropsy, R., and Daures, J. P., *Cross-sectional epidemiological survey of rheumatoid arthritis patients seen in private practice in France. Descriptive results (1629 cases).* Rev Rhum Engl Ed, 1998. 65:462–470.

121. Stastny, P., *Association of the B-cell alloantigen DRw4 with rheumatoid arthritis.* N Engl J Med, 1978. 298: 869–871.

122. Moore, C. P., and Wilkens, R. F., *The subcutaneous nodule: Its significance in the diagnosis of rheumatic disease.* Semin Arthritis Rheum, 1977. 7:63–79.

123. Belloch, I., Moragon, M., Jorda, E., Jiminez, A., Ramon, D., and Verdeguer, J. M., *Linear rheumatoid nodule.* Int J Dermatol, 1988. 27:645–646.

124. Chu, P., Connolly, K., and LeBoit, P. E., *The histopathologic spectrum of palisaded neutrophilic and granulomatous dermatitis in patients with collagen vascular disease.* Arch Dermatol, 1994. 130:1278–1283.

125. Lowe, L., Kornfeld, B., Clayman, J., and Golitz, L. E., *Rheumatoid neutrophilic dermatitis.* J Cutan Pathol, 1992. 19:48–53.

126. Vollersten, R. S., Conn, D. L., Ballard, D. J., Ilstrup, D. M., Kazmar, R. E., and Silverfield, J. C., *Rheumatoid vasculitis: Survival and associated risk factors.* Medicine, 1986. 65:365–375.

127. Hurd, E. R., *Extraarticular manifestations of rheumatoid arthritis.* Semin Arthritis Rheum, 1979. 8:151–176.

128. Sienknecht, C. W., Urowitz, M. B., Pruzanski, W., and Stein, H. B., *Felty's syndrome: Clinicopathological study of 27 patients.* Ann Rheum Dis, 1977. 36:500–507.

129. Sokoloff, L., McCluskey, R. T., and Bunim, J. J., *Vascularity of the early subcutaneous nodule of rheumatoid arthritis.* Arch Pathol, 1953. 55:475–495.

130. Sanchez, J. L., and Curz, A., *Rheumatoid neutrophilic dermatitis.* J Am Acad Dermatol, 1990. 22:922–925.

131. Higaki, Y., Yamashita, H., Sato, K., Higaki, M., and Kawashima, M., *Rheumatoid papules: A report on four patients with histopathologic analysis.* J Am Acad Dermatol, 1993. 28:406–411.

132. Jorizzo, J. L., and Daniels, J. C., *Dermatologic conditions reported in patients with rheumatoid arthritis.* J Am Acad Dermatol, 1983. 4:439–457.

133. Aherne, M. J., Bacon, P. A., Blake, D. R., Gallagher, P. J., Jones, D. B., Morris, C. J., and Potter, A. R., *Immunohistochemical findings in rheumatoid nodules.* Virchows Arch [A], 1985. 407:191–202.

134. Tikly, M., Bellingan, A., Lincoln, D., and Russell, A., *Risk factors for gout: A hospital-based study in urban black South Africans.* Rev Rheum Engl Ed, 1998. 65:225–231.

135. Lambert, W. C., *Cutaneous deposition disorders.* In *Pathology of the Skin,* E. R. Farmer and A. F. Hood, Eds. 1990, Appleton and Lange, East Norwalk, CT. pp. 432–450.

136. Roubenoff, R., *Gout and hyperuricemia.* Rheum Dis Clin North Am, 1990. 16:539–550.

137. Loghman-Adham, M., *Renal effects of environmental and occupational lead exposure.* Environ Health Perspect, 1997. 105:928–939.

138. Touart, D. M., and Sau, P., *Cutaneous deposition diseases. Part II.* J Am Acad Dermatol, 1998. 39:527–544.

139. Schlesinger, N., Gowin, K. M., Baker, D. G., Beutler, A. M., Hoffman, B. I., and Schumacher, H. R., Jr., *Acute gouty arthritis is seasonal.* J Rheumatol, 1998. 25:342–344.

140. Hadler, N. M., Franck, W. A., Bress, N. M., and Robinson, D. R., *Acute polyarticular gout.* Am J Med, 1974. 56:715–719.

141. O'Duffy, J. D., Hunder, G. G., and Kelley, P. J., *Decreasing prevalence of tophaceous gout.* Mayo Clin Proc, 1975. 50:227–228.

142. Yu, T.-F., *Secondary gout associatied with myeloproliferative disorders.* Arthritis Rheum, 1965. 8:765–771.

143. Seegmiller, J. E., *Skin manifestations of gout.* In *Dermatology in general medicine,* T. B. Fitzpatrick et al., Eds. 1993, McGraw-Hill, New York. pp. 1894–1900.

144. DeCastro, P., Jorizzo, J. L., Solomon, A. R., Lisse, J. R., and Daniels, J. C., *Coexistent systemic lupus erythematosus and tophaceous gout.* J Am Acad Dermatol, 1985. 13:650–654.

145. Malawista, S. E., Duff, G. W., Atkins, E., Cheung, H. S., and McCarty, D. J., *Crystal-induced pyrogen production: A further look at gouty inflammation.* Arthritis Rheum, 1985. 28:1039–1046.

146. Delaporte, E., Gaveau, D. J., Piette, F. A., and Bergoend, H. A., *Acute febrile neutrophilic dermatitis (Sweet's syndrome): Association with rheumatoid vasculitis.* Arch Dermatol, 1989. 125:1101–1104.

147. Stolman, L. P., Rosenthal, D., Yaworsky, R., and Horan, F., *Pyoderma gangrenosum and rheumatoid arthritis.* Arch Dermatol, 1975. 111:1020–1023.

148. Despaux, J., Manzoni, P., Toussirot, E., Auge, B., Cedoz, J. P., and Wendling, D., *Prospective study of the prevalence of bronchiectasis in rheumatoid arthritis using high-resolution computed tomography.* Rev Rhum Engl Ed, 1998. 65:453–461.

Diabetes Mellitus

Diabetes mellitus is a disease in which elevated serum glucose levels affect virtually every organ system. Although the initial lesion is located in the insulin-producing cells in the pancreas, the consequences of lowered or absent insulin levels are far reaching and frequently devastating. It has been estimated that up to 30% of patients with diabetes will experience cutaneous manifestations [1]. This chapter addresses cutaneous diseases that have been specifically associated with diabetes mellitus. It is beyond the scope of this volume to individually address the pathologic alterations found in other organ systems affected by diabetes. It should be noted that various eruptions, including pigmented purpuric dermatoses [2], oral lichen planus [3], dermatitis herpetiformis [4], alopecia areata universalis [5], and eruptive clear cell syringomas [6], have been associated with diabetes mellitus. They are not discussed here, however, owing to the tenuous nature of these relationships. Other processes such as erysipelas, erythrasma, and candidal infections, although frequently seen in association with diabetes, are not specifically related to diabetes and are not further addressed in this chapter.

Necrobiosis Lipoidica Diabeticorum

Epidemiology. Necrobiosis lipoidica diabeticorum (NLD) is usually associated with diabetes mellitus. In one large series, 65% of patients with NLD suffered from diabetes [7], and an additional 20% of patients had some level of glucose intolerance. It is a rare complication, however, occurring in about 0.3% of diabetic patients overall [8]. The female/male prevalence ratio is 3:1, and the average age of onset is 30 years in diabetic patients and 41 years in those without diabetes [8].

Cutaneous Findings. In the vast majority of cases, the onset of diabetes antedates the appearance of NLD; however, in approximately 15% of cases, the cutaneous lesions will appear first [9]. Early lesions appear as erythematous to violaceous papules or plaques with a fine scale or no scale. Necrobiosis lipoidica diabeticorum is seen most commonly on the pretibial surfaces of the lower extremities in patients with long-standing diabetes mellitus [10]. As the lesions progress, the surface becomes progressively atrophic. Indurated plaques develop, which ulcerate in about 30% of patients [7]. Nonulcerated, older lesions assume a yellow color. The periphery of the lesions remains erythematous, and telangiectasias may be present [8]. There may be some loss of hair in lesional skin [11]. Decreased sensitivity to light touch and heat has been reported in NLD lesions [11].

The legs are involved in 85% of cases, and presentation with multiple, bilateral lesions is common [12]. Necrobiosis lipoidica diabeticorum has also been described in other locations, including the scalp and face, back, nipple, forearms, and trunk [12–14]. Only 2% of patients will, however, have involvement of other sites in the absence of pretibial lesions [8]. Face and scalp lesions appear to be more prevalent among patients who do not have concomitant diabetes [15]. Lesions heal with scarring and atrophy. Only 17% of patients have complete resolution of lesions over an average of 11 years [7, 16].

Associated Disorders. There are several reports of coexisting necrobiosis lipoidica and granuloma annulare [17–20]. Some authors have questioned whether these may represent variants of the same process [18]. Rare cases of coexisting inflammatory bowel disease and necrobiosis lipoidica have been reported, as has a single case of necrobiosis arising after a jejunal bypass procedure [21–23]. Necrobiosis lipoidica has also been associated with ataxia telangiectasia in several patients [24].

Histologic Findings. Major histologic alterations are present in the midreticular dermis. The epidermis is normal to slightly atrophic. Characteristically, there is a large zone of degenerated collagen, which is often relatively pale staining (Fig. 3–1). Elastic tissue fibers are markedly diminished or absent. In these regions, the dermis appears hypocellular. Surrounding this affected zone is a palisade of histiocytes that may be mononuclear or multinucleated. Some of these cells may contain lipid in the cytoplasm, presumably accumulating from the breakdown products of dead cells, giving rise to the yellow color in clinically advanced lesions. Extracellular lipid may also be seen between degenerating collagen fibers [7]. Other scattered inflammatory cells, including lymphocytes and plasma cells, are present in varying numbers. Deep dermal nodules of perivascular lymphoid aggregates are found in up to 11% of patients [25]. In most cases, the papillary dermis is spared. The zone of altered collagen may extend down the fibrous septa between fat lobules in the subcutaneous fat. Endothelial cell proliferation and thickening of reticular dermal blood vessels are common findings in NLD (Fig. 3–2) [7]. Leukocytoclasia involving vessel walls is rarely seen [8]. This finding has been reported most commonly in early lesions [9, 26].

In another histologic variant, the zone of degenerating collagen is inapparent, and the reticular dermis is replete with well-formed, sarcoidal granulomas that consist of histiocytes, lymphocytes, and plasma cells (Fig. 3–3). Zones of necrosis may be present in the cen-

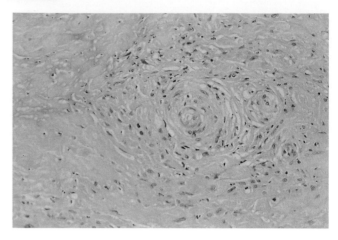

Fig. 3–2. Thickening of blood vessel walls in reticular dermis is characteristic of necrobiosis lipoidica diabeticorum.

ters of the granulomas, and differentiation from infectious etiologies becomes difficult. Vascular wall thickening is also present in these cases [7]. It has been suggested that these more granulomatous-appearing cases occur more frequently in lesions on sites other than the lower extremities. The following entities must be considered in the differential diagnosis of necrobiosis lipoidica diabeticorum:

- Epithelioid sarcoma
- Granuloma annulare
- Necrobiotic xanthogranuloma
- Rheumatoid nodule
- Sarcoidosis

Special Studies. In some studies, direct immunofluorescence has demonstrated the presence of granular de-

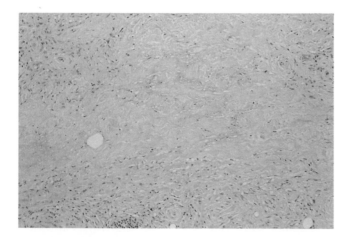

Fig. 3–1. Necrobiosis lipoidica diabeticorum shows a pale-staining area of collagen with a surrounding palisade of histiocytes.

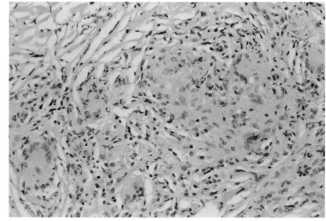

Fig. 3–3. Well-formed, sarcoidal-like granulomas are found in some cases of necrobiosis lipoidica diabeticorum.

posits of immunoglobulins (usually IgM) and complement (C3) in vessel walls in affected skin [7, 27]. Uninvolved skin also demonstrated immunoreactants within vessels in one study [28]. These studies found no differences in immunostaining between patients with type I and type II diabetes mellitus. Others have found vascular deposits of immune complexes to be a less constant finding [29, 30].

Pathogenesis. It has been suggested that vasculopathy is the underlying etiology for the cutaneous changes seen in patients with necrobiosis lipoidica diabeticorum. In up to one-third of cases, however, the characteristic vasculopathic changes are not observed [7]. It is reasonably well established that the onset of lesions of necrobiosis lipoidica is not closely related to the degree of blood glucose levels, and genetic factors do not appear to play a central role [8]. There has been a multitude of other explanations for the occurrence of these lesions, including immune mechanisms, abnormalities in leukocyte functions, abnormal lipids, and collagen. None have proved to be entirely satisfactory [8]. In some cases, trauma seems to be a precipitating event [29].

Disseminated Granuloma Annulare

Epidemiology. Granuloma annulare is a very common cutaneous disease that may occur with increased frequency in patients with diabetes mellitus. It is a self-limited process, and lesions resolve within several years in most cases. Granuloma annulare is more common in younger adults than in the elderly population and has a 2.5:1 female to male prevalence. There are two forms of the disease: localized granuloma annulare and disseminated or generalized granuloma annulare. Approximately 15% of patients with granuloma annulare have generalized lesions [31, 32]. The disseminated form of this disease has been reported to appear more frequently in patients with diabetes mellitus [33]. In one series, 21% of patients with disseminated granuloma annulare also had diabetes [34]. Other studies have failed to support this observation [32, 35]. There is an increased incidence of human leukocyte antigen (HLA) type Bw35 in patients with disseminated granuloma annulare that is not seen in patients with localized disease [36]. The average age of onset of disseminated granuloma annulare is 51.7 years [34], which is slightly later than that of the localized disease.

Cutaneous Findings. Asymptomatic, tan to erythematous macules and papules are present by the hundreds. Papules coalesce into annular or circinate plaques in about 33% of cases [34]. An annular distribution of the individual papules is more commonly seen in

women. Acral areas most commonly exhibit a symmetric pattern, but a similar eruption can also be seen to involve the trunk. Palms, soles, and mucous membranes are not commonly involved. The generalized form of the disease lasts for years to decades and may relapse subsequent to apparent resolution [37].

Associated Disorders. Other diseases have been less strongly associated with disseminated granuloma annulare. These include underlying malignancy, drug allergies, hypertension, obesity, arthritis, and autoimmune thyroid diseases, which all occurred in more than 10% of patients with the generalized eruption. Atopy, anemia, hyperuricemia, carpal tunnel syndrome, rheumatoid arthritis, systemic lupus erythematosus, and gout occurred in less than 10% of the same population [34]. In this study, however, no control population was studied to assess the true strength of these associations. There are also several reports of Hodgkin's disease and non-Hodgkin's lymphoma occurring in association with disseminated granuloma annulare [38–40]. Generalized granuloma annulare is also the most common form of the disease to develop in patients with human immunodeficiency virus infection [41].

Histologic Findings. Histologic changes in the disseminated form of granuloma annulare are identical to those seen in the localized form of the disease. Underlying a normal epidermis, there is an infiltrate of histiocytes and lymphocytes within the superficial portion of the reticular dermis (Figs. 3–4 and 3–5). These cells percolate between altered collagen bundles. The collagen bundles appear thinned and have increased amounts of acid mucopolysaccharides in well-developed foci. The inflammatory cells may aggregate around the degener-

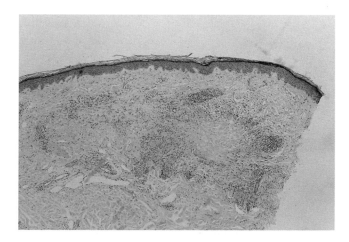

Fig. 3–4. Granuloma annulare demonstrates multiple small foci of granulomatous inflammation within the dermis.

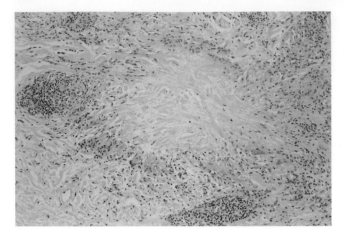

Fig. 3–5. A palisade of histiocytes surrounds degenerating collagen in the palisaded form of granuloma annulare.

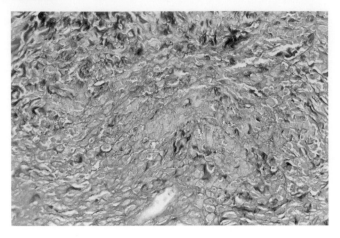

Fig. 3–6. A colloidal iron stain performed at pH 3.0 demonstrates abundant hyaluronic acid within a focus of collagenous degeneration in granuloma annulare.

ating collagen in a palisading pattern or may remain single and dispersed in an infiltrative pattern. According to some authors, the infiltrative pattern is far more common than the well-developed palisading form of the disease [42]. This is even more true for cases with generalized lesions of granuloma annulare [43]. A moderately intense perivascular lymphocytic infiltrate, composed of predominantly CD4+ T-helper cells [44], is also commonly seen. Some cases of granuloma annulare may also display scattered eosinophils and neutrophils [45]. Several studies have reported necrotizing vasculitis in very early lesions [46], but this remains controversial [42, 47]. The following entities must be considered in the differential diagnosis of granuloma annulare:

- Dermatofibroma
- Epithelioid sarcoma
- Kaposi's sarcoma, patch stage
- Necrobiosis lipoidica diabeticorum
- Rheumatoid neutrophilic dermatitis
- Rheumatoid nodule
- Tuberculosis

Special Studies. Increased amounts of hyaluronic acid can be highlighted with Alcian blue or colloidal iron stains performed at pH 3.0 (Fig. 3–6). No staining will be present if the study is performed at pH 0.4 [42, 47].

Direct immunofluorescence has proved to be of minimal utility in making a diagnosis of granuloma annulare. Fibrin is invariably present within the foci of degenerated collagen [46, 48], although other studies suggest that fibrin deposits may not always be seen in cases of disseminated granuloma annulare [43]. Some observers have demonstrated fibrin within blood vessel walls [30], but others have not found this to be the case [46, 48]. Complement deposition within vessel

walls and along the dermal–epidermal junction has been seen in a minority of cases, and IgM is infrequently observed in a similar location [30, 46].

Pathogenesis. The pathogenesis of granuloma annulare is unknown. Trauma [49], infectious processes [50], genetic predisposition [51], ultraviolet light exposure [34, 52], and insect bite reactions [53] have all been implicated as causative factors, largely without convincing supportive evidence. Dahl et al. [46] have suggested that vasculitis may play a role in the pathogenesis of granuloma annulare, but true vasculitis is rarely found. Others have suggested a lymphocyte-mediated hypersensitivity reaction [42]. After performing an electron microscopic study, investigators suggested that necrosis of histiocytes and fibroblasts leads to the release of lysosomal enzymes that causes the observed degeneration of the collagen [54].

Bullosis Diabeticorum

Epidemiology. This is a rare complication of long-standing diabetes mellitus [55].

Cutaneous Findings. Tense blisters form spontaneously without antecedent trauma [56]. Blisters range from millimeters to several centimeters in diameter [9]. The onset of blisters may be associated with a burning sensation. The usual site is on the feet and shins, although similar blisters limited to the hands have also been reported [55, 57]. As the blisters age, they darken in color due to hemorrhage and become flaccid and have been said to resemble burn blisters [56]. The blisters heal without scarring or other sequelae, but recurrence is frequent.

Associated Disorders. It has been suggested that this entity may be closely related to the bullous disorder of hemodialysis because most patients with bullosis diabeticorum and diabetes also suffer from chronic renal failure.

Histologic Findings. Several patterns of histologic change have been described in bullosis diabeticorum [58]. Some authors describe a relatively noninflammatory subepidermal blister with no keratinocyte necrosis or acantholysis (Fig. 3–7) [59, 60]. It has been suggested that subepidermal blister formation can be attributed to chronic renal failure. Others describe an intraepidermal spongiotic blister with marked surrounding spongiosis [61]. In rare cases, the blisters appear to be subcorneal in location. It remains unclear if there is a single, primary level of blister formation in this condition that is yet to be precisely classified or whether the disease has several different patterns of involvement. A minimal lymphohistiocytic inflammatory infiltrate may be present. Blood vessel walls are thickened in some cases, but this is more likely related to the underlying systemic vasculopathy than to any specific cutaneous disease process. The following entities must be considered in the differential diagnosis of bullosis diabeticorum:

- Bullous pemphigoid (cell poor)
- Epidermolysis bullosa
- Porphyria cutanea tarda
- Pseudoporphyria

Special Studies. Direct immunofluorescence studies have not demonstrated immunoreactants in the skin in most series [55]. In some patients, however, im-munoglobulins have been seen around papillary dermal blood vessels [60]. The blister occurs at the level of the lamina lucida as seen on electron microscopic examination and may be related to decreased numbers of hemidesmosomes and/or anchoring filaments [55, 58]. These observations pertain to the blisters that have a subepidermal cleavage plane on routine histologic sections. They clearly are not observable in all of the blistering processes that have been categorized in conjunction with bullosis diabeticorum.

Pathogenesis. The blisters do not appear to be trauma related, and infectious processes are not the cause [26]. It has been speculated that the neuropathy or microangiopathic changes may be responsible for the blister formation, but there is no substantial evidence for these hypotheses. Abnormal calcium and magnesium regulation secondary to chronic renal failure has also been implicated [58].

Scleredema Diabeticorum

Epidemiology. Scleredema diabeticorum occurs in obese, middle-aged adults with diabetes [10]. It is more common in patients with noninsulin-dependent diabetes (type II), occurring in 3% of these patients [62]. In these patients, the disease may persist for decades and is more prevalent among men. This contrasts with the form of scleredema that occurs in younger patients after acute infectious processes, is more likely to affect women, and usually resolves within 6 months to 2 years [63].

Cutaneous Findings. Scleredema presents as a symmetric, indurated, nonpitting plaque on the shoulders, neck, or upper back. The face can also be involved, which may result in difficulty smiling and opening the mouth [64]. Scleredema tends to be more diffuse when it occurs in conjunction with diabetes and may spread to involve the entire trunk [65]. Scleredema has also been reported on the thighs [66]. Involvement of genital and acral skin is rare [67].

Associated Disorders. Scleredema also may be seen after an acute infectious process, most commonly streptococcal in nature. Viral infections have also been reported to precede the onset of scleredema [68]. In some patients, scleredema develops in the absence of any associated diseases. Patients with scleredema occasionally experience systemic problems associated with cutaneous mucin deposition. These include electroencephalogram abnormalities, paraproteinemias [69–71] including multiple myeloma [72], rheumatoid arthritis [73], hepatosplenomegaly, and involvement of skeletal muscles.

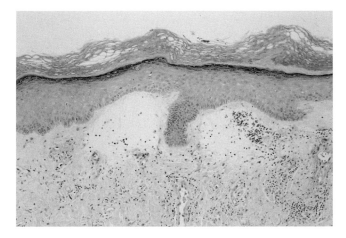

Fig. 3–7. Bullosis diabeticorum is often characterized by a noninflammatory subepidermal blister without necrosis or acantholysis.

Histologic Findings. The histologic findings in scleredema are localized primarily to the reticular dermis. The epidermis may display a slight effacement
of rete ridges and basilar hyperpigmentation. The
pronounced thickening of the reticular dermis is due
to increased glycosaminoglycans between the collagen bundles. The increased nonsulfated, acid mucopolysaccharides may be seen on routinely stained
sections and can be highlighted with Alcian blue or
colloidal iron stains. The increased amount of reticular dermal hyaluronic acid is most impressive in
early lesions and may be difficult to detect in biopsy
specimens taken from late, well-developed areas [68].
In some cases, increased mucin may not be detected
with special stains, but the widening of the interstices
between the collagen bundles is virtually always present (Fig. 3–8). This differentiates the cause of dermal
thickening from that of scleroderma in which the interstitial spaces between collagen bundles are decreased. There is not an appreciable increase in numbers of fibroblasts. Elastic fibers are fragmented and
may be reduced in number [74]. Some authors suggest that there may also be an increased number of
dermal mast cells [75]. Dermal appendages are not
destroyed in scleredema, in contrast to other sclerosing dermal processes [76]. The following entities must
be considered in the histologic differential diagnosis
of scleredema:

- Anasarca
- Connective tissue nevus (collagenoma)
- Morphea/progressive systemic sclerosis

Special Studies. Colloidal iron and Alcian blue stains
performed at neutral pHs enhance the staining properties of the hyaluronic acid (Fig. 3–9). Frozen sections also
may augment sensitivity in detecting increased amounts

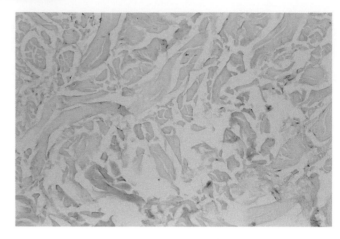

Fig. 3–9. Colloidal iron stain performed at pH 3.0 demonstrates increased acid mucopolysaccharides in the interstitial spaces of the reticular dermis in scleredema.

of reticular dermal mucin. Direct immunofluorescence
does not reveal immune complex deposition [64].

Pathogenesis. The pathogenesis of scleredema remains
unknown. Several lines of investigation suggest glycosylation of collagen that decreases its solubility or increased collagen hydration due to polyol accumulation,
if it plays a role [77, 78]. It has been shown that fibroblasts in scleredema produce increased levels of type
I procollagen mRNA in culture [71].

Diabetic Dermopathy

Epidemiology. Diabetic dermopathy is also known as
shin spots. It is believed to be the most common cutaneous manifestation of diabetes mellitus, occurring in
30%–60% of diabetic patients [79]. Similar cutaneous
changes were found in 20% of age-matched control patients without diabetes [80]. Diabetic dermopathy spots
are more prevalent in men [10]. The presence of lesions
does not appear to correspond to duration of disease
or level of glucose control [81].

Cutaneous Findings. Well-developed lesions of diabetic dermopathy appear as atrophic, hyperpigmented
oval patches on the pretibial regions. The eruption begins as flat-topped, red papules, which may or may not
have overlying scale [81]. Although lesions are usually
bilateral, they are not symmetric [82]. The shins are the
most commonly affected sites, but lesions have also
been described on the thighs, feet, and forearms [10].

Associated Disorders. There are no additional disorders associated with diabetes mellitus and diabetic dermopathy.

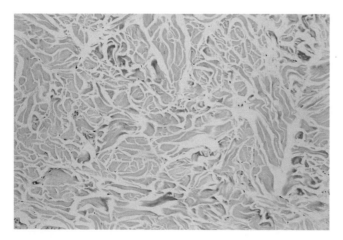

Fig. 3–8. Increased interstitial space is seen between collagen bundles in the reticular dermis in scleredema.

Histologic Findings. Histologic findings in diabetic dermopathy are subtle and generally nonspecific. A mildly spongiotic epidermis is seen overlying a slightly edematous papillary dermis. There is a slight perivascular lymphohistiocytic inflammatory infiltrate, and occasional extravasated erythrocytes may be present. As the lesions become fully developed, the edema diminishes and hemosiderin may be seen [83].

Special Studies. Special studies are not necessary to make a diagnosis of diabetic dermopathy.

Pathogenesis. It is believed that the lesions are a result of trauma. Postinflammatory hyperpigmentation and atrophy develop in skin with poor peripheral vascularization [26]. In support of this hypothesis, patients with diabetic dermopathy who were experimentally subjected to heat trauma developed additional lesions, whereas control patients with diabetes but no diabetic dermopathy did not develop lesions [84].

Eruptive Xanthomata

Epidemiology. Eruptive xanthomata occur in patients who have diabetes with concomitant hyperlipidemia [82].

Cutaneous Findings. The sudden eruption of crops of firm, nontender, yellow papules is characteristic of eruptive xanthomata. A rim of erythema may be observed. The papules can occur on any body surface, but are most commonly found on the buttocks and the extensor surfaces of extremities. They may also appear in the antecubital fossa and on lips and eyelids [85]. The lesions resolve quickly when serum lipid and glucose levels are brought under better control [82]. They may be pruritic or painful [85].

Associated Disorders. Eruptive xanthomata can be seen in association with several causes of hypertriglyceridemia, including myxedema, nephrotic syndrome, and inherited lipidemias [26]. The most frequent association is with type IV hyperlipoproteinemia (Frederickson classification). They are also associated with alcoholism, exogenous drugs such as corticosteroids, retinoids, and estrogens [85, 86]. Eruptive xanthomata may be seen in conjunction with hepatosplenomegaly, pancreatitis, and abdominal pain.

Histologic Findings. Eruptive xanthomata are characterized by a dermal infiltrate of abundant, foamy, lipid-laden macrophages admixed with lymphocytes and neutrophils localized primarily to the superficial reticular dermis (Fig. 3–10) [87]. Multinucleated and Touton giant cells are less pronounced than in other types of xanthomata, and the accompanying inflammatory infiltrate

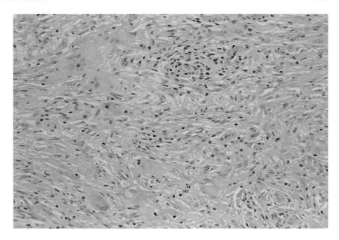

Fig. 3–10. Foamy histiocytes, occasional multinucleated giant cells, and an admixture of inflammatory cells are present within the dermis in eruptive xanthomas.

is more brisk. The infiltrate is initially perivascular and becomes more diffuse as the lesions develop [88]. In early lesions, intracytoplasmic lipid may be difficult to discern, but as the lesions develop the foamy cytoplasm becomes readily apparent [89]. Extracellular deposits of lipid may be seen in eruptive xanthomata.

Special Studies. Oil red O, scarlet red, and Sudan red all highlight the lipid within histiocytes in eruptive xanthomata. Because these stains require tissue that has not been fixed in formalin, however, they are rarely used and seldom required to make a diagnosis. The accumulated lipid is doubly refractile.

Pathogenesis. Adequate insulin levels are required for lipoprotein lipase to cleave free fatty acids to triglycerides. When insulin levels are insufficient, the enzyme will not properly function, leading to increased levels of serum triglycerides that result in eruptive xanthomata [26].

Yellow Skin

Epidemiology. Yellowing of the palms, soles, and face occurs in as many as 10% of patients with diabetes [90].

Cutaneous Findings. Many patients with diabetes will develop yellow palms, soles, and faces. The yellow color can be striking in some patients.

Associated Disorders. Carotenemia with subsequent development of yellow skin is associated with hypothyroidism and hepatic and renal diseases [91].

Histologic Findings. Histologic changes in diabetes-associated yellow skin have not been described.

Special Studies. Special studies are not required to make a diagnosis of diabetes-associated yellow skin.

Pathogenesis. Yellow skin in patients with diabetes may be caused by carotenemia. Unlike the situation in most cases of carotenemia that are due to ingestion of large amounts of carrots or other yellow vegetables, however, this does not appear to be the cause in patients with diabetes [91]. Studies suggest that, despite the yellow skin, serum carotene levels are normal in diabetic patients and that carotene is not the cause of the pigmentary changes [92]. Others hypothesize that nonenzymatic glycosylation of dermal collagen may lead to the color changes or "browning" of the collagen [26, 93].

References

1. Gilgor, R. S., and Lazarus, G. S., *Skin manifestations of diabetes mellitus.* In *Diabetes mellitus,* H. Rifkin and P. Raskin, Eds. 1981, RJ Brady Co., Bowie, MD, pp. 313–321.
2. Lithner, F., *Purpura, pigmentation and yellow nails of the lower extremities in diabetes.* Acta Med Scand, 1976. 199:203–208.
3. Albrecht, M., Banoczy, J., Dinya, E., and Tamas, G., Jr., *Occurrence of oral leukoplakia and lichen planus in diabetes mellitus.* J Oral Pathol, 1992. 21:364–366.
4. Reijonen, H., Ilonen, J., Knip, M., and Revuala, T., *Insulin-dependent diabetes mellitus associated with dermatitis herpetiformis: Evidence for heterogeneity of HLA-associated genes.* Tissue Antigens, 1991. 37:94–96.
5. Taniyana, M., Kushima, K., Ban, Y., Kaihara, M., Nagakura, H., Sekita, S., Katagiri, T., and Sueki, H., *Simultaneous development of insulin dependent diabetes mellitus and alopecia areata universalis.* Am J Med Sci, 1991. 301:269–271.
6. Kudo, H., Yonezawa, I., Ieka, A., and Miyachi, Y., *Generalized eruptive syringoma (letter).* Arch Dermatol, 1989. 125:1716–1717.
7. Muller, S. A., and Winkelmann, R. K., *Necrobiosis lipoidica diabeticorum: Histopathologic study of 98 cases.* Arch Dermatol, 1966. 94:1–10.
8. Lowitt, M. H., and Dover, J. S., *Necrobiosis lipoidica.* J Am Acad Dermatol, 1991. 25:735–748.
9. Braverman, I. M., *Skin Signs of Systemic Disease.* 1981, W. B. Saunders Company, Philadelphia, pp. 654–664.
10. Huntley, A. C., *The cutaneous manifestations of diabetes mellitus.* J Am Acad Dermatol, 1982. 7:427–455.
11. Binazzi, M., and Simonette, V., *Granuloma annulare, necrobiosis lipoidica, and diabetic disease.* Int J Dermatol, 1988. 27:576–579.
12. Kavanagh, G. M., Novelli, M., Hartog, M., and Kennedy, C. T. C., *Necrobiosis lipoidica—involvement of atypical sites.* Clin Exp Dermatol, 1993. 18:543–544.
13. Wilson Jones, E., *Necrobiosis lipoidica presenting on the face and scalp.* Trans St. Johns Hosp Dermatol Soc, 1971. 57:202–220.
14. Metz, G., and Metz, J., *Extracoporale Manifestation der Necrobiosis lipoidica. Isolierter Befall des Kopfes.* Hautzart, 1977. 28:359–363.
15. Mackey, J. P., *Necrobiosis lipoidica diabeticorum involving scalp and face.* Br J Dermatol, 1975. 93:729–730.
16. Wells, R. S., and Smith, M. A., *The natural history of granuloma annulare.* Br J Dermatol, 1963. 75:199–205.
17. Crosby, D. L., Woodley, D. T., and Leonard, D. D., *Concomitant granuloma annulare and necrobiosis lipoidica.* Dermatologica, 1991. 183:225–229.
18. Detwiler, S., and Smoller, B. R., *Immunohistochemical analysis of inflammatory infiltrate in concomitant granuloma annulare and necrobiosis lipoidica (abstract).* J Cutan Pathol, 1995. 22:58.
19. Cohen, I. J. K., *Necrobiosis lipoidica and granuloma annulare.* J Am Acad Dermatol, 1984. 10:123–124.
20. Schwartz, M. E., *Necrobiosis lipoidica and granuloma annulare. Simultaneous occurrence in a patient.* Arch Dermatol, 1982. 118:192–193.
21. DuBoulay, C., and Whorwell, P. J., *"Nodular necrobiosis": A new cutaneous manifestation of Crohn's disease?* Gut, 1982. 23:712–715.
22. Clegg, D. O., Zone, J. J., and Piepkorn, M. W., *Necrobiosis lipoidica associated with jejunoileal bypass surgery.* Arch Dermatol, 1982. 118:192–193.
23. Whorwell, P. J., Haboubi, N. Y., and DuBoulay, C., *Nodular necrobiosis in association with ulcerative colitis.* Gut, 1986. 27:1517.
24. Thibaut, S., Sass, U., Khoury, A., and Simonart, J.-M., *Ataxia-telangiectasia and necrobiosis lipoidca: An explanable association.* Eur J Dermatol, 1994. 4:509–513.
25. Alegre, V. A., and Winkelmann, R. K., *A new histopathologic feature of necrobiosis lipoidica diabeticorum: Lymphoid nodules.* J Cutan Pathol, 1988. 15:75–77.
26. Huntley, A. C., *Cutaneous manifestations of diabetes mellitus.* Dermatol Clin, 1989. 7:531–546.
27. Ullman, S., and Dahl, M. V., *Necrobiosis lipoidica: An immunofluorescence study.* Arch Dermatol, 1977. 113:1671–1673.
28. Quimby, S. R., Muller, S. A., and Schroeter, A. L., *The cutaneous immunopathology necrobiosis lipoidica diabeticorum.* Arch Dermatol, 1988. 124:1364–1371.
29. Laukkanen, A., Fraki, J. E., Vaatainen, N., Korhonen, T., and Naukkarinen, A., *Necrobiosis lipoidica: Clinical and immunofluorescent study.* Dermatologica, 1986. 172:89–92.
30. Nieboer, C., and Kasbeek, G. L., *Direct immunofluorescence in granuloma annulare, necrobiosis lipoidica and granulomatosis disciformis Miescher.* Dermatologica, 1979. 158:427–432.
31. Frenken, J. H., and Thije, O. J., *A really generalized granuloma annulare.* Dermatologica, 1967. 134:73–83.
32. Dicken, C. H., Carrington, S. G., and Winkelmann, R. K., *Generalized granuloma annulare.* Arch Dermatol, 1969. 99:556–563.
33. Goodfield, M. J. D., and Millard, L. G., *The skin in diabetes mellitus.* Diabetologica, 1988. 31:567–575.
34. Dabski, K., and Winkelmann, R. K., *Generalized gran-*

uloma annulare: Clinical and laboratory findings in 100 patients. J Am Acad Dermatol, 1989. 20:39–47.

35. Sibbald, R. G., and Schachter, R. K., *The skin and diabetes mellitus.* Int J Dermatol, 1984. 23:567–584.

36. Friedman-Birnbaum, R., Haim, S., Gideone, O., and Barzilai, A., *Histocompatibility antigens in granuloma annulare.* Br J Dermatol, 1978. 98:425–428.

37. Muhlbauer, J. E., *Granuloma annulare.* J Am Acad Dermatol, 1980. 3:217–230.

38. Barksdale, S. K., Perniciaro, C., Halling, K. C., and Strickler, J. G., *Granuloma annulare in patients with malignant lymphoma: Clinicopathologic study of thirteen new cases.* J Am Acad Dermatol, 1994. 31:42–48.

39. Harman, R. R. M., *Hodgkin's disease, seminoma of the testicle and widespread granuloma annulare.* Br J Dermatol, 1977. 97(suppl):50–51.

40. Schwartz, R. A., Hansen, R. C., and Lynch, P. J., *Hodgkin's disease and granuloma annulare.* Arch Dermatol, 1981. 117:185–186.

41. Toro, J. R., Chu, P., Ben Yen, T.-S., and LeBoit, P. E., *Granuloma annulare and human immunodeficiency virus infection.* Arch Dermatol, 1999. 135:1341–1346.

42. Umbert, P., and Winkelmann, R. K., *Histologic, ultrastructural, and histochemical studies of granuloma annulare.* Arch Dermatol, 1977. 113:1681–1686.

43. Dabski, K., and Winkelmann, R. K., *Generalized granuloma annulare: Histopathology and immunopathology.* J Am Acad Dermatol, 1989. 20:28–39.

44. Modlin, R. L., Vaccaro, S. A., Bottlieb, B., Gebhard, J. F., Linden, C. E., Forni, M., Meyer, P. R., Taylor, C. R., et al., *Granuloma annulare. Identification of cells in the cutaneous infiltrate by immunoperoxidase techniques.* Arch Pathol Lab Med, 1984. 108:379–382.

45. Silverman, R. A., and Rabinowitz, A. D., *Eosinophils in the cellular infiltrate of granuloma annulare.* J Cutan Pathol, 1985. 12:13–17.

46. Dahl, M. V., Ullman, S., and Goltz, R. W., *Vasculitis in granuloma annulare.* Arch Dermatol, 1977. 113: 463–467.

47. Charles, C. R., Johnson, B. L., and Damm, S. R., *Granuloma annulare.* Int J Dermatol, 1976. 15:655–665.

48. Umbert, P., and Winkelmann, R. K., *Granuloma annulare: Direct immunofluorescence study.* Br J Dermatol, 1976. 95:487–492.

49. Draheim, J. H., Johnson, L. C., and Helwib, E. B., *A clinicopathologic analysis of "rheumatoid" nodules occurring in 54 children.* Am J Pathol, 1959. 35:416–420.

50. Guill, M. A., and Goette, D. K., *Granuloma annulare at sites of healing herpes zoster.* Arch Dermatol, 1978. 114: 1383.

51. Goolamali, S. K., and Stevenson, C., *Granuloma annulare in identical twins.* Br J Dermatol, 1972. 86:636–637.

52. Dorval, J. C., Leroy, J. P., and Masse, R., *Granulomes annulaires disséminés après PUVA thérapie.* Acta Derm Venereol (Paris), 1979. 106:79–80.

53. Curwen, W., *Granuloma annulare, multiple, suggesting insect bite reaction.* Arch Dermatol, 1963. 88:355–356.

54. Charles, C. R., Cooper, P. H., and Helwig, E. B., *The fine structure of granuloma annulare.* Lab Invest, 1977. 36:444–451.

55. Toonstra, J., *Bullosis diabeticorum. Report of a case with a review of the literature.* J Am Acad Dermatol, 1985. 13:799–805.

56. Bodman, M., Friedman, S., and Clifford, L. B., *Bullosis diabeticorum. A report of two cases with a review of the literature.* J Am Podiatr Med Assoc, 1991. 81:561–563.

57. Collet, J. T., and Toonstra, J., *Bullosis diabeticorum: A case with lesions restricted to the hands.* Diabetes Care, 1985. 8:177–179.

58. Bernstein, J. E., Medinica, M., Soltani, K., and Griem, S. F., *Bullous eruption of diabetes mellitus.* Arch Dermatol, 1979. 115:324–325.

59. Basarab, T., Munn, S. E., McGrath, J., and Russell Jones, R., *Bullous diabeticorum. A case report and literature review.* Clin Exp Dermatol, 1995. 20:218–220.

60. James, W. D., Odom, R. B., and Goette, D. K., *Bullous eruption of diabetes mellitus. A case with positive immunofluorescence microscopy findings.* Arch Dermatol, 1980. 116:1191–1192.

61. Paltzik, R. L., *Bullous eruption of diabetes mellitus. Bullosis diabeticorum.* Arch Dermatol, 1980. 116:475–476.

62. Cole, G. W., Headley, J., and Skowsky, R., *Scleredema diabeticorum: a common and distinct cutaneous manifestation of diabetes mellitus.* Diabetes Care, 1983. 6:189–192.

63. Fleischmajer, R., Faludi, G., and Krol, S., *Scleredma and diabetes mellitus.* Arch Dermatol, 1970. 101:21–26.

64. Truhan, A. P., and Roenigk, H. H., *The cutaneous mucinoses.* J Am Acad Dermatol, 1986. 14:1–18.

65. Binkley, G. W., *Discussion of scleredema adultorum of Buschke, society transactions.* Arch Dermatol, 1969. 99:124–125.

66. Farrell, A. M., Branfoot, A. C., Moss, J., Papadaki, L., Woodrow, D. F., and Bunker, C. B., *Scleredema diabeticorum of Buschke confined to the thighs.* Br J Dermatol, 1996. 134:1113–1115.

67. Greenberg, L. M., Geppert, C., Worthen, H. G., and Good, R. A., *Scleredema "adultorum" in children: Report of three cases with a histochemical study and review of the world literature.* Pediatrics, 1963. 32:1044–1054.

68. Venencie, P. Y., Powell, F. C., Su, W. P. D., and Perry, H. O., *Scleredema: A review of thirty-three cases.* J Am Acad Dermatol, 1984. 11:128–134.

69. McFadden, N., Ree, K., Soyland, E., and Larsen, T. E., *Sclerema adultorum associated with a monoclonal gammopathy and generalized hyperpigmentation.* Arch Dermatol, 1987. 123:629–632.

70. Ohta, A., Uitto, J., Oikarinen, A. I., Palatsi, R., Mitrane, M., Bancila, E. A., Seiboid, J. R., and Kim, H. C., *Paraproteinemia in patients with scleredema. Clinical findings and serum effects on skin fibroblasts in vitro.* J Am Acad Dermatol, 1987. 16:96–107.

71. Oikarinen, A. I., Ala-Kokko, L., Palatsi, R., Peltonen, L., and Uitto, J., *Scleredema and paraproteinemia.* Arch Dermatol, 1987. 123:226–229.

72. Kovary, P. M., Vakilzadeh, F., Macher, E., Zaun, H., Merk, H., and Goertz, G., *Monoclonal gammopathy in scleredema: Observations in three new cases.* Arch Dermatol, 1981. 117:536–539.

73. Miyagawa, S., Dohi, K., Tsuruta, S., and Shirai, T., *Scle-*

redema of Buschke associated with rheumatoid arthritis and Sjörgren's syndrome. Br J Dermatol, 1989. 121:517–520.

74. Holubar, K., and Mach, K. W., *Scleredema (Buschke). Histological and histochemical investigations.* Acta Derm Venereol, 1967. 47:102–110.

75. Cohn, B. A., Wheeler, C. E., and Briggman, R. A., *Scleredema adultorum of Buschke and diabetes mellitus.* Arch Dermatol, 1970. 101:27–35.

76. Fleischmajer, R., and Lara, J. V., *Scleredema. A histochemical and biochemical study.* Arch Dermatol, 1965. 92:643–652.

77. Buckingham, B. A., Uitto, J., Sandborg, C., Keenst, T., Roe, T., Costin, G., Kaufman, F., Bernstein, B., et al., *Scleredema-like changes in insulin dependent diabetes mellitus: Clinical and biochemical studies.* Diabetes Care, 1984. 7:163–169.

78. Eaton, P. R., *The collagen hydration hypothesis: A new paradigm for the secondary complications of diabetes mellitus.* J Chronic Dis, 1986. 39:753–766.

79. Bernstein, J. E., *Cutaneous manifestations of diabetes mellitus.* Curr Concepts Skin Dis, 1980. 1:3–10.

80. Feingold, K. R., and Elias, P. M., *Endocrine-skin interactions.* J Am Acad Dermatol, 1987. 17:921–940.

81. Bauer, M., and Levan, N. E., *Diabetic dermangiopathy. A spectrum including pretibial pigmented patches and necrobiosis lipoidica diabeticorum.* Br J Dermatol, 1970. 83:528–535.

82. Perez, M. I., and Kohn, S. R., *Cutaneous manifestations of diabetes mellitus.* J Am Acad Dermatol, 1994. 30:519–531.

83. Binkley, G. W., Giraldo, B., and Stoughton, R. B., *Diabetic dermopathy—a clinical study.* Cutis, 1967. 3:955–958.

84. Lithner, F., *Cutaneous reactions of the extremities of diabetics to local thermal trauma.* Acta Med Scand, 1975. 198:319–325.

85. Cruz, P. D., East, C., and Bergstresser, P. R., *Dermal, subcutaneous and tendon xanthomas: Diagnostic markers for specific lipoprotein disorders.* J Am Acad Dermatol, 1988. 19:95–111.

86. Braun-Falco, O., and Eckert, F., *Macroscopic and microscopic structure of xanthomatous eruptions.* Curr Probl Dermatol, 1991. 20:54–62.

87. Crowe, M. J., and Gross, D. J., *Eruptive xanthoma.* Cutis, 1992. 50:31–32.

88. Cooper, P. H., *Eruptive xanthoma: A microscopic simulant of granuloma annulare.* J Cutan Pathol, 1986. 13:207–215.

89. Archer, C. B., and MacDonald, D. M., *Eruptive xanthomata in type V hyperlipoproteinemia associated with diabetes mellitus.* Clin Exp Dermatol, 1984. 9:312–316.

90. Jelinek, J. E., *The skin in diabetes mellitus: Cutaneous manifestations, complications and associations.* In *Year Book of Dermatology*, A. Kopf and R. Andrade, Eds. 1970, Year Book Medical Publishers, Chicago, pp. 5–35.

91. Lascari, A. D., *Carotenemia. A review.* Clin Pediatr (Phila), 1981. 20:25–29.

92. Hoerer, E., Dreyfuss, F., and Herzberg, M., *Carotenemia, skin color and diabetes mellitus.* Acta Diabetol Lat, 1975. 12:202–207.

93. Monnier, V. M., and Cerami, A., *Nonenzymatic browning in vivo: Possible process for aging of long-lived proteins.* Science, 1981. 211:491–493.

CHAPTER
4

Vasculitis

The spectrum of vasculitis is broad and ranges from conditions involving only the skin to those that destroy vessels in many organs. Although inflammation and destruction of blood vessel walls may be confined to a limited distribution, they also can be seen throughout multiple organ systems. For this reason, vasculitis does not fit neatly into a discussion of skin diseases as they relate to individual organ systems. It is difficult to organize vasculitides into a classification system that successfully discriminates between all of the different types. The Chapel Hill Consensus Conference Classification defines three major subclasses of vasculitis based on the caliber of the vessels predominantly affected: *(1)* small-vessel vasculitis, including leukocytoclastic vasculitis, Wegener's granulomatosis, Churg-Strauss syndrome, microscopic polyarteritis, Henoch-Schönlein purpura, and essential cryoglobulinemia; *(2)* medium-vessel vasculitis, including polyarteritis nodosa and Kawasaki's disease; and *(3)* large-vessel vasculitis, which includes giant cell arteritis and Takayasu's arteritis (both of which rarely involve the skin and are not further addressed) [1]. Henoch-Schönlein purpura is discussed in Chapter 8.

SMALL-VESSEL VASCULITIDES

Leukocytoclastic Vasculitis

Epidemiology. Leukocytoclastic vasculitis is a disease that affects patients of all ages, genders, and races with the same frequency. Approximately 10% of cases oc-

cur in children [2]. Inflammation of small-caliber vessels may occur in any anatomic location. In some cases, the disease is concentrated primarily in the cutaneous vasculature, whereas in other situations vessels throughout the body are similarly affected. In one series, 20% of patients with cutaneous lesions of leukocytoclastic vasculitis demonstrated signs of systemic involvement. If vasculitis is limited to the skin, the mortality rate is very low. Mortality increases when systemic involvement is present. In about two-thirds of cases, a precipitating cause for vasculitis can be identified. In one large series, the most common triggering antigens were drugs, infectious agents, and underlying malignancies [3].

Cutaneous Lesions. The clinical presentation of leukocytoclastic vasculitis is quite variable. Lesions are most common on the lower extremities, but they can appear at any body site. The classic, well-formed lesion is described as a "palpable purpura" [4]. Some lesions appear more urticarial, however, and are not obviously hemorrhagic. Older lesions are frequently ulcerated. Less commonly, the lesions can exhibit a more livedoid or reticulate pattern. Nodules also can occur in some situations. Papules, pustules, vesicles, bullae, and petechiae have all been described in patients with leukocytoclastic vasculitis. Lesions can persist for up to 2 years [3].

Clinically similar lesions that must be distinguished from cutaneous vasculitis include pigmented purpuric eruptions, actinic (or sun-damage-related) purpura, and dermal hemorrhage secondary to platelet or coagulation abnormalities.

Associated Disorders. Leukocytoclastic vasculitis is commonly associated with a wide range of systemic diseases. In one series, 12% of patients with leukocytoclastic vasculitis also had rheumatoid arthritis, 8% suffered from some type of malignancy, 6% had lupus erythematosus, and 3% had cryoglobulinemia [5]. In the same series, drug reactions precipitated the vasculitis in 13% of patients, and infections were present in 9%. The infectious agents included bacteria, fungi, and viruses [5]. Hepatitides B and C have been implicated [6, 7]. There is a strong association between patients with leukocytoclastic vasculitis secondary to essential mixed cryoglobulinemia and hepatitis C infection [3]. Other types of cryoglobulinemia induce vascular occlusion, but usually without an inflammatory process [8]. *Mycoplasma pneumoniae* infection has presented with cutaneous vasculitic lesions [9], and similar lesions have appeared after administration of the pneumococcal vaccine [10]. Leukocytoclastic vasculitis has also been seen in association with ulcerative colitis and cystic fibrosis [11, 12]. Rare cases of sarcoidosis have manifested with cutaneous lesions of leukocytoclastic vasculitis (see Chapter 6) [13].

Histologic Features. Leukocytoclastic vasculitis is defined as transmural neutrophilic infiltration of small blood vessel walls, leading to the destruction of these vessels and accumulation of fibrin in the vessel walls (Fig. 4–1). Most commonly, inflammatory infiltrate consisting primarily of neutrophils, with scattered eosinophils and lymphocytes, is concentrated around the small postcapillary venules of the superficial vascular plexus [14, 15]. Karyorrhectic debris may be extensive. Endothelial cell swelling and destruction, extravasated erythrocytes, and fibrin deposition are present in the walls of affected vessels. Thrombi may be extensive or relatively rare. Deeper vessels may also be involved, but are rarely involved in the absence of vasculitis in the superficial vascular plexus. It has been suggested that patients with involvement of deeper vessels are more likely to have systemic disease [5]. In later lesions, the neutrophilic infiltrate is less pronounced and lymphocytes predominate, making the histologic diagnosis a bit more difficult.

Special Studies. Direct immunofluorescence may be helpful in confirming a diagnosis of leukocytoclastic vasculitis and is positive in approximately 85% to 92% of biopsy specimens [3, 16]. The ideal specimen to study is from a newly developed lesion. Immunoglobulins and complement are deposited within affected vessel walls during the first 24–48 hours in most cases. IgG and IgM are the most commonly seen immunoglobulins, although IgA may also be present in drug-induced vasculitides and in Henoch-Schönlein purpura (see Chapter 8). Fibrin may be seen within the vessel walls and in the surrounding dermal collagen. Immunoreactants are less likely in older lesions; however, some authors have found immune complex deposition in a high percentage of very late, well-developed lesions [16].

Circulating antineutrophil cytoplasmic antibodies may be seen in about 20% of patients, and cryoglobulins may be present in up to one-fourth [3].

Pathogenesis. Leukocytoclastic vasculitis is a circulating immune complex–mediated disease. It is thought to be similar to the experimental Arthus reaction. Excess circulating antigen–antibody complexes deposit in vessel walls of postcapillary venules. Neutrophils, which

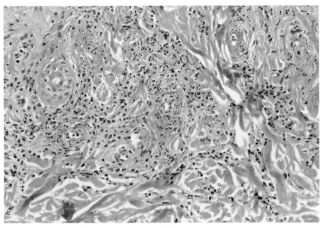

A

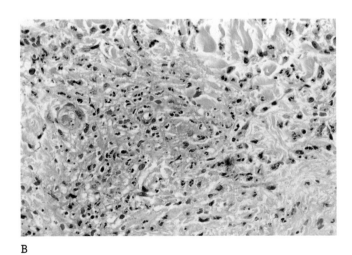

B

Fig. 4–1. *A.* Leukocytoclastic vasculitis is characterized by a neutrophilic infiltrate surrounding and destroying small vessels within the dermis. In *B*, Neutrophils with extravasated erythrocytes and fibrin are present around damaged dermal blood vessels in leukocytoclastic vasculitis.

express adhesion molecules, adhere to endothelial cells, infiltrate the vessel walls, and release lytic enzymes [17]. The membrane attack complex released by the neutrophil disrupts endothelial cell integrity. Cytokines released by neutrophils and disrupted endothelial cells play a central role in causing tissue destruction, as do the free oxygen radicals generated by infiltrating neutrophils. Adhesion molecules are now known to play a major role in the cellular trafficking of this process [18].

Wegener's Granulomatosis

Epidemiology. Wegener's granulomatosis is an idiopathic inflammatory disease that occurs primarily in middle-aged people, with no gender preference. In one study, the mean age at presentation was 49.5 years [19]. It is unusual in children, but has been reported [20]. The disease has a high morbidity rate, but due to aggressive treatment modalities the mortality rate has declined in recent years.

Cutaneous Lesions. Cutaneous lesions are present in approximately 30%–50% of patients with Wegener's granulomatosis [21, 22]. They are more likely in patients with the disseminated form of the disease than with the more limited form. In as many as 62% of patients, cutaneous lesions may be the first manifestation of Wegener's granulomatosis [19]. The manifestations themselves vary. Purpuric macules and papules are most prevalent on the extremities. Truncal involvement is also common. Other lesions most common on the elbows and knees consist of discrete papules that are often necrotic and ulcerated. Irregularly shaped ulcers with ragged edges, especially on the shins, occur commonly. Mucosal ulcerations may also be seen, and gin-

gival hyperplasia has been reported in these patients. Other presentations include pustules, nodules, hemorrhagic bullae, and a livedo reticularis pattern [23]. It has been suggested that the subset of Wegener's granulomatosis patients with necrotizing vasculitis in the skin may have the worst prognosis [21, 24]; others have not found this to be the case [23].

Associated Disorders. Wegener's granulomatosis often involves the upper and lower respiratory tracts with necrotizing granulomas and the kidneys with a segmental necrotizing glomerulonephritis. With systemic vasculitis present, other organ systems including the nervous system, the heart, and the eye, can be involved [25, 26].

Histologic Features. Several different histologic patterns may be seen in cutaneous lesions of Wegener's granulomatosis. These include palisading granulomas, necrotizing vasculitis, and granulomatous vasculitis. Necrotizing vasculitis is the most common histologic pattern, being present in 80% of cases in one series [19]. In these cases, the histologic differences between Wegener's granulomatosis and other causes of leukocytoclastic vasculitis are not distinguishable. Necrotizing vasculitis usually involves small vessels, but may also be seen in medium-sized vessels. The finding of granulomatous vasculitis is more specific for Wegener's granulomatosis, but is an extremely uncommon finding (Fig. 4–2). Palisaded extravascular granulomas (Churg-Strauss granulomas) [27], when present, may appear very epithelioid and sarcoidal or may be characterized by central caseating necrosis and appear more tuberculoid. These were seen in about 10% of patients with cutaneous disease in one study and correspond to

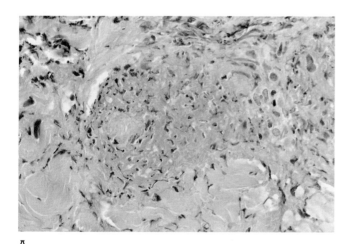
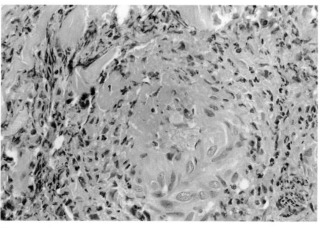

A B

Fig. 4–2. *A,* Wegener's granulomatosis is often characterized by the presence of a leukocytoclastic vasculitis. *B,* In rare cases of Wegener's granulomatosis, granulomatous vasculitis is identified. Note the palisade of histiocytes, including one multinucleated giant cell, within the wall of a dermal blood vessel.

the clinical observation of papules and nodules [19]. Some authors have suggested that the presence of granulomas in skin biopsy material is more common in patients without active disease [24]. Eosinophils and plasma cells can be present in and around the foci of granulomatous inflammation. It is unusual to see more than a single pattern of involvement in a single biopsy specimen [23]. In a subset of patients, the changes observed are nonspecific and do not reflect the underlying disease process.

Special Studies. Serum IgG antineutrophilic cytoplasmic autoantibodies have been shown to be a very sensitive marker for Wegener's granulomatosis and are found in only a limited range of conditions [28]. These antibodies can be found with indirect immunofluorescence studies.

Direct immunofluorescence studies on lesional skin demonstrate immunoglobulin and complement deposition in affected vessel walls in a pattern identical to that seen in other forms of leukocytoclastic vasculitis [23].

Pathogenesis. Antineutrophil cytoplasmic autoantibodies are found in up to 90% of patients with Wegener's granulomatosis [29, 30]. It has been suggested that antineutrophilic cytoplasmic autoantibodies may play a pathogenic role in triggering leukocyte activation and degranulation in these patients [31, 32].

It has also been suggested that the vasculitis seen in Wegener's granulomatosis may be cell mediated rather than humoral. This is based on a study that revealed T cells and monocytes in vessel walls and the absence of immunoglobulins in the affected blood vessel walls [33]. Others have suggested that vascular involvement in other organs, including the skin, appears histologically different and may have a different etiology [34].

Churg-Strauss Allergic Granulomatosis

Epidemiology. Churg-Strauss allergic granulomatosis is a systemic vasculitis, also known as *allergic granulomatous angiitis*, and is most common in people with a history of asthma and very high peripheral eosinophil counts [35]. It affects men and women approximately equally and most commonly presents in patients between the ages of 20 and 40 years [36]. It is an exceedingly rare type of vasculitis that accounted for only 1.3% of all cases of vasculitis in one large series [37].

Cutaneous Lesions. Cutaneous lesions are seen in up to 70% of patients with Churg-Strauss syndrome [38]. Extremities are the most common site of involvement, but the back and abdomen are also frequently involved. Macules and papules, and less commonly deep-seated

nodules, are reported. Papulovesicles have also been reported. Purpura is common and may be associated with necrosis and ulcerations. Nodules persist for months and tend to heal with scarring [39]. Livedo reticularis and periorbital edema have also been described [38].

Associated Disorders. Patients will often develop constitutional symptoms, including fever, malaise, and weakness. Necrotizing vasculitis with abundant eosinophils has been described in many organs, including the lungs, kidneys, gastrointestinal tract, heart, muscles, and central nervous system [36]. The lungs are the most severely affected and account for most of the morbidity of this disease. Allergic rhinitis may be the earliest presenting symptom in these patients. Later, severe asthma may develop. Renal involvement has been reported in up to 84% of patients with Churg-Strauss syndrome [40]. Focal segmental glomerulonephritis is the most common form of renal involvement. Gastrointestinal symptoms include peritonitis, obstruction, and cholecystitis. Mitral valve regurgitation has been reported in patients with heart involvement, as has vasculitis affecting the coronary arteries [41]. Myocardial fibrosis may be a long-term complication [42]. Arthritis, obstructive uropathy, splenomegaly, and transient lymphadenopathy have also been reported [36]. Unlike the situation with polyarteritis nodosa, hepatitis B and human immunodeficiency virus are not associated with Churg-Strauss syndrome [36].

Histologic Features. Histologic features of Churg-Strauss syndrome include tissue eosinophilia, granulomatous inflammation, and necrotizing vasculitis (Figs. 4–3 and 4–4). The vast majority of biopsy specimens will not show all of these patterns of involvement. The vasculitis mainly involves small vessels, with abundant

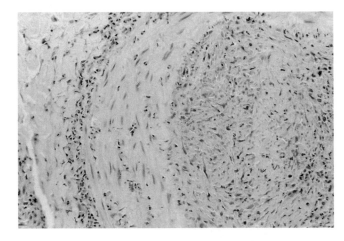

Fig. 4–3. Churg-Strauss disease demonstrates transmural inflammation and thrombosis of a medium-sized dermal blood vessel.

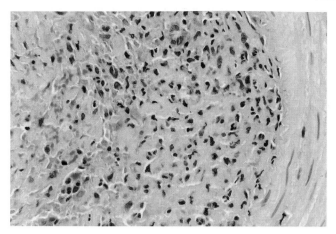

Fig. 4–4. Abundant eosinophils, admixed with neutrophils, are present in the inflammatory infiltrate within the wall of this vessel affected by Churg-Strauss disease.

eosinophil infiltrates, destruction of the vessel wall, and fibrinoid deposits. In some cases, a predominance of neutrophils may be present in the vessel walls. In addition, large numbers of eosinophils may be present in the interstitial reticular dermis. In florid cases, dense clusters of eosinophils are present around a central zone of degenerating collagen, forming a granulomatous area [43]. These granulomas can occur either adjacent to or separate from areas of vasculitis. Larger vessels may also be affected.

Special Studies. Direct immunofluorescence studies demonstrate granular deposits of immunoglobulins and complement in the walls of affected vessels. In addition, circulating IgE immune complexes have been demonstrated in these patients and may play a role in causing the vasculitis [44]. Antineutrophil cytoplasmic antibodies are positive in about half of the patients with Churg-Strauss syndrome [45]. This number is probably higher when patients with only active disease are counted.

Pathogenesis. Patients with Churg-Strauss syndrome have elevated serum levels of soluble interleukin-2 receptors and eosinophil cationic protein. This suggests that eosinophils and T lymphocytes are activated in these patients and are presumably responsible for the endothelial cell damage and vasculitis that occurs [45].

Behçet's Disease

Epidemiology. Behçet's disease is a chronic, relapsing systemic disease that has a high prevalence in Japan and the Middle East [46]. The disease is most common in young to middle-aged males. It is rare in children. There is a strong association between Behçet's disease and human leukocyte antigen (HLA) type B51 [47]. Others report a strong association with HLA-B12 [48]. It has been proposed that a diagnosis can be made based on a complex of symptoms that include oral aphthosis and any two of the following: uveitis, genital aphthae, cutaneous vasculitis, synovitis, and meningoencephalitis [49]. Cutaneous pathergy has also been included as a diagnostic feature [50]. The overall mortality rate is about 2%–4%.

Cutaneous Lesions. Cutaneous manifestations of Behçet's disease are widely varied, although painful aphthous ulcers are found in all cases. These last 1 to 2 weeks and heal without scarring. Skin changes are present in 64% of patients with Behçet's disease [51]. Many patients present with palpable, purpuric lesions. Blisters and ulceration may develop. Other patients may have erythema nodosum-like subcutaneous nodules [46]. Sweet's syndrome-like and pyoderma gangrenosum-like eruptions have also been described, as have papulopustular lesions [52, 53]. Pathergic, sterile pustules often develop at the sites of recent, minor trauma.

Associated Disorders. Patients with Behçet's disease also suffer recurrent genital and oral ulcerations, as well as uveitis and arthralgias. Less commonly, there may be vascular involvement of the central nervous system and gastrointestinal tract ulcerations [46]. Dyspnea, cough, and other respiratory symptoms may occur. Epididymitis has also been reported [48].

Histologic Features. It is difficult to adequately classify Behçet's disease based on histologic findings, as these changes are quite varied from one case to another. In one study, approximately 50% of biopsy specimens from patients with cutaneous lesions attributed to Behçet's disease demonstrated a vasculitis. In a minority of these patients, the lesions demonstrated characteristic changes of leukocytoclastic vasculitis, including transmural infiltration of venular walls by neutrophils, fibrinoid necrosis, and endothelial cell destruction. Extravasated erythrocytes were present. In the other group of patients, the inflammatory infiltrate was composed of lymphocytes infiltrating the vessel walls, associated with fibrinoid necrosis [54]. Vasculitic changes may involve arterioles as well as venules and can affect vessels of any size [55]. Other authors have found vasculitis to be present in a much lower percentage of cases [51].

Biopsy specimens from oral aphthous ulcers show nonspecific changes secondary to the mucosal disruption. A polymorphous infiltrate of neutrophils, lymphocytes, and macrophages is present.

Erythema nodosum-like lesions most commonly demonstrate a septal inflammatory infiltrate in which lymphocytes can be seen throughout the walls of affected vessels, accompanied by fibrinoid necrosis. In rare cases, a lobular panniculitis may be seen [56].

Special Studies. Direct immunofluorescence studies may demonstrate deposits of immunoglobulins and complement in the affected walls, but this is only seen in a few patients [54].

Pathogenesis. Behçet's disease is now thought to be an immunologically mediated systemic vasculitis; however, the precipitating factors that induce these inflammatory lesions are unknown. Although some authors report circulating immune complexes in patients with Behçet's disease [57], others have not found evidence for this [54].

MEDIUM-VESSEL VASCULITIDES

Polyarteritis Nodosa. Polyarteritis nodosa is best thought of as a group of vasculitides that affect medium-sized vessels and that demonstrate a range of clinical and histologic changes.

Systemic (Classic)

Epidemiology. Polyarteritis is a disease that usually occurs in middle-aged patients, but has been described in children and in elderly patients [58]. There is a 2:1 male predominance in some studies [59]. In one study, the 5 year survival rate was only 55% despite aggressive treatment with immunosuppressive therapies. Twenty percent of the patients in this series died within 1 year of initial presentation [59]. Gastrointestinal crises are the main cause of death in patients with polyarteritis nodosa.

Cutaneous lesions. The skin is affected in about 25% of cases of polyarteritis nodosa [60]. Cutaneous lesions vary from palpable purpura to ulcerations. Macules and papules are common. Less commonly, nodules may be present. Rarely, vesicles and urticaria may be the only cutaneous signs. The lower extremities are the most common site of involvement, but lesions may occur at any location.

Associated disorders. Patients with classic, or systemic, polyarteritis nodosa often have involvement of many internal organs. The kidneys are most frequently involved, followed by liver, heart, adrenals, gastrointestinal tract, joints, spleen, lungs, and central nervous system. Constitutional symptoms include weight loss, fever, anorexia, and fatigue [59].

Hepatitis B infection has been found in some patients with systemic polyarteritis, and it has been suggested that this virus may be the precipitating cause of the immune complex–mediated disease [61, 62]. Hepatitis C has also been associated [63]. Cryoglobulins have been demonstrated in some patients [59], as has hairy cell leukemia [64, 65]. A patient with human immunodeficiency virus infection and polyarteritis nodosa has been reported [66]. In children, there has been an association between polyarteritis nodosa and streptococcal infection [67]. Associated autoimmune diseases such as inflammatory bowel disease and lupus erythematosus have also been reported to coexist with polyarteritis nodosa [68, 69].

Histologic features. The characteristic histologic change is a necrotizing vasculitis of the medium-sized muscular arteries (Fig. 4–5). Smaller caliber arteries can also be involved [70]. Affected vessels are infiltrated by neutrophils and demonstrate destruction of the vessel wall. There is endothelial cell disruption and fibrin deposition (Fig. 4–6). Thrombi may be present. In some

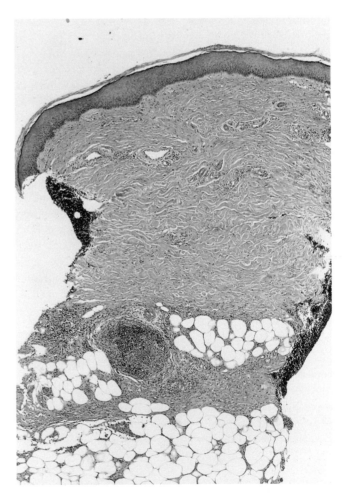

Fig. 4–5. Polyarteritis nodosa demonstrates a necrotizing vasculitis of medium-sized muscular arteries, commonly located at the junction between the deep reticular dermis and the subcutaneous fat.

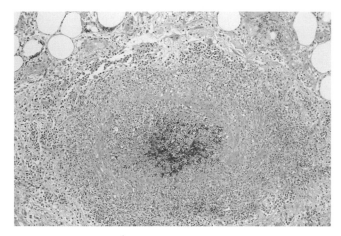

Fig. 4–6. Arteries affected by polyarteritis nodosa are overrun by neutrophils and fibrin and demonstrate extravasated erythrocytes and thrombosis.

cases, elastic tissue stains are helpful in demonstrating destruction of the internal elastic lamina in affected medium-seized vessels. Involvement of the medium-sized vessels in the deep reticular dermis and subcutaneous fat is the most specific histologic change, but similar changes in the smaller, more superficially located vessels are frequently the only histologic findings. In these cases, it may not be possible to distinguish polyarteritis nodosa from other types of leukocytoclastic vasculitis.

Special studies. Direct immunofluorescence studies demonstrate immunoglobulin and complement deposits in affected vessels. Lesions less than 48 hours old are most likely to be positive. Patients often have elevated levels of antineutrophil cytoplasmic antibodies.

Pathogenesis. Polyarteritis nodosa is a circulating immune complex–mediated disease. In most cases, the inciting antigen remains unknown, but in some patients the precipitating antigen can be identified.

Benign Cutaneous Polyarteritis Nodosa

Epidemiology. The existence of localized cutaneous polyarteritis nodosa as a discrete entity is quite controversial [71, 72]. Certainly, there is a form of polyarteritis nodosa that appears to preferentially affect the cutaneous vasculature, causing less serious systemic disease. Whether these patients truly have limited cutaneous disease and not a systemic process is still uncertain [73–75].

In one series, there was a female predominance of 1.7:1 in patients with primarily cutaneous polyarteritis nodosa [73]. This variant of the disease appears to affect primarily middle-aged adults. The course of cutaneous polyarteritis is often chronic and relapsing, lasting for years. This form of the disease is rare in children

[76]. Transplacental transmission has been reported to occur [77].

Cutaneous lesions. The lesions in cutaneous polyarteritis are usually described as painful, erythematous to violaceous subcutaneous nodules that measure 0.5–1.5 cm in diameter. They often appear in crops intermittently for years. The lower extremities are the usual site of lesions, but they can appear at any location. Papules, plaques, pustules, and vesicles may be present [74]. Livedo reticularis, accompanied by nodules and ulcers, occurs in 50%–80% of patients [73]. The most characteristic histologic changes can be found in samples taken from these nodules. Ulcerations and gangrene have been described. Patients also present with systemic symptoms such as fever, arthralgias, and arthritis. Sensory disturbances and neuropathies may be present [73].

Associated disorders. Cutaneous polyarteritis has been associated with hepatitis B by some authors [75], whereas others have not found this association [73]. Hepatitis C has also been associated [78]. Some patients have coexisting inflammatory bowel disease and rheumatoid arthritis [79]. In some patients, there is an antecedent history of streptococcus infection [73].

Histologic features. The histologic findings are those of a necrotizing vasculitis of medium-sized muscular arteries, usually located primarily in the deep reticular dermis and in the subcutaneous fat. Transmural neutrophils are present, along with fibrin deposits and endothelial cell destruction (Fig. 4–7). Eosinophils may be present in small numbers in up to one-third of cases [73]. The inflammation may be focal, and serial sections may be necessary to locate the

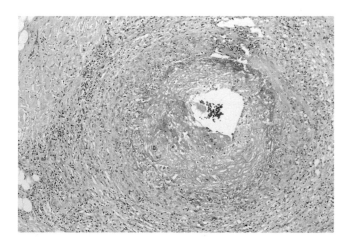

Fig. 4–7. Benign cutaneous polyarteritis nodosa demonstrates a histologic pattern similar to that in classic polyarteritis nodosa, with medium-sized muscular arteries displaying transmural neutrophilic infiltration, fibrin deposition, and extravasation of erythrocytes.

areas of inflammation. Elastic tissue stains may demonstrate destruction of the internal elastic lamina. In other cases, the artery may be so destroyed that this study is unhelpful. In late lesions, the vascular lumina of destroyed vessels may be largely obliterated and surrounded by fibrosis. Rare cases will also demonstrate leukocytoclastic vasculitis of the small vessels in the superficial vascular plexus [73].

Special studies. Unlike the situation in the microscopic (see later) and classic forms of polyarteritis nodosa, most patients with the limited cutaneous form do not have demonstrable levels of circulating antineutrophil cytoplasmic antibodies [73].

Direct immunofluorescence shows strong granular staining with immunoglobulins and complement within the affected vessel walls in the vast majority of cases.

Pathogenesis. Benign cutaneous polyarteritis nodosa is a circulating immune complex–mediated disease. In most cases, the inciting antigen remains unknown, but in some patients the precipitating antigen can be identified.

Microscopic Polyarteritis Nodosa

Epidemiology. Microscopic polyarteritis is a rare, systemic neutrophil-mediated vasculitis that is most common in middle-aged men. Patients present with prodromal symptoms of fever, malaise, and arthralgias [80]. The diagnosis is made only after other vasculitic processes have been excluded. The 5 year survival rate is 65% [81]. Mortality, when it occurs, is related to renal failure and pulmonary hemorrhage.

Cutaneous lesions. The skin is affected in 30%–40% of patients with microscopic polyarteritis nodosa [81, 82]. Lesions are usually described as splinter hemorrhages, purpuric macules, and papules that appear identical to those in patients with leukocytoclastic vasculitis. Ulcerations are common. Unlike the other forms of polyarteritis nodosa, however, tender, erythematous nodules have not been described in this condition [81].

Associated disorders. The microscopic form of polyarteritis primarily involves the kidneys. Involvement of the lungs and central nervous system has been reported [80]. Patients may develop hemoptysis. Other symptoms include abdominal pain, arthritis, oral ulcerations, ocular involvement, pericarditis and arrhythmias, and peripheral neuropathies. Unlike in the other types of polyarteritis described in this chapter, there does not seem to be a relationship between microscopic polyarteritis and hepatitis B or C infection.

Histologic features. Unlike leukocytoclastic vasculitis (described earlier), which affects primarily postcapillary venules, the inflammatory reaction in microscopic polyarteritis primarily destroys small arterioles in the reticular dermis. Both smaller and larger vessels can be similarly affected; however, medium-sized arteries are not inflamed, unlike the situation with other types of polyarteritis nodosa. The inflammatory infiltrate is primarily neutrophilic, with scattered numbers of lymphocytes and eosinophils. Fibrin deposition is present within vessel walls, and endothelial cell destruction may occur [81]. Secondary changes of ulceration and a more diffuse inflammatory infiltrate can be seen in more fully developed lesions.

Special studies. Patients with microscopic polyarteritis have demonstrable levels of circulating antineutrophilic antibodies of the antimyeloperoxidase type. This is a highly specific finding, and the presence of these antibodies is strongly supportive of this diagnosis [83]. The relationship between the titer of these circulating antibodies and disease activity remains controversial [84].

Pathogenesis. The pathogenesis of microscopic polyarteritis remains unknown.

Kawasaki's Disease (Mucocutaneous Lymph Node Syndrome)

Epidemiology. Kawasaki's disease is an acute, self-limited, but serious systemic disease that occurs most commonly in younger children [85]. Although it has been reported in adults, it is quite rare in patients over the age of 40 years [86]. The disease displays seasonal variation, being more prevalent in the winter and spring. The overall mortality rate is approximately 0.5%, with death occurring within 3–4 weeks after onset of symptoms [86].

Cutaneous lesions. The most common cutaneous manifestations include a polymorphous exanthem consisting largely of erythematous macules and patches with scale, accompanied by peeling of the hands and feet, along with acral swelling and erythema, conjunctivitis, and dry, erythematous lips [86]. Pustules superimposed on erythematous urticarial plaques in a symmetric distribution along the trunk have been described in a small group of patients with Kawasaki's disease [87]. A distinctive, desquamative, periorificial eruption has been reported in two-thirds of patients with Kawasaki's disease. The eruption occurs early in the course of the disease and may be a useful aid in early diagnosis [88].

Associated disorders. Patients with Kawasaki's disease usually present with cardiac abnormalities, including coronary artery aneurysms, myocarditis, and thromboses, which may lead to death. Coronary artery aneurysms occur in up to 20% of patients [89]. Patients also experience prolonged fevers, mucositis, and cervical lymphadenopathy [85]. Patients with Kawasaki's disease often have thrombocytosis.

Histologic features. Biopsy specimens from the usual exanthematous eruptions demonstrate perivascular edema and vasodilation, which are nonspecific histologic changes [90]. Histologic changes in the coronary arteries and other organs may include a necrotizing vasculitis of medium-sized muscular arteries that is indistinguishable from polyartcritis nodosa. These findings occur only rarely, if at all, in the skin [76, 91]. In patients with pustular lesions, the histologic changes demonstrate intraepidermal spongiform collections of neutrophils [87].

Special studies. Special studies are not required to make a diagnosis of Kawasaki's disease.

Pathogenesis. The pathogenesis of Kawasaki's disease remains obscure. Most investigators believe that an infectious agent, perhaps a bacterial superantigen, triggers an immune complex–mediated systemic vasculitis [85]. It has been suggested that extracellular products from oral *Streptococcus viridans* species may play a role in the etiology of this condition, as these organisms were cultured from a significant number of patients with Kawasaki's disease. These products have been shown to increase capillary permeability and increase swelling and erythema [92]. Interleukin-1α and tumor necrosis factor are present in acute cutaneous lesions, with lesser amounts of interleukin-2 and gamma interferon-γ [90].

References

1. Jennette, J. C., Falk, R. J., Andrassy, K., Bacon, P. A., Churg, J., Gross, W. L., Hagen, E. C., Hoffman, G. S., et al., *Nomenclature of systemic vasculitides: The proposal of an international conference.* Arthritis Rheum, 1994. 37:187–192.
2. Resnick, A. H., and Esterly, N. B., *Vasculitis in children.* Int J Dermatol, 1985. 24:139.
3. Sais, G., Vidaller, A., Jucgla, A., Servitje, O., Condom, E., and Peyri, J., *Prognostic factors in leukocytoclastic vasculitis: A clinicopathologic study of 160 patients.* Arch Dermatol, 1998. 134:309–315.
4. Lotti, T., Ghersetich, I., Comacchi, C., and Jorizzo, J. L., *Cutaneous small-vessel vasculitis.* J Am Acad Dermatol, 1998. 39:667–687.
5. Sanchez, N. P., Van Hale, H. M., and Su, W. P. D., *Clinical and histopathologic spectrum of necrotizing vasculitis.* Arch Dermatol, 1985. 121:220–224.
6. von Kobyletzki, G., Stucker, M., Hoffman, K., Pohlau, D., Hoffman, V., and Altmeyer, P., *Severe therapy-resistant necrotizing vasculitis associated with hepatitis C virus infection: Successful treatment of the vasculitis with extracoporeal immunoadsorption.* Br J Dermatol, 1998. 138:718–719.
7. Dienstag, J. L., Rhodes, A. R., Bhan, A. K., Dvorak, A.

M., Mihm, M. C., Jr., and Wands, J. R., *Urticaria associated with acute viral hepatitis type B: Studies of pathogenesis.* Ann Intern Med, 1978. 89:34–40.
8. McCluskey, R. T., and Fienberg, R., *Vasculitis in primary vasculitides, granulomatoses and connective tissue diseases.* Hum Pathol, 1983. 14:305–315.
9. Perez, C., Meondoza, H., Henandez, R., Valcayo, A., and Gurach, R., *Leukocytoclastic vasculitis and polyarthritis associated with Mycoplasma pneumoniae infection.* Clin Infect Dis, 1997. 25:154–155.
10. Fox, B. C., and Peterson, A., *Leukocytoclastic vasculitis after pneumococcal vaccination.* Am J Infect Control, 1998. 26:365–366.
11. Gorevic, P. D., Levo, Y., Kassab, H., Kohn, R., Meltzer, M., Prose, P., and Franklin, E. C., *Mixed cryoglobulinemia: An immune complex disease often associated with hepatitis B.* Trans Assoc Am Phys, 1977. 90:167–172.
12. Soter, N. A., Mihm, M. C., Jr., and Colten, H. R., *Cutaneous necrotizing vasculitis in a patient with cystic fibrosis.* J Pediatr, 1979. 95:197–201.
13. Garcia-Porrua, C., Gonzalez-Gay, M. A., Garcia-Pais, M. J., and Blanco, R., *Cutaneous vasculitis: An unusual presentation of sarcoidosis in adulthood.* Scand J Rheumatol, 1998. 27:80–82.
14. Soter, N. A., Mihm, M. C., Jr., Gigli, I., Dvorak, H. F., and Austen, K. F., *Two distinct cellular patterns in cutaneous necrotizing angiitis.* J Invest Dermatol, 1976. 66:344–350.
15. Fauci, A. S., Haynes, B. F., and Katz, P., *The spectrum of vasculitis: Clinical, pathologic, immunologic, and therapeutic considerations.* Ann Intern Med, 1978. 89:660–676.
16. Grunwald, M. H., Avinoach, I., Amichai, B., and Halevy, S., *Leukocytoclastic vasculitis—correlation between different histologic stages and direct immunofluorescence results.* Int J Dermatol, 1997. 36:349–352.
17. Sais, G., Vidaller, A., Jucgla, A., Condom, E., and Peyri, J., *Adhesion molecule expression and endothelial cell activation in cutaneous vasculitis: An immunohistologic and clinical study in 42 patients.* Arch Dermatol, 1997. 133:443–450.
18. Claudy, A., *Pathogenesis of leukocytoclastic vasculitis.* Eur J Dermatol, 1998. 8:75–79.
19. Daoud, M. S., Gibson, L. E., DeRemee, R. A., Specks, U., el-Azhar, R. A., and Su, W. P. D., *Cutaneous Wegener's granulomatosis: Clinic, histopathologic, and immunopathologic features of thirty patients.* J Am Acad Dermatol, 1994. 31:605–612.
20. Rottem, M., Fauci, A. S., Hallahan, C. W., Kerr, G. S., Lebovics, R., Leavitt, R. Y., and Hoffman, G. S., *Wegener granulomatosis in children and adolescents: Clinical presentation and outcome.* J Pediatr, 1993. 122:26–31.
21. Hu, C. H., O'Loughlin, S., and Winkelmann, R. K., *Cutaneous manifestations of Wegener's granulomatosis.* Arch Dermatol, 1977. 113:175–182.
22. Frances, C., Du, L. T. H., Piette, J.-C., Saada, V., Boisnic, S., Wechsler, B., Bletry, O., and Godeau, P., *Wegener's granulomatosis. Dermatologic manifestations in*

75 cases with clinicopathologic correlation. Arch Dermatol, 1994. 130:861–867.

23. Frunza Patten, S., and Tomecki, K. J., *Wegener's granulomatosis: Cutaneous and oral mucosal disease.* J Am Acad Dermatol, 1993. 28:710–718.

24. Barksdale, S. K., Hallahan, C. W., Kerr, G. S., Fauci, A. S., Stern, J. B., and Travis, W. D., *Cutaneous pathology in Wegener's granulomatosis. A clinocpathologic study of 75 biopsies in 46 patients.* Am J Surg Pathol, 1995. 19:161–172.

25. DeRemee, R. A., *In search of the ELK.* Semin Respir Med, 1989. 10:109–100.

26. Fauci, A. S., Haynes, B. F., Katz, P., and Wolff, S. M., *Wegener's granulomatosis: Prospective clinical and therapeutic experience with 85 patients for 21 years.* Ann Intern Med, 1983. 98:76–85.

27. Cohen Tervaert, J. W., van der Woude, F. J., Fauci, A. S., Ambrus, J. L., Velosa, J., Keane, W. F., Meijer, S., van der Giessen, M., et al., *Association between active Wegener's granulomatosis and anticytoplasmic antibodies.* Arch Intern Med, 1989. 149:2461–2465.

28. Kerr, G. S., Fleisher, T. A., Hallahan, C. W., Leavitt, R. Y., Fauci, A. S., and Hoffman, G. S., *Limited prognostic value of changes in antineutrophilic cytoplasmic antibody titer in patients with Wegener's granulomatosis.* Arthritis Rheum, 1993. 36:365–371.

29. Specks, U., Wheatley, C. L., McDonald, T. J., Rohrback, M. S., and DeRemee, R. A., *Anticytoplasmic autoantibodies in the diagnosis and follow-up of Wegener granulomatosis.* Mayo Clin Proc, 1989. 94:28–36.

30. van der Woude, F. J., Rasmussen, N., Lobatto, S., Wiik, A., Permin, H., van Esla, L. A., van der Giessen, M., and van der Hem, G. K., *Autoantibodies against neutrophils and monocytes: Tool for diagnosis and marker of disease activity in Wegener's granulomatosis.* Lancet, 1985. 1:425–429.

31. Jennette, J. C., and Falk, R. J., *Anti-neutrophilic cytoplasmic autoantibodies: New insight into cresentic glomerulonephritis, pulmonary-renal syndrome and systemic vasculitis.* AKF Nephrol Lett, 1989. 6:11–18.

32. Falk, R. J., Terrell, R. S., Charles, L. A., and Jenette, J. C., *Anti-neutrophil cytoplasmic autoantibodies induce neutrophils to degranulate and produce oxygen radicals in vitro.* Proc Natl Acad Sci USA, 1990. 87:4115–4119.

33. Gephardt, G. N., Ahmad, M., and Tubbs, R. R., *Pulmonary vasculitis (Wegener's granulomatosis). Immunohistochemical study of T and B cell markers.* Am J Med, 1983. 74:700–704.

34. Yoshikawa, Y., and Watanabe, T., *Pulmonary lesions in Wegener's granulomatosis: A clinicopathologic study of 22 autopsy cases.* Hum Pathol, 1986. 17:401–410.

35. Churg, J., and Strauss, L., *Allergic granulomatosis, allergic angiitis and periarteritis nodosa.* Am J Pathol, 1951. 27:277–301.

36. Schwartz, R. A., and Churg, J., *Churg-Strauss syndrome.* Br J Dermatol, 1992. 127:199–204.

37. Lie, J. T., *The classification of vasculitis and a reappraisal of allergic granulomatosis and angiitis (Churg-Strauss syndrome).* Mt. Sinai J Med., 1986. 53:429–439.

38. Crotty, C. P., DeRemee, R. A., and Winkelmann, R. K., *Cutaneous clinicopathologic correlation of allergic granulomatosis.* J Am Acad Dermatol, 1981. 5:571–581.

39. Lanham, J. G., Elkon, K. B., Pusey, C. D., and Hughes, G. R., *Systemic vasculitis with asthma and eosinophilia: A clinical approach to the Churg-Strauss syndrome.* Medicine, 1984. 63:65–81.

40. Clutterbuck, E. J., Evans, D. J., and Pusey, C. D., *Renal involvement in Churg-Strauss syndrome.* Nephrol Dial Transplant, 1990. 5:161–167.

41. Leung, W. H., Wong, K. K., Lau, C. P., Wong, C. K., Cheng, C. H., and So, K. F., *Myocardial involvement in Churg-Strauss syndrome: The role of endomyocardial biopsy.* J Rheumatol, 1989. 16:828–831.

42. Morgan, J. M., Raposo, L., and Gibson, D. G., *Cardiac involvement in Churg-Strauss syndrome shown by echocardiography.* Br Heart J, 1989. 62:462–466.

43. Churg, J., and Churg, A., *Idiopathic and secondary vasculitis: a review.* Mod Pathol, 1989. 2:144–160.

44. Manger, B. J., Krapf, F. E., Gramatzki, M., Nusslein, H. G., Burmester, G. R., Krauledat, P. B., and Kalden, J. R., *IgE-containing circulating immune complexes in Churg-Strauss vasculitis.* Scand J Immunol, 1985. 21: 369–373.

45. Schmitt, W. H., Csernok, E., Kobayashi, S., Klingenborgm, A., Reinhold-Keller, E., and Gross, W. L., *Churg-Strauss syndrome. Serum markers of lymphocyte activation and endothelial damage.* Arthritis Rheum, 1998. 41:445–452.

46. Shimizu, T., Erlich, G. E., and Inaba, G., *Behçet's disease (Behcet's syndrome).* Semin Arthritis Rheum, 1979. 8:223–260.

47. Mizoguchi, M., Matsuki, K., Mochizuki, M., Watanabe, R., Ogawa, K., Harada, S., Hino, H., Amagai, M., et al., *Human leukocyte antigen in Sweet's syndrome and its relationship to Behçet's syndrome.* Arch Dermatol, 1988. 124:1069–1073.

48. Arbesfeld, S. J. and Kurban, A. K., *Behçet's disease. New perspectives on an enigmatic syndrome.* J Am Acad Dermatol, 1988. 19:767–779.

49. O'Duffy, J. D., and Goldstein, N. P., *Neurologic involvement in seven patients with Behçet's disease.* Am J Med, 1976. 61:170–178.

50. Disease, International Study Group for Behçet's disease, *Criteria for diagnosis of Behçet's disease.* Lancet, 1990. 335:1078–1080.

51. Balabanova, M., Calamia, K. T., Perniciaro, C., and O'Duffy, J. D., *A study of the cutaneous manifestations of Behçet's disease in patients from the United States.* J Am Acad Dermatol, 1999. 41:540–545.

52. Armas, J. B., Davies, J., Davis, M., Lovell, C., and McHugh, N., *Atypical Behçet's disease with peripheral erosive arthropathy and pyoderma gangrenosum.* Clin Exp Rheumatol, 1992. 10:177–180.

53. Mizoguchi, M., Chikakane, K., Goh, K., Asahina, Y., and Masuda, K., *Acute febrile neutrophilic dermatosis (Sweet's syndrome) in Behçet's disease.* Br J Dermatol, 1987. 116:727–734.

54. Chen, K. R., Kawahara, Y., Miyakawa, S., and

Nishikawa, T., *Cutaneous vasculitis in Behçet's disease: A clinical and histopathologic study of 20 patients.* J Am Acad Dermatol, 1997. 36:689–696.

55. Lie, J. T., *Vascular involvement in Behçet's disease: Arterial and venous and vessels of all sizes.* J Rheumatol, 1992. 19:341–343.

56. Chun, S. I., Su, W. P. D., Lee, S., and Rogers, R. S. I., *Erythema nodosum-like lesions in Behçet's syndrome: A histopathologic study of 30 cases.* J Cutan Pathol, 1989. 16:259–265.

57. Jorizzo, J. L., Hudson, R. D., Schmalstieg, F. C., Daniels, J. C., Apisarnthanarax, P., Henry, J. C., Gonzalez, E. B., Ichikawa, Y., et al., *Behçet's syndrome: Immune regulation, circulating immune complexes, neutrophil migration, and colchicine therapy.* J Am Acad Dermatol, 1984. 10:205–214.

58. Jones, S. K., Lane, A. T., Golitz, L. E., and Weston, W. L., *Cutaneous periarteritis nodosa in a child.* Am J Dis Child, 1985. 139:920–922.

59. Cohen, R. D., Conn, D. L., and Ilstrup, D. M., *Clinical features, prognosis and response to treatment in polyarteritis.* Mayo Clin Proc, 1980. 55:146–155.

60. Ketron, L. W., and Bernstein, J. C., *Cutaneous manifestations of periarteritis nodosa.* Arch Dermatol Syphilol, 1939. 40:929–944.

61. Michalak, T., *Immune complexes of hepatitis B surface antigen in the pathogenesis of periarteritis nodosa. A study of seven necropsy cases.* Am J Pathol, 1978. 90:619–632.

62. Trepco, C. G., Zuckerman, A. J., Bird, R. C., and Prince, A. M., *The role of circulating hepatitis B antigen/antibody immune complexes in the pathogenesis of vascular and hepatic manifestations in polyarteritis nodosa.* J Clin Pathol, 1974. 27:863–868.

63. Carson, C. W., Conn, D. L., Czaja, A. J., Wright, J. L., and Brecher, M.E., *Frequency and significance of antibodies to hepatitis C virus in polyarteritis nodosa.* J Rheumatol, 1993. 20:304–309.

64. Lie, J. T., *Isolated polyarteritis of testis in haircy-cell leukemia.* Arch Pathol Lab Med, 1988. 112:646–647.

65. Krol, T., Robinson, J., Bekeris, L., and Messmore, H., *Hairy cell leukemia and a fatal periarteritis nodosa-like syndrome.* Arch Pathol Lab Med, 1983. 107:583–585.

66. Gherardi, R., Lebargy, F., Gaulard, P., Mhiri, C., Bernaudin, J. F., and Gray, F., *Necrotizing vasculitis and HIV replication in peripheral nerves (letter).* N Engl J Med, 1989. 321:685–686.

67. Sheth, A. P., Olson, J. C., and Esterly, N. B., *Cutaneous polyarteritis nodosa in childhood.* J Am Acad Dermatol, 1994. 31:561–566.

68. Raimer, S. S., and Sanchez, R. L., *Vasculitis in children.* Semin Dermatol, 1992. 11:48–56.

69. Volk, D. M., and Owen, L. G., *Cutaneous polyarteritis nodosa in a patient with ulcerative colitis.* J Pediatr Gastroenterol Nutr, 1986. 5:970–972.

70. Moskowitz, R. W., Baggenstoss, A. H., and Slocum, C. H., *Histopathologic classification of periarteritis nodosa: A study of 56 cases confirmed at necropsy.* Mayo Clin Proc, 1963. 38:345–357.

71. Diaz-Perez, J. L., and Winkelmann, R. K., *Cutaneous periarteritis nodosa.* Arch Dermatol, 1974. 110:407–414.

72. Thomas, R. H. M., and Black, M. M., *The wide clinical spectrum of polyarteritis nodosa with cutaneous involvement.* Clin Exp Dermatol, 1983. 8:47–59.

73. Daoud, M. S., Hutton, K. P., and Gibson, L. E., *Cutaneous periarteritis nodosa: A clinicopathologic study of 79 cases.* Br J Dermatol, 1997. 136:706–713.

74. Fisher, I., and Orkin, M., *Cutaneous form of periarteritis nodosa—an entity?* Arch Dermatol, 1964. 89:180–189.

75. Minkowitz, G., Smoller, B. R., and McNutt, N. S., *Benign cutaneous polyarteritis nodosa: Relationship to systemic polyarteritis nodosa and hepatitis B infection.* Arch Dermatol, 1991. 127:1520–1523.

76. Siberry, G. K., Cohen, B. A., and Johnson, B., *Cutaneous polyarteritis nodosa. Reports of two cases in children and review of the literature.* Arch Dermatol, 1994. 130:884–889.

77. Seabury Stone, M., Olson, R. R., Weismann, D. N., Giller, R. H., and Goeken, J. A., *Cutaneous vasculitis in the newborn of a mother with cutaneous polyarteritis nodosa.* J Am Acad Dermatol, 1993. 28:101–105.

78. Cacaoub, P., Lunel-Fablani, F., and Du, L. T., *Polyarteritis nodosa and hepatitis C virus infection (letter).* Ann Intern Med, 1992. 116:605–606.

79. Gudbjornsson, B., and Hallgren, R., *Cutaneous polyarteritis nodosa associated with Crohn's disease.* J Rheumatol, 1990. 17:386–390.

80. Homas, P. B., David-Bajar, K. M., Fitzpatrick, J. E., West, S. G., and Tribelhorn, D. R., *Microscopic polyarteritis. Report of a case with cutaneous involvement and antimyeloperoxidase antibodies.* Arch Dermatol, 1992. 128:1223–1228.

81. Savage, C. O., Winearls, C. G., Evans, D. J., Rees, A. J., and Lockwood, C. M., *Microscopic polyarteritis: Presentation, pathology and prognosis.* Q J Med, 1985. 56:467–483.

82. Rodgers, H., Guthrie, J. A., Brownjohn, A. M., and Turney, J. H., *Microscopic polyarteritis: Clinical features and treatment.* Postgrad Med J, 1989. 65:515–518.

83. Falk, R. J., and Jennette, J. C., *Anti-neutrophil cytoplasmic antibodies with specificity for myeloperoxidase in patients with systemic vasculitis and idiopathic necrotizing and crescentic glomerulonephritis.* N Eng J Med, 1988. 318:1651–1657.

84. Savage, C. O. S., Winearls, C. G., Jones, S., Marshall, P. D., and Lockwood, C. M., *Prospective study of radioiimmunoassay for antibodies against neutrophil cytoplasm in diagnosis of systemic vasculitides.* Lancet, 1987. 1:1389–1393.

85. Wortmann, D. W., and Nelson, A. M., *Kawasaki syndrome.* Rheum Dis Clin North Am, 1990. 16:363–375.

86. Landing, B. H., and Larson, E. J., *Pathologic features of Kawasaki disease (mucocutaneous lymph node syndrome).* Am J Cardiovasc Pathol, 1987. 1:218–229.

87. Kimura, T., Miyazawa, H., Watanabe, K., and Moriya, T., *Small pustules in Kawasaki disease. A clinicopathologic study of four patients.* Am J Dermatopathol, 1988. 10:218–223.

88. Friter, B. S., and Lucky, A. W., *The perineal eruption of Kawasaki syndrome.* Arch Dermatol, 1988. 124:1805–1810.

89. Hicks, R. V., and Melish, M. E., *Kawasaki syndrome.* Pediatr Clin North Am, 1986. 33:11151–1175.

90. Sato, N., Sagawa, K., Sasaguri, Y., Intoue, O., and Kato, H., *Immunopathology and cytokine detection in the skin lesions of patients with Kawasaki disease.* J Pediatr, 1993. 122:198–203.

91. Kawasaki, T., Kosaki, F., Okawa, S., Shigematsu, I., and Yanagawa, H., *A new infantile acute febrile mucocutaneous lymph node syndrome (MLNS) prevailing in Japan.* Pediatrics, 1974. 54:271–276.

92. Ohkuni, H., Todome, Y., Mizuse, M., Ohtani, N., Suzuki, H., Igarashi, H., Hashimoto, Y., Ezaki, T., et al., *Biologically active extracellular products of oral viridans streptococci and the aetiology of Kawasaki disease.* J Med Microbiol, 1993. 39:352–362.

PART II

Diseases Involving the Skin and Limited Other Organ Systems

CHAPTER 5

Gastrointestinal and Hepatic Diseases

There are many cutaneous disorders that have associated gastrointestinal manifestations. For organizational simplicity, these disorders are divided into processes that primarily affect the intestinal tract, the liver, and the pancreas.

INTESTINAL DISORDERS AND ASSOCIATED CUTANEOUS DISEASES

Dermatitis Herpetiformis

Epidemiology. Dermatitis herpetiformis is a multisystem disease that primarily affects the skin. It is invariably associated with a gluten-sensitive enteropathy that affects the small intestine. An association with human leukocyte antigen (HLA) types A1, B8, DR3, and DQw2 has been reported [1]. It is more common in the white population of the United States than in American blacks and Asians [2]. The disease usually presents in the second or third decade, but may appear at any age [3].

Cutaneous Lesions. Patients present with intensely pruritic, grouped (hence *herpetiform*) vesicles and papules, most commonly on the extensor surfaces of extremities. Elbows and knees are frequently involved. Often, it is difficult to find intact vesicles because the pruritus leads to scratching and erosion.

Associated Disorders. The most common gastrointestinal disorder associated with dermatitis herpetiformis is a gluten-sensitive enteropathy that resembles mild celiac sprue. Most patients have no gastrointestinal symptoms, but up to 30% have mild steatorrhea, and as many as 10% suffer from bloating, diarrhea, and malabsorption [1].

Patients with dermatitis herpetiformis frequently have gastric hypochlorhydria, and most suffer from gastric atrophy. The incidence of autoimmune thyroid disease is also increased in patients with dermatitis herpetiformis. These relationships are probably due to the HLA-B8 and -DR3 haplotype seen in some patients with dermatitis herpetiformis.

There is a slightly increased risk for gastrointestinal lymphoma in patients with long-standing dermatitis herpetiformis and associated gluten-sensitive enteropathy [4]. In most cases, the lymphomas are B-cell lymphomas of the "maltoma" type [5]. There is also a slight increased risk of other malignancies [6].

Histologic Features. Lesional skin is characterized by small subepidermal blisters. Within the papillary dermal tips, small neutrophilic abscesses are seen in well-formed lesions (Figs. 5–1 and 5–2). Earlier lesions may have less discrete collections of neutrophils. The epidermis remains intact, and keratinocyte necrosis is not prominent. There is often a slight lymphohistiocytic infiltrate present around the vessels of the superficial vascular plexus. Although usually not abundant, occasional eosinophils may be seen in some cases. The

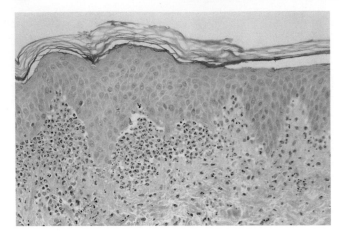

Fig. 5–1. Dermatitis herpetiformis: an early lesion shows dense collections of neutrophils at the papillary dermal tips.

following entities must be considered in the histologic differential diagnosis of dermatitis herpetiformis:

- Bullous lupus erythematosus
- Cicatricial pemphigoid
- Epidermolysis bullosa acquisita
- Linear IgA bullous dermatosis

Biopsy specimens from the small intestine display histologic changes of celiac sprue, even in patients who are clinically asymptomatic. The villi are markedly attenuated. There is an increased lymphocytic and plasmacellular infiltrate within the epithelium and lamina propria. The jejunum is most commonly involved. These changes have been well described. Avoidance of dietary wheat results in reversal of the gastrointestinal changes as well as resolution of the cutaneous lesions, but the diet is arduous.

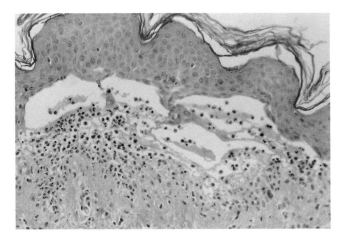

Fig. 5–2. Dermatitis herpetiformis with a subepidermal blister and abundant neutrophils within the blister cavity.

Special Studies. Direct immunofluorescence studies are helpful in confirming the diagnosis of dermatitis herpetiformis and in differentiating it from other subepidermal blisters with neutrophilic infiltrates. Granular deposits of IgA are present within the papillary dermal tips in perilesional skin, uninvolved skin, and mucosal surfaces [7]. It has been shown that the autoantibodies are directed against tissue transglutaminase that is present in both the gut mucosa and the cutaneous basement membrane zone [8]. Normal-appearing perilesional skin has the highest likelihood of revealing positive immunostaining results. Biopsy specimens from lesional skin are less commonly positive, probably due to enzymatic digestion from neutrophils. Occasional deposits of C3 may be present, but other immunoreactants are usually not seen. It is unknown how the polyclonal IgA deposits arrive and bind within the skin.

Serologic studies have demonstrated that circulating levels of antitissue transglutaminase levels can be used to discriminate between dermatitis herpetiformis and other autoimmune blistering diseases [8]. This test, however, is not yet widely available.

Pathogenesis. It remains unknown what triggers the development of cutaneous lesions in dermatitis herpetiformis. It has been suggested that patients with certain HLA haplotypes such as A1 or B8 may have an increased immunologic susceptibility to gluten, inducing mucosal inflammation and production of IgA, and binding to the skin. This could lead to the subsequent release of cytokines, leading to neutrophil chemotaxis and development of cutaneous lesions [9, 10]. Indeed, a gluten-free diet reverses both the cutaneous and gastrointestinal manifestations.

Pyoderma Gangrenosum

Epidemiology. Pyoderma gangrenosum is a disease that is most common in young to middle-aged adults, although cases have been reported in children and the elderly. It occurs in otherwise healthy people, although it also is commonly associated with inflammatory bowel disease and hematopoietic malignancies. It has been reported in immunosuppressed patients, including those with human immunodeficiency virus (HIV) infection [11]. The incidence of pyoderma gangrenosum is difficult to assess, in part due to the clinical and histologic overlap with other neutrophilic dermatoses such as Sweet's syndrome [12, 13]. It is estimated that approximately 50% of patients with pyoderma gangrenosum have some associated underlying disease [14].

Cutaneous Lesions. Pyoderma gangrenosum can be present at any site, but it is most common on the trunk and lower extremities. Lesions arise as small pustules, with surrounding erythema that coalesce to form ulcers in most but not all cases. The relationship between pustular lesions of pyoderma gangrenosum and those seen in subcorneal pustular dermatosis and in the bowel-related dermatitis/arthritis syndrome is not yet fully understood. Bullous lesions of pyoderma gangrenosum have been described. In these cases, clinical overlap with lesions classified as Sweet's syndrome occurs. A more vegetative, superficial variant also exists. The classic, fully developed ulcers have well-defined borders with characteristic overhanging margins and a border of erythema. The lesions are very painful. A characteristic, but poorly understood phenomenon of pyoderma gangrenosum is that of "pathergy," wherein lesions are localized to sites of skin damaged by trauma or surgery. Thus, superficial debridement is generally contraindicated. Pathergy is also seen in patients with other neutrophilic dermatoses and with Behçet's syndrome. In all cases, it exacerbates previously existing lesions [11].

Associated Disorders. Approximately 33% of patients with pyoderma gangrenosum have associated inflammatory bowel disease [15]. Chronic ulcerative colitis and Crohn's disease are equally associated. Less than 5% of all patients with inflammatory bowel disease, however, suffer from pyoderma gangrenosum. Either pyoderma gangrenosum or the inflammatory bowel disease may present first, and the diseases do not run parallel courses. The classic ulcerative and pustular variants of pyoderma gangrenosum are most strongly associated with the presence of inflammatory bowel disease.

About one-third of patients with ulcerative pyoderma gangrenosum suffer from asymmetric, seronegative arthritis involving large joints. Other types of arthritis such as rheumatoid arthritis, osteoarthritis, and Felty's syndrome have been associated with pyoderma gangrenosum.

Congenital, acquired, and iatrogenic immunosuppression have been associated with lesions of pyoderma gangrenosum. This relationship is seen most commonly in patients with HIV infection and in patients immunosuppressed secondary to renal or bone marrow transplantation.

Leukemia is the most common malignant neoplasm associated with pyoderma gangrenosum, but this still remains a rare association. The onset of these cutaneous lesions conveys an especially bad prognosis for leukemia patients [16]. Multiple myeloma, polycythemia vera, and Waldenström's macroglobulinemia have also been associated, as have Hodgkin's disease and other lymphomas. IgA monoclonal gammopathy is seen in up to 10% of patients with pyoderma gangrenosum [17]. In only rare cases does this progress to multiple myeloma. Solid organ tumors including carcinomas of the colon, breast, prostate, bronchus, and ovaries have been associated with pyoderma gangrenosum [11].

Histologic Features. Histologic changes in pyoderma gangrenosum are variable and nonspecific. Some authors have described intraepidermal pustules as an early change, but others do not recognize this as an invariable, or even common, finding [11]. Some investigators have suggested that a vasculitic process underlies the changes seen [18], and both lymphocytes and neutrophils are implicated by various other observers. Certainly, in the central portion of the lesion, underlying the ulcer, there is a marked neutrophilic infiltrate that resembles a dermal abscess. More lymphocytes and fewer neutrophils are seen at the periphery of the lesions. In some cases, there appears to be vascular wall disruption with infiltration of the walls by either lymphocytes or neutrophils. Pseudoepitheliomatous hyperplasia may be present in the vegetative lesions, and the overhanging margin can sometimes be seen microscopically, as evidenced by an intact epidermis overlying the dense dermal inflammatory infiltrate (Figs. 5–3 and 5–4). Dermal necrosis may be focal or widespread.

Special Studies. Some authors have reported immunoglobulins within the vessel walls of lesional skin, but others have not observed this [19].

Bowel-Associated Dermatitis/Arthritis Syndrome

Epidemiology. Bowel-associated dermatitis/arthritis syndrome is an unusual condition that is probably identi-

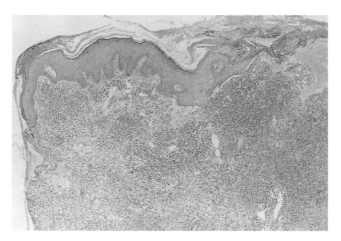

Fig. 5–3. Pyoderma gangrenosum with a dense, mixed dermal inflammatory infiltrate. An intact overlying epidermis from the edge of an ulcer is present in this biopsy specimen.

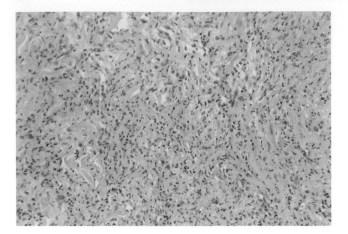

Fig. 5–4. Pyoderma gangrenosum has a dense dermal infiltrate with an admixture of inflammatory cells.

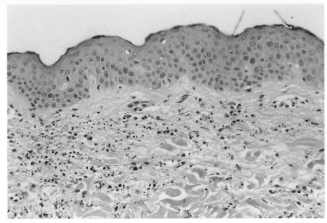

Fig. 5–5. Bowel-bypass syndrome is characterized by neutrophilic dermatitis. Leukocytoclasis can be seen.

cal to the bowel-bypass syndrome, but it occurs in patients without a history of bowel-bypass surgery. It has been reported in patients with ulcerative colitis, Crohn's disease, and diverticulosis [20].

Cutaneous Findings. The trunk and upper extremities are most commonly involved, but lesions may occur at any site. The most common presentation is that of small, pruritic pustules and vesicles [20]. Less commonly, deep-seated nodules similar to those seen in erythema nodosum may be present [21].

Associated Disorders. Patients may have multiple types of gastrointestinal disorders including ulcerative colitis, Crohn's disease, and diverticulosis. Patients who have had ileal-bypass operations for morbid obesity may present with identical cutaneous findings. Cryoglobulinemia has also been associated with this syndrome [22]. In addition to the cutaneous manifestations, patients usually present with fever, malaise, and arthralgias [23].

Histologic Features. The histologic findings show a dense neutrophilic dermatosis that is histologically indistinguishable from Sweet's disease. Minimal, if any, vascular destruction is present, but fibrin may be identified [23]. Leukocytoclasis may be present (Fig. 5–5). Eosinophils and lymphocytes are seen in increased numbers in older lesions. A septal panniculitis that is histologically identical to early lesions of erythema nodosum may be seen in deep-seated nodular lesions. The following entities must be considered in the differential diagnosis:

- Leukocytoclastic vasculitis
- Pyoderma gangrenosum
- Rheumatoid neutrophilic dermatitis
- Sweet's syndrome

Special Studies. Direct immunofluorescence studies have revealed variable results, with some authors describing immunoglobulin and complement deposits in vessel walls and along the dermal–epidermal junction and other authors finding no such deposits [20].

Pathogenesis. It has been suggested that the deposition of immune complexes containing bacterial antigens is responsible for the findings [24].

Cutaneous Crohn's Disease

Epidemiology. Crohn's disease may manifest itself in the skin in several forms [25]. Cutaneous involvement of some type may occur in up to 25% of cases and almost always presents after the gastrointestinal symptoms appear [26]. The skin has been reported to be the most common extraintestinal organ to be affected in patients with Crohn's disease [27].

Cutaneous Findings. Perianal fistulas and fissures are the most common cutaneous manifestation of Crohn's disease and may be seen in up to 36% of patients [28]. They are more likely to occur in patients with involvement of the large bowel than in those with disease restricted to the small intestine. Frequently, the cutaneous lesions will appear as erythematous plaques surrounding the anus. Another cutaneous manifestation is so-called metastatic Crohn's disease, which demonstrates cutaneous pathology similar to that seen in the gastrointestinal tract at skin sites distant from the primary disease. These lesions often appear, particularly in flexural regions, as erythematous plaques that ulcerate [27]. In other patients, "metastatic" lesions may clinically resemble erythema nodosum [29]. A series of case reports further enhances the range of lesions that "metastatic" Crohn's disease can resemble, including factitial lesions, acne, cellulitis, hidradenitis suppurativa, and seborrheic dermatitis [25].

Associated Disorders. Patients with Crohn's disease can develop zinc deficiency and subsequent acrodermatitis enteropathica (Chapter 6). Striae may also develop on the abdominal skin, presumably due to the frequent weight changes that these patients experience as the course of their disease waxes and wanes, as well as corticosteroid therapy. Pyoderma gangrenosum, erythema nodosum, and Sweet's syndrome may be seen in patients with Crohn's disease. Rare cases of epidermolysis bullosa acquisita, a subepidermal blistering disease, have been associated with Crohn's disease [30]. Other cutaneous conditions associated with Crohn's disease include palmar erythema, erythema multiforme, and digital acropachy.

Histologic Features. The histologic findings of cutaneous lesions in patients with Crohn's disease resemble those of intestinal Crohn's disease in most cases (Fig. 5–6). Sarcoidal-type granulomas are present within the dermis, not in particular association with vessels or cutaneous appendages [31]. Multinucleated giant cells are present. The differential diagnosis includes sarcoidosis, foreign body giant cell reaction, and infection. Definitive diagnosis is usually only possible in concert with a clinical history of Crohn's disease.

In some cases, granulomatous inflammation may be more deeply situated within the subcutaneous fat, giving the appearance of an erythema nodosum-type of reaction pattern. Rare cases with a diffuse neutrophilic inflammatory infiltrate resembling Sweet's syndrome have also been described in patients with cutaneous Crohn's disease [32].

Special Studies. Direct immunofluorescence plays no role in the diagnosis of most cases of cutaneous Crohn's disease. In the rare patient with Crohn's disease and associated epidermolysis bullosa acquisita, however, linear depositions of IgG and C3 along the dermal–epidermal junction may be present. Polarization microscopy may be helpful in excluding granulomas secondary to foreign material.

Degos' Disease (Malignant Atrophic Papulosis)

Epidemiology. Degos' disease is a rare disorder involving the skin, gastrointestinal tract, and central nervous system. In most cases, the cutaneous eruption

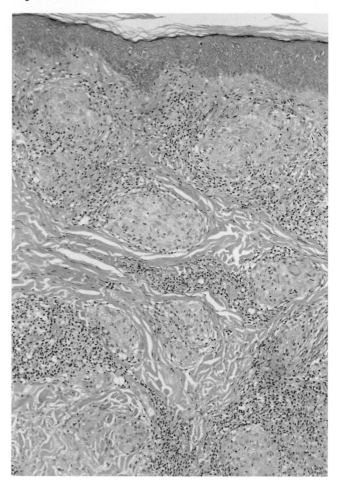

Fig. 5–6. Cutaneous Crohn's disease with sarcoidal granulomas admixed with inflammatory cells throughout the dermis.

marks the earliest clinical change. Vascular thrombosis leading to infarction in the intestinal tract or in the central nervous system frequently leads to death. Peritonitis secondary to bowel infarction is the most common cause of death. The disease is most common in young adults, with a mean age in the fourth decade, and may begin insidiously [33]. The disease is most prevalent in whites [34].

Cutaneous Findings. Multiple, atrophic, porcelain-white papules appear on the trunk and extremities, sparing the palms, soles, scalp, and face. Lesions begin as yellow-pink papules and rapidly become white and centrally depressed. Individual lesions rarely exceed 1 cm in diameter. The lesions are neither painful nor pruritic. Similar-appearing lesions may be present on the genital and buccal mucosal surfaces [34].

Associated Disorders. Intestinal lesions appear eventually in virtually all patients and frequently are a main reason for the poor prognosis of this disease. Rarely, intestinal lesions may precede the onset of cutaneous lesions. Clinical signs of intestinal disease are often vague initially and include slight dyspepsia, diarrhea and constipation, and abdominal distention. On endoscopic examination, atrophic white patches can be seen throughout the intestinal mucosa. These white areas of infarction are sharply demarcated. In some patients, there may be no clinical suggestion of gastrointestinal involvement until a catastrophic infarction leads to an acute abdomen and death. Although the small intestine is the most frequent site of intestinal involvement, the stomach and large intestine may also be involved.

The central nervous system can also be affected by the same vaso-occlusive process resulting in cerebrovascular accidents. Less commonly, other internal organs may show similar lesions that become apparent only at time of postmortem examination.

Histologic Features. Histologic features are those of a minimally inflammatory, thrombotic process involving the small vessels within the dermis. There is secondary

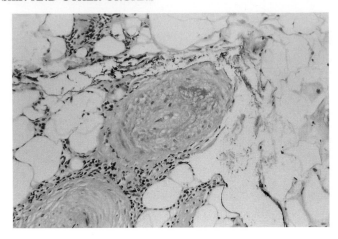

Fig. 5–8. Degos' disease with a thrombosed arteriole and minimal inflammatory infiltrate.

dermal necrosis, mucinous degeneration, and overlying epidermal atrophy in well-developed lesions (Fig. 5–7). Basal vacuolization may be present. The infarcted areas appear wedge shaped, corresponding to the tissue previously supplied by the destroyed blood vessel. Affected vessel walls may appear thickened and edematous and contain fibrin. Arterioles are the most commonly affected vessels (Fig. 5–8). Only rare lymphocytes are seen, and neutrophils are not a common feature [35]. The following entities must be considered in the differential diagnosis:

- Cryoglobulinemia
- Lichen sclerosis et atrophicus
- Livedoid vasculitis
- Morphea/progressive systemic sclerosis
- Protein C or S deficiency
- Septic emboli

Special Studies. Only scattered reports of direct immunofluorescence findings are available, and they suggest the occasional presence of slight deposits of C3 within vessel walls. Immunoglobulins are usually not seen [36].

Pathogenesis. The most common hypothesis is that Degos' disease is a primary coagulopathy [37]. No consistent abnormality in coagulation has, however, been found. Other authors believe the disease to be a primary vasculitis [38]. Others have suggested that the disease represents a lymphocyte-mediated vasculitis [35]. It must be concluded that the pathogenesis of this disease remains unknown.

Peutz-Jehgers Syndrome

Epidemiology. Peutz-Jehgers syndrome is a rare, autosomal dominantly inherited genodermatosis charac-

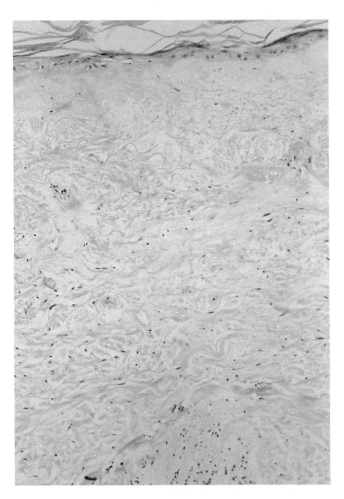

Fig. 5–7. Degos' disease with an atrophic epidermis and mucinous degeneration of affected dermis.

terized by cutaneous lesions and gastrointestinal polyps.

Cutaneous Findings. Hyperpigmented macules are present in and around the mouth and can also be present on acral surfaces. The buccal mucosa is a frequent location for hyperpigmented lesions, as is the vermillion border of the lips. In most cases, the brown or black macules are apparent within the first 2 years of life.

Associated Disorders. Hamartomatous polyps of the gastrointestinal tract are the cause of the most common symptomatic presentation of patients with Peutz-Jehgers syndrome, who often present with intussusception and intestinal bleeding. The polyps are most commonly found in the jejunum, but are also common in the stomach and ileum. They are less frequently found in the colon. Similar hamartomatous polyps have been described in the upper airways and in the genitourinary tract. Malignant degeneration of the gastrointestinal polyps is rare. Patients have an increased risk for nongastrointestinal carcinomas [39].

Histologic Features. The histologic findings of the hyperpigmented macules are indistinguishable from those of lentigo simplex. The epidermis may show slight elongation of the rete ridges, and the basal keratinocytes have increased amounts of melanin (Fig. 5–9). Melanocytes may appear slightly enlarged, but are not significantly increased in number [40].

Special Studies. Special studies are not required to make a diagnosis of Peutz-Jehgers syndrome.

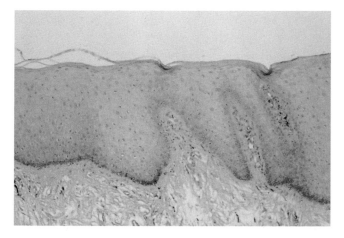

Fig. 5–9. Hyperpigmented macule in a patient with Peutz-Jehger syndrome showing the increased melanin within basal keratinocytes without increased numbers of melanocytes.

HEPATIC DISEASES AND ASSOCIATED CUTANEOUS DISORDERS

Porphyrias

Epidemiology. The porphyrias represent a category of acquired or inherited enzyme deficiencies in porphyrin metabolism that result in elevated breakdown products. All of the subtypes except for acute intermittent porphryia have cutaneous manifestations (Table 5–1).

Cutaneous Findings. Although each of the porphyrias involves the skin to differing degrees, the fundamental processes are the same for each of the conditions. The hepatic porphyrias, such as porphyria cutanea tarda, variegate porphyria, and hereditary coproporphyria have similar cutaneous presentations. The lesions are generally photodistributed. Patients develop fragile skin with vesicles and bullae in sun-exposed areas, which heal with scarring and milia formation giving a "weather-beaten" appearance. Hypertrichosis is common and is most pronounced on the face. Pigmentary changes may occur, and in later lesions sclerodermatous thickening may become apparent. Alopecia has also been reported in patients with porphyria. The erythropoietic subtypes of porphyria present with burning, erythema, and edema ("smarting reaction"), which occur immediately after exposure to sunlight [41]. These patients also get small erosions.

Associated Disorders. The most common associations with acquired porphyrias are diseases involving liver damage, including cirrhosis (usually due to increased ethanol intake) and metastatic carcinomas, and hepatocellular carcinoma. Porphyrias have also been described in patients with increased estrogen levels, including a rare condition seen in patients taking oral contraceptives. Porphyria cutanea tarda has been described in HIV-positive patients [42], as well as in patients with hepatitides B [43] and C [44]. It remains unclear whether the blistering, porphyria-like cutaneous eruptions that develop after prolonged exposure to tanning beds or in patients receiving hemodialysis because of chronic renal failure are best categorized as porphyrias or pseudoporphyrias [45–47]. The clinical and histologic features of the pseudoporphyrias are virtually indistinguishable from those of the true porphyrias, and care must be taken to exclude a cause of pseudoporphyria before making an unequivocal diagnosis of porphyria.

Histologic Features. Characteristic histologic changes are those of a minimally inflammatory subepidermal blister (Fig. 5–10). The epidermis may be acanthotic, with overlying hyperkeratosis. Segmented eosinophilic structures known as "caterpillar bodies," which are

Table 5–1. Porphyrias with Cutaneous Manifestations [69]

Type of Porphyria	Inheritance	Enzyme Defect	Symptoms	Laboratory Abnormality
Porphyria cutanea tarda	Sporadic AD Acquired	Uroporphyrinogen decarboxylase	Blisters Milia Scarring Hypertrichosis	Elevated urinary uroporphyrin Urinary and stool isocoproporphyrins
Congenital erythropoietic porphyria	AR	Uroporphyrinogen III synthetase	Severe photosensitivity Edema Erythema	Elevated uroporphyrin Coproporphyrin in urine and stool
Erythropoietic protoporphyria	AD	Ferrochelatase	Crusted lesions Scarring Waxy thickening of skin	Normal urine Elevated coproporphyrin in stool and urine Elevated protoporphyrin in blood, stool
Hepatoerythropoietic porphyria	AR	Uroporphyrinogen decarboxylase	Extreme photosensitivity Erythema Edema Vesicles Scarring Hypertrichosis Scleroderma-like changes	Increased uroporphyrins in stool and urine Increased coproporphyrin and isocoproporthyrin in stool Increased protoporphyrin in blood
Variegate porphryia	AD	Protoporphyrinogen oxidase	Like PCT Often mild	Increased aminolevulinic acid and porphobilinogen during attacks Increased protoporphyrinogen and coproporphyrinogen in stool
Hereditary coproporphyria	AD	Coproporphyrinogen oxidase	Like PCT	Increased coproporphyrins in stool and urine

AD = autosomal dominant; AR = autosomal recessive; PCT = porphyria cutanea tarda.

made from degenerating bits of basement membrane material, may be seen in the blister roofs [48]. Homogeneous eosinophilic deposits that stain positive with periodic acid–Schiff are found around vessels of the superficial vascular plexus, as well as along the

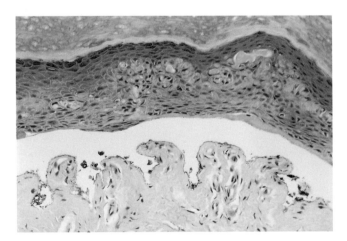

Fig. 5–10. Porphyria cutanea tarda is characterized by a noninflammatory subepidermal blister. Eosinophilic "caterpillar bodies" are seen within the roof of the blister, and festooning of the dermal papillae is prominent.

dermal–epidermal junction in most cases (Fig. 5–11). These deposits have been shown to be type IV collagen and laminin [49]. When present, the blister occurs at a level above the lamina densa, as type IV collagen and laminin have been shown to be present on the floor of the blister cavity [50]. Festooning of the papillary dermal tips is a common finding [51]. When present, the inflammatory reaction consists of scattered perivascular lymphocytes. Later lesions may demonstrate dermal sclerosis [52]. The histologic changes in the erythropoietic subtypes are less specific and may demonstrate only mild papillary dermal edema. Increased basement membrane components may be seen around blood vessels, but there is no blister formation.

In some cases, sclerodermatous changes develop with prolonged disease. The dermal collagen is markedly thickened. Cutaneous appendages are decreased in number. Clinical history is the best way to distinguish between sclerodermatoid porphyria and progressive systemic sclerosis or morphea.

Special Studies. Direct immunofluorescence studies may be helpful in distinguishing cutaneous porphyria from one of the other minimally inflammatory conditions with subepidermal blisters [53]. Immunoglobulins, most com-

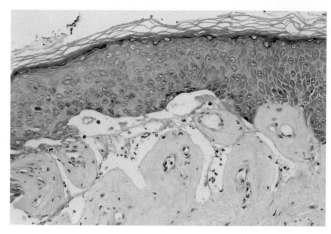

Fig. 5–11. Porphyria cutanea tarda with prominent thickening of the papillary dermal blood vessel walls.

monly IgM and C3, are found on the walls of blood vessels in the superficial perivascular plexus, and there is frequently staining with IgG and C3 at the dermal–epidermal junction [51]. The staining pattern is thickened and linear, as opposed to the granular depositions seen in leukocytoclastic vasculitis. It should be noted that a similar staining pattern can be seen in pseudoporphyria syndromes related to drugs, hemodialysis, or exposure to ultraviolet A light tanning salons [54–56].

Pathogenesis. In porphyria cutanea tarda and in erythropoietic porphyria, reduplication of basement membranes and fibrillar deposits on the vessel walls have been described [49]. It has been postulated that ultraviolet light plays a major role in the development of cutaneous lesions secondary to the absorption properties of increased the porphyrins [57].

Hemochromatosis

Epidemiology. The skin becomes a site for excess deposition of hemosiderin in patients with greatly increased amounts. This process occurs in patients with hemochromatosis.

Cutaneous Findings. Clinical findings include a characteristic "bronze" hyperpigmentation that is accentuated in sun-exposed areas [58]. Hyperpigmentation is seen in more than 90% of patients with hemochromatosis [59]. As iron stores are depleted with therapy, the hyperpigmentation will reverse.

Associated Disorders. As hemosiderin deposits accumulate in other organs, a range of clinical manifestations may become apparent. These include congestive heart failure, arrhythmias, diabetes mellitus, and cirrhosis. There is also an association of vitiligo in patients with hemochromatosis [60].

Histologic Features. Histologic features include an increased amount of dermal pigment, located both within macrophages and extracellularly among collagen bundles. Most of the pigment is seen in the vicinity of the superficial vascular plexus and in the basement membrane surrounding cutaneous appendages. Small amounts of golden-brown pigment may also be seen within the epidermis. There is increased melanin within basal keratinocytes.

Special Studies. Iron stains will label the golden-brown pigment within the dermis and in some cases within the epidermis.

Pathogenesis. The hyperpigmentation of the skin is due primarily to increased melanin production that is not directly due to iron deposits. In patients with both hemochromatosis and vitiligo, there is no hyperpigmentation in the vitiliginous areas. This finding suggests that melanocytes and not the iron deposits are responsible for producing the clinical pigmentation [60]. It is not known how the deposition of iron (as well as other metals) increases melanin production in the skin.

Terry's nails refers to nails that are abnormally white except for the most distal section of the nail. They are associated with cirrhosis in most cases, but have been observed in a wide range of conditions including congestive heart failure and adult-onset diabetes mellitus [61]. Histologic examination reveals only telangiectatic blood vessels [62].

PANCREATIC DISEASES AND ASSOCIATED CUTANEOUS DISORDERS

Pancreatic Panniculitis

Epidemiology. Patients with pancreatitis or pancreatic carcinoma are predisposed to develop associated cutaneous lesions. Less than 2% of patients with pancreatic disease will develop them.

Cutaneous Findings. Subcutaneous nodules may be asymptomatic or tender and tend to occur on the buttocks, thighs, and distal extremities. There may be no overlying surface change, or superficial ulceration may be present.

Associated Disorders. Pancreatic panniculitis is associated with acute pancreatitis. Less commonly, cutaneous lesions may be present in patients with pancreatic carcinoma of either the islet cell type or the acinic type [63, 64]. Patients may also present with arthritis or a leukemoid reaction, abdominal pain, and ascites.

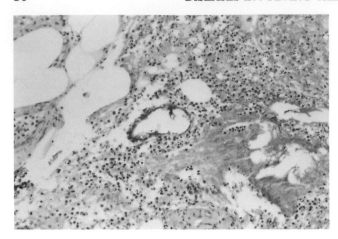

Fig. 5–12. Pancreatic panniculitis demonstrates a dense, neutrophilic lobular infiltrate with abundant necrosis and calcification.

Histologic Features. Pancreatic panniculitis is characterized by a neutrophil-mediated lobular panniculitis (Fig. 5–12). The fatty lobules are overrun by a dense infiltrate of neutrophils that do not appear to destroy surrounding blood vessels [65]. Extensive fat necrosis is present. Ghost cells, corresponding to necrotic adipocytes, may be seen in early lesions. Secondary calcification is commonly seen in more advanced lesions. Older lesions have pigment-laden macrophages and fibrosis [66]. In other cases, the inflammatory infiltrate may be rather sparse, leaving the necrotic adipocytes as the main diagnostic feature.

Special Studies. No special studies are necessary to make a diagnosis of pancreatic panniculitis.

Pathogenesis. Increased serum levels of lipase and trypsin result in enzymatic digestion of fat throughout the body, including the subcutis. The necrotic fat is rapidly infiltrated by neutrophils. Saponification of the degenerating fat leads to calcification [67]. Others have postulated an immunologic mechanism for the fat necrosis [68].

NOTE: α_1 antitrypsin deficiency is discussed in Chapter 6.

References

1. Hall, R. P., *Dermatitis herpetiformis.* J Invest Dermatol, 1992. 99:873–881.
2. Hall, R. P., Clark, R. E., and Ward, F. E. *Dermatitis herpetiformis in two American blacks: HLA type and clinical characteristics.* J Am Acad Dermatol, 1989. 21:436–439.
3. Buckley, D. B., English, J., Molloy, W., Doyle, C. T., and Whelton, M. J. *Dermatitis herpetiformis: A review of 119 cases.* Clin Exp Dermatol, 1983. 8:477–487.
4. Swerdlow, A. J., Whittaker, S., Carpenter, L. M., and English, J. S. C. *Mortality and cancer incidence in patients with dermatitis herpetiformis: A cohort study.* Br J Dermatol, 1993. 129:140–144.
5. Bose, S. K., Lacour, J. P., Bodokh, I., and Ortonne, J. P. *Malignant lymphoma and dermatitis herpetiformis.* Dermatology, 1994. 188:177–181.
6. Leonard, J. N., Tucker, W. F. G., Fry, J. S., Coulter, C. A., Boylston, A. W., McMinn, R. M., Haffenden, G. P. et al., *Increased incidence of malignancy in dermatitis herpetiformis.* BMJ 1983. 286:16.
7. Pazderka Smith, E., and Zone, J. J., *Dermatitis herpetiformis and linear IgA bullous dermatosis.* Dermatol Clin 1993. 11:511–526.
8. Rose, C., Dieterich, W., Brocker, E.-B., Schuppan, D., and Zillikens, D., *Circulating autoantibodies to tissue transglutaminase differentiate patients with dermatitis herpetiformis from those with linear IgA disease.* J Am Acad Dermatol, 1999. 41:957–961.
9. Katz, S. L., Hall, R. P., Lawley, T. M., and Strober, W., *Dermatitis: The skin and the gut.* Ann Intern Med, 1980. 93:857–874.
10. Graeber, M., Baker, B. S., Garioch, J. J., Valdimarsson, H., Leonard, J. N., and Fry, L., *The role of cytokines in the generation of skin lesions in dermatitis herpetiformis.* Br J Dermatol, 1993. 129:530–532.
11. Powell, F.C., Su, W. P. D., and Perry, H. O., *Pyoderma gangrenosum: Classification and management.* J Am Acad Dermatol, 1996. 34:395–409.
12. Benton, E. C., Rutherford, D., and Hunter, J. A., *Sweet's syndrome and pyoderma gangrenosum associated with ulcerative colitis.* Acta Derm Venereol (Stockh), 1985. 65:77–80.
13. Callen, J. P., *Acute febrile neutrophilic dermatosis (Sweet's syndrome) and the related conditions of "bowel bypass" syndrome and bullous pyoderma gangrenosum.* Dermatol Clin, 1985. 3:153–63.
14. Hickman, J. G., and Lazarus, G. S., *Pyoderma gangrenosum: A reappraisal of associated systemic diseases.* Br J Dermatol, 1980. 102:235–237.
15. Levitt, M. D., Ritchie, J. K., Lennard-Jones, J. E., and Phillips, R. K. *Pyoderma gangrenosum in inflammatory bowel disease.* Br J Surg, 1991. 78:676–678.
16. Perry, H. O., and Winkelmann, R. K., *Bullous pyoderma gangrenosum and leukaemia.* Arch Dermatol, 1972. 106:901–905.
17. Powell, F. C., Schroeter, A. L., Su, W. P. D., and Perry, H. O., *Pyoderma gangrenosum and monoclonal gammopathy.* Arch Dermatol, 1983. 119:468–472.
18. Thompson, D. M., Main, R. A., Beck, J. S., and Albert-Recht, F., *Studies on a patient with leukocytoclastic vasculitis, "pyoderma gangrenosum" and paraproteinemia.* Br J Dermatol, 1973. 88:117–125.
19. Powell, F. C., Schroeter, A. L., Perry, H. O., and Su, W. P. D., *Direct immunofluorescence in pyoderma gangrenosum.* Br J Dermatol, 1983. 108:287–293.
20. Dicken, C. H., *Bowel-associated dermatitis-arthritis syn-*

drome: *Bowel bypass syndrome without bowel bypass.* J Am Acad Dermatol, 1986. 14:792–796.

21. Kennedy, C., *The spectrum of inflammatory skin lesions following jejuno-ileal bypass for morbid obesity.* Br J Dermatol, 1981. 105:425–436.

22. Utsinger, P. D., *Systemic immune complex disease following intestinal bypass surgery: Bypass disease.* J Am Acad Dermatol, 1980. 2:488–495.

23. Morrison, J. G. L., and Fourie, E. D., *A distinctive skin eruption following small-bowel by-pass surgery.* Br J Dermatol, 1980. 102:467–471.

24. Ely, P. H., *The bowel bypass syndrome: A response to bacterial peptidoglycans.* J Am Acad Dermatol, 1980. 2:473–487.

25. Burgdorf, W., *Cutaneous manifestations of Crohn's disease.* J Am Acad Demratol, 1981. 5:689–695.

26. Samitz, M. H., Dana, A. S., Jr., and Rosenberg, P., *Cutaneous vasculitis in association with Crohn's disease.* Cutis, 1970. 6:51–56.

27. McCallum, D. I., and Gray, W. M., *Metastatic Crohn's disease.* Br J Dermatol, 1976. 95:551–554.

28. Rankin, G. B., Watts, H. D., Melnyk, C. S., and Kelley, M. L., Jr., *National cooperative Crohn's disease study: Extraintestinal manifestations and perianal complications.* Gastroenterology, 1979. 77:914–920.

29. Witkowski, J. A., Parish, L. C., and Lewis, J. E., *Crohn's disease—non-caseating granulomas on the legs.* Acta Derm Venereol (Stockh), 1977. 57:181–183.

30. Livden, J. K., Nisen, R., Thunold, S., and Schjonsby, H., *Epidermolysis bullosa acquisita and Crohn's disease.* Acta Derm Venereol, 1978. 58:241–244.

31. Billings, J. K., Ellis, C. N., and Milgraum, S. S., *Cutaneous granuloma formations in Crohn's disease.* JAMA, 1986. 255:2661.

32. Smoller, B.R., Weishar, M., and Gray, M. H., *An unusual cutaneous manifestation of Crohn's disease.* Arch Pathol Lab Med, 1990. 114:609–610.

33. Degos, R., *Malignant atrophic papulosis.* Br J Dermatol, 1979. 100:213–235.

34. Magrinat, G., Kerwin, K. S., and Gabriel, D. A., *The clinical manifestations of Degos' syndrome.* Arch Pathol Lab Med, 1989. 113:354–362.

35. Soter, N. A., Murphy, G. F., and Mihm, M. C., Jr., *Lymphocytes and necrosis of the cutaneous microvasculature in malignant atrophic papulosis: A refined light microscopic study.* J Am Acad Dermatol, 1982. 7:620–630.

36. Muller, S. A., and Landry, M., *Exchange autografts in malignant atrophic papulosis (Degos' disease).* Mayo Clin Proc, 1974. 49:884–888.

37. Degos, R., *Malignant atrophic papulosis: A fatal cutaneo-intestinal syndrome.* Br J Dermatol, 1966. 66:304–307.

38. Strole, W. E., Jr., Clark, W. H., Jr., and Isselbacher, K. J., *Progressive arterial occlusive disease (Kohlmeier-Degos).* N Engl J Med, 1967. 276:195–201.

39. Giardello, F. M., Welsh, S. B., Hamilton, S. R., Offerhaus, G. J., Gittelson, A. M., Booker, S. V., Krush, A. J., et al., *Increased risk of cancer in the Peutz-Jeher syndrome.* N Eng J Med, 1987. 116:1511–1514.

40. Yamada, K., Matsukawa, A., Hori, Y., and Kukita, A., *Ultrastructural studies on pigmented macules in Peutz-Jehger syndrome.* J Dermatol (Tokyo), 1981. 8:367–377.

41. Epstein, J. H., Tuffannelli, D. L., and Epstein, W. L., *Cutaneous changes in the porphyrias.* Arch Dermatol, 1973. 107:689–698.

42. Hogan, D., Card, R. T., Ghadially, R., McSheffrey, J. B., and Lane, P., *Human immunodeficiency virus infection and porphyria cutanea tarda.* J Am Acad Dermatol, 1989. 20:17–20.

43. Rocchi, E., Gibertini, P., Cassanelli, M., Pietranglo, A., Jensen, J., and Ventura, E., *Hepatitis B virus infection in porphyria cutanea tarda.* Liver, 1986. 6:153–157.

44. LaCour, J. P., Bodokh, I., Castanet, J., Bekri, S., and Ortonne, J. P., *Porphyria cutanea tarda and antibodies to hepatitis C.* Br J Dermatol, 1993. 128:121–123.

45. Murphy, G. M., Wright, J., Nicholls, D. S. H., McKee, P. H., Messenger, A. G., Hawk, J. L., and Levene, G. M., *Sunbed-induced pseudoporphyria.* Br J Dermatol, 1989. 120:555–562.

46. Stenberg, A., *Pseudoporphyria and sunbeds.* Acta Derm Venereol, 1990. 70:354–356.

47. Poh-Fitzpatrick, M. B., Masullo, A. S., and Grossman, M. E., *Porphyria cutanea tarda associated with chronic renal disease and hemodialysis.* Arch Dermatol, 1980. 116:191–195.

48. Egbert, B. M., LeBoit, P. E., McCalmont, T., Hu, C. H., and Austin, C., *Caterpillar bodies: Distinctive basement membrane containing structures in blisters of porphyria.* Am J Dermatopathol, 1993. 15:199–202.

49. Wolff, K., Hongismann, H., Rauschmeier, W., Schuler, G., and Perchlaner, R., *Microscopic and fine structural aspects of porphyrias.* Acta Derm Venereol Suppl (Stockh), 1982. 100:17–28.

50. Dabski, C., and Beutner, E. H., *Studies of laminin and type IV collagen in blisters of porphyria cutanea tarda and drug-induced pseudoporphryia.* J Am Acad Dermatol, 1991. 25:28–32.

51. Maynard, B., and Peters, M. S., *Histologic and immunofluorescence study of cutaneous porphyrias.* J Cutan Pathol, 1991. 19:40–47.

52. Freidman, S.J., and Doyle, J. A., *Sclerodermoid changes of porpyhria cutanea tarda: possible relationship to urinary uroporphyrin levels.* J Am Acad Dermatol, 1985. 13:70.

53. Cormane, R. H., Szabo, E., and Hoo, T. T., *Histopathology of the skin in acquired and hereditary porphyria cutanea tarda.* Br J Dermatol, 1971. 85:531.

54. Judd, L. E., Henderson, D. W., and Hill, D. C., *Naproxen-induced pseudoporphyria: A clinical and ultrastructural study.* Arch Dermatol, 1986. 122:451–454.

55. Gilchrest, B., Rowe, J. W., and Mihm, M. C., Jr., *Bullous dermatosis of hemodialysis.* Ann Intern, 1975. 83:480–483.

56. Epstein, J. H., Tuffanelli, D. L., Seibert, J. S., and Epstein, W. L., *Porphyria-like cutaneous changes induced by tetracycline hydrochloride photosensitization.* Arch Dermatol, 1976. 112:661–666.

57. Dermatology, Photobiology Task Force of the American Academy of Dermatology. *Risks and benefits from high-intensity ultraviolet A sources for cosmetic purposes.* J Am Acad Dermatol. 1986. 12:380–381.

58. Milder, M. S., Cook, J. D., Stray, S., and Finch, C. A., *Idiopathic hemochromatosis: An interim report.* Medicine (Baltimore), 1980. 59:34–49.

59. Cawley, E. P., Hsu, Y. T., Wood, B. T., and Weary, P. E., *Hemochromatosis and the skin.* Arch Dermatol, 1969. 100:1–6.

60. Perdrup, A., and Poulsen, H., *Hemochromatosis and vitiligo.* Arch Dermatol, 1964. 90:34–37.

61. Scher, R.K., and Daniel, C. R. I., *Nails: Therapy, Diagnosis, Surgery.* 1990, W. B. Saunders, Philadelphia, pp. 177.

62. Holzberg, M., and Walker, H. K., *Terry's nails: Revised definition and new correlations.* Lancet, 1984. 1:896–899.

63. Lee, M.-S., Lowe, P. M., Nevell, D. F., Fryer, J., and Le Guay, J., *Subcutaneous fat necrosis following traumatic pancreatitis.* Austral J Dermatol, 1995. 36:196–198.

64. Detlefs, R. L., *Drug-induced pancreatitis presenting as subcutaneous fat necrosis.* J Am Acad Dermatol, 1985. 13:305–307.

65. Cannon, J. R., Pitha, J. V., and Everett, M. A., *Subcutaneous fat necrosis in pancreatitis.* J Cutan Pathol, 1979. 6:501–506.

66. Hughes, P. S. H., Apisarntharax, P., and Mullins, J. F., *Subcutaneous fat necrosis associated with pancreatic disease.* Arch Dermatol, 1975. 111:506–510.

67. Forstrom, L., and Winkelmann, R. K., *Acute, generalized panniculitis with amylase and lipase in skin.* Arch Dermatol, 1975. 111:497–502.

68. Berman, B., Conteas, C., Smith, B., Leong, S., and Hornveck, L., 3rd, *Fatal pancreatitis presenting with subcutaneous fat necrosis.* J Am Acad Dermatol, 1987. 17:359–364.

69. Young, J. W., and Conte, E. T., *Porphyrias and porphyrins.* Int J Dermatol, 1991. 30:399–406.

Pulmonary and Skin Diseases

Sarcoidosis

Epidemiology. There is wide regional variation in the incidence of sarcoidosis. Up to 200 persons per 100,000 are afflicted in some communities in the United States, but the overall incidence is closer to 20 persons per 100,000 [1]. Young adult women have the highest likelihood of developing sarcoidosis, with a 10:1 female to male predominance [2]. In the United States, the highest incidence is seen in black patients. This subgroup also experiences the most fulminant course, with the most atypical cutaneous manifestations [3–5]. Human leukocyte antigen (HLA) type A1B8 has been associated with Löfgren's syndrome and acute sarcoidosis [6]. Patients with HLA-B8 may have an increased incidence of sarcoidosis, and those with HLA-B13 may be at risk for a more chronic, persistent form of the disease [7, 8]. The overall mortality rate of sarcoidosis is 3%–6%, and it is usually related to cardiac, respiratory, or renal involvement.

Cutaneous Features. Cutaneous manifestations occur in up to one-third of patients with sarcoidosis [9, 10] and have been divided into specific and nonspecific eruptions. In one series, as many as 25% of patients with cutaneous sarcoidosis had disease limited to the skin [11]. It has been suggested that patients with cutaneous sarcoidosis have a worse prognosis than do those in whom no cutaneous eruption is present. Other authors suggest that in otherwise healthy patients in whom the initial presentation of sarcoidosis is in the skin, the prognosis does not appear to be adverse [12]. Patients with an acute and severe onset often experience complete resolution of the disease.

Cutaneous sarcoidosis has many clinical appearances. The most common specific clinical presentations include lupus pernio, chronic erythematous plaques or nodules spanning the nasal bridge and malar region, erythematous plaques in other sites, and dermal nodules within previous scars. There may be one cutaneous lesion or hundreds. *Lupus pernio* is an old term that has no relationship to either lupus erythematosus or perniosis. It is used, by general consensus, for sarcoidosis that primarily involves the midface. Lupus pernio progresses to scarring and telangiectasias and rarely resolves. It is frequently associated with upper respiratory involvement [13]. Less commonly, other cutaneous lesions may resolve with slightly depressed scars. Lupus pernio may occur at other body sites and may lead to digital mutilation [13].

Papules are less commonly seen and may be suggestive of more limited disease [11]. They frequently occur on the extremities, buttocks, and shoulders and may take on a serpiginous distribution. Midfacial papules have been reported in a child with cutaneous sarcoidosis [14]. This is noteworthy because sarcoidosis is rare in children. Papules may demonstrate keratotic plugging, believed to be a form of transepidermal elimination [15]. In other patients, the papules may be tiny and appear lichenoid. An asymptomatic eruption of macules and papules involving the face, trunk, and extremities has been reported to herald the onset of sarcoidosis [10, 16]. Sarcoidosis manifesting as several subcutaneous nodules is known as *Darier and Roussy sarcoidosis*. In this form of the disease, oval or round, skin-colored or violaceous nodules are present on the lower extremities.

Onset of cutaneous sarcoidosis has been associated with Koebner's phenomenon in some circumstances. Sarcoidal granulomas have developed at the sites of cutaneous venipuncture [17, 18] and following facial trauma [19]. Scar-associated sarcoidosis clinically resembles keloid formation at the sites of previous injury.

There are nonspecific cutaneous eruptions associated with sarcoidosis. Acquired ichthyosis, usually of the lower extremities, occurs in this setting [20]. Erythroderma has been reported, as have hypopigmented macules and papules [21]. Less commonly, ulcerative and psoriasiform forms of the disease have been observed, as has a scarring alopecia [13, 22–24]. A morpheaform eruption of the trunk and extremities has been reported in three females with sarcoidosis

Löfgren's syndrome, characterized by hilar adenopathy, fever, polyarthralgias, uveitis, and erythema nodosum, tends to resolve spontaneously and has an excellent prognosis [25]. The cutaneous eruption is clinically, as well as histologically, indistinguishable from erythema nodosum not associated with sarcoidosis.

Rare cases of isolated cutaneous sarcoidosis involving the vulva, neck, and face have been reported [26].

Associated Disorders. Sarcoidosis has been associated with progressive systemic sclerosis and systemic lupus erythematosus [27, 28], as well as with Sjögren's syndrome [29] and with primary biliary cirrhosis [30]. Cases of coexisting necrobiosis lipoidica, granuloma annulare, and sarcoidosis have been described [31]. Leukocytoclastic vasculitis commonly occurs in conjunction with cutaneous sarcoidosis in children. This association is rarely found in adults [32]. There is also one report of porphyria cutanea tarda occurring in a patient with sarcoidosis [33]. Cutaneous sarcoidosis has also appeared after interferon-α treatment in a patient with chronic myelogenous leukemia [34]. Rare cases of necrotizing sarcoid granulomatosis have been associated with crescentic glomerulonephritis, Hashimoto's thyroiditis, and pulmonary hemorrhage [35].

Sarcoidosis affects many other organ systems. Patients frequently have lymphadenopathy and splenomegaly. Cardiac abnormalities such as complete heart block, papillary muscle dysfunction, congestive heart failure, pericarditis, and arrhythmias can be seen [36], as well as abnormal liver function tests and musculoskeletal involvement [37]. Hypercalcemia and hypercalciuria may be seen in patients with sarcoidosis [38].

Histologic Features. The classic histologic features of sarcoidosis are similar to those in other affected organs. Throughout the dermis and into the subcutaneous fat, there is a dense infiltrate of well-formed, "naked" granulomas (Fig. 6–1). Collections of tightly aggregated epithelioid histiocytes are surrounded by relatively sparse

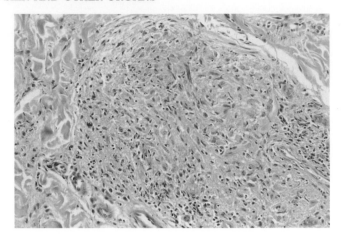

Fig. 6–1. Sarcoidal granuloma with abundant epithelioid histiocytes and a thin rim of lymphocytes.

collections of lymphocytes. In the usual cases, there is no caseation and only rarely a focus of fibrinoid necrosis in the centers of the granulomas. Asteroid bodies and Schaumann bodies may be present, but are not specific for sarcoidosis. The granulomas are evenly dispersed throughout the papillary and reticular dermis and do not show any predilection for cutaneous appendages or blood vessels. Simmilar epithelioid granulomas are present lower in the dermis and in the subcutaneous fat in Darier and Roussy sarcoidosis. In one series, granulomatous angiitis was seen in 30% of patients with cutaneous sarcoidosis [39]. Most other authors do not, however, recognize vasculitis as a significant component of the histologic features of sarcoidosis. The following entities must be considered in the differential diagnosis:

- Blastomycosis
- Crohn's disease
- Cryptococcosis
- Foreign body granulomatous reaction
  - Berylliosis
  - Zirconiosis
- Granulomatous rosacea
- Lupus miliaris disseminatum faciei
- Sporotrichosis
- Tuberculosis
- Wegener's granulomatosis

A rare variant of sarcoidosis that appears with epithelioid granulomas and central coagulative necrosis in conjunction with angiitis and glomerulonephritis has been described [40]. In this unusual variant, granulomas may become confluent throughout the dermis. They develop central necrosis with suppuration. Small-vessel leukocytoclastic vasculitis or granulomatous vasculitis may be seen in this pattern of cutaneous involvement [41].

Special Studies. Direct immunofluorescence studies are rarely performed in studies of cutaneous sarcoidosis. In one study, investigators found deposits of IgM, IgA, or complement in the dermal vessel walls or along the dermal–epidermal junction in about half of their cases. In the same study, 25% of biopsy specimens taken from clinically normal skin showed a similar staining pattern [42]. The authors suggest that circulating immune complexes may play a role in the development of cutaneous granulomas in sarcoidosis. The immunostaining results, however, appear too inconstant to provide strong evidence for this assertion, and direct immunofluorescence is not generally recommended.

In most cases, it is essential to perform special histochemical stains to look for infectious agents before arriving at a diagnosis of sarcoidosis. It is also important to polarize the tissue sections in search of foreign material as a possible cause for a granulomatous dermatitis; however, polaroscopic findings must be interpreted cautiously. Birefringent crystals may be present as a byproduct of histiocyte metabolism. In addition, foreign material such as silica from previous trauma may serve as a nidus for sarcoidal inflammation. It is best to avoid potential sites of previous trauma when performing a biopsy to confirm or exclude a diagnosis of sarcoidosis.

Pathogenesis. The cause of sarcoidosis remains unknown. Although infectious agents have repeatedly been implicated, none have been proved. There has also been speculation that agents such as zirconium and beryllium are responsible for the disease, but there is no convincing evidence for this. It is generally believed that sarcoidosis is a cell-mediated process that may have some autoimmune characteristics [43]. There are increased numbers of antigen-presenting Langerhans cells and CD4+ T-helper lymphocytes at the sites of cutaneous granulomas suggesting that these cells play a major role in the pathogenesis of sarcoidosis [44, 45]. An oligoclonal proliferation was documented in early reactions to Kveim-Siltzbach injection in patients with sarcoidosis. This was interpreted to be evidence in favor of an immune response to a specific antigen [46].

Lymphomatoid Granulomatosis

Epidemiology. Lymphomatoid granulomatosis is an angiocentric lymphoma (see Chapter 10). It primarily affects middle-aged adults and is twice as common in men as in women. It has a mortality rate of 70%–90%, and this is usually due to respiratory failure. In one large series, the median survival was only 14 months [47]. Patients less than 25 years of age tend to have a worse prognosis [47]. Lymphomatoid granulomatosis has also been reported in children [47].

Cutaneous Features. From 40% to 60% of patients with lymphomatoid granulomatosis display cutaneous manifestations of their disease [48]. The cutaneous lesions most commonly appear concomitantly [47], but in rare cases they can precede pulmonary symptoms. Skin findings have been reported to antedate onset of pulmonary symptoms by as much as 8–9 years [49, 50]. Multiple scattered, erythematous nodules are the most common clinical presentation. Erythematous or violaceous, well-circumscribed plaques ranging from 0.5 to 8.0 cm are also seen. An annular configuration has been described, and individual lesions may display necrosis, ulceration, and bulla formation [51]. A diffuse eruption of macules and papules occurs less commonly [52]. A folliculitis-like eruption is also reported [48]. Ichthyosiform eruptions and plaques resembling necrobiosis lipoidica diabeticorum occur rarely [53], and in one case an angioedema-like presentation has been reported [54].

Associated Disorders. The lungs are the most common site of involvement with the angiocentric lymphoma known as *lymphomatoid granulomatosis*. The central nervous system and renal system are each involved in about 30% of patients with lymphomatoid granulomatosis [51]. Lymphomatoid granulomatosis can also involve the musculoskeletal system [55], peripheral nervous system [56], ocular system [57], and gastrointestinal tract [58, 59].

Lymphomatoid granulomatosis has been reported in patients with immunodeficiency disorders such as Wiskott-Aldrich syndrome [60] and acquired immunodeficiency syndrome and human immunodeficiency virus [61] and after transplantation [62].

Histologic Features. The most characteristic histologic feature of lymphomatoid granulomatosis is a dense, dermal infiltrate of atypical lymphocytes. The infiltrate is angiocentric, involving arteries and veins in the dermis and the subcutis, and may also be periappendageal [63]. Neural infiltration by the atypical lymphocytes is also a common finding [51]. There is little, if any, epidermotropism. The atypical lymphocytes are present within the walls of affected vessels and often result in vascular destruction with fibrinoid necrosis (Fig. 6–2). In these cases, there may be widespread necrosis within the dermis and in the overlying epidermis. There is a polymorphous population of small and large lymphocytes. The lymphocytes have indented and lobulated nuclei that are

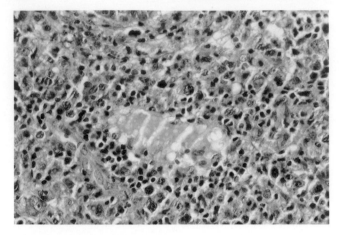

Fig. 6–2. Angiocentric lymphoma with atypical cells permeating walls of affected vessels.

somewhat different from the cerebriform-appearing cells characteristic of mycosis fungoides [64]. The nuclei may be vesicular and have conspicuous nucleoli in some cases. Rare eosinophils and plasma cells may be seen. The following entities must be considered in the histologic differential diagnosis:

- Leukocytoclastic vasculitis
- Lymphoma (other forms)
- Lymphomatoid papulosis
- Wegener's granulomatosis

Special Studies. Gene rearrangement studies have revealed clonal populations of B cells in at least 60% of these cases [65, 66]. Other cases have demonstrated clonal T-cell proliferations. In situ hybridization studies have been helpful in identifying Epstein-Barr virus in the infected B lymphocytes [66].

Pathogenesis. The pathogenesis of lymphomatoid granulomatosis is uncertain. It has been established that this disease is an angiocentric lymphoma. Early reports suggested that the process might be an angiocentric T-cell lymphoma, given the predominance of T cells present in immunolabeling studies [67, 68]. Epstein-Barr virus was localized to the cells within these lesions [67, 69, 70]. It was subsequently demonstrated that the Epstein-Barr virus was infecting B lymphocytes, and lymphomatoid granulomatosis has therefore been reclassified as a T-cell-rich, B-cell lymphoproliferative disorder [65, 66, 71, 72].

α_1-Antitrypsin Deficiency

Epidemiology. α_1-Antitrypsin deficiency is caused by a recessively inherited mutation. Approximately 1 in 2500 persons living in the United States has a ho-

mozygous deficiency resulting in decreased serum enzyme levels. Up to 80% of patients suffering from this form develop severe emphysema by the fourth to sixth decades [73]. Only a minority of patients with α_1-antitrypsin deficiency, however, ever develop cutaneous manifestations [74, 75].

Cutaneous Features. Subcutaneous, erythematous, indurated nodules begin on the lower extremities and are characteristically tender. Widespread nodules may be present on the trunk. The cutaneous eruption is chronic, with repeated appearance of newer foci of involvement concurrent with the disappearance of older nodules. The nodules frequently ulcerate spontaneously and drain.

Associated Disorders. Panlobular emphysema is the most common complication seen in patients with α_1-antitrypsin deficiency. Liver damage is present in about 10% of affected patients, leading to cirrhosis. Hepatocellular carcinoma develops in 2%–3% of these patients [76]. Patients also suffer from aneurysms [77]. Fibromuscular dysplasia was seen in 33% of patients with α_1-antitrypsin deficiency in one series [78].

α_1-Antitrypsin deficiency may occur in association with severe psoriasis involving more than 20% of the total body surface [79]. Some authors have associated Marhsall's syndrome (a pediatric illness characterized by Sweet's disease followed by cutis laxa) with α_1-antitrypsin deficiency [80]. It should be noted, however, that dermal neutrophilic infiltrate has been recognized as an early histologic change in α_1-antitrypsin activity. This calls into question the exact nature of Marshall's syndrome [81]. Rare cases of patients with α_1-antitrypsin deficiency and connective tissue abnormalities have also been reported [82].

Histologic Features. It has been suggested that the earliest histologic change in α_1-antitrypsin deficiency-induced skin disease is the percolation of individual neutrophils and splaying dermal collagen bundles [81]. This occurs in the presence of only mild inflammation within the subcutaneous fat. Progressive involvement of the dermis results in the destruction of the dermal collagen and extension of the disease into the subcutaneous fat [75]. A lobular neutrophilic panniculitis is the characteristic pattern of well-developed α_1-antitrypsin deficiency disease. Foci of necrotic panniculi abut large areas of entirely normal panniculi. The affected areas are necrotic and are infiltrated by sheets of neutrophils (Fig. 6–3). Lymphocytes and extravasated erythrocytes are more abundant at the periphery of the affected areas. Secondary inflammation of surrounding blood vessel walls has been described, but primary leukocytoclastic vasculitis is not a feature of this disease. Late

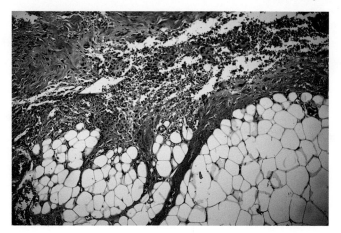

Fig. 6–3. α_1-Antitrypsin deficiency with a marked neutrophilic infiltrate within the lobules of the subcutaneous fat.

foci of panniculitis demonstrate abundant lipophages and multinucleated giant cells [83].

Special Studies. Direct immunofluorescence studies show weak, inconstant deposits of C3 and IgM in blood vessels in both the dermis and panniculus. It is likely that these are associated with secondary vascular damage and not a primary immune complex–mediated process [83].

Pathogenesis. Neutrophils are able to release elastase and collagenase in the absence of normal regulatory controls in patients deficient in α_1-antitrypsin. This results in destruction of dermal collagen and elastic tissue fibers [77].

Cystic Fibrosis–Associated Dermatosis

Epidemiology. Cutaneous eruptions are uncommon in patients with cystic fibrosis [84]. They are believed to be related to nutritional deficiencies of proteins, zinc, and essential fatty acids. In rare instances, the appearance of cutaneous eruptions may precede any other signs or symptoms of cystic fibrosis [85].

Cutaneous Features. The cutaneous manifestations of cystic fibrosis are similar to those of acrodermatitis enteropathica [86]. Unlike eruptions in acrodermatitis enteropathica, however, eruptions in cystic fibrosis tend to have a predilection for the lower extremities, in addition to a periorificial distribution. Earliest changes include the appearance of erythematous, scaling papules that progress to desquamating plaques. Alopecia has also been reported, occurring in association with the eruption [85].

A vesiculobullous eruption located on the extremi-

ties and associated with hepatobiliary disease has also been reported in patients with cystic fibrosis. In this report, the pustules became necrotic and resulted in atrophic scars [87].

Associated Disorders. Patients with cystic fibrosis may have recurrent episodes of leukocytoclastic vasculitis, concurrent with exacerbations of pulmonary disease [88]. Other patients with cystic fibrosis experience purpura on the lower extremities in association with elevated mixed cryoglobulins [89].

Histologic Features. The histologic findings are similar to those of acrodermatitis enteropathica and other nutritional deficiencies. The characteristic pallor and necrolysis of the upper third of the epidermis seen in these entities is not, however, seen in cystic fibrosis–associated dermatitis, but only a few patients have been reported. This makes it difficult to arrive at a precise, definitive histologic diagnosis. There is mild acanthosis of the epidermis with an overlying confluent, thick, parakeratotic scale. The granular layer is diminished to absent. Slight spongiosis and a mild superficial perivascular lymphocytic inflammatory infiltrate are present [85] (Fig. 6–4). The following entities must be considered in the histologic differential diagnosis:

- Acrodermatitis enteropathica
- Necrolytic migratory erythema
- Pellagra

Special studies. No additional special studies have been proposed to aid in making or confirming a diagnosis of cystic fibrosis–related dermatosis.

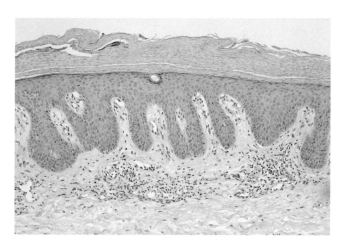

Fig. 6–4. Cystic fibrosis–associated dermatosis shows psoriasiform epidermal hyperplasia, dense overlying parakeratosis, and a slight perivascular lymphocytic infiltrate.

Pathogenesis. Cutaneous eruption associated with cystic fibrosis has been shown to rapidly resolve with nutritional supplementation and pancreatic enzymes. This suggests that the disease may be due to diminished levels of zinc, protein, and essential fatty acids [85].

Pachydermoperiostosis

Epidemiology. Pachydermoperiostosis, or clubbing of the fingers, can be an inherited, idiopathic disorder, or it can be acquired later in life. In its inherited form, it generally appears after puberty and affects all fingernails and toenails [90]. Younger children can, however, be similarly affected [91]. The acquired form is more common in males [92].

Cutaneous Features. Pachydermoperiostosis presents as a symmetric clubbing of the fingernails and toenails. It may also occur unilaterally. Nail plates are distended and curve downward due to increased amounts of soft tissue between the nail bed and the bone.

Associated Disorders. The acquired form of pachydermoperiostosis is associated with pulmonary, mediastinal, and bronchial disorders. These can be infectious or neoplastic in nature. It has also been associated with cardiovascular disease, myelofibrosis [93], cirrhosis, and chronic gastrointestinal disorders [94–96]. Pachydermoperiostosis also occurs in association with cutis verticis gyrata [97], and it has been associated with palmoplantar keratoderma [98]. When the presentation of pachydermoperiostosis is asymmetric, an underlying vascular abnormality is almost always the cause.

Histologic Features. Dermal collagen bundles are markedly thickened and extend into the subcutaneous fat. Increased fibroblasts are present, accompanied by increased dermal hyaluronic acid [90].

Special Studies. Alcian blue or colloidal iron stains performed at pH 2.5 will demonstrate increased hyaluronic acid.

Pathogenesis. The pathogenesis of pachydermoperiostosis remains unknown. Increased vascular pressure, altered nerve reflexes, and toxins released by tumors have all be implicated without much supporting evidence [99, 100]. Increased sensitivity to circulating sex steroids may be responsible for causing the soft tissue hypertrophy [101].

Yellow Nail Syndrome

Epidemiology. The yellow nail syndrome is characterized by a triad of symptoms including yellow discolored nails, lymphedema, and pleural effusions. The usual onset is during middle age, and the syndrome is slightly more common in women [102]. There are rare reports of childhood cases [103]. Yellow nail syndrome has also been reported in patients with congenital lymphedema syndrome [104].

Cutaneous Features. Nails are yellow and grow at a slow rate [105]. Dystrophic nails have also been described in some patients. Patients with the yellow nail syndrome frequently have pitting edema of the ankles [106].

Associated Disorders. Yellow nail syndrome has been associated with a large number of underlying pulmonary conditions, including pneumocystis pneumonia [107], giant cell interstitial pneumonitis [108], rhinosinusitis [109], and empyema [110]. Rheumatoid arthritis has been associated with the yellow nail syndrome. In these patients, there was evidence of concurrent pulmonary involvement [111]. Similarly, pleural effusions were present in a patient with yellow nail syndrome and xanthogranulomatous pyelonephritis [112]. Pericardial effusions have been associated with the syndrome [113].

Yellow nail syndrome has been associated with several types of malignancy, including carcinoma of the larynx [114], breast [108], and gallbladder [115]. In most of these cases, lung involvement was also documented. The yellow nail syndrome was also seen in a patient after penicillamine therapy [116].

Histologic Features. In affected nails, the nail matrix and bed are characterized by dense fibrous tissue that replaces the normal subungual stroma. Numerous ectatic lymphatic vessels are present [105].

Special Studies. Special stains are not helpful in making a diagnosis of yellow nail syndrome.

Pathogenesis. The pathogenesis of yellow nail syndrome appears to involve impaired lymphatic drainage [102]. It has been suggested that primary stromal sclerosis leads to lymphatic obstruction in the pleura and nail beds [105]. Lymphatic impairment does not appear to be the primary defect [106].

References

1. James, D. G., Nevill, E., and Castairs, L. S., *Bone and joint sarcoidosis.* Semin Arthritis Rheum, 1976. 6:53–81.
2. Hanno, R., and Callen, J. P., *Sarcoidosis: A disorder with prominent cutaneous features and their interrela-*

tionships with systemic disease. Med Clin North Am, 1980. 64:847–866.

3. Sartwekkm, O. E., *Racial differences in sarcoidosis.* Ann NY Acad Sci, 1976. 278:368–370.

4. Siltzbach, L. E., James, D. G., Neville, E., Turiaf, J., Battesti, J. P., Sharma, O. P., Hosoda, Y., Mikami, R., et al., *Course and prognosis of sarcoidosis around the world.* Am J Med, 1974. 57:847–852.

5. James, D. G., Siltzbach, L. E., Sharma, O. P., and Castairs, L. S., *A tale of two cities: A comparison of sarcoidosis in London and New York.* Arch Intern Med, 1969. 123:187–191.

6. Brewerton, D. A., Cockburn, C., James, D. G., and Neville, E., *HLA antigens in sarcoidosis.* Clin Exp Immunol, 1977. 27:227–229.

7. James, D. G., and Williams, W. J., *Immunology of sarcoidosis.* Am J Med, 1982. 72:5–8.

8. Olenchock, S. A., Heise, E. R., Marx, J. J., Jr., Mentnech, M. S., Mull, J. C., Spureon, D. E., Hancock, J. S., Elliott, J. A., et al., *HLA-B8 in sarcoidosis.* Ann Allergy, 1981. 47:151–153.

9. Callen, J. P., *Sarcoidosis.* In *Dermatologic Signs of Internal Disorders,* R. L. Dobson and B. Thieis, Eds. 1980, Year Book Medical Publishers, Inc., Chicago, pp. 311–332.

10. James, D. G., *Dermatological aspects of sarcoidosis.* Q J Med, 1959. 28:108–124.

11. Veien, N. K., Stahl, D., and Brodthagen, H., *Cutaneous sarcoidosis in Caucasians.* J Am Acad Dermatol, 1987. 16:534–540.

12. Hanno, R., Needelman, A., Eiferman, R. A., and Callen, J. P., *Cutaneous sarcoidal granulomas and the development of systemic sarcoidosis.* Arch Dermatol, 1981. 117:203–207.

13. Sharma, O. P., *Cutaneous sarcoidosis: Clinical features and management.* Chest, 1972. 61:320–325.

14. Gupta, A. K., Goldfarb, M. T., and Rasmussen, J. E., *Papular midfacial eruption in a child. Cutaneous sarcoidosis.* Arch Dermatol, 1989. 125:1704–1705.

15. Hagari, Y., Kambe, N., Shimao, S., Sutoh, Y., and Ikeda, H., *Cutaneous sarcoidosis showing multiple papular eruptions with keratotic plugs.* J Dermatol, 1989. 16:321–324.

16. Burov, E. A., Kantor, G. R., and Isaac, M., *Morpheaform sarcoidosis: Report of three cases.* J Am Acad Dermatol, 1998. 39:345–348.

17. MacGregor, G., *Cutaneous sarcoidosis in venipuncture sites.* BMJ, 1973. 1(849):357.

18. Hancock, B. W., *Cutaneous sarcoidosis in blood donation venepuncture sites.* BMJ, 1972. 4(842):706–708.

19. Lewis, F. M., and Harrington, C. I., *Lupus pernio following facial trauma.* Clin Exp Dermatol, 1993. 18:476–477.

20. Banse-Kupin, L., and Pelachyk, J. M., *Ichthyosiform sarcoidosis. Report of two cases and a review of the literature.* J Am Acad Dermatol, 1987. 17:616–620.

21. Clayton, R., Breathnack, A., Martin, B., and Feiwel, M., *Hypopigmented sarcoidosis in the Negro: Report of eight cases with ultrastructural observations.* Br J Dermatol, 1977. 96:119–125.

22. Cronin, E., *Skin changes in sarcoidosis.* Postgrad Med, 1959. 46:507–509.

23. Elgart, M.L., *Cutaneous lesions of sarcoidosis.* Primary Care, 1978. 5:249–262.

24. Greer, K. E., Harman, L. E., Jr., and Kayne, A. L., *Unusual cutaneous manifestations of sarcoidosis.* South Med J, 1977. 70:666–668.

25. James, D. G., Thomson, A. D., and Wilcox, A., *Erythema nodosum as manifestation of sarcoidosis.* Lancet, 1956. 2:218–221.

26. Klein, P. A., Appel, J., and Callen, J. P., *Sarcoidosis of the vulva: A rare cutaneous manifestation.* J Am Acad Dermatol, 1998. 39:281–283.

27. Needleman, S. W., Silber, R. A., Von Brecht, J. H., and Goeken, J. A., *Systemic lupus erythematosus complicated by disseminated sarcoidosis: Report of a case associated with circulating immune complexes.* Am J Clin Pathol, 1982. 78:105–107.

28. Wiesenhutter, C. W., and Sharma, O. P., *Is sarcoidosis an autoimmune disease?: Report of four cases and review of the literature.* Semin Arthritis Rheum, 1979. 9:124–144.

29. Miyaya, M., Takase, Y., Kobayashi, H., Kokubun, M., Yoshimura, A., Katsure, Y., Nishimaki, T., and Kasukawa, R., *Primary Sjögren's syndrome complicated by sarcoidosis.* Intern Med, 1998. 37:174–178.

30. Sherman, S., Nieland, N. S., and Van Thiel, D. H., *Sarcoidosis and primary biliary cirrhosis. Coexistence in a single patient.* Dig Dis Sci, 1988. 33:368–374.

31. Gudmundsen, K., Smith, O., Dervan, P., and Powell, F. C., *Necrobiosis lipoidica and sarcoidosis.* Clin Exp Dermatol, 1991. 16:287–291.

32. Garcia-Porrua, C., Gonzalez-Gay, M. A., Garcia-Pais, M. J., and Blanco, R., *Cutaneous vasculitis: An unusual presentation of sarcoidosis in adulthood.* Scand J Rheumatol, 1998. 27:80–82.

33. Mann, R. J., and Harman, R. R. M., *Porphyria cutanea tarda and sarcoidosis.* Clin Exp Dermatol, 1982. 7:619–623.

34. Yavorkovsky, L. L., Carrum, G., Bruce, S., and McCarthy, P. L., Jr., *Cutaneous sarcoidosis in a patient with Philadelphia-positive chronic myelogenous leukemia treated with interferon-alpha.* Am J Hematol, 1998. 58:80–81.

35. Shintaku, M., Mase, K., Ohtsuki, H., Yasumizu, R., Yasunaga, K., and Ikehara, S., *Generalized sarcoidlike granulomas with systemic angiitis, crescentic glomerulonephritis and pulmonary hemorrhage.* Arch Pathol Lab Med, 1989. 113:1295–1298.

36. Veinot, J. P., and Johnston, B., *Cardiac sarcoidosis—an occult cause of sudden death: A case report and literature review.* J Forens Sci, 1998. 43:715–717.

37. Kerdel, F. A., and Moschella, S. L., *Sarcoidosis. An updated review.* J Am Acad Dermatol, 1984. 11:1–19.

38. Zax, R. H., and Callen, J. P., *Sarcoidosis.* Dermatol Clin, 1989. 7:505–515.

39. Takemura, T., Shishiba, T., Akiyama, O., Oritsu, M., Matsui, Y., and Eishi, Y., *Vascular involvement in cutaneous sarcoidosis.* Pathol Int, 1997. 47:84–89.

40. Liebow, A. A., *Pulmonary angiitis and granulomatosis.* Am Rev Respir Dis, 1973. 108:1–18.

41. Rolfes, D. B., Weiss, M. A., and Sanders, M. A., *Necrotizing sarcoid granulomatosis with suppurative features.* Am J Clin Pathol, 1984. 82:602–607.

42. Ullman, S., Halberg, P., Stahl, D., and Veien, N. K., *Cutaneous sarcoidosis: An immunofluorescence study.* Acta Derm Venereol, 1983. 63:343–346.

43. Kataria, Y. P., and Holter, J. F., *Immunology of sarcoidosis.* Clin Chest Med, 1997. 18:719–739.

44. Martin, A. G., Kleinhenz, M. E., and Elmets, C. A., *Immunohistologic identification of antigen-presenting cells in cutaneous sarcoidosis.* J Invest Dermatol, 1986. 86:625–629.

45. Buechner, S. A., Winkelmann, R. K., and Banks, P. M., *T-cell subsets in cutaneous sarcoidosis.* Arch Dermatol, 1983. 119:728–732.

46. Klein, J. T., Horn, T. D., Forman, J. D., Silver, R. F., Teirstein, A. S., and Moller, D. R., *Selection of oligoclonal V beta-specific T cells in the intradermal response to Kveim-Siltzbach reagent in individuals with sarcoidosis.* J Immunol, 1995. 154:1450–1460.

47. Katzenstein, A. L. A., Carrington, C. B., and Liebow, A. A., *Lymphomatoid granulomatosis.* Cancer, 1979. 43:360–373.

48. Carlson, K. K., and Gibson, L. E., *Cutaneous signs of lymphomatoid granulomatosis.* Arch Dermatol, 1991. 127:1693–1698.

49. Liebow, A. A., Carrington, C. R. B., and Friedman, P. J., *Lymphomatoid granulomatosis.* Hum Pathol, 1972. 3:457–458.

50. Holden, C. A., Wells, R. S., and MacDonald, D. M., *Cutaneous lymphomatoid granulomatosis.* Clin Exp Med, 1982. 7:449–454.

51. Jambrosic, J., From, L., Assad, D. A., Lipa, M., Sibbald, R.G., and Walter, J.B., *Lymphomatoid granulomatosis.* J Am Acad Dermatol, 1987. 17:621–631.

52. James, W. D., Odom, R. B., and Katzenstein, A. L., *Cutaneous manifestations of lymphomatoid granulomatosis. Report of 44 cases and a review of the literature.* Arch Dermatol, 1981. 117:196–202.

53. Akagi, M., Taniguchi, S., Okzaki, M., Imamura, S., Kitaichi, M., Matsui, Y., and Oshima, Y., *Necrobiosis-like skin manifestation in lymphomatoid granulomatosis (Liebow).* Dermatologica, 1987. 174:84–92.

54. Torrelo, A., Martin, M., Rocamora, A., Allegue, F., and Ledo, A., *Lymphomatoid granulomatosis presenting as angioedema.* Postgrad Med J, 1992. 68:366–368.

55. Ralston, S. H., McVicar, R., Finlay, A. Y., Morton, R., and Pitkeathly, D. A., *Lymphomatoid granulomatosis presenting with polyarthritis.* Scott Med J, 1988. 33:373–374.

56. Garcia, C. A., Hackett, E. R., and Kirkpatrick, L. L., *Multiple mononeuropathy in lymphomatoid granulomatosis: Similarity to leprosy.* Neurology, 1978. 28:731–733.

57. Kinyoun, J. L., Kalina, R. E., and Klein, M. L., *Choroidal involvement in systemic necrotizing vasculitis.* Arch Ophthalmol, 1987. 105:939–942.

58. Rattinger, M. D., Dunn, T. L., Christian, C. D., Jr., Donnell, R. M., Collins, R. D., O'Leary, J. P., and Flexner, J. M., *Gastrointestinal involvement in lymphomatoid granulomatosis. Report of a case and review of the literature.* Cancer, 1983. 51:694–700.

59. Rubin, L. A., Little, A. H., Kolin, A., and Keystone, E. C., *Lymphomatoid granulomatosis involving the gastrointestinal tract. Two case reports and a review of the literature.* Gastroenterology, 1983. 84:829–833.

60. Ilowite, N. T., Fligner, C. L., Ochs, H. D., Brichacek, B., Harada, S., Haas, J. E., Purtilo, D. T., and Wedgewood, R. J., *Pulmonary angiitis with atypical lymphoreticular infiltrates in Wiskott-Aldrich syndrome: Possible relationship to lymphomatoid granulomatosis and EBV infection.* Clin Immunol Immunopathol, 1996. 41:479–484.

61. Mittal, K., Neri, A., Feiner, H., Schinella, R., and Alfonso, F., *Lymphomatoid granulomatosis in the acquired immunodeficiency syndrome. Evidence of Epstein-Barr virus infection and B-cell clonal selection without myc rearrangement.* Cancer, 1990. 65:1345–1349.

62. Swerdlow, S. H., *Post-transplant lymphoproliferative disorders: A morphologic, phenotypic and genotypic spectrum of disease.* Histopathology, 1992. 20:373–385.

63. MacDonald, D. M., and Sarkany, I., *Lymphomatoid granulomatosis.* Clin Exp Dermatol, 1976. 1:163–173.

64. Sumiyoshi, Y., Kikuchi, M., Oshima, K., Masuda, Y., Takeshita, M., and Okamura, T., *A case of histiocytic necrotizing lymphadenitis with skin and bone involvement.* Virchows Arch [A], 1992. 420:275–279.

65. Jaffe, E. S., and Wilson, W. H., *Lymphomatoid granulomatosis: Pathogenesis, pathology and clinical implications.* Cancer Surv, 1997. 30:233–248.

66. Madison McNiff, J., Cooper, D., Howe, G., Crotty, P. L., Tallini, G., Crouch, J., and Eisen, R. N., *Lymphomatoid granulomatosis of the skin and lung. An angiocentric T-cell-rich B-cell lymphoproliferative disorder.* Arch Dermatol, 1996. 132:1464–1470.

67. Tsai, T.-F., Su, I.-J., Lu, Y.-C., Cheng, A.-L., Yeh, H.-P., Hsieh, H.-C., Tien, H.-F., Chen, J.-S., et al., *Cutaneous angiocentric T-cell lymphoma associated with Epstein-Barr virus.* J Am Acad Dermatol, 1992. 26:31–38.

68. Chan, J. K. C., Ng, C. S., Ngan, K. C., Hui, P. K., Lo, S. T., and Lau, W. H., *Angiocentric T-cell lymphoma of the skin.* Am J Surg Pathol, 1988. 12:861–876.

69. Su, I. J., Hsieh, H. C., Lin, K. H., Uen, W. C., Kao, C. L., Chen, C. J., Cheng, A. L., Kadin, M. E., et al., *Aggressive peripheral T-cell lymphomas containing Epstein-Barr viral DNA: A clinicopathologic and molecular analysis.* Blood, 1991. 77:799–808.

70. Angel, C. A., Slater, D. N., Royds, J. A., Nelson, S. N. P., and Bleehen, S. S., *Epstein-Barr virus in cutaneous lymphomatoid granulomatosis.* Histopathology, 1994. 25:545–548.

71. Guinee, D., Jaffe, E., Kingma, J. D., Fishback, N., Wallberg, K., Krishnan, J., Fizzera, G., Travis, W., et al., *Pulmonary lymphomatoid granulomatosis: Evidence for a proliferation of Epstein-Barr virus infected B-lymphocytes with a prominent T-cell component and vasculitis.* Am J Surg Pathol, 1994. 18:753–764.

72. Nicholson, A. G., Wotherspoon, A. C., Diss, T. C., Singh, N., Butcher, D. N., Pan, L. X., Isaacson, P. G., and Corrin, B., *Lymphomatoid granulomatosis: Evidence that some cases represent Epstein-Barr virus-associated B-cell lymphoma.* Histopathology, 1996. 29: 317–324.

73. Buist, A. S., *α_1-Antitrypsin deficiency—diagnosis, treatment and control: identification of patients.* Lung, 1990. 168(suppl):543–551.

74. Smith, K. C., Pittelkow, M. R., and Su, W. P. D., *Panniculitis associated with severe α_1-antitrypsin deficiency: Treatment and review of the literature.* Arch Dermatol, 1987. 123:1655–1661.

75. Hendrick, S. J., Silverman, A. K., Solomon, A. R., and Headington, J. T., *α_1-antitrypsin deficiency associated with panniculitis.* J Am Acad Dermatol, 1988. 18:684–692.

76. Zhou, H., and Fischer, H. P., *Liver carcinoma in PiZ alpha-1 antitrypsin deficiency.* Am J Surg Pathol, 1998. 22:742–748.

77. Shields, R. C., and Su, W. P. D., *35-Year-old woman with ulcerating skin lesions.* Mayo Clin Proc, 1996. 71:59–62.

78. Schievink, W. I., Bjornsson, J., Parisi, J. E., and Prakash, U. B. S., *Arterial fibromuscular dysplasia associated with severe α_1-antitrypsin deficiency.* Mayo Clin Proc, 1994. 69:1040–1043.

79. Heng, M. C., Moy, R. L., and Lieberman, J., *Alpha-1 antitrypsin deficiency in severe psoriasis.* Br J Dermatol, 1985. 112:129–133.

80. Hwang, S. T., Williams, M. L., McCalmont, T. H., and Frieden, I. J., *Sweet's syndrome leading to acquired cutis laxa (Marshall's syndrome) in an infant with alpha-1 antitrypsin deficiency.* Arch Dermatol, 1995. 131: 1175–1177.

81. Geller, J. D., and Su, W. P. D., *A subtle clue to the histopathologic diagnosis of early α_1-antitrypsin deficiency panniculitis.* J Am Acad Dermatol, 1994. 31: 241–245.

82. Schandevyl, W., Hennebert, A., Leblanc, G., de Coster, A., Yernault, J. C., Achten, G., Ledoux, M., and Buneaux, J. J., *Alpha-1 antitrypsin deficiency of the Pi100 type and connective tissue defect.* In *L'alpha-1-antitrypsin et le systeme Pi.* 1976, INSERM, Paris, pp. 97–107.

83. Su, W. P. D., Smith, K. C., Pittelkow, M. R., and Winkelmann, R. K., *Alpha 1 antitrypsin deficiency panniculitis: A histopathologic and immunopathologic study of four cases.* Am J Dermatopathol, 1987. 9:483–490.

84. Hansen, R. C., Lemen, R., and Revsin, B., *Cystic fibrosis manifesting with acrodermatitis enteropathica-like eruption.* Arch Dermatol, 1983. 119:51–55.

85. Darmstadt, G. L., Schmidt, C. P., Wechsler, D. S., Tunnessen, W. W., and Rosenstein, B. J., *Dermatitis as a presenting sign of cystic fibrosis.* Arch Dermatol, 1992. 128:1358–1364.

86. Goskowicz, M., and Eichenfield, L. F., *Cutaneous findings of nutritional deficiencies in children.* Curr Opin Pediatr, 1993. 5:441–445.

87. Magro, C. M., and Crowson, A. N., *A distinctive eruption associated with hepatobiliary disease.* Int J Dermatol, 1966. 36:837–844.

88. Fradin, M. S., Kalb, R. E., and Grossman, M. E., *Recurrent cutaneous vasculitis in cystic fibrosis.* Pediatr Dermatol, 1987. 4:108–111.

89. Garty, B. Z., Scanlin, T., Goldsmith, D. P., and Grunstein, M., *Cutaneous manifestations of cystic fibrosis: Possible role of cryoglobulins.* Br J Dermatol, 1989. 121:655–658.

90. Hambrick, G. W. J., and Carter, D. M., *Pachdermoperiostosis.* Arch Dermatol, 1966. 94:594–608.

91. Sinha, G. P., Curtis, P., Haigh, D., Lealman, G. T., Dodds, W., and Bennett, C. P., *Pachydermoperiostosis.* Br J Rheumatol, 1997. 36:1224–1227.

92. Rimoin, D. L., *Pachydermoperiostosis (idiopathic clubbing and periostosis).* N Engl J Med, 1965. 272:923.

93. Fontenay-Roupie, M., Dupuy, E., Berrou, E., Tobelem, G., and Bryckaert, M., *Increased proliferation of bone marrow–derived fibroblasts in primitive hypertrophic osteoarthropathy with severe myelofibrosis.* Blood, 1995. 85:3229–3238.

94. Shim, Y. W., and Suh, J. S., *Primary hypertrophic osteoarthropathy accompanied by Crohn's disease: A case report.* Yonsei Med J, 1997. 38:319–322.

95. Vogl, A., Blumenfeld, S., and Gutner, L. B., *Diagnostic significance of pulmonary hypertrophic osteoarthropathy.* Am J Med, 1955. 18:51–65.

96. Compton, R. F., Sandborn, W. J., Yang, H., Lindor, N. M., Tremaine, W. J., Davis, M. D., Khalil, A. A., Tountas, N. A., et al., *A new syndrome of Crohn's disease and pachydermoperiostosis in a family.* Gastroenterology, 1997. 112:241–249.

97. Beauregard, S., *Cutis verticis gyrata and pachydermoperiostosis. Several cases in the same family. Initial results of the treatment of pachyderma with isotretinoin.* Ann Dermatol Venereol, 1994. 121:134–137.

98. Barraud-Klenovsek, M. M., Lubbe, J., and Burg, G., *Primary digital clubbing associated with palmoplantar keratoderma.* Dermatology, 1997. 194:302–305.

99. Black, L. F., *Neoplasms of the lung.* In *Textbook of Medicine,* P. B. Beeson, W. McDermott, and J. B. Wyngaarden, Eds. 1979, W. B. Saunders Company, Philadelphia.

100. Altman, B. B., *Hypertrophic osteoarthropathy.* In *Arthritis and Allied Conditions,* J. L. Hollander and D. J. McCarty, Jr., Eds. 1989, Lea & Febiger, Philadelphia, pp. 1360–1370.

101. Bianchi, L., Lubrano, C., Carrozzo, A. M., Iraci, S., Tomassoli, M., Spera, G., and Nini, G., *Pachydermoperiostosis: Study of epidermal growth factor and steroid receptors.* Br J Dermatol, 1995. 132:128–133.

102. Nordkild, P., Kromann-Andersen, H., and Struve-Christensen, E., *Yellow nail syndrome—the triad of yellow nails, lymphedema and pleural effusions. A review of the literature and a case report.* Acta Med Scand, 1986. 219:221–227.

103. Magid, M., Esterly, N. B., Prendiville, J., and Fujisaki, C., *The yellow nail syndrome in an 8–year-old girl.* Pediatr Dermatol, 1987. 5:90–93.

104. Govaert, P., Leroy, J. G., Pauwels, R., Vanhaesebrouck, P., De Praeter, C., Van Kets, H., and Goeteyn, M., *Peri-

natal manifestations of maternal yellow nail syndrome. Pediatrics, 1992. 89:1016–1018.

105. DeCoste, S. D., Imber, M. J., and Baden, H. P., *Yellow nail syndrome.* J Am Acad Dermatol, 1990. 22:608–611.

106. Bull, R. H., Fenton, D. A., and Mortimer, P. S., *Lymphatic function in the yellow nail syndrome.* Br J Dermatol, 1996. 134:307–312.

107. Chernosky, M. E., and Finley, V. K., *Yellow nail syndrome in patients with acquired immunodeficiency disease.* J Am Acad Dermatol, 1985. 13:731–736.

108. Gupta, A. K., Davies, G. M., and Haberman, H. F., *Yellow nail syndrome.* Cutis, 1986. 37:371–374.

109. Varney, V. A., Cumberworth, V., Sudderick, R., Durham, S. R., and Mackay, I. S., *Rhinitis, sinusitis and the yellow nail syndrome: a review of symptoms and response to treatment in 17 patients.* Clin Otolaryngol, 1994. 19:237–240.

110. Lodge, J. P., Hunter, A. M., and Saunders, N. R., *Yellow nail syndrome associated with empyema.* Clin Exp Dermatol, 1989. 14:328–329.

111. Mattingly, P. C., and Bossingham, D. H., *Yellow nail syndrome in rheumatoid arthritis: Report of three cases.* Ann Rheum Dis, 1979. 38:475–478.

112. Danenberg, H. D., Eliashar, R., Flusser, G., Rosenmann, E., and Chajek-Shaul, T., *Yellow nail syndrome and xanthogranulomatous pyelonephritis.* Postgrad Med J, 1995. 71:110–111.

113. Wakasa, M., Imaizumi, T., Suyama, A., Takeshita, A., and Nakamura, M., *Yellow nail syndrome associated with chronic pericardial effusion.* Chest, 1987. 92:366–367.

114. Guin, J. D., and Elleman, J. H., *Yellow nail syndrome. Possible association with malignancy.* Arch Dermatol, 1979. 115:734–735.

115. Burrows, N. P., and Jones, R. R., *Yellow nail syndrome in association with carcinoma of the gall bladder.* Clin Exp Dermatol, 1991. 16:471–473.

116. Ilchyshyn, A., and Vickers, C. F., *Yellow nail syndrome associated with penicillamine therapy.* Acta Derm Venereol, 1983. 63:554–555.

CHAPTER

7

Cardiac and Skin Diseases

Relatively few diseases have as their primary manifestations cardiac symptoms in conjunction with cutaneous manifestations. Amyloidosis is a multisystem disease that affects these two organs, as well as many others, but because cardiac involvement is frequently the most devastating, it is addressed in this chapter. LEOPARD and Carney's syndromes involve the heart in addition to the manifold cutaneous changes, and cholesterol emboli often emanate from the heart and give rise to presenting cutaneous manifestations.

Amyloidosis

Amyloidosis is a category of diseases that are characterized by the deposition of distinct eosinophilic material. Some forms of amyloidosis are associated with underlying conditions. It is important to note that two of the most common forms that involve the skin, lichen amyloidosis and macular amyloidosis, are not associated with systemic processes. These conditions are related to degenerating keratinocytes and thus are addressed only briefly in this volume.

Epidemiology. Primary systemic amyloidosis is a disease that is almost always related to underlying plasma cell dyscrasias and/or multiple myeloma. In some cases, the plasma cell disorder remains occult. There is considerable overlap in the clinical features of those patients with myeloma and those patients with primary systemic amyloidosis and no obvious plasma cell dyscrasia [1]. Only 15% of patients with multiple myeloma will develop amyloidosis [2]. Primary systemic amyloidosis tends to occur in middle-aged to elderly patients with a mean age of 65 years, and it is

more common in men [3]. Death is typically caused by cardiac and renal failure secondary to amyloid infiltration [2, 4]. The median survival for patients with multiple myeloma and amyloidosis is only 5–6 months [3, 4]. Based on a single case study, it has been suggested that patients with kappa light chain paraproteinemia may have a more benign clinical course [5].

Primary cutaneous nodular amyloidosis is a limited cutaneous disease in which amyloid deposits appear in the dermis in conjunction with a localized plasmacytoma [6]. A small percentage of these patients will develop overt systemic multiple myeloma. The other forms of primary cutaneous amyloidosis, lichen amyloidosis and macular amyloidosis, are limited exclusively to the skin and have no systemic associations. Secondary systemic amyloidosis rarely, if ever, leads to clinically apparent cutaneous disease [7, 8].

Mucocutaneous Features. Primary systemic amyloidosis has cutaneous involvement in 30% to 40% of cases [9, 10]. The most common findings are purpura, petechiae, and ecchymoses [4]. "Pinch purpura" around the eyes is a common cutaneous manifestation, as is periorbital purpura following a Valsalva maneuver or vomiting. Similar purpuric areas may be present on other flexural surfaces and usually arise secondary to mild trauma [2]. Cutaneous manifestations of primary systemic amyloidosis may also include waxy, smooth, yellow papules and nodules that may resemble xanthomas [11]. Occasionally these can be translucent and appear vesicular. Less commonly, they may develop into plaques [12]. On the fingers or toes, the amyloid deposition may lead to loss of mobility and contractures [2]. Rare cutaneous presentations include sclerodermatous infiltration [13], bullous lesions [14], alopecia [15], and cutis laxa [16].

Secondary systemic amyloidosis related to familial Mediterranean fever may present with urticaria, vasculitic nodules, or erysipelas-like lesions on the legs [17].

The gingiva are occasionally infiltrated in the systemic amyloidoses and may serve as a site for sampling to make a diagnosis. Rectal mucosa can also be biopsied for this purpose.

Associated Disorders. Patients with primary amyloidosis related to plasma cell abnormalities have a range of nonspecific symptoms, including fatigue, paresthesias, hoarseness, weight loss, and orthostatic hypotension leading to syncope. More specific signs and symptoms include angina, arrhythmias, carpel tunnel syndrome, hepatomegaly, and edema [2]. Cardiac infiltration leading to death occurs in up to 40% of patients with primary myeloma-related amyloidosis [3]. Macroglossia is seen in a minority of cases and can be papular, nodular, diffuse, or plaque-like [4]. Claudication may occur secondary to amyloid deposition around blood vessels. Peripheral neuropathy is also seen in some patients. Amyloid deposits can also be found in the gastrointestinal tract leading to malabsorption or hemorrhage. Less commonly, sicca syndrome [18] can be present, as can a rheumatoid arthritis–like condition [19].

Histologic Features. In primary systemic amyloidosis, masses of amyloid are present within the papillary dermis. These may lead to effacement of the rete ridges. More infiltrative lesions may have larger deposits of amyloid, extending into the reticular dermis or into the subcutaneous fat. Amyloid deposits characteristically center around blood vessels, arrector pili muscles, and pilosebaceous units and within the lamina propria of eccrine structures (Fig. 7–1). In the subcutis, amyloid may surround individual adipocytes. The amyloid deposits appear as homogeneous eosinophilic masses, often with a dry, fissured appearance, similar to that of "cracked pavement" (Fig. 7–2). There is no associated inflammatory response in most cases [8, 20].

In rare cases where the skin is affected in secondary systemic amyloidosis, the amyloid deposits are found centered on blood vessels and adnexal structures in the lower dermis and around individual adipocytes in the subcutis. No deposits are seen within the papillary dermis [21].

Lichen amyloidosis and macular amyloidosis demonstrate cutaneous deposits of similar-appearing eosinophilic material. These deposits are smaller, however, and are confined to the papillary dermis. In many

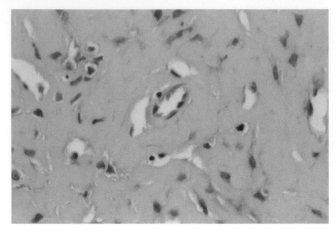

Fig. 7–1. Dense homogenous deposits of eosinophilic material are seen around dermal blood vessels in primary systemic amyloidosis.

cases, degenerating keratinocytes can be found in the overlying epidermis.

Special Studies. A variety of techniques exist for the demonstration of amyloid in tissue sections. These special techniques will accentuate amyloid deposits, regardless of the type of amyloid present. These include the Congo red stain, which demonstrates the characteristic apple green birefringence, as well as a crystal violet stain with its metachromatic staining properties.

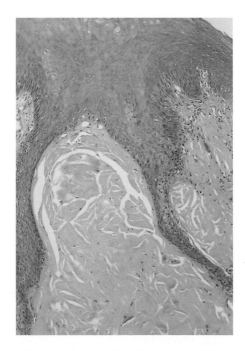

Fig. 7–2. Amyloid deposits have the appearance of "cracked pavement."

The thioflavin T stain requires immunofluorescence in order to demonstrate amyloid deposits and is therefore less useful in most situations. In electron microscopic studies, amyloid fibrils characteristically appear as 7.5–10 nm rigid fibrils with hollow cores arranged in β-pleated sheets [22], but such studies are rarely performed in routine diagnostic work.

Immunopathologic studies are helpful in documenting clonality in the plasma cell population for cases in which abundant plasma cells are apparent within the skin. Kappa and lambda light chain restriction by the infiltrating plasma cells is easily identified on routinely fixed tissue sections. Lambda light chains are more commonly found in amyloid depositions than are kappa chains [19].

Pathogenesis. Primary systemic amyloidosis is caused by the deposition of amyloid fibrils, which are composed of degenerating light chain proteins known as AL amyloid. An overabundance of these proteins produced by an aberrant population of plasma cells results in deposition in multiple organs in the body, including the skin. Light chain proteins identical to those giving rise to the amyloid deposits can be found in the urine or blood of affected patients [23].

Secondary systemic amyloidosis is caused by the deposition of AA proteins secondary to conditions with long-standing chronic inflammation, such as rheumatoid arthritis, familial Mediterranean fever, and the Muckle-Wells syndrome (acute episodic fevers, arthritis, abdominal pain, and urticaria). The exact nature of the proteins is less well defined than in the primary systemic form of the disease [24].

As was alluded to in the beginning of this section, the amyloid deposits seen in lichen amyloidosis and macular amyloidosis are due to keratin breakdown products [25]. These diseases are limited to the skin and have no systemic amyloid deposition.

Carney's Complex

Epidemiology. Approximately 150 patients worldwide have been diagnosed with Carney's complex [26]. Carney's complex has an autosomal dominant inheritance pattern [27]. Cardiac myxomas are the most serious manifestation of the complex and are responsible for the deaths of up to one-fourth of affected patients [28]. Other patients succumb to metastases from psammomatous melanotic schwannoma [29].

Cutaneous Features. Pigmented lesions associated with Carney's complex include multiple lentigines along with blue nevi, ephelides, and melanocytic nevi [30]. The lentigines are diffuse throughout the skin surface and can involve the conjunctiva and vermillion border of the lips in up to one-half of patients [28]. Intraoral lesions may also be found. The blue nevi associated with Carney's complex are more commonly seen on the face, trunk, and extremities and are less frequent on the hands and feet [31]. They appear as darkly pigmented, small (less than 1 cm), dome-shaped papules.

Cutaneous myxomas in Carney's complex are most commonly found in the external ear canal, nipples, and eyelids. They often present in patients during the second and third decades of life and are multiple in up to 70% of cases [32]. These lesions may recur after initial attempts at excision [30]. Up to one-half of patients with Carney's complex will demonstrate cutaneous myxomas. In most of these patients, the cutaneous tumors appear before the diagnosis of similar cardiac neoplasms [32]. Similar myxomas have also been observed in the oral cavities of these patients [28].

Associated Disorders. Myxomas are present within the heart and breast, in addition to the previously described cutaneous myxomas [30]. Cardiac myxomas are the most serious component of Carney's complex, and they are frequently multiple in affected patients [33].

Lesions of the breast have been found in 21% of patients with Carney's complex [34]. Myxoid fibroadenomas of the breast have been reported [27]. Ductal adenomas with tubular features have also been described in association with Carney's complex [35].

Endocrine abnormalities include Cushing's syndrome caused by primary pigmented nodular adrenocortical disease, acromegaly due to growth-hormone–producing pituitary adenomas, and sexual precocity due to calcifying Sertoli cell tumors [30]. The Sertoli cell tumors can be bilateral in this patient population [36]. There can also be an increased incidence of thyroid abnormalities, including hyperplasia and carcinoma [37].

Psammomatous and pigmented schwannomas occur in the upper gastrointestinal tract and sympathetic nerve chains in patients with Carney's complex. Similar neoplasms rarely affect the skin of these patients [30].

There is a single case report of sarcoidosis developing in a patient with Carney's complex [38]. It appears that this association may be fortuitous.

Histologic Features. The lentigines observed in Carney's complex are histologically identical to sporadic lentigines (Fig. 7–3). Hyperpigmentation of the basal layer of the epidermis is evident, with a slight increase in the number of normal-appearing melanocytes. Rete ridges are elongated. There is no pagetoid scatter of the melanocytes, and no cytologic atypia is detected [39].

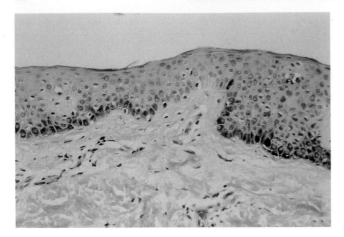

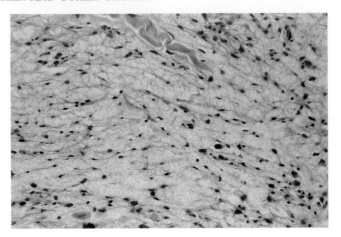

Fig. 7–3. Lentigines seen in Carney's complex demonstrate increased basal layer melanin without a significant increase in numbers of melanocytes.

Fig. 7–5. Spindle-shaped cells are seen coursing within abundant myxoid stroma in cutaneous myxoma.

The following entities must be considered in the histologic differential diagnosis of lentigo simplex:

- Becker's nevus
- Café-au-lait macule
- Ephelide
- Large cell acanthoma
- Nevus spilus
- Pigmented actinic keratosis
- Seborrheic keratosis, reticulated type

Other pigmented lesions frequently seen in Carney's complex include junctional and compound melanocytic nevi and ephelides. All of these appear histologically identical to their similar, sporadically occurring counterparts [39].

Histologic features of the cutaneous myxomas in-

clude a sharply circumscribed tumor arising in the dermis or subcutaneous fat characterized by paucicellularity, abundant myxoid stroma, and prominent capillaries (Figs. 7–4 and 7–5). Large lesions are sometimes multilobular. Rarely, an epithelial component is recognized within the myxoid dermal neoplasm [32]. The following entities must be considered in the histologic differential diagnosis of a cutaneous myxoma:

- Myxoid dermatofibroma
- Myxoid liposarcoma
- Myxoid malignant fibrous histiocytoma
- Myxoid melanoma
- Nodular fasciitis
- Neurofibroma
- Neurothekeoma
- Papular mucinosis
- Schwannoma

Epithelioid blue nevi have been described as part of Carney's complex. These dermal tumors are characterized by two types of cells. The first is an intensely pigmented, fusiform population of cells. A less pigmented population of polygonal and spindle-shaped cells, with vesicular nuclei and single prominent nucleoli, is also present (Fig. 7–6). The melanocytes are distributed throughout the dermis singly, in small groups, and in linear arrays [31]. Epithelioid blue nevus may occur as one component of a combined pattern nevus in patients with Carney's complex.

Psammomatous melanotic schwannomas rarely involve the skin. The histologic features are those of a pseudoencapsulated tumor within the dermis composed of epithelioid to spindle-shaped cells lacking nuclear atypia. The tumor cells are strongly positive for S100 protein and HMB-45 and should not be confused with malignant melanoma cells [40].

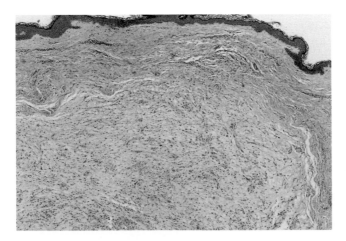

Fig. 7–4. Cutaneous myxoma is characterized by a sharply demarcated dermal tumor composed of spindle-shaped cells.

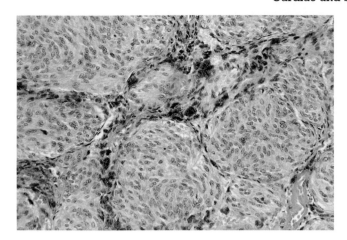

Fig. 7–6. A biphasic population of nonpigmented epithelioid nevus cells and interspersed, densely pigmented spindle cells are present within the dermis of epithelioid cellular blue nevi seen in Carney's complex.

Special Studies. Flow cytometric studies from patients with Carney's complex have revealed tetraploid patterns of DNA abnormalities in cardiac myxomas [41]. This tetraploid pattern was associated with a high rate of local recurrence. The abnormal DNA patterns were not seen in a group of patients with sporadic cardiac myxomas.

Pathogenesis. Linkage analysis studies suggest that a 2p16 chromosomal defect is present in patients with Carney's complex. It is thought that this defect plays a major role in altering the structure of telomeres in replicating chromosomes in these patients [42]. The defective gene does not, however, appear to have a tumor suppressor function [43].

LEOPARD Syndrome

Epidemiology. LEOPARD syndrome is inherited as a autosomal dominant trait, and the name is an acronym for a syndrome characterized by multiple lentigines (L), electrocardiographic abnormalities (E), ocular hypertelorism (O), pulmonary stenosis (P), abnormalities of genitalia (A), growth retardation (R), and sensorineural deafness (D) [44]. It has been suggested that LEOPARD syndrome is transmitted by affected fathers, but mothers have also been implicated [45]. Most patients with LEOPARD syndrome have a normal life expectancy. Rare patients may succumb to respiratory insufficiency [46].

Cutaneous Features. The most salient cutaneous feature of LEOPARD syndrome is the appearance of numerous 1–5 mm dark brown lentigines, which tend to spare mucosal surfaces. They are present in highest densities on the neck and upper trunk and often are more sparsely distributed along the face, acral surfaces, and

genitalia. The lentigines appear at birth or shortly thereafter. In addition to the characteristic widespread lentigines, darker café-au-lait spots may be present [44]. In a single patient, steatocystoma multiplex and hyperelastic skin were reported to coexist [47].

Associated Disorders. Electrocardiographic abnormalities include a pulmonary systolic ejection murmur (without a click) and an S1, S2, S3 pattern [44]. Atrial septal defects and cardiomyopathy have been reported, as have hypospadias, cryptorchidism and absence of one ovary [44, 48]. Mandibular prognathism, pectus carinatum and excavatum, and other skeletal anomalies have been described in these patients, along with premature cataracts that arise during the third decade [49]. Less common findings include macroglossia, dental anomalies such as supernumerary teeth, megacolon, clitoral hypertrophy, and anal ectopy [50, 51]. Patients can also suffer from primary pulmonary hypertension [52]. Psychoses have also been described, but may not be genetically related [53]. Central nervous system anomalies, including parietal lobe atrophy and a Chiara I malformation, have been reported [54, 55]. Co-occurrence of LEOPARD syndrome and Werner's syndrome has been reported in a single patient [56]. About 85% of patients with the LEOPARD syndrome are below the 25th percentile for both height and weight [44].

Histologic Features. The histologic features of the lentigines seen in LEOPARD syndrome are not specific and resemble those of lentigo simplex (Fig. 7–3). The epidermis shows slight elongation of rete ridges, and there is increased melanin within the basal keratinocytes. The number of melanocytes is increased within the lesional skin, but the melanocytes are not atypical and no pagetoid upward spread is seen. There is no associated increased solar elastosis.

Similarly, the café-au-lait macules seen in patients with LEOPARD syndrome have no histologic features that distinguish them in any way from those occurring in patients with neurofibromatosis or other conditions.

Special Studies. Electron microscopy of lentigines in LEOPARD syndrome reveals giant melanosomes, similar in appearance to those in café-au-lait spots arising as part of neurofibromatosis [57]. This finding has subsequently been shown to be nonspecific and can occur in a wide range of conditions. Accumulations of melanin in membrane-bound structures of Langerhans' cells have been associated with LEOPARD syndrome [58].

Pathogenesis. Some linkage studies have excluded the possibility that LEOPARD syndrome is related to the neurofibromatosis type 1 locus [59]. Other studies suggest that a missense mutation in exon 18 of the neurofibromatosis type 1 gene may be responsible in some cases [60]. Most investigators believe that LEOPARD syndrome is a neural crest defect, perhaps with some associated mesodermal abnormality [51, 61].

Cholesterol Emboli

Epidemiology. Cholesterol emboli are predominantly seen in elderly males with a mean age of 72 years and with histories of hypertension and atherosclerotic coronary artery disease. The incidence has been estimated at 6 per 1 million people [62]. In most cases, an invasive therapeutic procedure precedes and triggers the appearance of cholesterol emboli [63]; however, spontaneous embolization does occur [64, 65]. Cholesterol embolization has also been reported after thrombolytic therapy and after chest compressions from cardiopulmonary resuscitation efforts [66]. The mortality rate following the appearance of cholesterol emboli is 70%–80%, and is most frequently due to cardiac and renal embolization [63, 67].

Cutaneous Features. Cutaneous findings are present in 35% of patients with cholesterol emboli [63, 67]. Livedo reticularis involving the lower part of the body is the most frequent cutaneous manifestation of cholesterol embolization, occurring in up to one-half of all patients [67, 68]. The toes are most commonly involved. Livedo reticularis may be painful [69] and in rare cases may be position dependent [70]. Less common cutaneous presentations include gangrene, cyanosis as evidenced by purple toes, intractable ulceration [71], and nodules and purpura, all of which occur in more than 10% of patients with cholesterol emboli [67].

Associated Disorders. Patients with cutaneous manifestations of cholesterol emboli frequently have involvement of other organ systems. Atherosclerotic coronary artery disease is present in about half of these patients, and renal failure may be seen in up to one-third. Aortic aneurysms were seen in one-fourth of patients in the same series [63]. Although less common, cerebrovascular accidents may occur as a result of cholesterol emboli [72], and pleural effusions are occasionally observed [73]. Abdominal pain is also reported in some patients [68]. Gastrointestinal bleeding and intestinal perforation may result from cholesterol emboli [63, 74].

Nonspecific findings include fever, weight loss, myalgias, and headaches. Elevation of blood pressure occurs in most affected patients, and elevated sedimentation rates are also commonly seen [65]. Cholesterol emboli have been reported in patients taking coumarin [75].

Histologic Features. Crystal-shaped spaces are seen within the blood vessels of the dermis and subcuta-

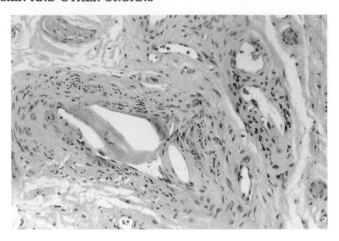

Fig. 7–7. Needle-like spaces are found within vessels in biopsy specimen containing cholesterol emboli.

neous fat. These spaces remain after cholesterol is extracted from the tissue from routine processing. The needle-like spaces are entirely intravascular and provoke minimal, if any, inflammatory response in early lesions (Fig. 7–7). Vessels ranging from 100 to 200 μm in diameter, which are found in the lower parts of the dermis and in the subcutis, are the usual sites of emboli. In older lesions, an acute inflammatory response, often with giant cells, may develop around the cholesterol clefts [76]. The diagnostic findings may be focal, and multiple levels through the paraffin tissue block may be required to make the diagnosis. Cutaneous biopsy tissue was confirmatory in 92% of cases in one series [67].

Special Studies. There are no special studies that are reported to help diagnose cholesterol emboli.

Pathogenesis. Cholesterol-laden, atherosclerotic plaques are dislodged from large-caliber vessels, either spontaneously or secondary to angioinvasive procedures. These small fragments of tissue circulate within the arterial system until they arrive at a vessel whose diameter is not large enough to permit passage. The cholesterol emboli remain lodged in these small-caliber vessels, causing obstruction of blood flow and infarction of tissue supplied by this vascular bed.

Miscellaneous Conditions

Kawasaki's disease is associated with aneurysms of the coronary arteries. This is discussed more fully in Chapter 4. Neonatal lupus erythematosus is associated with heart block. A discussion of this relationship can be found in Chapter 1. Myocarditis has been associated with Lyme disease, and this relationship is covered more fully in Chapter 17.

References

1. Kyle, R. A., and Gertz, M. A., *Primary systemic amyloidosis: Clinical and laboratory features in 474 cases.* Semin Hematol, 1995. 32:45–59.

2. Breathnach, S. M., *Amyloid and amyloidosis.* J Am Acad Dermatol, 1988. 18:1–16.

3. Kyle, R. A., and Greipp, P. R., *Amyloidosis (AL): Clinical and laboratory features in 229 cases.* Mayo Clin Proc, 1983. 58:665–683.

4. Kyle, R. A., and Bayrd, E. D., *Amyloidosis: Review of 236 cases.* Medicine, 1975. 54:271–299.

5. Wallis, M. S., and Sough, D. B., 4th, *Extended survival of patients with primary systemic amyloidosis.* Cutis, 1992. 49:193–195.

6. Husby, G., Sletten, K., Blumenkrantz, N., and Danielsen, L., *Characterization of an amyloid fibril protein from localized amyloidosis of the skin as lambda immunoglobulin light chains of variable subgroup I (A lambda I).* Clin Exp Immunol, 1981. 45:90–96.

7. Brownstein, M. H., and Helwig, E. B., *Systemic amyloidosis complicating dermatoses.* Arch Dermatol, 1970. 102:1–7.

8. Brownstein, M. H., and Helwig, E. B., *The cutaneous amyloidoses: II. Systemic forms.* Arch Dermatol, 1970. 102:20–28.

9. Barth, W. F., Willerson, J. T., Waldmann, T. A., and Decker, J. L., *Primary amyloidosis. Clinical, immunochemical and immunoglobulin metabolism studies in fifteen patients.* Am J Med, 1969. 47:259–273.

10. Rubinow, A., and Cohen, A. S., *Skin involvement in generalized amyloidosis: A study of clinically involved and uninvolved skin in 50 patients with primary and secondary amyloidosis.* Ann Intern Med, 1978. 88:781–785.

11. Chapman, R. S., Neville, E. A., and Lawson, J. W., *Xanthoma-like skin lesions as a presenting feature in primary systemic amyloidosis.* Br J Clin Pract, 1973. 27:271–273.

12. Branat, K., Cathart, E. S., and Cohen, A. S., *A clinical analysis of the course and prognosis of forty-two patients with amyloidosis.* Am J Med, 1968. 44:955–969.

13. Leach, W. B., Vassar, P. S., and Calling, C. F. A., *Primary systemic amyloidosis presenting as scleroderma.* Can Med Assoc J, 1960. 83:263–265.

14. Robert, C., Aractingi, S., Prost, C., Verola, O., Blanchet-Bardon, C., Blanc, F., et al., *Bullous amyloidosis.* Medicine, 1994. 24:124–138.

15. Wheeler, G. E., and Barrows, G. H., *Alopecia universalis: A manifestation of occult amyloidosis and multiple myeloma.* Arch Dermatol, 1981. 117:818–826.

16. Newton, J. A., McKee, P. H., and Black, M. M., *Cutis laxa associated with amyloidosis.* Clin Exp Dermatol, 1986. 11:87–91.

17. Sohar, E., Gafni, J., Pras, M., and Heller, H., *Familial Mediterranean fever: A survey of 470 cases and a review of the literature.* Am J Med, 1967. 43:227–253.

18. Inazumi, T., Hakuno, M., Yamada, H., Tanaka, M., Naka, W., Tajima, S., et al., *Characterization of the amyloid fibril from primary localized cutaneous nodular amyloidosis associated with Sjögren's syndrome.* Dermatology, 1994. 189:125–128.

19. Lambert, W. C., *Cutaneous deposition disorders.* in *Pathology of the Skin,* E. R. Farmer and A. F. Hood, Eds. 1990, Appleton and Lange, East Norwalk, CT, pp. 432–450.

20. Westermark, P., *Amyloidosis of the skin: A comparison between localized and systemic amyloidosis.* Acta Derm Venereol (Stockh), 1979. 80:341–345.

21. Westermark, P., *Occurrence of amyloid deposits in the skin in secondary systemic amyloidosis.* Acta Path Microbiol Scand (Sect A), 1972. 80:718–720.

22. Shirahama, T., and Cohen, A. S., *High-resolution electron microscopic analysis of the amyloid fibril.* J Cell Biol, 1967. 33:679–708.

23. Terry, W. D., Page, D. L., Kimura, S., Isobe, T., Osserman, E. F., and Glenner, G. G., *Structural identity of Bence-Jones and amyloid fibril proteins in a patient with plasma cell dyscrasia and amyloidosis.* J Clin Invest, 1973. 52:1276–1281.

24. Linke, R. P., Heilmann, K. L., Nathrath, W. B. J., and Eulitz, M., *Identification of amyloid A protein in a sporadic Muckle-Wells syndrome.* Lab Invest, 1983. 48:698–704.

25. Kumakiri, M., and Hashimoto, K., *Histogenesis of primary localized cutaneous amyloidosis: Sequential change of epidermal keratinocytes to amyloid via filamentous degeneration.* J Invest Dermatol, 1979. 73:150–162.

26. Carney, J. A., *The Carney complex (myxomas, spotty pigmentation, endocrine overactivity, and schwannomas).* Dermatol Clin, 1995. 13:19–26.

27. Carney, J. A., Hruska, L. S., Beauchamp, G. D., and Gordon, H., *Dominant inheritance of the complex of myxomas, spotty pigmentation and endocrine overactivity.* Mayo Clin Proc, 1986. 61:165–172.

28. Cook, C. A., Lund, B. A., and Carney, J. A., *Mucocutaneous pigmented spots and oral myxomas: The oral manifestations of the complex of myxomas, spotty pigmentation, and endocrine overactivity.* Oral Surg Oral Med Oral Pathol, 1987. 63:175–183.

29. Radin, R., and Kempf, R. A., *Carney complex: Report of three cases.* Radiology, 1995. 196:383–386.

30. Carney, J. A., *Carney complex: The complex of myxomas, spotty pigmentation, endocrine overactivity, and schwannomas.* Semin Dermatol, 1995. 14:90–98.

31. Carney, J. A., and Ferreiro, J. A., *The epithelioid blue nevus. A multicentric familial tumor with important associations, inlcuding cardiac myxoma and psammomatous melanotic schwannoma.* Am J Surg Pathol, 1996. 20:259–272.

32. Carney, J. A., Headington, J. T., and Su, W. P. D., *Cutaneous myxomas. A major component of the complex of myxomas, spotty pigmentation, and endocrine overactivity.* Arch Dermatol, 1986. 122:790–798.

33. McCarthy, P. M., Piehler, J. M., Schaff, H. V., Pluth, J. R., Orszulak, T. A., Vidaillet, H. J., Jr., and Carney, J. A., *The significance of multiple, recurrent, and "complex" cardiac myxomas.* J Thorac Cardiovasc Surg, 1986. 91:389–396.

34. Carney, J. A., and Toorkey, B. C., *Myxoid fibroadenoma and allied conditions (myxomatosis) of the breast. A heritable disorder with special associations including cardiac*

and cutaneous myxomas. Am J Surg Pathol, 1991. 15: 713–722.

35. Carney, J. A., and Toorkey, B. C., *Ductal adenoma of the breast with tubular features. A probable component of the complex of myxomas, spotty pigmentation, endocrine overactivity, and schwannomas.* Am J Surg Pathol, 1991. 15:722–731.

36. Noszian, I. M., Balon, R., Eitelberger, F. G., and Schmid, N., *Bilateral testicular large-cell calcifying Sertoli cell tumor and recurrent cardiac myxoma in a patient with Carney's complex.* Pediatr Radiol, 1995. 25(suppl 1):S236–S237.

37. Statakis, C. A., Courcoutsakis, N. A., Abati, A., Filie, A., Doppman, J. L., Carney, J. A., and Shawker, T., *Thyroid gland abnormalities in patients with the syndrome of spotty skin pigmentation, myxomas, endocrine overactivity and schwannomas.* J Clin Endrocrinol Metab, 1997. 82:2037–2043.

38. Akama, H., Tanaka, H., Yamada, H., Oshima, H., Ichikawa, Y., Yoshida, T., Kawai, S., and Ikeda, Y., *Cushing's syndrome due to primary adrenocortical nodular dysplasia, cardiac myxomas, and spotty pigmentation, complicated by sarcoidosis.* Intern Med, 1992. 31:1329–1334.

39. Carney, J. A., Gordon, H., Carpenter, P. C., Shenoy, B. V., and Go, V. L. W., *The complex of myxomas, spotty pigmentation, and endocrine overactivity.* Medicine, 1985. 64:270–283.

40. Utiger, C. A., and Headington, J. T., *Psammomatous melanotic schwannoma. A new cutaneous marker for Carney's complex.* Arch Dermatol, 1993. 129:202–204.

41. McCarthy, P. M., Schaff, H. V., Winkler, H. Z., Lieber, M. M., and Carney, J. A., *Deoxyribonucleic acid ploidy pattern of cardic myxomas. Another predictor of biologically unusual myxomas.* J Thorac Cardiovasc Surg, 1989. 98:1083–1086.

42. Stratakis, C. A., Jenkins, R. B., Pras, E., Mitsiadis, C. S., Raff, S. B., Stalboerger, P. G., Tsigos, C., Carney, J. A., et al., *Cytogenetic and microsatellite alterations in tumors from patients with the syndrome of myxomas, spotty skin pigmentation, and endocrine overactivity (Carney complex).* J Clin Endocrinol Metab, 1996. 81: 3607–3614.

43. Chrousos, G. P., and Statakis, C. A., *Carney complex and the familial lentiginous syndromes: Link to inherited neoplasias and developmental disorders, and genetic loci.* J Intern Med, 1998. 243:573–579.

44. Gorlin, R. J., Anderson, R. C., and Moller, J. H., *The Leopard (multiple lentigines) syndrome revisited.* Birth Defects Orig Artic Ser, 1971. 7:110–115.

45. Seuanez, H., Mane-Garzon, F., and Kolski, R., *Cardiocutaneous syndrome (the "LEOPARD" syndrome). Review of the literature and a new family.* Clin Genet, 1976. 9:266–276.

46. Peter, J. R., and Kemp, J. S., *LEOPARD syndrome: Death because of chronic respiratory insufficiency.* Am J Med Genet, 1990. 37:340–341.

47. Mochizuki-Osawa, M., Terui, T., Kato, T., and Tagami, H., *LEOPARD syndrome associated with steatocystoma multiplex and hyperelastic skin. Report of a Japanese case.* Acta Derm Venereol, 1995. 75:323–324.

48. Coppin, B. D., and Temple, I. K., *Multiple lentigines syn-*

drome (LEOPARD syndrome or progressive cardiomyopathic lentiginosis. J Med Genet, 1997. 34:582–586.

49. Howard, R. O., *Premature cataracts associated with generalized lentigo.* Trans Am Ophthalmol Soc, 1979. 77: 121–132.

50. Ho, I. C., O'Donnell, D., and Rodrigo, C., *The occurrence of supernumerary teeth with isolated, nonfamilial leopard (multiple lentigines) syndrome: Report of a case.* Spec Care Dentist, 1989. 9:200–202.

51. Peixoto, M. A., Perpetuo, F. O., de Souza, R. P., Miranda, D., and Loures, C. G., *Leopard syndrome, a neural crest disorder: A case report.* Arq Neuropsiquiatr, 1981. 39:214–222.

52. Blieden, L. C., Schneeweiss, A., and Neufeld, H. N., *Primary pulmonary hypertension in leopard syndrome.* Br Heart J, 1981. 46:458–460.

53. Loyd, D. W., Tsuang, M. T., and Benge, J. W., *A study of a family with leopard syndrome.* J Clin Psychiatry, 1982. 43:113–116.

54. Agha, A., and Hashimoto, K., *Multiple lentigines (Leopard) syndrome with Chiara I malformation.* J Dermatol, 1995. 22:520–523.

55. Garty, B. Z., Scanlin, T., Goldsmith, D. P., and Grunstein, M., *Cutaneous manifestations of cystic fibrosis: Possible role of cryoglobulins.* Br J Dermatol, 1989. 121:655–658.

56. Lazarov, A., Finkelstein, E., Avinoach, I., Kachko, L., and Halevy, S., *Diffuse lentiginosis in a patient with Werner's syndrome—a possible association with incomplete leopard syndrome.* Clin Exp Dermatol, 1995. 20:46–50.

57. Bhawan, J., Purtilo, D. T., Riordan, J. A., Saxena, V. K., and Edelstein, L., *Giant and "granular melanosomes" in Leopard syndrome: An ultrastructural study.* J Cutan Pathol, 1976. 3:207–216.

58. Fryer, P. R., and Pope, F. M., *Accumulation of membrane-bound melanosomes occurs in Langerhans cells of patients with the Leopard syndrome.* Clin Exp Dermatol, 1992. 17:13–15.

59. Ahlbom, B. E., Dahl, N., Zetterqvist, P., and Anneren, G., *Noonan syndrome with cafe-au-lait spots and multiple lentigines syndrome are not linked to the neurofibromatosis type 1 locus.* Clin Genet, 1995. 48:85–89.

60. Wu, R., Legius, E., Robberecht, W., Dumoulin, M., Cassiman, J. J., and Fryns, J. P., *Neurofibromatosis type I gene mutation in a patient with features of LEOPARD syndrome.* Hum Mutat, 1996. 8:51–56.

61. Nordlund, J. J., Lerner, A. B., Braverman, I. M., and McGuire, J. S., *The multiple lentigines syndrome.* Arch Dermatol, 1973. 107:259–261.

62. Moolenaar, W., and Lamers, C. B., *Cholesterol crystal embolization in the Netherlands.* Arch Intern Med, 1996. 156:653–657.

63. Fine, M. J., *Cholesterol crystal embolization: A review of 221 cases in the English literature.* Angiology, 1987. 38:769–784.

64. Badawi, G., Jebara, V. A., el-Rassi, I., Tabet, G., el-Ayle, N., Ashoush, R., el-Asmar, B., Arid, J., et al., *Spontaneous cholesterol embolization—a rare event.* J Med Liban, 1993. 41:95–98.

65. Rosman, H. S., Davis, T. P., Reddy, D., and Goldstein,

S., *Cholesterol embolization: Clinical findings and implications.* J Am Coll Cardiol, 1990. 15:1296–1299.

66. Geraets, D. R., Hoehns, J. D., Burke, T. G., and Grover-McKay, M., *Thrombolytic-associated cholesterol emboli syndrome: Case report and literature review.* Pharmacotherapy, 1995. 15:441–450.

67. Falanga, V., Fine, M. J., and Kapoor, W. N., *The cutaneous manifestations of cholesterol crystal embolization.* Arch Dermatol, 1986. 122:1194–1198.

68. Kalter, D. C., Rudolph, A., and McGavran, M., *Livedo reticularis due to multiple cholesterol emboli.* J Am Acad Dermatol, 1985. 13:235–242.

69. Williams, H. C., and Pembroke, A. C., *Livedo reticularis and massive thoracoabdominal aneurysm.* Clin Exp Dermatol, 1994. 19:353–355.

70. Sheehan, M. G., Condemi, J. J., and Rosenfeld, S. I., *Position dependent livedo reticularis in cholesterol emboli syndrome.* J Rheumatol, 1993. 20:1973–1974.

71. Davies, D. J., and Thurasingham, K., *Intractable leg ulceration caused by cutaneous cholesterol embolism.* Med J Aust, 1992. 157:267–268.

72. Pascual, M., Baumgartner, J. M., and Bounameaux, H., *Stroke secondary to multiple spontaneous cholesterol emboli.* Vasa, 1991. 20:74–77.

73. Kollef, M. H., McCormack, M. T., Kristo, D. A., and Reddy, V. V., *Pleural effusion in patients with systemic cholesterol embolization.* Chest, 1993. 103:792–795.

74. Dahlberg, P. J., Frencentese, D. F., and Cogbill, T. H., *Cholesterol embolism: Experiences with 22 histologically proven cases.* Surgery, 1989. 105:737–746.

75. Park, S., Schroeter, A. L., Park, Y. S., and Forston, J., *Purple toes and livedo reticularis in a patient with cardiovascular disease taking coumadin. Cholesterol emboli associated with coumadin therapy.* Arch Dermatol, 1993. 129:777.

76. Borrego, L., Gil, R., Mazuecos, A., Ruiz, R., Lopez, J. L., and Iglesias, L., *Cholesterol embolism to the skin.* Clin Exp Dermatol, 1992. 17:424–426.

CHAPTER
8

Renal and Skin Diseases

Cutaneous eruptions can be seen in patients with acute renal disease and renal failure and in patients with chronic renal disease. The cutaneous presentations are quite different and are addressed separately in this chapter.

ACUTE RENAL DISEASES

Henoch-Schönlein Purpura

Epidemiology. Henoch-Schönlein purpura is a disease that is relatively common in children, but can occur rarely in people of any age. It is defined as a nonthrombocytopenic purpura with cutaneous vascular deposits of IgA. In the pediatric population, less than 2% of patients develop serious complications and long-term morbidity [1]. When present, the most common adverse sequela is end-stage renal disease. Henoch-Schönlein purpura also occurs in children less than 2 years of age and appears to have an excellent prognosis in this very young population [2]. Complete recovery was observed in 93.9% of children and 89.2% of adults in one large study [3].

Cutaneous Features. The cutaneous eruption in Henoch-Schönlein purpura is similar in appearance to other types of leukocytoclastic vasculitis. The skin is affected in more than 50% of patients with Henoch-Schönlein purpura [4]. Petechiae, purpuric macules, and papules and ecchymoses are present on any body site, with a predilection for the lower extremities. In very young children, the face is a common site for purpura [2]. Edema caused by acute renal failure is also a common cutaneous presentation. Hemorrhagic vesicles and bullae may be seen on the skin and mucosal surfaces [5, 6]. Koebner's phenomenon has been described in one patient with Henoch-Schönlein purpura [7].

Associated Disorders. Renal involvement is more common in adults than in children with Henoch-Schönlein purpura [3]. The usual clinical presentation of the renal disease is hematuria. In one study, 23% of affected patients had IgA glomerulonephritis on biopsy and another 26% had abnormal urinalyses [8]. In the same study, involvement of the kidneys was more common in patients with purpura of the upper body and a history of a recent infectious process.

The gastrointestinal tract is affected in up to 33% of adults with Henoch-Schönlein purpura [8]. Patients present with colicky abdominal pain. The small bowel is the most common site of gastrointestinal involvement, although colonic involvement has been reported [9, 10]. Small bowel infarction may lead to death in patients with Henoch-Schönlein purpura [11]. Hydrops of the gallbladder has also been reported in some patients with Henoch-Schönlein purpura [12].

Joints are involved in about 20% of adult patients with Henoch-Schönlein purpura [8]. Symptomatic joint involvement appears to be more common in adult patients than in children [3].

Rare cases of hemorrhage involving the pleura occur in Henoch-Schönlein purpura [13]. Pulmonary edema, interstitial fibrosis and fibrinoid thrombosis were found at autopsy in another patient with this disease [14].

Rare cases of orchitis mimicking testicular torsion have been reported in patients with Henoch-Schönlein purpura [15]. Cardiac and neurologic manifestations have also been reported [16, 17]. Involvement of the kidneys, joints, and gastrointestinal tract is uncommon in infants and very young children with Henoch-Schönlein purpura [2].

Henoch-Schönlein purpura has been reported in association with other systemic diseases, including prostate cancer [18], breast cancer [19, 20], and diabetic nephropathy [21]. It has been reported to recur in patients after renal transplantation [22]. It has also been reported to occur after a wide range of infectious processes, including hepatitis B [23], salmonella [24], staphylococcal endocarditis [25], and disseminated tuberculosis [26] and with gastric *Helicobacter pylori* infection [27]. Henoch-Schönlein purpura has also been reported in a child with concurrent post-streptococcal acute glomerulonephritis [28].

Rare cases have been described in patients after streptokinase treatment [29] and after taking cefuroxime and diclofenac [30]. There is also a report of the disease occurring after cocaine ingestion [31].

Histologic Features. Routine histologic sections demonstrate features of vasculitis that are not distinguishable from other types of leukocytoclastic vasculitis. Small, postcapillary venules in the superficial vascular plexus show transmural infiltration with neutrophils (Fig. 8–1). Fibrin is present, and destruction of the lumen of affected vessels and endothelial cells may be apparent. Extravasated erythrocytes are present within the dermis. A similar-appearing leukocytoclastic vasculitis has been reported in affected mucosa from the gastrointestinal tract [32].

Special Studies. Direct immunofluorescence studies reveal IgA and complement deposits within small ves-

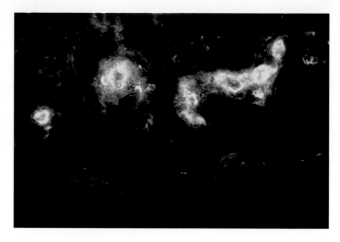

Fig. 8–2. Deposits of IgA are seen in affected vessels in Henoch-Schönlein purpura.

sel walls in the skin and gastrointestinal tract and in the mesangium of kidneys [33] (Fig. 8–2). From 75% to 80% of biopsy specimens demonstrate these immune complexes, and the sensitivity is highest in early lesions [34, 35]. Similar IgA deposits have been reported to occur in the superficial cutaneous vessels in apparently normal skin of patients with Henoch-Schönlein purpura [35]. Similar perivascular immune complexes have been reported in patients with IgA nephropathy and in patients with alcoholic liver disease. In another study [34], IgA deposits were as likely to be found in biopsy specimens from normal skin as in those from purpuric lesions. It has been reported that while IgA deposits are present in vessels in patients with alcoholic liver disease, skin biopsy specimens from these patients also demonstrate similar deposits in the basement membrane of eccrine secretory coils, a finding not associated with Henoch-Schönlein purpura [36]. Demonstration of increased serum levels of C5b–9 (terminal complement complex) correlates with presence of deposits in cutaneous vessel walls on direct immunofluorescence examination and with disease activity [37].

Both anticardiolipin antibodies and antineutrophilic cytoplasmic antibodies have been reported in patients with Henoch-Schönlein purpura [38, 39].

Pathogenesis. Circulating IgA immune complexes have been proposed to play a primary role in the pathogenesis of Henoch-Schönlein purpura [33]. High levels of circulating IgA immune complexes have been described in these patients [4]. It has further been suggested that the circulating IgA and the IgA in vascular deposits are of the secretory type [40]. Tumor necrosis factor, interleukin-1, and interleukin-6 may also play a role in mediating the inflammation associated with this disease [41].

It has been speculated that Henoch-Schönlein purpura and IgA nephropathy may be closely related en-

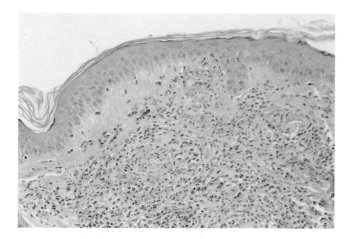

Fig. 8–1. Henoch-Shönlein purpura is characterized by a neutrophilic vasculitis involving small postcapillary venules.

tities. In one adult patient, investigators documented progression from IgA nephropathy to Henoch-Schön-lein purpura [42]. In another report, Human leukocyte antigen (HLA) types B35 and D4 were commonly expressed by a father with Henoch-Schönlein purpura and his son with IgA nephropathy [43].

In some cases, increased plasma IgE levels were found in patients with Henoch-Schönlein purpura. In this study, investigators postulated that in some cases an inmmunoallergy leading to stimulation of IgE-sensitized mast cells in the presence of IgA circulating immune complexes might give rise to the cutaneous and intestinal manifestations [44].

Hemolytic Uremic Syndrome

Epidemiology. Hemolytic uremic syndrome is a systemic thrombotic microangiopathy. It can occur in sporadic or epidemic forms and can be inherited [45]. The overall incidence is about 2.1 cases/100,00 persons per year [46]. The disease is most common in children, especially the epidemic form [45]. There is a seasonal peak, with most cases occurring between June and September. The overall mortality rate from the acute disease is less than 5% [45].

Cutaneous Features. The cutaneous manifestations of hemolytic uremic syndrome resemble other hypercoagulable states. There are cutaneous infarctions of distal body sites. Hemorrhagic lesions secondary to vascular occlusion and blisters caused by epidermal necrosis may be present.

Associated Disorders. Hemolytic uremic syndrome has been associated with infectious agents such as *Escherichia coli* [47], *Shigella* [48], *Salmonella, Pneumococcus,* and viruses. It has also been associated with malignant neoplasms, pregnancy, and exposures to radiation, mitomycin, and cyclosporine [45]. Approximately 90% of affected children will present with bloody diarrhea. Malignant hypertension, glomerulonephritis, and transplant rejection are also frequently seen [45]. Hemolytic anemia is present [49].

In the acute phase of the illness, patients have hypertension, edema, and anuria as part of the acute renal failure. Neurologic involvement as manifested by strokes and cortical blindness, although infrequent, does occur at this stage of the disease. The renal failure resolves in most patients, but progresses to end-stage renal failure in about one-third of cases [45].

Histologic Features. Skin biopsy specimens reveal fibrin thrombi within small vessels of affected skin (Fig. 8–3). Vessel wall thickening of affected capillaries and

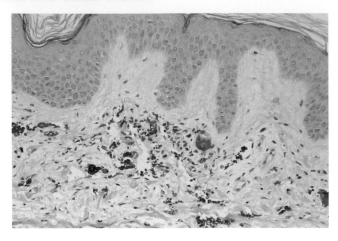

Fig. 8–3. Hemolytic uremic syndrome is characterized by noninflammatory thrombosis of many dermal blood vessels.

arterioles is present, and endothelial cells are swollen and may separate from the basement membrane [49]. There is minimal inflammation surrounding the vessels in early lesions, but a secondary inflammatory response may be seen in later ones. The following entities must be considered in the differential diagnosis of hemolytic uremic syndrome:

- Cryoglobulinemia
- Disseminated intravascular coagulation
- Livedoid vasculitis
- Lupus anticoagulant syndrome
- Protein C or protein S deficiency
- Septic emboli

Special Studies. Special studies are not usually necessary to make the diagnosis of hemolytic uremic syndrome; however, multiple levels of tissue may be necessary to find the vascular occlusions. Direct immunofluorescence reveals fibrin within affected vessels, but immunoglobulins are not ordinarily detected.

Pathogenesis. It is believed that tumor necrosis factor-α may cause neutrophil adhesion to vascular walls, with subsequent release of cytokines. This then leads to the observed vascular thrombosis [47].

Impetigo Contagiosa with Subsequent Acute Post-Streptococcal Glomerulonephritis

Epidemiology. Impetigo contagiosa, caused by the group A β-hemolytic streptococci *Streptococcus pyogenes* is seen most frequently in children and young adults. There is some seasonal variation in incidence, with most cases occurring in the late summer and autumn [50, 51]. Impetigo is the most common cutaneous infection in children [52, 53]. Bullous impetigo, caused by *Staphylococcus aureus,* is far more common than is impetigo contagiosa and is not related to the development of renal disease [54]. The infection may arise secondary to mild trauma. As many as 11% of cases of impetigo contagiosa may be followed by acute glomerulonephritis, as determined by low serum complement levels and abnormal urinalyses [55]. High rates of endemic group A streptococcal infection with subsequent glomerulonephritis are seen in Aboriginal communities in Australia [56].

Approximately 90% of acute post-streptococcal glomerulonephritis occurs in children. In children, the renal disease is usually self-limited and resolves without sequelae. When seen in adults, up to 25% of patients develop hypertension and chronic renal failure. In one series, the fatality rate in the acute disease among children was 1.3% [57]. In the same series, none of the other children developed any long-term complications.

Cutaneous Features. Streptococcal infections of the skin can occur at any location but are most common on the legs. The arms, face, and trunk are less commonly involved [58]. Small, erythematous papules develop into vesicles and pustules. Rapidly, vesicles rupture and form thick yellow crusts surrounded by a rim of erythema. Central clearing may be apparent in older lesions. Because the progression through the various stages is very rapid, patients will simultaneously have lesions at all phases of development. The eruption usually resolves within 2–4 weeks.

Deeper cutaneous streptococcal infections, known as *ecthyma,* occur mainly on the legs. Crust formation is much more pronounced, and lesions last for 4–8 weeks. Ulceration and scarring often follow [59]. Rarely, staphylococci may be the causative organism in ecthyma.

Associated Disorders. Patients with atopic dermatitis have an increased incidence of cutaneous streptococcal infections [60]. This predisposes these patients to higher rates of acute post-streptococcal glomerulonephritis in some settings [61]. *Streptococcus pyogenes*–induced impetigo contagiosa does not predispose patients to streptococcal-induced rheumatic fever.

Histologic Features. Histologic changes of impetigo contagiosa consist of a subcorneal blister filled with neutrophils (Fig. 8–4). Rare acantholytic cells may be seen within the blister cavity. The surrounding epidermis is spongiotic, and additional neutrophils may be present. Within the superficial dermis, there is a mixed

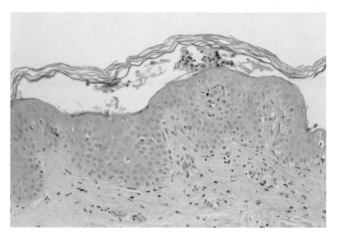

Fig. 8–4. Impetigo contagiosa demonstrates subcorneal neutrophilic abscesses.

inflammatory infiltrate with abundant neutrophils. The following entities must be considered in the differential diagnosis of impetigo contagiosa:

- Acute generalized exanthematous pustulosis
- Candidiasis
- Dermatophytosis
- Pustular psoriasis
- Subcorneal pustular dermatosis of Sneddon and Wilkinson

Ecthyma has similar, but more pronounced, histologic changes. In well-developed lesions, dermal edema and vascular dilation become more apparent. Neutrophils are present throughout the affected dermis.

Special studies. Tissue Gram stains such as the Brown-Brenn stain may be helpful in highlighting organisms within the tissue sections.

Antistreptolysin O titers are helpful in confirming the diagnosis of streptococcal infection, as is tissue culture. Anti-DNAase B titers are also helpful. Circulating antizymogen antibodies have been shown to be more predictive of acute post-streptococcal glomerulonephritis than the antistreptolysin O or anti-DNAase levels [62].

Pathogenesis. Several different strains, including serotypes 49-14, NT-14 [63], and T4 (M60) [55], of *Streptococcus* are associated with acute glomerulonephritis. The incidence and levels of circulating immune complexes in patients with acute post-streptococcal glomerulonephritis are no different from those of patients with cutaneous streptococcal infections and no renal sequelae. This suggests that trapping of circulating immune complexes probably does not play a central role in the development of acute post-streptococcal glomerulonephritis [64].

CHRONIC RENAL DISEASE

Calciphylaxis

Epidemiology. Cutaneous calciphylaxis is seen almost exclusively in patients with hyperparathyroidism and end-stage renal disease requiring dialysis [65]. In one series, approximately 90% of affected patients had chronic renal failure [66]. Most patients have an elevated calcium × phosphate product exceeding 6.5 mmol^2/L^2 [65]. Rare patients have been described to have calciphylaxis with normal calcium [67] and parathormone levels [68]. This disease is associated with severe morbidity and a very high mortality rate [69]. Some patients have shown improvement with parathyroidectomy, but may not have improved overall survival rates [70].

Cutaneous Features. The lower legs are the most frequently involved site, but thighs, abdomen, and buttocks can also be affected [71, 72]. The earliest cutaneous changes, which appear suddenly, include mottling of the skin that resembles livedo reticularis and that can be painful. These areas undergo necrosis and ulceration. The necrosis may extend deeply into the skeletal muscles [73]. Bullae may be apparent. Other common cutaneous manifestations include plaques and subcutaneous nodules. Gangrene of the fingers and toes has also been described [74]. The disease progresses rapidly.

Associated Disorders. In addition to the cutaneous regions with zonal necrosis, infarction of the central nervous system, bowel, and myocardium have been reported in calciphylaxis [75].

Calciphylaxis has rarely been described in association with other hypercalcemic conditions such as primary hyperparathyroidism, hypercalcemia of malignancy, and multiple myeloma [76]. Excessive intake of vitamin D can rarely cause calciphylaxis [69].

Histologic Features. The major histologic finding is calcification of the media of small- and medium-sized vessels in the deep dermis and subcutaneous fat (Fig. 8–5). Vessels with diameters of approximately 100 μm are mainly affected [66]. Secondary thrombosis may be present, and intimal hyperplasia is often seen. Later lesions demonstrate necrosis of the surrounding panniculus and dermis [65]. Minimal inflammation is seen. A giant cell reaction may be seen exclusively limited to the regions of calcium deposition [66]. Changes associated with calciphylaxis are most prominent in vessels with a smaller diameter than those primarily affected in atherosclerosis.

Special Studies. A von Kossa stain can be performed to highlight the calcium phosphate deposits, but this is unnecessary in most cases. The deposits are readily apparent on routine histologic sections; however, they may be very focal. Deep samples are often necessary, and multiple levels through the tissue sections may be required to demonstrate the calcifications. Ossification is not present.

Pathogenesis. Seyle [77] initially defined calciphylaxis as "a condition of induced systemic hypersensitivity in which tissues respond to appropriate challenging agents with local calcification." Sensitizers such as parathormone, vitamin D, and dihydrotochysterol (vitamin D analogue) are believed to play a role in this process, especially when serum levels of calcium and phosphate

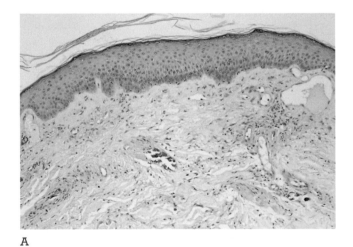

A

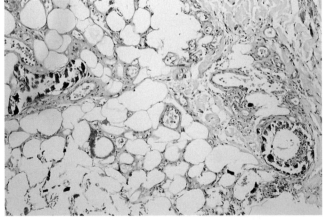

B

Fig. 8–5. Small vessels within the dermis (A) and subcutaneous fat (B) have intramural calcium in calciphylaxis secondary to renal failure.

are normal [65]. Others believe this concept to be inconsistent with the pathophysiology of chronic renal failure and thus probably not valid [70]. Endovascular fibrosis with vascular calcification is thought by some to be the cause of ischemia in calciphylaxis [73].

Metastatic calcification due to elevated calcium and phosphate levels may also be responsible for the vascular deposits of calcium in these patients.

Reactive Perforating Disorders of Diabetes and Renal Failure

There is much discussion in the literature about perforating disorders associated with chronic renal disease [78]. Certain writers believe that perforating folliculitis, reactive perforating collagenosis, and Kyrle's disease are all variants of the same process [79], while others believe each to be a discrete entity. Patterson [78] has suggested a classification scheme that would group Kyrle's disease, perforating folliculitis, and the acquired form of reactive perforating collagenosis into a single grouping of "acquired perforating diseases," leaving elastosis perforans serpiginosa and the inherited form of reactive perforating collagenosis as separate, discrete entities. In any case, they are all somewhat similar clinically as well as histologically. The entity known as *reactive perforating collagenosis* is the one most closely associated with chronic renal failure and is described in depth in this chapter.

Epidemiology. Reactive perforating collagenosis can be inherited or acquired. When inherited, it appears in childhood, whereas the acquired form is most commonly seen in adults. The mean age of onset in adults is about 55–60 years [80]. It is believed that cutaneous lesions in both forms arise in response to minor trauma [81].

The inherited form of reactive perforating collagenosis may have a genetic predisposition. There is a 2:1 male-to-female ratio in these patients [82, 83].

The acquired form of the disease occurs equally in men and women. In one series, 72% of patients with reactive perforating collagenosis had diabetes mellitus, and 68% had some type of nephropathy, most of whom were receiving dialysis [80]. There is some suggestion of seasonal variation, with lesions more likely to occur in the winter months [82] and less likely in the summer months [81, 84]. The disease appears to be more common in black patients [85].

Cutaneous Features. Multiple, recurrent, umbilicated 5–10 mm papules and nodules occur in crops and last for 6–8 weeks. They resolve spontaneously, leaving hyperpigmented macules. The extensor surfaces are the most commonly involved sites in reactive perforating collagenosis. The upper and lower extremities are frequently affected, and the trunk is also a common site of involvement. Fewer lesions are seen on the face and scalp. Pruritus is a major symptom in most affected patients [80]. Linear lesions [82] and Koebner's phenomenon [86] have been described in reactive perforating collagenosis.

Associated Disorders. Reactive perforating collagenosis has also been associated with hypo- and hyperthyroidism, Hodgkin's disease, non-Hodgkin's lymphoma, liver disease, and hypertension [80]. Reactive perforating collagenosis has been described in patients with acquired immunodeficiency syndrome [87], and lesions have been associated with acne vulgaris [84] and insect bites [81].

Histologic Features. Histologic features include a central channel that is occluded with parakeratotic keratin, degenerating strands of vertically oriented collagen, scattered neutrophils, and degenerating epidermal material. There is surrounding epidermal hyperplasia, which may be "psuedoepitheliomatous," and at the base of the central crater the epidermis is markedly thin to absent (Fig. 8–6). Immediately deep to the point where the collagen is extruded through the epidermis, there may be a pronounced inflammatory infiltrate with abundant neutrophils, histiocytes, and lymphocytes. The collagen in this location is more basophilic than the surrounding, uninvolved collagen. There is no apparent association with hair follicles in most cases classified as reactive perforating collagenosis. The following entities must be considered in the histologic differential diagnosis of reactive perforating collagenosis:

- Elastosis perforans serpiginosum
- Kyrle's disease
- Lichen simplex chronicus
- Perforating calcific elastosis
- Perforating folliculitis
- Perforating granuloma annulare

Special Studies. Masson's trichrome will highlight the degenerating collagen fibers present within the epidermal canal and in the hyperkeratotic plug. Elastic tissue stains are usually negative in these sites [80].

Pathogenesis. It is believed by some that, in response to minor trauma, the collagen within the dermal papillae degenerates [86]. This degenerating collagen is transepidermally eliminated [88]. It has been shown that types I and III collagen are being eliminated [89]. It is noteworthy that lesions do not develop in response to deep trauma [82]. Others are less convinced that trauma plays a central role in the pathogenesis of this disorder [90]. The four perforating disorders may represent dif-

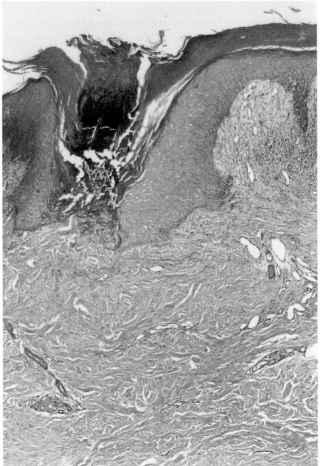

A

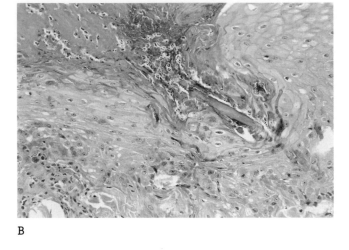

B

Fig. 8–6. Perforating disorders demonstrate a central area of epidermal invagination, pseudoepitheliomatous hyperplasia *(A)* and transepidermal elimination of degenerating collagen *(B)*.

ferent time points in the same pathologic process, with elastic fibers eliminated earlier and degenerating collagen later in the course of the disease [79].

Pruritus of Chronic Renal Failure

Epidemiology. Pruritus affects 50%–90% of patients with chronic renal failure receiving dialysis [91]. It can be mild and focal or generalized and severe and does not appear to correlate with length of time receiving dialysis.

Cutaneous Features. Patients complain of itching. No primary skin lesion typifies uremic patients. Excoriations are evident as secondary changes. Xerosis is also a common finding.

Associated Disorders. Pruritus is associated with end-stage renal disease due to any cause.

Histologic Features. There are no specific histologic changes found in primary lesions. The changes that are

usually observed are secondary ones as a result of scratching and are not specific for pruritus associated with renal failure. Acute excoriations, with disruption of the epidermis and a mixed inflammatory infiltrate, may be present. In long-standing lesions, changes of prurigo nodularis or lichen simplex chronicus may be seen, with hyperkeratosis, acanthosis, hypergranulosis, and papillary dermal fibrosis.

Special Studies. No special studies are indicated on histologic sections to make a diagnosis of pruritus associated with chronic renal failure.

Pathogenesis. The pathogenesis of pruritus associated with chronic renal failure remains unknown. It has been suggested that elevated aluminum levels in patients undergoing long-term dialysis may be responsible for the pruritus [92]. Others have reported that increased rates of mast cell proliferation and subsequent release of histamine may play a central role in this process [93, 94]; however, other workers have found no differences in numbers of cutaneous mast cells in hemodialysis patients with and without pruritus [95]. Elevated levels of prostaglandin E_2 have been reported in these patients and implicated in the pathogenesis of the pruritus [96].

Half-and-Half Nails

The condition known as half-and-half nails is characterized by nails that have a normal to white proximal half and an abnormal, brown discoloration on their distal halves [97]. It has been demonstrated that this increased pigment is due to melanin [98]. Histologic changes have not been described for this entity.

Post-Transplant Lymphoproliferative Disorder

Epidemiology. Post-transplant proliferative disorder (PTLD) occurs in 1%–2% of patients receiving solid organ transplants [99]. The incidence appears to be approximately the same independent of type of organ transplanted and is closely related to immunosuppression and infection with Epstein-Barr virus. Post-transplant lymphoproliferative disorders represent up to 50% of post-transplantation tumors in the pediatric population, but account for only 15% of such tumors in adults [100]. Onset of PTLD follows organ transplantation by an average of 8–9 months [101]. Post-transplant lymphoproliferative disorders represent a heterogeneous group of lymphoid proliferations that range from those that cause minimal disease to rapidly fatal cases. Although difficult to assess, the overall mortality rate is quite high [102], with an overall survival rate of 5 months in one series [101].

Cutaneous Features. Although tumors caused by PTLD can occur in any location within the body, these growths are often detected initially in the skin. The tumors appear as erythematous, firm dermal nodules with no overlying surface changes.

Associated Disorders. Patients with PTLD present with a infectious mononucleosis-like syndrome [99]. Some patients have persistent fever, adenopathy, and pulmonary infiltrates [103]. The central nervous system, lungs, and bone marrow are involved in up to one-fourth of patients [104]. Post-transplant lymphoproliferative disorder has rarely been reported in patients after autologous bone marrow transplantation [103].

Histologic Features. Most PTLDs demonstrate the features of high-grade, non-Hodgkin's lymphomas. Some of them have a Burkitt's lymphoma-type appearance, and others resemble those of diffuse large cell lymphomas [105]. A diffuse infiltrate of lymphocytes is present throughout the dermis, usually sparing the epidermis and papillary dermis. In most cases, there is a polymorphous population of lympoid cells, with large, transformed cells admixed with immunoblastic lymphocytes and occasional plasmacytoid differcntiation [106]. The lymphocytes are large, with vesicular nuclei with irregular margins and irregularly prominent nucleoli. Individual cell necrosis is prominent, and the mitotic rate is high.

In other patients, the PTLD demonstrates more of a benign, reactive lymphoid hyperplasia. In these cases, the polymorphous mix of lymphocytes lacks the significant cytologic atypia and high mitotic rate described above.

Special Studies. Lymphocyte immunophenotyping is helpful in confirming a diagnosis in many cases. In most cases, PTLD has been attributed to a polyclonal or monoclonal proliferation of B cells. In approximately 10% of cases, T-cell proliferations have been detected [101, 107]. bcl-2 expression is present in neoplastic lymphocytes in most cases [108]. With in situ hybridization techniques, Epstein-Barr virus can be detected within the tumor cells.

Pathogenesis. Post-transplant lymphoproliferative disorder has been associated Epstein-Barr virus infection in immunosuppressed patients [99]. Alterations in the interferon-α and p16 genes on chromosome 9p have been described in many of the cases [109].

NOTE: Staphylococcal scalded skin syndrome (SSSS) is discussed in Chapter 17.

References

1. Robson, W. L., and Leung, A. K., *Henoch-Schönlein purpura.* Adv Pediatr, 1994. 41:163–194.
2. Al-Sheyyab, M., El-Shanti, H., Ajlouni, S., Sawalha, D., and Daoud, A., *The clinical spectrum of Henoch-Schönlein purpura in infants and young children.* Eur J Pediatr, 1995. 154:969–972.
3. Blanco, R., Martinez-Taboada, V. M., Rodriguez-Valverde, V., Garcia-Fuentes, M., and Gonzalez-Gay, M. A., *Henoch-Schönlein purpura in adulthood and childhood: Two different expressions of the same syndrome.* Arthritis Rheum, 1997. 40:859–864.
4. Wenner, N. P., and Safai, B., *Circulating immune complexes in Henoch-Schönlein purpura.* 1983. Int J Dermatol(22).
5. Garland, J. S., and Chusid, M. J., *Henoch-Schoenlein purpura: Association with unusual vesicular lesions.* Wis Med J, 1985. 84:21–23.
6. Wananukul, S., Pongprasit, P., and Korkij, W., *Henoch Schönlein purpura presenting as hemorrhagic vesicles and bullae: Case report and literature review.* Pediatr Dermatol, 1995. 12:314–317.

7. Green, S. T., and Natarajan, S., *The Koebner phenomenon in anaphylactoid purpura.* Cutis, 1986. 38:56–57.

8. Tancrede-Bohin, E., Ochonisky, S., Vignon-Pennamen, M. D., Flageul, B., Morel, P., and Rybojad, M., *Schönlein-Henoch purpura in adult patients. Predictive factors for IgA glomerulonephritis in a retrospective study of 57 cases.* Arch Dermatol, 1997. 133:438–442.

9. Cappell, M. S., and Gupta, A. M., *Colonic lesions associated with Henoch-Schönlein purpura.* Am J Gastroenterol, 1990. 85:1186–1188.

10. Di Febo, G., Gizzi, G., Biasco, G., and Miglioli, M., *Colonic involvement in adult patients with Henoch-Schönlein purpura.* Endoscopy, 1984. 16:36–39.

11. Chan, J. C., Li, P. K., Lai, F. M., and Lai, K. N., *Fatal adult Henoch-Schönlein purpura due to small intestinal infarction.* J Intern Med, 1992. 232:181–184.

12. McCrindle, B. W., Wood, R. A., and Nussbaum, A. R., *Henoch-Schönlein syndrome. Unusual manifestations with hydrops of the gallbladder.* Clin Pediatr (Phila), 1988. 27:254–256.

13. Hammoudeh, M., and Qaddoumi, N. K., *Pleural haemorrhage in Henoch Schönlein purpura.* Clin Rheumatol, 1993. 12:538–539.

14. Marandian, M. H., Ezzati, M., Behvad, A., Moazzami, P., and Rakhchan, M., *Pulmonary involvement in Schönlein-Henoch purpura.* Arch Fr Pediatr, 1982. 39:255–257.

15. O'Regan, S., and Robitaille, P., *Orchitis mimicking testicular torsion in Henoch-Schönlein's purpura.* J Urol, 1981. 126:834–835.

16. Raimer, S.S., and Sanchez, R. L., *Vasculitis is children.* Semin Dermatol, 1992. 11:48–56.

17. Heng, M. C. Y., *Henoch-Schönlein purpura.* Br J Dermatol, 1985. 112:235–240.

18. Garcias, V. A., and Herr, H. W., *Henoch-Schönlein purpura associated with cancer of prostate.* Urology, 1982. 19:155–158.

19. Hughes, R. A., Bottomley, D. M., Keat, A. C., and Drury, A., *Henoch-Schonelein purpura occurring in association with carcinoma of the breast.* Eur J Med, 1993. 2:310–312.

20. Maestri, A., Malacarne, P., and Santini, A., *Henoch-Schönlein syndrome associated with breast cancer. A case report.* Angiology, 1995. 46:625–627.

21. Orfila, C., Lepert, J. C., Modesto, A., Pipy, B., and Suc, J. M., *Henoch-Schönlein purpura in a patient with diabetic nephropathy.* Am J Kindey Dis, 1994. 24:509–514.

22. Nast, C. C., Ward, H. J., Koyle, M. A., and Cohen, A. H., *Recurrent Henoch-Schönlein purpura following renal-transplantation.* Am J Kidney Dis, 1987. 9:39–43.

23. Maggiore, G., Martini, A., Grifeo, S., De Giacomo, C., and Scotta, M. S., *Hepatitis B virus infection and Schönlein-Henoch purpura.* Am J Dis Child, 1984. 138:681–682.

24. Zucchini, A., and Manfredi, R., *Schöenlein-Henoch syndrome and Salmonella infection: A new association?* Minerva Pediatr, 1992. 44:559–563.

25. Montoliu, J., Miro, J. M., Campistol, J. M., Trilla, A., Mensa, J., Torras, A., and Revert, L., *Henoch-Schönlein purpura complicating staphylococcal endocarditis in a heroin addict.* Am J Nephrol, 1987. 7:137–139.

26. Han, B. G., Choi, S. O., Shin, S. J., Kim, H. Y., Jung, S. H., and Lee, K. H., *A case of Henoch-Schönlein purpura in disseminated tuberculosis.* Korean J Int Med, 1995. 10:54–59.

27. Reinauer, S., Megahed, M., Goerz, G., Ruzicka, T., Borchard, F., Susanto, F., and Reinauer, H., *Schönlein-Henoch purpura associated with gastric Helicobacter pylori infection.* J Am Acad Dermatol, 1995. 33:876–879.

28. Onisawa, S., Morishima, N., and Ichimura, T., *Concurrent poststreptococcal acute glomerulonephritis and Schönlein-Henoch purpura.* Acta Paediatr Jpn, 1989. 31:487–492.

29. Zillioz, A. P., Domoto, D. T., Hutcheson, P. S., Tasi, C. C., and Slavin, R. G., *Henoch-Schönlein purpura due to streptokinase.* J Clin Immunol, 1993. 13:415–423.

30. Escudero, A., Lucas, E., Vidal, J. B., Sanchez-Guerrero, I., Martinez, A., Illan, F., and Ramos, J., *Drug-related Henoch-Schönlein purpura.* Allergol Immunopathol (Madr), 1996. 24:22–24.

31. Chevalier, X., Rostoker, G., Larget-Piet, B., and Gherardi, R., *Schoenlein-Henoch purpura with necrotizing vasculitis after cocaine snorting.* Clin Nephrol, 1995. 43:348–349.

32. Park, S. H., Kim, C. J., Seo, J. K., and Park, K. W., *Gastrointestinal manifestations of Henoch-Schönlein purpua.* J Korean Med Sci, 1990. 5:101–104.

33. Stevenson, J. A., Leong, L. A., Cohen, A. H., and Border, W. A., *Henoch-Schönlein purpura: simultaneous demonstration of IgA deposits in involved skin, intestine and kidney.* Arch Pathol Lab Med, 1982. 106:192–195.

34. Van Hale, H. M., Gibson, L. E., and Schroeter, A. L., *Henoch-Schönlein vasculitis: Direct immunofluorescence study of uninvolved skin.* J Am Acad Dermatol, 1986. 15:665–670.

35. Hene, R. J., Velthuis, P., van de Wiel, A., Klepper, D., Dorhout Mees, E. J., and Kater, L., *The relevance of IgA deposits in vessel walls of clinically normal skin. A prospective study.* Arch Intern Med, 1986. 146:745–749.

36. Saklayen, M. G., Schroeter, A. L., Nafz, M. A., and Jalil, K., *IgA deposition in the skin of patients with alcoholic liver disease.* J Cutan Pathol, 1996. 23:12–18.

37. Kawana, S., and Nishiyama, S., *Serum SC5b-9 (terminal complement complex) level, a sensitive indicator of disease activity in patients with Henoch-Schönlein purpura.* Dermatology, 1992. 184:171–176.

38. Burrows, N. P., and Lockwood, C. M., *Antineutrophil cytoplasmic antibodies and their relevance to the dermatologist.* Br J Dermatol, 1995. 132:173–181.

39. Burden, A. D., Gibson, I. W., Rodger, R. S. C., and Tillman, D. M., *IgA anticardiolipin antibodies associated with Henoch-Schönlein purpura.* J Am Acad Dermatol, 1994. 31:857–860.

40. Kaneko, F., Mori, N., and Miura, Y., *Secretory IgA in Schönlein-Henoch purpura.* Dermatologica, 1984. 169:318–323.

41. Besbas, N., Saatci, U., Ruacan, S., Ozen, S., Sungur, A., Bakkaloglu, A., and Elnahas, A. M., *The role of cytokines in Henoch Schönlein purpura.* Scan J Rheumatol, 1997. 26:456–460.

42. Araque, A., Sanchez, R., Alamo, C., Torres, N., and Praga, M., *Evolution of immunoglobulin A nephropathy into Henoch-Schönlein purpura in an adult patient.* Am J Kidney Dis, 1995. 25:340–342.

43. Montoliu, J., Lens, X. M., Torras, A., and Revert, L., *Henoch-Schönlein purpura and IgA nephropathy in father and son.* Nephron, 1990. 54:77–79.

44. Davin, J. C., Pierard, G., Dechenne, C., Grossman, D., Nagy, J., Quacoe, M., Malaise, M., Hall, M., et al., *Possible pathogenic role of IgE in Henoch-Schönlein purpura.* Pediatr Nephrol, 1994. 8:169–171.

45. Repetto, H. A., *Epidemic hemolytic-uremic syndrome in children.* Kidney Int, 1997. 52:1708–1719.

46. Su, C., and Brandt, L. J., *Escherichia coli O157:H7 infection in humans.* Ann Intern Med, 1995. 123:698–714.

47. Remuzzi, G., and Ruggenenti, P., *The hemolytic uremic syndrome.* Kidney Int, 1995. 47:2–19.

48. Koster, F., Levin, J., Walker, L., Tunk, K. S. K., Gilman, R. H., Rahaman, M. M., Majid, M. A., Islam, A., et al., *Hemolytic-uremic syndrome after Shigellosis.* N Engl J Med, 1978. 298:927–933.

49. Remuzzi, G., and Ruggenenti, P., *The hemolytic uremic syndrome.* Kidney Int, 1998. 53 (Suppl 66):S54–S57.

50. Dillon, H. C., Jr., *Impetigo contagiosa: Suppurative and non-suppurative complications: I. Clinical, bacteriologic, and epidemiologic characteristics of impetigo.* Am J Dis Child, 1968. 115:530–541.

51. Wannamaker, L. W., *Differences between streptococcal infectons of the throat and of the skin.* N Eng J Med, 1970. 282:23–31.

52. Hayden, G. E., *Skin disease encountered in a pediatric clinic.* Am J Dis Child, 1985. 139:36–38.

53. Darmstadt, G. L., and Lane, A. T., *Impetigo: An overview.* Pediatr Dermatol, 1994. 11:293–303.

54. Tunneson, W. W., Jr., *Cutaneous infections.* Pediatr Clin North Am, 1983. 30:515–532.

55. el Tayeb, S. H., Nasr, E. M., and Sattallah, A. S., *Streptococcal impetigo and acute glomerulonephritis in children in Cairo.* Br J Dermatol, 1978. 98:53–62.

56. Gardiner, D. L., and Sriprakash, K. S., *Molecular epidemiology of impetiginous group A streptococcal infections in aboriginal communities of northern Australia.* J Clin Microbiol, 1996. 34:1448–1452.

57. Sanjad, S., Tolaymat, A., Whitworth, J., and Levin, S., *Acute glomerulonephritis in children: A review of 153 cases.* South Med J, 1977. 70:1202–1206.

58. Ferrieri, P., Dajani, A. S., and Wannamaker, L. W., *Natural history of impetigo: I. Site sequence of acquisition and familial patterns of spread of cutaneous streptococci.* J Clin Invest, 1972. 51:2851–2862.

59. Tunneson, W. W., Jr., *Practical aspects of bacterial skin infections in children.* Pediatr Dermatol, 1985. 2:255–265.

60. Adachi, J., Endo, K., Fukuzumi, T., Tanigawa, N., and Aoki, T., *Increasing incidence of streptococcal impetigo in atopic dermatitis.* J Dermatol Sci, 1998. 17:45–53.

61. Kobayashi, S., Ikeda, T., Okada, H., Suzuki, Y., Ishii, M., Ohtake, T., Oda, T., and Hishida, A., *Endemic occurrence of glomerulonephritis associated with streptococcal impetigo.* Am J Nephrol, 1995. 15:356–360.

62. Parra, G., Rodriguez-Iturbe, B., Batsford, S., Vogt, A., Mezzano, S., Olavarria, F., Exeni, R., Laso, M., et al., *Antibody to streptococcal zymogen in the serum of patients with acute glomerulonephritis: A multicentric study.* Kidney Int, 1998. 54:509–517.

63. Margolis, H. S., Lum, M. K., Bender, T. R., Elliott, S. L., Fitzgerald, M. A., and Harpster, A. P., *Acute glomerulonephritis and streptococcal skin lesions in Eskimo children.* Am J Dis Child, 1980. 134:681–685.

64. Mezzano, S., Olavarria, F., Ardiles, L., and Lopez, M. I., *Incidence of circulating immune copmlexes in patients with acute poststreptococcal glomerulonephritis and in patients with streptococcal impetigo.* Clin Nephrol, 1986. 26:61–65.

65. Ivker, R. A., Woosley, J., and Briggaman, R. A., *Calciphylaxis in three patients with end-stage renal disease.* Arch Dermatol, 1995. 131:63–68.

66. Fischer, A. H., and Morris, D. J., *Pathogenesis of calciphylaxis: Study of three cases with literature review.* Hum Pathol, 1995. 26:1055–1064.

67. Fox, R., Barnowsky, L. H., and Cruz, A. B., *Post-renal transplant calciphylaxis.* J Urol, 1983. 129:362–363.

68. Massry, S. G., Gordon, A., Coburn, J. W., Kaplan, L., Franklin, S. S., Maxwell, M. H., and Kleeman, C. R., *Vascular calcification and peripheral necrosis in a renal transplant patient: Reversal of lesions following subtotal parathyroidectomy.* Am J Med, 1970. 49:416–422.

69. Dahl, P. R., Winkelmann, R. K., and Connolly, S. M., *The vascular calcification-cutaneous necrosis syndrome.* J Am Acad Dermatol, 1995. 33:53–58.

70. Hafner, J., Keusch, G., Wahl, C., Sauter, B., Hurlimann, A., von Weizsaker, F., Krayenbuhl, M., Biedermann, K., et al., *Uremic small-artery disease with medial calcification and intimal hyperplasia (so-called calciphylaxis): A complication of chronic renal failure and benefit from parathyroidectomy.* 1995. 33:954–962.

71. Richens, G., Piepkorn, M. W., and Krueger, G. G., *Calcifying panniculitis associated with renal failure: A case of Selye's calciphylaxis in man.* J Am Acad Dermatol, 1982. 6:537–539.

72. Lugo-Somolinos, A., Sanchez, J. L., Mendez-Coll, J., and Joglar, F., *Calcifying panniculitis associated with polycystic kidney disease and chronic renal failure.* J Am Acad Dermatol, 1990. 22:743–747.

73. Richardson, J. A., Herron, G., Reitz, R., and Layzer, R., *Ischemic ulcerations of skin and necrosis of muscle in azotemic hyperparathyroidism.* Ann Intern Med, 1969. 71:129–138.

74. Winkelmann, R. K., and Keating, F. R., *Cutaneous vascular calcification, gangrene and hyperparathyroidism.* Br J Dermatol, 1970. 83:263–268.

75. Adrogue, H. J., Frazier, M. R., Zeluff, B., and Suki, W. N., *Systemic calciphylaxis revisited.* Am J Nephrol, 1981. 1:177–183.

76. Harris, T., and Schapiro, B., *Calciphylaxis.* Med Surg Dermatol, 1996. 3:387–389.

77. Seyle, H., *Calciphlyaxis.* 1962, Chicago: University of Chicago Press.

78. Patterson, J. W., *The perforating disorders.* J Am Acad Dermatol, 1984. 10:561–581.

79. Rapini, R. P., Hebert, A. A., and Drucker, C. R., *Acquired perforating dermatosis: Evidence for combined transepidermal elimination of both collagen and elastic fibers.* Arch Dermatol, 1989. 125:1074–1078.

80. Faver, I. R., Daoud, M. S., and Su, W. P. D., *Acquired reactive perforating collagenosis. Report of six cases and review of the literature.* J Am Acad Dermatol, 1994. 30:575–580.

81. Bovenmeyer, D. A., *Reactive perforating collagenosis: Experimental production of the lesion.* Arch Dermatol, 1970. 102:213–217.

82. Kanan, M. W., *Familial reactive perforating collagenosis and intolerance to cold.* Br J Dermatol, 1974. 91:405–414.

83. Rotta, O., *Reactive perforating collagenosis: Report of 3 cases.* Dermatologica, 1983. 166:308–310.

84. Cullen, S. I., *Successful treatment of reactive perforating collagenosis with tretinoin.* Cutis, 1979. 23:187–193.

85. Hood, A. F., Hardegen, G. L., Zarate, A. R., Nigra, T. P., and Gelfand, M. C., *Kyrle's disease in patients with chronic renal failure.* Arch Dermatol, 1982. 118:85–88.

86. Poliak, S. C., Lebwohl, M. G., Parris, A., and Prioleau, P. G., *Reactive perforating collagenosis associated with diabetes mellitus.* N Engl J Med, 1982. 306:81–84.

87. Bank, D. E., Cohen, P. R., and Kohn, S. R., *Reactive perforating collagenosis in a setting of double disaster: Acquired immunodeficiency syndrome and end-stage renal disease.* J Am Acad Dermatol, 1989. 21:371–374.

88. Mehregan, A. H., Scjwartz, E. D., and Livingood, C. S., *Reactive perforating collagenosis.* Arch Dermatol, 1967. 96:277–282.

89. Zelger, B., Hintner, H., Aubock, J., and Fritsch, P. O., *Acquired perforating dermatosis.* Arch Dermatol, 1991. 127:695–700.

90. Cochran, R. J., Tucker, S. B., and Wilkin, J. K., *Reactive perforating collagenosis of diabetes mellitus and renal failure.* Cutis, 1983. 31:55–58.

91. Robertson, K. E., and Mueller, B. A., *Uremic pruritis.* Am J Health Syst Pharm, 1996. 53:2159–2170.

92. Friga, V., Linos, A., and Linos, D. A., *Is aluminum toxicity responsible for uremic pruritis in chronic hemodialysis patients?* Nephron, 1997. 75:48–53.

93. Dimkovic, N., Djukanovic, L., Radmilovic, A., Bojic, P., and Juloski, T., *Uremic pruritis and skin mast cells.* Nephron, 1992. 61:5–9.

94. Leong, S. O., Tan, C. C., Lye, W. C., Lee, E. J., and Chan, H. L., *Dermal mast cell density and pruritis in end-stage renal failure.* Ann Acad Med Singapore, 1994. 23:327–329.

95. Klein, L. R., Klein, J. B., Hanno, R., and Callen, J. P., *Cutaneous mast cell quantity in pruritic and nonpruritic hemodialysis patients.* Int J Dermatol, 1988. 27:557–559.

96. Peck, L. W., *Essential fatty acid deficiency in renal failure: Can supplements really help?* J Am Diet Assoc, 1997. 97(Suppl 2):S150–S153.

97. Scher, R. K., and Daniel, C. R. I., *Nails: Therapy, Diagnosis, Surgery.* 1990, W. B. Saunders Company, Philadelphia. pp. 181–183.

98. Leyden, J. J., and Wood, M. G., *The half and half nail.* Arch Dermatol, 1972. 105: pp. 591–592.

99. Caillard, S., Heibel, F., Benaicha, M., and Moulin, B., *Post-transplantation lymphomas and Epstein-Barr virus.* Nephrologie, 1998. 19:481–488.

100. Penn, I., *De novo malignancies in pediatric organ transplant recipients.* Pediatr Transplant, 1998. 2:56–63.

101. LeBlond, V., Sutton, L., Dorent, R., Davi, F., Bitker, M. O., Gabarre, J., Charlotte, F., Ghoussoub, J. J., et al., *Lymphoproliferative disorders after organ transplantation: A report of 24 cases observed in a single center.* J Clin Oncol, 1995. 13:961–968.

102. Mamzer-Brunel, M. F., Bourquelot, P., Hermine, O., Legendre, C., and Kreis, H., *Treatment and prognosis of post-transplant lymphoproliferative disease.* Ann Transplant, 1997. 2:42–48.

103. Hanke, R. J., Greiner, T. C., Smir, B. N., Vose, J. M., Tarantolo, S. R., Bashir, R. M., and Bierman, P. J., *Epstein-Barr virus–associated lymphoproliferative disorder after autologous bone marrow transplantation: Report of two cases.* Bone Marrow Transplant, 1998. 21:1271–1274.

104. Morrison, V. A., Dunn, D. L., Manviel, J. C., Gajl-Peczalska, K. J., and Peterson, B. A., *Clinical characteristics of post-transplant lymphoproliferative disorders.* Am J Med, 1994. 97:14–24.

105. Niedobitek, G., Mutimer, D. J., Williams, A., Whitehead, L., Wilson, P., Rooney, N., Young, L. S., and Hubscher, S. G., *Epstein-Barr virus infection and malignant lymphomas in liver transplant recipients.* Int J Cancer, 1997. 73:514–520.

106. Dusenbery, D., Nalesnik, M. A., Locker, J., and Swerdlow, S. H., *Cytologic features of post-transplant lymphoproliferative disorder.* Diagn Cytopathol, 1997. 16:489–496.

107. Goral, S., Felgar, R., and Shappell, S., *Posttransplantation lymphoproliferative disorder in a renal allograft recipient.* Am J Kidney Dis, 1997. 30:301–307.

108. Chetty, R., Biddolph, S., Kaklamanis, L., Cary, N., Stewart, S., Giatromanolaki, A., and Gatter, K., *bcl-2 protein is strongly expressed in post-transplant lymphoproliferative disorders.* J Pathol, 1996. 180:254–258.

109. Wood, A., Anugs, B., Kestevan, P., Dark, J., Notarianni, G., Miller, S., Howard, M., Proctor, S., et al., *Alpha interferon gene deletions in post-transplant lymphoma.* Br J Haematol, 1997. 98:1002–1003.

CHAPTER
9

Diseases of the Nervous System and the Skin

Neurofibromatosis

Epidemiology. There are various subtypes of neurofibromatosis, each of which has a characteristic inheritance pattern and clinical presentation. Type I neurofibromatosis is also known as von Recklinghausen's disease. It has an autosomal dominant inheritance pattern and occurs with an incidence of 1:3000 to 1:5000 [1]. There is a high rate of spontaneous mutations. Type I neurofibromatosis accounts for 85%–90% of all cases of neurofibromatosis. The diagnosis is based on the presence of at least two of the following criteria: more than 6 café-au-lait macules larger than 5 mm in children (or 15 mm in adults); at least two neurofibromas or one plexiform neurofibroma; axillary or inguinal freckling; optic nerve glioma; two or more Lisch's nodules; distinctive bone lesions; or a parent, sibling, or child with diagnostic criteria for neurofibromatosis type I [2].

Type II neurofibromatosis is much less common, with an incidence of 1:50,000 [3]. Neurofibromatosis type II has a mean age of onset of about 20 years [4]. It has an autosomal dominant inheritance pattern [5]. The diagnosis is based on either the presence of bilateral VIIIth cranial nerve schwannomas or a first-degree relative with type II neurofibromatosis in addition to two of the following: dermal neurofibromas, plexiform neurofibromas, schwannomas, gliomas, meningiomas, or cataracts.

Type III neurofibromatosis is a variant of the disease in which there are features of both types I and II.

This form of the disease appears to be inherited, but the pattern of inheritance has not yet been established.

Type IV neurofibromatosis is a variant of the disease in which lesions are limited to the presence of café-au-lait macules and cutaneous neurofibromas. The inheritance pattern is variable.

Segmental neurobfibromatosis, or type V neurofibromatosis, is a rare subtype. It occurs more commonly in women than in men and has a mean age of onset of 28 years. The cervical or thoracic dermatome is most commonly affected, and lesions are unilateral [6]. A family history of neurofibromatosis cannot be elicited in more than 90% of patients [6].

Type VI neurofibromatosis is characterized solely by the presence of multiple café-au-lait macules, with no other signs or symptoms of the disease. Type VII neurofibromatosis presents with late-onset neurofibromas. Type VIII neurofibromatosis is a miscellaneous category in which patients have neurofibromas, but do not otherwise fit neatly into one of the aforementioned categories.

Cutaneous Features. Neurofibromas are a very common cutaneous manifestation of neurofibromatosis. They usually appear around the onset of puberty and continue to appear throughout the remainder of the affected patient's life. They are usually pedunculated, asymptomatic, soft tumors that can range from several millimeters to multiple centimeters in diameter. They are usually the same color as the surrounding skin or may be slightly hyperpigmented and do not generally have any overlying surface changes. A characteristic "button hole" sign helps make the clinical diagnosis. Rare lesions that appear more plaque-like and atrophic but have the histologic features of neurofibroma have also been reported [7]. Plexiform neurofibromas are most commonly congenital and are clinically apparent early in life. These present as a large, deep swelling in the dermis or subcutaneous tissue. The overlying epidermis may be hyperpigmented and atrophic. These lesions can be painful. When hyperpigmentation is present overlying a plexiform neurofibroma that extends to the midline, there is often involvement of the spinal cord [8]. Neurofibromas may occur as sporadic growths, unassociated with any other findings of neurofibromatosis.

Schwannomas are also common cutaneous tumors in patients with neurofibromatosis. Unlike neurofibromas, these lesions can be tender or painful. They have no characteristic appearance on the skin, except when a direct relationship to an underlying nerve can be identified. Otherwise, schwannomas appear as ill-defined, deep-seated nodules. They are most common on the head, neck, and extremities [9]. Plexiform schwannomas are very rare but may occur with type II neurofibromatosis [10].

Café-au-lait macules are the most common cutaneous manifestation of neurofibromatosis. They are present in up to 82% of patients by the age of 4 years and in up to 99% of all affected individuals with type I neurofibromatosis [11]. They are light brown-tan colored flat lesions that are sharply demarcated. Café-au-lait macules are seen in patients with type II neurofibromatosis but are less common. They also, not infrequently, a sporadic finding, unassociated with neurofibromatosis.

Axillary or inguinal freckling is present in 70%–80% of adults with neurofibromatosis type I. Freckling does not usually occur in patients with other types of neurofibromatosis.

Lisch's nodules, which are collections of melanocytes present within the iris, occur primarily in patients with type I neurofibromatosis and may be present in more than 90% of adults with the disease [12]. They appear by puberty and increase in size with age. They are usually asymptomatic. Cataracts are present in up to 50% of patients with type II neurofibromatosis and may precede the onset of other cutaneous lesions.

Juvenile xanthogranulomas have been reported to occur with increased frequency in patients with type I neurofibromatosis. In addition, it has been shown that in patients with this association there is an increased risk of juvenile chronic myelogenous leukemia [13].

Although there are scattered isolated reports of nevus spilus [14], melanoma [15], and other melanotic lesions [16] occurring in patients with neurofibromatosis, no clear-cut association has been identified.

In one large study, 97% of children under the age of 6 years with type I neurofibromatosis had café-au-lait spots, 81% had freckling of the axilla or inguinal regions, 30% had Lisch's nodules, and 15% demonstrated neurofibromas [17].

Approximately 60% of patients with neurofibromatosis type II have cutaneous neoplasms. Café-au-lait macules were present in about one-third of the patients in this series, but less than 5% had more than six such lesions. The most common cutaneous neoplasm in this group of patients was the schwannoma, followed by neurofibromas [18]. The presence of multiple angiofibromas has been reported in a patient with type II neurofibromatosis [19].

Neurofibromatosis type V, or segmental neurofibromatosis, manifests with café-au-lait spots in about one-fourth of patients, axillary freckling in about 10% of patients, and neurofibromas in the skin [6].

Localized hypertrichosis, often overlying a cutaneous neurofibroma, has been a presenting feature in patients with neurofibromatosis [20]. Other associated cutaneous neoplasms that have been reported in patients with neurofibromatosis include multiple subungual glomus tumors [21], primary cutaneous meningiomas [22], and Merkel cell carcinomas [23, 24]. Multiple granular cell tumors have also been reported in a child with type I neurofibromatosis [25].

Pruritus has been described as a feature of neurofibromatosis. The itching can be present in skin overlying neurofibromas and in skin that has been recently traumatized. This finding may be related to increased numbers of mast cells within the skin of these patients [8].

Associated Disorders. Patients with neurofibromatosis type I are often of short stature, with 16% of affected children below the 2nd percentile and 50% below the 25th percentile. Macrocephaly and macroglossia are common findings in these patients. Mild mental retardation may be found in 30%–40% of patients with type I neurofibromatosis [26].

Vestibular schwannomas are present in almost 99% of patients with neurofibromatosis type II [4]. Almost half of these patients also have meningiomas, and cataracts are present in about 80% [4]. Other spinal tumors are seen in two-thirds of patients with type II neurofibromatosis, and other central nervous system tumors are present in about 20% [4].

A relationship between neurofibromatosis and childhood chronic myelogenous leukemia has been reported by several groups [27]. Acute lymphoblastic leukemia has also been described in a patient with neurofibromatosis who also had an optic glioma and multiple xanthogranulomas [28]. The association of acute lymphoblastic leukemia and neurofibromatosis has also been observed in a child with multiple juvenile xanthogranulomas [29].

Orthopedic manifestations include scoliosis, kyphosis, and tibial bowing. Other bone lesions include absence of the greater wing of the sphenoid bone leading to exophthalmos. Coexistence of neurofibromatosis type I and multiple sclerosis has been described in several patients [30]. Precocious puberty has also been reported in a child with neurofibromatosis [31].

Increased risk of neoplasms is reported in patients with type I neurofibromatosis. These tumors include rhabdomyosarcomas, fibrosarcomas [32], and Wilms' tumors, and the neural tumors and leukemias described earlier. Familial occurrence of pheochromocytoma has also been associated with type I neurofibromatosis [33]. Hypertension secondary to renal vascular stenosis has been reported in several patients with type I neurofibromatosis.

Histologic Features

Café-au-lait macules. Café-au-Lait macules are characterized by densely pigmented melanocytes and increased melanin within basal keratinocytes. There is no significant increase in number of melanocytes (Fig. 9–1). Although some reports suggest that increased numbers of macromelanosomes are helpful in making the diagnosis of café-au-lait macules [34], subsequent studies have found them to be a nonspecific finding [35]. The following entities must be considered in the histologic differential diagnosis of café-au-lait macules:

- Becker's nevus
- Dermatofibroma (surface)
- Ephelid
- Labial melanotic macule
- Lentigo simplex
- Seborrheic keratosis

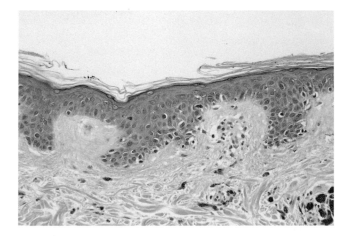

Fig. 9–1. A café-au-lait macule is characterized by increased melanin in basal keratinocytes with no appreciable increase in numbers of melanocytes.

Neurofibroma. Neurofibromas are dermal neoplasms. The epidermis is unremarkable or may be somewhat compressed by the dermal tumor. A grenz zone is usually present (Fig. 9–2 A). The tumor is composed of bland-appearing spindle-shaped cells that course in a myxoid stroma (Fig. 9–2 B). The tumor cells, which consist of mixed numbers of axons and Schwann's cells, have thick, wavy, spindle-shaped nuclei and small amounts of cytoplasm (Fig. 9–2 C). Increased thin-walled blood vessels are present within the lesion. Mast cells are also readily identified. Although reasonably well circumscribed, these neoplasms are not encapsulated. Cutaneous neurofibromas are centered in the dermis, but may extend into the underlying subcutaneous fat. At least 10 different histologic variants of neurofibroma, including epithelioid, cellular, myxoid, glandular, xanthomatized, and neurofibromas with foci of rhabdomyoma have been described [36]. As lesions become older, the nuclei of the tumor cells become focally enlarged and atypical; however, mitotic figures are not found in such cases. These lesions are referred to as *ancient* or *bizarre* neurofibromas. The following entities must be considered in the histologic differential diagnosis of neurofibroma:

- Leiomyoma
- Malignant peripheral nerve sheath tumor
- Neurothekeoma
- Neurotized nevus
- Palisaded encapsulated neuroma
- Schwannoma
- Trichodiscoma

Plexiform neurofibroma. Plexiform neurofibromas are often larger and more cellular than other cutaneous neurofibromas. They are usually centered deeper than the skin or subcutaneous fat, but can arise in these superficial locations. In some areas they appear similar to other neurofibromas, but grow in and around an enlarged, distorted nerve (Fig. 9–3). Multiple fascicles of neural tissue are separated by bands of fibrous tissue. The presence of increased numbers of mitotic figures is suggestive of malignant transformation [37]. Mitoses should be evaluated in the context of growth pattern, nuclear anaplasia, and cellularity in order to assess for likelihood of malignant behavior. Many observers believe that the presence of a single plexiform neurofibroma is pathognomonic for the diagnosis of neurofibromatosis. Others believe that plexiform lesions can occur in patients with no other evidence of the disease [38].

Schwannoma. Schwannomas are encapsulated tumors that are more common in deeper locations than in the skin. The tumors are surrounded by a perineurial capsule. When found in the skin, however, they are usually located in the mid-dermis, underlying flattened

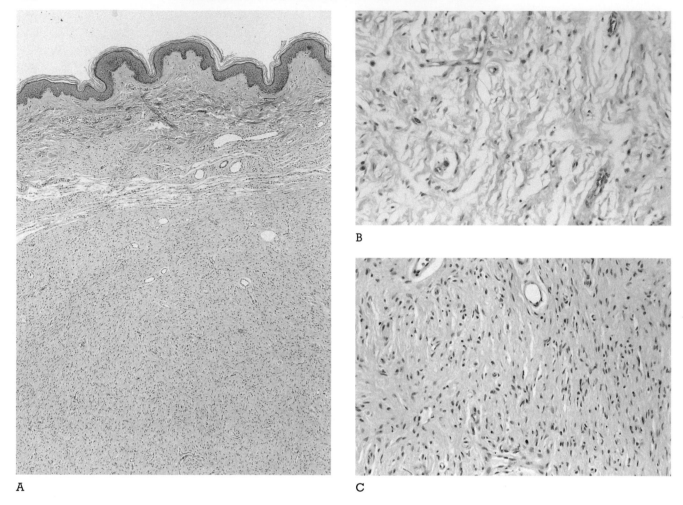

Fig. 9–2. *A,* Neurofibromas are located in the dermis and do not involve the epidermis. A grenz zone is often present. *B,* Spindle-shaped cells course within myxoid stroma in neurofibromas. *C,* Neurofibroma cells are spindle shaped and have small amounts of eosinophilic cytoplasm.

epidermis. The tumor nodule consists of areas with increased cellularity and a more dense, eosinophilic stroma, referred to as *Antoni A areas,* admixed with less cellular areas with a more myxoid-appearing stroma and increased vascularity, referred to as *Antoni B areas* (Fig. 9–4 *A*). The tumor is composed of spindle-shaped, wavy cells that form palisading arrangements known as *Verocay bodies* within the Antoni A areas (Fig. 9–4 *B*). Many variants of schwannoma, including plexiform, ancient, cellular, melanotic, epithelioid, angiomatoid, granular, and pacinian, have been described [37].

Plexiform schwannomas are very rare neoplasms and are not usually associated with neurofibromatosis, unlike plexiform neurofibromas [39]. Multiple nodules, separated by compressed fibrous tissue, are present in the dermis. Antoni A areas predominate in these lesions. These lesions are not associated with malignant degeneration [37].

Ancient schwannomas are typical schwannomas that have undergone changes including cytologic atypia with bizarre nuclear pleomorphism, calcification, cystic degeneration, hemorrhage, and fibrosis. Increased cellularity is not seen in these lesions, which helps to differentiation them from malignant foci in cellular schwannomas [37].

Cellular schwannomas are more cellular than the usual schwannoma, have occasional typical mitotic figures, and also display some degree of cytologic atypia. Necrosis is not a feature of these lesions. They tend, however, to remain encapsulated and behave in a benign fashion [40].

Lisch's nodules. Lisch's nodules are clusters of densely pigmented spindle-shaped melanocytes and nests of more epithelioid-shaped cells present in the submucosa of the iris.

Malignant peripheral nerve sheath tumors. Malignant peripheral nerve sheath tumors, also known as *neu-*

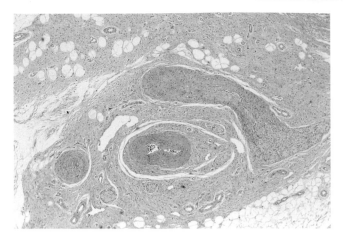

Fig. 9–3. Large nerve bundles are present within the neural proliferation in plexiform neurofibromas.

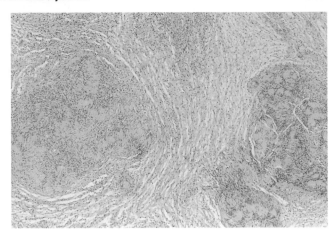

A

rofibrosarcomas or *malignant schwannomas*, are rare tumors that are associated with type I neurofibromatosis in 50% of cases [41]. Only 2%–3% of patients with neurofibromatosis will, however, develop one of these neoplasms [42]. These tumors are most common in adulthood, and the lower extremities are a common site. They can arise de novo, but more commonly are associated with long-standing neurofibromas [43]. Histologic features consist of a proliferation of spindle-shaped cells that have areas of dense cellularity alternating with paucicellular, myxoid areas located primarily in the subcutis or deep dermis (Fig. 9–5 A). The tumors tend to be asymmetric and poorly circumscribed. Zones of necrosis may be present in a minority of cases. Nuclear atypia and pleomorphism are seen, and mitoses, including atypical forms, can be focally abundant [43] (Fig. 9–5 B).

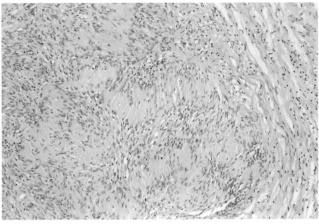

B

Fig. 9–4. *A*, Antoni A and Antoni B areas are present in many schwannomas. *B*, Verocay bodies are clearly distinguished in Antoni A areas of schwannoma.

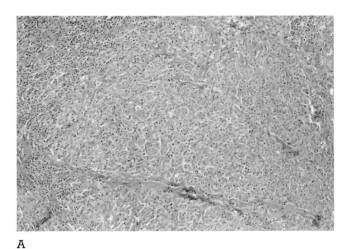

A

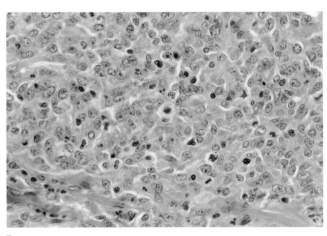

B

Fig. 9–5. *A*, Malignant schwannoma is characterized by sheets and nests of epithelioid cells. *B*, Marked cytologic atypia and mitotic activity are seen in most malignant schwannomas.

Special Studies. No special studies are ordinarily necessary to make a histologic diagnosis of the cutaneous lesions of neurofibromatosis. Occasionally, a Masson's trichrome stain may be helpful in distinguishing the collagen of a schwannoma from the smooth muscle of a leiomyoma with a pseudo-palisading appearance. Additionally, an S100 protein antibody stain can also be used to distinguish these two entities.

Pathogenesis. The gene for neurofibromatosis type I is located on chromosome 17q11.2 [30, 44]. The gene product may interact with a ras-like gene to inhibit cell growth. When the gene is defective, its inhibitory properties may be lost, leading to inappropriate cell growth. Loss of heterozygosity of chromosome 22 and ring chromosome formation have been associated with neurofibromatosis II [23, 24]. The gene locus resides on 22q12 [5] and may be associated with a tumor suppressor gene that results in tumorigenesis when it is lost.

Tuberous Sclerosis

Epidemiology. Tuberous sclerosis is inherited in an autosomal dominant manner. Up to 75% of cases may arise from spontaneous mutation. The prevalence of the disease varies from 1/6000 to 1/170,000, depending on the population studied [45, 46]. The disease occurs with equal frequency in men and women and across all races [47]. The gene for tuberous sclerosis is located on chromosome 9q34 [48]. Chromosome 16p13 has also been implicated in equal numbers of patients with tuberous sclerosis [49].

Cutaneous Features. Cutaneous manifestations are present in as many as 96% of patients with tuberous sclerosis [50]. Hypomelanotic macules and forehead plaques tend to occur in younger patients, while angiofibromas and periungual fibromas appear later.

Hypopigmented macules, known as *ash leaf spots,* are present at birth in up to 90% of patients with tuberous sclerosis. These are best viewed with a Wood's light. They are usually 1–3 cm in diameter. Similar-appearing small hypopigmented macules may also be present.

Shagreen patches are orange-pink plaques that are most commonly found on the back. The skin surface has increased markings. Shagreen patches occur in about 40% of patients with tuberous sclerosis.

Angiofibromas, also known as *adenoma sebaceum,* are skin-colored papules or nodules that are most prevalent on the midportion of the face. These are symmetrically distributed on the nose and cheeks. More than half of all patients with tuberous sclerosis will develop these facial lesions during childhood or early adulthood.

Periungual fibromas, also known as Koenen's papules, are seen in up to 20% of patients with tuberous sclero-

sis and usually do not appear before puberty. They are smooth, firm nodules that appear around the nail plate.

The forehead plaque is described as a soft red or yellow plaque and has been observed to be the presenting sign of tuberous sclerosis [51]. It occurs in about one-fourth of affected patients [52].

Café-au-lait macules have also been described in patients with tuberous sclerosis [47]. Widespread angiokeratomas were reported in a patient with tuberous sclerosis and no evidence of Fabry's disease [53].

Associated Disorders. Involvement of many organ systems has been documented in patients with tuberous sclerosis. The central nervous system is the most commonly affected organ system. Its involvement may manifest with seizures in infancy in up to 90% of patients [54], mental retardation in about half of affected patients [55], and neoplasms including retinal astrocytomas in about 10%–15% of cases [11]. Patients with seizure are often of subnormal intelligence, while those without seizure are of normal intelligence [56].

Renal angiomyolipomas are present in at least half of the patients with tuberous sclerosis [57]. They may be asymptomatic or may cause hematuria, proteinuria, and abdominal pain. There is also an association with infantile polycystic disease [58].

Hamartomas in the liver are seen more commonly in affected females [59]. Cardiac rhabdomyomas are common in children and may lead to arrhythmias or emboli, but often regress without treatment [60]. Smooth muscle hamartomas may be seen in the lungs [47].

Dental pits are a common and highly specific finding in patients with tuberous sclerosis [61]. Other dental anomalies may also be seen [11].

Histologic Features. Ash leaf spots and the smaller 1–3 mm hypopigmented macules seen in tuberous sclerosis have a similar histologic appearance. According to some observers, there is a decrease in the number of melanocytes. The melanocytes that are present have fewer than normal numbers of melanosomes [62]. Others report normal numbers of melanocytes and attribute the hypopigmentation to the decrease in numbers of melanosomes [63].

Shagreen patches are connective tissue hamartomas. They are characterized by an abnormal pattern of collagen distribution within the reticular dermis (Fig. 9–6 A). The bundles of collagen are often increased in size, and they stain with increased eosinophilia than the surrounding background collagen. The bundles may be oriented in a more vertical direction, traveling almost perpendicular to the skin surface, than the normal horizontal orientation. Elastic tissue fibers may be decreased in number in lesional skin (Fig. 9–6 B). This can be a difficult diagnosis to make histologically, and

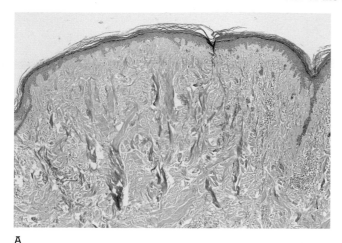
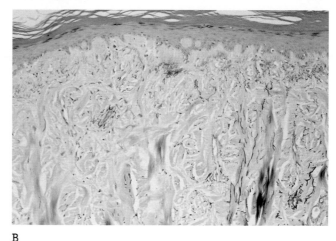

A

B

Fig. 9–6. *A,* A shagreen patch demonstrates the same histologic features as a connective tissue nevus, with markedly increased dermal collagen. *B,* Elastic tissue fibers are diminished in a shagreen patch, as is demonstrated by the Verhoeff-van Gieson stain.

many biopsy specimens may appear essentially normal. The following entities must be considered in the histologic differential diagnosis of shagreen patches:

- Connective tissue nevus (sporadic)
- Morphea/progressive systemic sclerosis
- Normal back skin

Angiofibromas are another common cutaneous manifestation of tuberous sclerosis. These lesions have the same histologic findings as fibrous papules. The epidermis is thinned, with effacement of rete ridges. In some cases, there may be a slight increase in number of melanocytes. The melanocytes are often slightly enlarged. The papillary and reticular dermis is replaced with densely fibrotic collagen. Coursing between the collagen bundles are increased numbers of spindle-shaped cells, some of which have a stellate appearance and can be quite enlarged (Fig. 9–7 *A*). Blood vessels are ectatic but have no changes in the endothelial cells (Fig. 9–7 *B*). Periappendageal fibrosis is present in many cases and may have a concentric configuration. Appendageal atrophy may be present in long-standing lesions. The following entities must be considered in the histologic differential diagnosis of angiofibroma:

- Capillary hemangioma
- Fibrous papule
- Multinucleate cell angiohistiocytoma
- Neurotized nevus
- Perifollicular fibroma
- Trichodiscoma

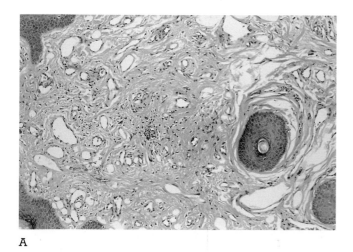
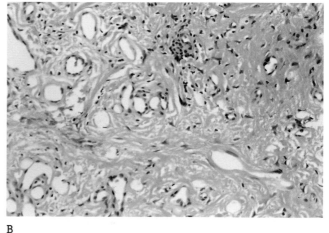

A

B

Fig. 9–7. *A,* An angiofibroma is characterized by increased dermal collagen, ectatic vessels, perifollicular fibrosis, and stellate fibroblasts. *B,* Stellate fibroblasts and vascular ectasia are prominent in many angiofibromas.

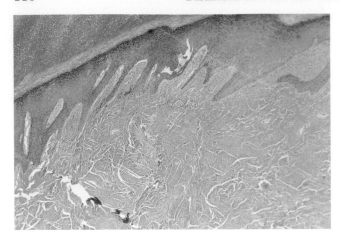

Fig. 9–8. A subungual fibroma is characterized by dense collagen bundles throughout the dermis.

Periungual fibromas are similarly collagenomas. They appear similar to shagreen patches, with thick bundles of dense collagen and diminished elastic tissue fibers (Fig. 9–8).

Special Studies. It is sometimes difficult to evaluate the amount of epidermal melanin present within lesions clinically thought to be ash leaf spots. In this circumstance, a Fontana stain for melanin is often helpful. No other special studies are required to diagnose the cutaneous lesions associated with tuberous sclerosis.

Pathogenesis. Many hypotheses have been put forth to explain the findings in tuberous sclerosis. These include dysregulation of paracrine growth factors [64], disruption of neuronal migration [65], and defective catecholamine synthesis [66]. Tuberin, a gene product of the defective 16p13 chromosome, is important in regulation of cell growth and is believed to be involved in the pathogenesis of the tumors found in patients with tuberous sclerosis [63].

Refsum's Syndrome

Epidemiology. Refsum's syndrome is inherited in an autosomal recessive manner [67]. This slowly progressive disease results in death due to respiratory failure. Cardiac arrhythmias can also occur and may be fatal [67].

Cutaneous Features. Ichthyosis is present in patients with Refsum's syndrome [68]. It is of limited distribution [67]. The ichthyosis appears as small white scales or, in some cases, may resemble ichthyosis vulgaris. The scales may not be apparent until adulthood.

Associated Disorders. Night blindness due to retinitis pigmentosa often occurs during childhood and may

progress with age [67]. Recurrent segmental demyelinization of motor units can occur, resulting in weakness and progressive loss of motor function. Ataxia can be present [69]. Nerve deafness may also be present [67].

Histologic Features. Routine histologic sections reveal skin with overlying hyperkeratosis and usually hypogranulosis [67]. Mild hypergranulosis has also been described. Acanthosis is usually present. The keratohyaline granules are normal [70]. Lipid-containing vacuoles may be seen within basal keratinocytes on routine light microscopy. These vacuoles are easily detected with electron microscopy [68].

Special Studies. The diagnosis of Refsum's disease can be confirmed by finding excess phytanic acid in the triglyceride portion of serum lipids [67]. A stain for neutral lipids will stain the vacuoles present within the basal keratinocytes, but frozen tissue is required to perform this procedure [68].

Pathogenesis. Accumulation of phytanic acid has been implicated as the defect in patients with Refsum's disease [71]. This accumulation is due to a defect in fibroblast α-oxidation of phytanic acid [71, 72] as a result of a deficiency in phytanoyl-CoA hydroxylase [73].

Sjögren-Larsson Syndrome

Epidemiology. Sjögren-Larsson syndrome is a rare, inherited neurocutaneous disorder in which patients have ichthyosis, mental retardation, and spastic diplegia or tetraplegia [74]. It has an autosomal recessive inheritance pattern [75]. Linkage to the short arm of chromosome 17 has also been reported in some affected kindreds [76, 77].

Cutaneous Features. The degree of ichthyosis does not appear to correlate with severity of neurologic symptoms [78]. Patients are born with slight to moderate, generalized ichthyosis, with some tendency to spare the face [79]. The ichthyosis becomes fully developed during infancy. Changes are most pronounced in the neck, flexural surfaces, and lower abdomen. In these regions, the scaling can become hyperpigmented. Erythroderma is rare. There are no changes described in the hair or nails or in the ability to sweat [79].

Associated Disorders. Sjögren-Larsson syndrome is associated with eye problems, including maculopathies and astigmatisms, that can lead to decreased visual acuity [80]. All patients with the syndrome who are more than 1 year of age display glistening dots in their fundi [78]. In addition to the motor defects, other neurologic deficits have been reported, including speech defects, seizures, mental retardation, and pyramidal tract disorders. One patient with Sjögren-Larsson syndrome was reported to have an associated Dandy-Walker malformation [81].

Histologic Features. Histologic changes include marked hyperkeratosis with slight follicular prominence. Hypergranulosis is also present. The epidermis is diffusely acanthotic and may be papillomatous. A slight lymphohistiocytic inflammatory infiltrate is seen in the dermis [82, 83]. Electron microscopy reveals abnormal lamellar inclusions in the cytoplasm of cells within the stratum corneum. In addition, increased numbers of mitochondria are present in the basal keratinocytes of affected skin [84]. It is not possible to make an unequivocal diagnosis of Sjögren-Larsson syndrome based solely on histopathologic findings. Special studies demonstrating altered enzyme activity are necessary (see later).

Special Studies. Frozen sections of skin can be assayed for the presence of fatty aldehyde dehydrogenase activity [85]. A deficiency in this enzyme provides strong support for the diagnosis of Sjögren-Larsson syndrome [86]. This technique is not widely performed.

Pathogenesis. Patients with Sjögren-Larsson syndrome suffer from a defect in the activity of the fatty aldehyde dehydrogenase enzyme. The defect arises from point mutation [74]. Ceramides 1 and 6 are both deficient in patients with Sjögren-Larsson syndrome, which serves to disrupt the normal skin barrier function in these patients [87]. In the same patients, glucosylceramides have been demonstrated to be deficient in neural tissues [87].

Rud's Syndrome.

Patients who were previously diagnosed as having Rud's syndrome have now been reclassified as having one of several different congenital ichthyotic syndromes. This heterogeneous group of patients has a constellation of ichthyosis, hypogonadism, small stature, mental retardation, epilepsy, and, rarely, retinitis pigmentosa. It is now believed that all of these patients are better regarded as having one of the other neurocutaneous syndromes [88]. As previously described, Rud's syndrome had an autosomal recessive inheritance pattern and was characterized by lamellar ichthyosis that could be erythrodermic [67].

KID Syndrome.

KID syndrome is a neurocutaneous disorder originally described in 1981 in which patients were described as having the triad of keratitis,

ichthyosis, and deafness [89]. It has subsequently been suggested that the cutaneous changes are not those of ichthyosis [90].

Epidemiology. KID syndrome is a rare, probably inherited syndrome that is characterized by an ectodermal defect. The skin and the central nervous system are affected. The mode of inheritance is not fully understood. Vertical transmission of KID syndrome has been reported, as has transmission to two half siblings by an unaffected mother, suggesting some form of autosomal dominant transmission [91–93]. An autosomal recessive mode of inheritance has also been reported [94]. Other cases appear to arise spontaneously [95].

Cutaneous Features. The cutaneous findings in KID syndrome have been described as a distinctive pattern of fine scaling with follicular hyperkeratotic spines and a reticulated pattern of hyperkeratosis on the palms and soles [89]. In other patients, the hyperkeratosis is more diffuse and leads to an erythrodermic appearance [92]. These changes have been described as being an erythrokeratoderma and have been found in up to 89% of patients with KID syndrome [90]. Others have described the diffuse clinical changes as being similar to a heavy-grain leather-like keratoderma [96]. In the same series, 79% of affected patients had alopecia [90]. The reticulated hyperkeratosis of the palms and soles is seen in about half of patients with KID syndrome [90]. A similar process may be found on the face. Later lesions are described as verrucous, brown-yellow plaques [93]. Peribuccal grooves have also been reported [96].

Associated Disorders. Frequent cutaneous infections are present in 50%–75% of patients with KID syndrome [89, 93]. Bacterial, [89, 93], fungal [97], and disseminated viral infections have been reported in these patients [98].

The corneal epithelium is involved with a vascularizing keratitis in patients with KID syndrome [89]. This defect occurs in up to 95% of patients with the syndrome [90]. Photophobia is common.

The inner ear is also affected, causing neurosensory hearing loss in patients with KID syndrome [89]. The deafness is a feature in 90% of patients with the syndrome [90]. It is caused by a defect in the cochleosaccular region of the temporal bone [99]. Deafness may be total and present at birth or may develop during childhood [100]. Other central nervous system anomalies such as cerebellar hypoplasia have been reported, but occur much less frequently [101].

In one affected family, progressive cirrhosis has also been reported in association with KID syndrome [93]. This was described as a micronodular cirrhosis with abundant Mallory's hyaline and increased copper storage. Rare patients with KID syndrome have been reported with arthropathies and musculoskeletal problems [102]. Hyperhidrosis and growth retardation have also been reported [93, 96, 97, 100, 103, 104]. In rare cases, multiple squamous cell carcinomas have been reported in patients with KID syndrome, occasionally resulting in death from metastatic disease [96, 105].

Histologic Features. Histologic changes in the skin of patients with KID syndrome include orthokeratotic hyperkeratosis, papillomatosis, and slight acanthosis. Rare foci of parakeratosis may be present. The granular layer is preserved. Rare follicular plugs and similar plugs obstructing the acrosyringia may be present [106]. The dermis may have a minimal increase in the number of perivascular lymphocytes [100]. There are no changes in the apocrine structures [101], and a focal decrease in the numbers of eccrine structures is variably seen [96, 100]. Dyskeratosis of the corneal epithelium with subsequent corneal atrophy are present with slight lymphocytic infiltrates [107].

Special Studies. There are no special studies currently available to aid in making the diagnosis of KID syndrome.

Pathogenesis. The pathogenesis of KID syndrome is currently unknown.

Vogt-Koyanagi-Harada Syndrome

Epidemiology. Vogt-Koyanagi-Harada syndrome is a rare disorder that affects pigmented tissue, including the skin, eyes, and occasionally the ears. The disease is strongly associated with several human leukocyte antigen (HLA) subtypes, including HLA-DR4 in Japanese and Mexican patients [108] and white patients [109] and HLA-DR1 and HLA-DQ4 [110]. The disease has also been reported in identical twins [111]. The authors note a difference in onset of 16 years between the twins and suggest that exogenous factors may also play a role in the development of the disease. The disease usually develops in adolescents and young adults, but has been reported in young children as well [112].

Cutaneous Features. Vitiligo is the most common manifestation of Vogt-Koyanagi-Harada syndrome [113]. An erythematous, edematous eruption preceding the vitiligo has also been reported in some patients [114]. Halo nevi have been seen in association with vitiligo [115]. A periocular distribution to the vitiligo is frequently seen.

Associated Disorders. Patients with Vogt-Koyanagi-Harada syndrome have bilateral diffuse uveitis, which

is often associated with central nervous system and auditory anomalies [116]. Approximately half the patients will develop long-term visual impairment secondary to cataracts, glaucoma, and subretinal neovascular membranes [116]. Other patients have been described with tonic pupils, anesthesia of the corneas, and inability to accommodate [117]. Angle closure glaucoma has also been reported [118].

Vogt-Koyanagi-Harada syndrome is an autoimmune disease that has been associated with a number of other autoimmune processes, including hypothyroidism, diabetes mellitus [119], primary adrenal insufficiency, hypoparathyroidism, Graves' disease, alopecia universalis [120], and Hashimoto's thyroiditis [121]. It has also been reported in a patient with psoriasis [122], in a patient with a positive rheumatoid factor [123], in patients with Hodgkin's disease [124, 125], and after bone marrow transplantation [126]. Non-Hodgkin's B-cell lymphoma has been reported to develop in the eye of a patient with Vogt-Koyanagi-Harada syndrome [127].

Histologic Features. Histologic features of the skin in Vogt-Koyanagi-Harada syndrome are indistinguishable from those in vitiligo. A loss of melanocytes occurs in affected areas (Fig. 9–9 *A*). There is a loss of melanin pigment within the keratinocytes [128] (Fig. 9–9 *B*). A sparse lymphocytic inflammatory infiltrate may be present around the superficial vascular plexus, as well as around hair follicles and sweat glands in early, edematous lesions [129]. A more pronounced infiltrate has been described in patients with marked erythema [114]. There is minimal, if any, melanin pigment present in the dermis. In the eye, a non-necrotizing, diffuse granulomatous infiltrate is present in patients with uveitis [116].

Special Studies. A Fontana stain for melanin can be helpful in highlighting the change in melanin provided that comparison with normally pigmented epidermis is available. In some cases, an immunostain against S100 protein may be useful in determining numbers of melanocytes.

Pathogenesis. Vogt-Koyanagi-Harada syndrome is thought to be an autoimmune process directed against melanocytes [116]. A parallel process is implicated in the destruction of melanocytes within the skin and in visual and cochlear pigment-producing cells derived from the neural crest. Immunohistochemical studies reveal a cutaneous infiltrate of CD4+, CD29+ HLA-DR+ memory T-helper cells [130]. These T-helper cells express the Fas antigen, and this may represent the immunopathologic mechanism of this disease [131]. Smaller numbers of CD8+ T cells and B cells are present in the infiltrate. It has been suggested that a cell-mediated immune response is pivotal in the pathogen-

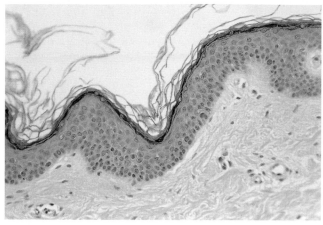
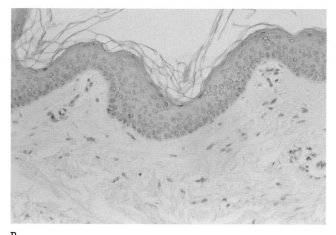

A   B

Fig. 9–9. *A,* Vitiligo, as seen in Vogt-Koyanangi-Hirada syndrome, has a marked decrease in melanocytes within affected epidermis. *B,* A Fontana melanin stain demonstrates complete lack of melanin in vitiliginous skin from a patient with Vogt-Koyanangi-Hirada syndrome.

esis of the vitiligo [129]. Epstein-Barr virus has been recovered from the vitreous of a patient with Vogt-Koyanagi-Harada syndrome, but this does not appear to be an invariable association [132].

Rubinstein-Taybi Syndrome

Epidemiology. Rubinstein-Taybi syndrome is a rare heritable multisystem disease that occurs in about 1 in 300,000 births and with equal incidence in boys and girls [133]. Autosomal dominant transmission has been reported [134]. In most monozygotic twins, if one is affected, the other is similarly affected [135].

Cutaneous Features. The major cutaneous finding in patients with Rubinstein-Taybi syndrome is the spontaneous appearance of keloids, which are often enormous [136–139]. Keloids appear in only about 5% of patients with the syndrome [136]. The appearance of multiple pilomatricomas is less commonly associated with this syndrome [140, 141]. Rare cases of piebaldism have also been reported in association with Rubinstein-Taybi syndrome [142]. Abnormal dermatoglyphic patterns have been described in these patients [143].

Associated Disorders. Rubinstein-Taybi syndrome is a multisystem disorder with a broad range of presentations. Patients often have broad, short terminal phalanges of the thumbs and halluces. They may also have a beaked nose, abnormal slanting of the palpebral fissures, hypertelorism, and a grimacing smile. These patients tend to be small and have marked retardation of mental, motor, and social skills. There is a characteristic stiff gait. In men, delay or absence of testicular descent may be present [144].

Cardiac anomalies affect about one-third of patients with Rubinstein-Taybi syndrome. These include atrial septal defects, ventricular septal defects, patent ductus arteriosus, coarctation of the aorta, pulmonic stenosis, and bicuspid aortic valves [145].

Tumors of the central nervous system, including oligodendroglioma, medulloblastoma [146], granular cell tumor [147], neuroblastoma, and meningioma are seen in patients with Rubinstein-Taybi syndrome [148]. Nasopharyngeal rhabdomyosarcomas [149], leiomyosarcomas, seminomas and embryonal carcinomas, odontomas, choristomas, and dermoid cysts have also been associated [148]. Other disorders rarely associated with the Rubinstein-Taybi syndrome include congenital glaucoma [150], thymic hypoplasia [151], acute leukemia [152], hypoplastic kidneys [153], and skeletal anomalies [154].

Histologic Features. The histologic findings of the keloids in Rubinstein-Taybi syndrome are indistinguishable from those of keloids in other clinical settings. A flattened epidermis is compressed by a nodule of collagen in the dermis. Collagen bundles are thickened and more eosinophilic than surrounding normal collagen (Fig. 9–10). Increased fibroblasts may be present in early lesions. Later lesions are relatively paucicellular.

Special Studies. There are no special studies that help make the diagnosis of Rubinstein-Taybi syndrome.

Pathogenesis. A chromosomal deletion of 16p13.3 is found in approximately 12% of patients with Rubinstein-Taybi syndrome. There are no apparent clinical differences between those with the syndrome who have

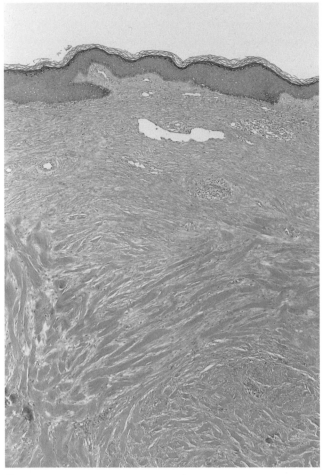

A

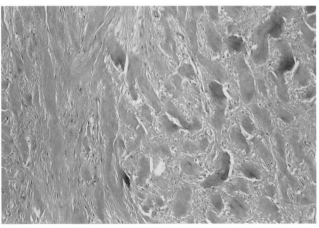

B

Fig. 9–10. *A*, A keloid is characterized by haphazardly oriented bundles of thick collagen within the dermis. *B*, Higher magnification of a keloid demonstrates the markedly thickened and very eosinophilic collagen bundles.

the chromosomal defect and those with the syndrome who do not display this aberration [155]. It is not yet clear what the role of this chromosomal deletion and its subsequent genetic alterations plays in the pathogenesis of this disease.

Myotonic Dystrophy

Epidemiology. Myotonic dystrophy is the most commonly inherited neuromuscular disease. It is inherited in an autosomal dominant manner [156]. Myotonic dystrophy can be present at birth or can be acquired later in life. Longevity is diminished, with most patients dying before age 65 years. Death is most frequently due to pneumonia and cardiac arrhythmias [157].

Cutaneous Features. The most frequent cutaneous association with myotonic dystrophy is the presence of pilomatricomas [158–163]. The clinical appearance of these lesions is similar to that of spontaneously occurring pilomatricomas. Deep dermal, firm bluish nodules with no surface changes are seen, most commonly on the upper extremities and the face and scalp.

Other cutaneous changes found in patients with myotonic dystrophy include generalized cutis marmorata [164], cutis verticis gyrata [165], and Raynaud's syndrome [164]. Multiple basal cell carcinomas have also been reported in a patient with myotonic dystrophy [166], as has the constellation of myotonic dystrophy and pilomatricomas in a patient with a family history of melanoma [161].

Associated Disorders. Patients with myotonic dystrophy have a characteristic facies, with muscular paresis and atrophy. They tend to have slurred speech and below normal intelligence [164]. Medullary carcinoma of the thyroid has been described in a patient with myotonic dystrophy and multiple pilomatricomas [167].

Several defects in the immune system have been described in patients with myotonic dystrophy. Abnormal granulocyte function has been reported [168], as has an abnormal contact sensitization response [169].

Histologic Features. The pilomatricomas that occur in myotonic dystrophy are indistinguishable from sporadically occurring neoplasms. Pilomatricomas are located within the dermis and may extend into the underlying subcutaneous fat (Fig. 9–11 *A*). They are composed of two populations of cells (Fig. 9–11 *B*). There is a population of basaloid cells that have a high nuclear:cytoplasmic ratio and are mitotically active (Fig. 9–11 *C*). These cells undergo abrupt keratinization in the central portion of the cystic cavity often formed by the tumor. Other cells present in the neoplasm have been described as "ghost cells." These cells, which are dead, retain the architectural features of mature keratinocytes while losing their nuclei and are a characteristic feature of these lesions. Calcification is common, as is a marked granulomatous inflammatory reaction to the keratinized ghost cells making contact with the dermis.

Special Studies. There are no special studies required to make the diagnosis of pilomatricoma.

Pathogenesis. Myotonic dystrophy has been shown to be caused by increased numbers of cytosine-thymine-guanine nucleotide repeats on the long arm of chromosome 19 [170]. It is not known what the relationship is between multiple pilomatricomas and myotonic dystrophy.

Sneddon's Syndrome

Epidemiology. Sneddon's syndrome is defined as the constellation of cutaneous livedo reticularis and cerebrovascular accidents. Its incidence has been estimated to be about 4 cases per year per 1 million people [171].

Cutaneous Features. The cutaneous manifestation of Sneddon's syndrome consists of erythematous patches in a livedoid or net-like pattern on the lower legs or frequently generalized [172].

Associated Disorders. Other organs are often involved in Sneddon's syndrome. Vascular occlusion is present in the central nervous system and can also be seen in the heart, leading to myocardial infarction and valvulopathies. Cerebrovascular accidents are the most common central nervous system finding, but psychiatric disturbances have also been described in these patients [173]. Venous thrombosis, arterial hypertension, and fetal death have also been reported. Similar vascular lesions have been reported in the kidney [174].

Autoimmune diseases occur in about 20% of patients diagnosed with Sneddon's syndrome. Schellong et al. [175] suggest dividing patients with this syndrome into a primary group, in whom no other etiologies for vascular thrombosis are present, and a secondary group, in whom etiologic agents may be present to explain the vascular obstructions. Another patient with essential thrombocythemia was reported to have Sneddon's syndrome and would probably fit into the group of patients with secondary Sneddon's syndrome [176]. Similarly, a group of 10 patients with circulating lupus anticoagulant and symptoms of Sneddon's syndrome would be classified as having the secondary type of disease [177].

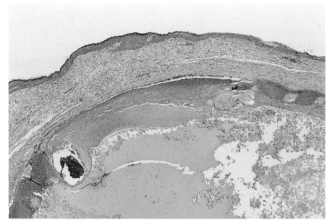

A

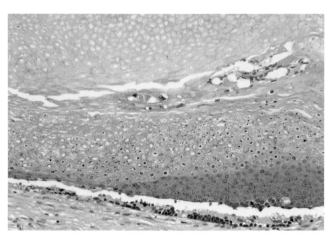

B

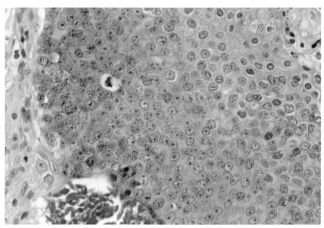

C

Fig. 9–11. *A*, Pilomatricoma is a sharply demarcated dermal neoplasm. *B*, Basaloid cells and "ghost cells" are immediately adjacent in pilomatricomas. *C*, Abundant mitoses and immature-appearing keratinocytes are present within the basaloid component of pilomatricoma.

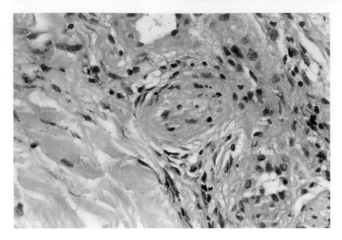

Fig. 9–12. Sneddon's syndrome is characterized by occluded dermal blood vessels in the absence of significant inflammation.

A single patient with coexisting annular atrophic lichen planus and Sneddon's syndrome has been reported [171]. Another patient with the syndrome also had shortening of his fingers and toes [173].

Histologic Features. Histologic changes in Sneddon's syndrome include endothelial cell proliferation within the intima of affected vessels with production of fibromucinous matrix [172]. Fibrin also accumulates in vessel walls. This progression leads to vascular obstruction and ultimately to the obliteration of the dermal arterioles [178] and deterioration of the internal elastic lamina [171] (Fig. 9–12).

Special Studies. No special studies are necessary to make the diagnosis of Sneddon's syndrome.

Pathogenesis. The pathogenesis of Sneddon's syndrome remains unknown [175].

Hypomelanosis of Ito (Incontinentia Pigmenti Achromians)

Epidemiology. Hypomelanosis of Ito was seen in about 1 in 8000 to 1 in 10,000 unselected patients in a children's hospital [179]. This is a disease that is present at birth or shortly thereafter and affects boys and girls approximately equally [180]. Up to 94% of patients with hypomelanosis of Ito have extracutaneous abnormalities [179]. About half of these patients have significant mental retardation, and many others show lesser degrees of decreased mentation. Only 22% have normal intelligence [180]. There is little evidence of an inherited basis for the disease, but, rather, it appears that the disease may arise from a chromosomal mo-

saicism. [181]. In some cases, an autosomal dominant inheritance pattern has been described [179]. A wide range of chromosomal mosaicisms have been described, with no obvious consistent pattern. A subset of female patients has been described in whom a balanced X; autosome translocation is present [182]. In another series, only 3 of 19 patients with hypomelanosis of Ito had chromosomal abnormalities [183].

Cutaneous Features. The characteristic cutaneous changes seen in hypomelanosis of Ito are generalized, hypopigmented patches on the trunk and extremities. Many patients display linear streaks of hypopigmentation that have a swirling appearance [184]. The trunk and proximal extremities are the most commonly affected sites. Pigmentary changes are present in up to 97% of affected patients during childhood.

Other cutaneous lesions were found in about one-third of patients in one large series. These included café-au-lait spots, angiomatous hamartomas, nevus marmorata, nevus of Ota, mongolian spots, and heterochromias of the hair and irises [179]. Rare cases of hypertrichosis associated with the hypopigmented streaks following the lines of Blashko have been reported [185]. Hypomelanosis of Ito coexisted in one patient with palmoplantar keratoderma [186].

Associated Disorders. Patients with hypomelanosis of Ito display a wide range of associated disorders of the central nervous system. These include arteriovenous malformations [187], brain tumors such as medulloblastoma [188], epilepsy in about half of patients [179], mental retardation, and autism [180]. Sensorineural deafness has also been reported in these patients [189]. Macrocephaly and microcephaly also occur in patients with hypomelanosis of Ito [179].

Less commonly, anomalies of organ systems other than the skin and central nervous system may be affected. Defects in the musculoskeletal system such as ectrodactyly, cleft lip, and cleft palate occur [190]. Hemifacial hypoplasia has also been reported in these patients [191]. Hemihypertrophy, syndactyly, and scoliosis have been associated [181]. Hypomelanosis of Ito has been associated with precocious puberty [192]. Genital anomalies, congenital heart disease, and abnormalities of the teeth may also be seen [179]. There is a report of a patient with hypomelanosis of Ito with segmental glomerular disease [193]. It is not yet established if this represents a fortuitous occurrence.

Histologic Features. Hypopigmented areas demonstrate melanocytes with shortened dendritic processes and decreased amounts of melanin [194]. In rare cases, a reduction in the number of melanocytes along the basal layer of the epidermis can be detected on routine histologic sections [195]. In most cases, the numbers of melanocytes appear to be normal and the hypopigmentation appears to be related to decreased basal keratinocyte melanin [184]. There is no inflammatory infiltrate, and no pigment incontinence is seen within the dermis [184]. Electron microscopic studies reveal only rare cytoplasmic projections and poorly formed organelles [195, 196].

Special Studies. In cases in which it is difficult to adequately evaluate numbers of melanocytes, an S100 stain can be useful. In cases in which melanin pigment changes are not readily apparent, a Fontana stain for melanin may help. In most cases, these special studies are not necessary to make the diagnosis. Karyotyping to detect mosaicisms may be helpful in the full workup of these patients [197].

Pathogenesis. It has been suggested that hypomelanosis of Ito reflects a biochemical defect in all tissues derived from the near-ectodermal anlage [194].

Incontinentia Pigmenti

Epidemiology. Incontinentia pigmenti is an X-linked dominant genodermatosis that is usually lethal in boys. Two forms of the condition have been described and termed incontinentia pigmenti type I and type II [198].

Although incontinentia pigmenti is far more common in girls, it does rarely occur in boys and is usually more severe in boys [199]. These children are afflicted with type II incontinentia pigmenti. Gonadal mosaicisms have been reported in affected boys [200]. Sex chromosome aneuploidy is more likely to be present in these patients, as is a higher rate of mental retardation, than in the general population [199]. There is an increased association with Klinefelter's syndrome and incontinentia pigmenti [201, 202]. Patients with neonatal seizures have a poor prognosis for normal development [203].

Cutaneous Features. Cutaneous changes are present in approximately 95% of patients with incontinentia pigmenti. The classic disease has three stages of evolution. The initial phase of the disease is characterized by vesicles and bullae and usually presents within the first 2 weeks of life; it is almost always present within the first year. In some patients, the cutaneous lesions may begin in utero, and these patients are born displaying later changes. Vesicles are present on an erythematous base and are predominantly on the extremities. In some patients, vesicles may have a linear distribution. The vesicles are not distributed in a dermatomal pattern and may cross the midline. They may pattern along

Blaschko's lines. Vesicles progress into pustules and usually resolve within 1–4 weeks. The vesicles may be pruritic, but are most commonly asymptomatic.

The next phase of the disease is characterized by verrucous epidermal papules and plaques, which range from 0.5 to 1.0 cm in diameter. These usually present between the second and sixth weeks of life and are arranged in a linear configuration with a predilection for the extremities [204]. The verrucous papules clinically may resemble common verrucae. The development of the verrucous papules may overlap with the vesicular phase of the process. Proliferation of the verrucous papules may continue into teenage years [203]. Verrucous lesions do not necessarily occur in all patients who have the initial vesicles and bullae.

The final stage manifests as hyperpigmented streaks and whorls that follow the lines of Blaschko. The hyperpigmentation peaks between the third and fourth months of life and are present primarily on the trunk. No antecedent inflammation is reported in most patients. These pigmented whorls progress for a few years and tend to fade throughout the remainder of life.

Subtle hypochromatic and atrophic linear streaks may be present late in the course [205]. Less common cutaneous manifestations include periungual and subungual hyperkeratotic tumors, which can be painful [206]. These tumors may cause lytic changes in the underling terminal phalanges [207]. They usually arise late in the course of the disease. They have been described as clinically resembling keratoacanthomas, squamous cell carcinomas, or subungual fibromas [208]. Alopecia has been described in up to 38% of patients with incontinentia pigmenti [204].

Associated Disorders. Systemic manifestations, as summarized in Table 9–1, are present in up to 80% of patients with incontinentia pigmenti [209]. Peripheral blood eosinophilia is present in most patients with incontinentia pigmenti. From 25% to 50% of patients with incontinentia pigmenti suffer from neurologic deficits [210]. A fatal encephalopathy with generalized seizures can occur in patients with incontinentia pigmenti [211]. Other reported central nervous system anomalies include hypoplasia of the corpus callosum, enlargement of the lateral ventricles, and periventricular white matter lesions [212]. Retinal disease, including ischemia with neovascularization and retinal detachment, have been reported as causes of blindness [213]. Optic atrophy and cerebral infarction have also contributed to blindness in some of these patients [213]. Hypopigmented lesions in the retinal pigment epithelium have been reported [214]. Keratitis of the cornea is found in some patients with incontinentia pigmenti [215]. Iris hypoplasia is also associated with inconti-

Table 9–1. Disorders Associated with Incontinentia Pigmenti

Organ System	Disorder	Percentage Affected
Central nervous system	Fatal encephalopathy	25–50
	Hypoplasia of corpus callosum	
	Enlargement of lateral ventricles	
	Cerebral infarction	
	Periventricular white matter lesions	
Ocular anomalies	Retinal detachment	35%
	Blindness	
	Retinal ischemia and neovascularization	
	Optic atrophy	
	Hypopigmented lesions in retina	
	Keratitis of cornea	
	Iris hypoplasia	
	Nasolacrimal duct obstruction	
Dental anomalies	Anodontia	
	Mild pegging	
	Cleft lip and palate	
Sweating abnormalities		
Childhood malignancies	Rhabdoid tumors of the kidney	
Hematologic anomalies	Peripheral eosinophilia	

nentia pigmenti [216], as is nasolacrimal duct obstruction [217]. Overall, up to 35% of patients with incontinentia pigmenti experience some type of eye problem.

Many types of dental anomalies, including an-odontia and mild pegging, have been described in patients with incontinentia pigmenti [218]. Cleft lip and palate have also been reported in these patients [209]. There appears to be an increased association between incontinentia pigmenti and focal abnormalities in sweat production [219, 220]. Incontinentia pigmenti may be related to a higher incidence of childhood malignancies, including rhabdoid tumors of the kidney [221].

Histologic Features. Incontinentia pigmenti has several clinical stages with accompanying specific histologic characteristics. The initial vesicular stage is characterized by the presence of an intraepidermal vesicle surrounded by abundant spongiosis. Eosinophils are present within the blister cavity and in the surrounding epidermis (Fig. 9–13 *A*). Individually necrotic keratinocytes are present at all layers of the epidermis (Fig. 9–13 *B*). Lymphocytes and histiocytes are also present within the epidermis and in the papillary dermis. The following entities must be considered in the histologic differential diagnosis of early lesions of incontinentia pigmenti:

- Contact dermatitis
- Dermatophytosis
- Erythema toxicum neonatorum
- Neonatal pustular melanosis
- Pemphigus vulgaris

The second, verrucous stage of incontinentia pigmenti is characterized by psoriasiform epidermal hyperplasia and papillomatosis. There is overlying parakeratosis and hyperkeratotic orthokeratosis. Increased mitoses may be present within the epidermis. Abundant necrotic keratinocytes are present at this stage. A slight perivascular lymphocytic infiltrate is present, and scattered melanophages are seen within the papillary der-

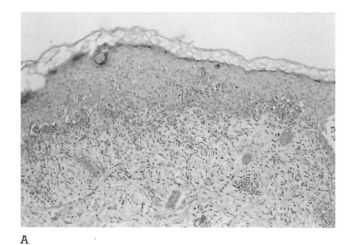

A

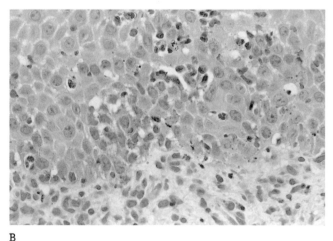

B

Fig. 9–13. *A,* Incontinentia pigmenti is characterized by epidermal spongiosis and exocytosis of eosinophils in the epidermis. *B,* Intraepidermal eosinophils and scattered dyskeratotic cells are found in early lesions of incontinentia pigmenti.

mis. The following entities must be considered in the histologic differential diagnosis of midstage lesions of incontinentia pigmenti:

- Acanthosis nigricans
- Epidermal nevus
- Verruca vulgaris

The last stage of incontinentia pigmenti is that of hyperpigmented streaks along Blaschko's lines. The histologic features are those of postinflammatory hyperpigmentation. There is a slight decrease in the amount of epidermal pigment, with increased amounts of melanin pigment present within melanophages in the papillary dermis [222]. Rarely, hypopigmented areas may be seen as well. These areas demonstrate focally decreased numbers of melanocytes, epidermal atrophy, and reduced numbers of cutaneous appendages in affected areas, along with increased numbers of degenerated keratinocytes within the papillary dermis [222].

Special Studies. No special studies are usually necessary to establish a histologic diagnosis of incontinentia pigmenti.

Pathogenesis. A chromosomal defect at Xp11.21 has been described in patients with type I incontinentia pigmenti [223]. The chromosomal defect has been localized to Xq28 in most cases of type II disease [224].

Increased levels of leukotriene B_4 have been demonstrated in lesional skin in patients with the vesicular stage of incontinentia pigmenti. Leukotriene B_4 is believed to play a role in the chemotaxis of eosinophils into the epidermis [225]. Eosinophil granule major basic protein has been found within the tissue of lesional skin, suggesting that eosinophil degranulation plays a role in the pathogenesis of the cutaneous blisters [226]. The relationships between the genetic mutations and the observed clinical, histologic, and biochemical findings have not yet been explained.

References

1. Huson, S. M., Compston, D. A. S., Clark, P., and Harper, P. S., *A genetic study of von Recklinghausen neurofibromatosis in southeast Wales I. Prevalence, fitness, mutation rate, and effect of parental transmission on severity.* J Med Genet, 1989. 26:704–711.
2. Conference, N. I. C., *Neurofibromatosis.* Arch Neurol, 1988. 45:575–578.
3. Evans, D. G. R., Huson, S. M., Donnai, D., Neary, W., Blair, V., Teare, D., Newton, V., Stachan, T., et al., *A genetic study of type 2 neurofibromatosis in the United Kingdom. I. Prevalence, mutation rate, fitness, and confirmation of maternal effect on severity.* J Med Genet, 1992. 29:841–846.
4. Parry, D. M., Elderidge, R., Kaiser-Kupfer, M. I., Bouzas, E. A., Pikus, A., and Patronas, N., *Neurofibromatosis 2 (NF2): Clinical characteristics of 63 affected individuals and clinical evidence for heterogeneity.* Am J Med Genet, 1994. 52:450–461.
5. Honda, M., Arai, E., Sawada, S., Ohta, A., and Niimura, M., *Neurofibromatosis 2 and neurilemmomatosis gene are identical.* J Invest Dermatol, 1995. 104:74–77.
6. Hager, C. M., Cohen, P. R., and Tschen, J. A., *Segmental neurofibromatosis: Case reports and review.* J Am Acad Dermatol, 1997. 37:864–869.
7. Pique, E., Olivares, M., Farina, M. C., Martin, L., Sarasa, J. L., Campos, J. M., and Requena, L., *Pseudoatrophic macules: A variant of neurofibroma.* Cutis, 1996. 57:100–102.
8. Riccardi, V. M., *Cutaneous manifestations of neurofibromatosis: Cellular interaction, pigmentation and mast cells.* Birth Defects, 1981. 17:129–145.
9. Enzinger, F. M., and Weiss, S. W., *Soft Tissue Tumors.* 1988, CV Mosby, St. Louis, pp. 719–780.
10. Val-Bernal, J. F., Figols, J., and Vazquez-Barquero, A., *Cutaneous plexiform schwannoma associated with neurofibromatosis type 2.* Cancer, 1995. 76:1181–1186.
11. Zvulunov, A., and Esterly, N. B., *Neurocutaneous syndromes associated with pigmentary skin lesions.* J Am Acad Dermatol, 1995. 32:915–935.
12. Lewis, R. A., and Riccardi, V. M., *Von Recklinghausen neurofibromatosis: Incidence of iris hamartoma.* Ophthalmology, 1981. 88:348–354.
13. Zvulunov, A., Barak, Y., and Metzker, A., *Juvenile xanthogranuloma, neurofibromatosis, and juvenile myelogenous leukemia. World statistical analysis.* Arch Demratol, 1995. 131:904–908.
14. Selvang, E., Thune, P., and Larsen, T. E., *Segmental neurofibromatosis presenting as a giant naevus spilus (letter).* Acta Derm Venereol, 1994. 74:327.
15. Rutten, A., and Goos, M., *Nevus spilus with malignant melanoma in a patient with neurofibromatosis (letter).* Arch Dermatol, 1990. 126:539–540.
16. Allegue, F., Espana, A., Fernandez-Garcia, J. M., and Ledo, A., *Segmental neurofibromatosis with contralateral lentiginosis.* Clin Exp Dermatol, 1989. 14:448–450.
17. Obringer, A. C., Meadows, A. T., and Zackai, E. H., *The diagnosis of neurofibromatosis-1 in the child under the age of 6 years.* Am J Dis Child, 1989. 143:717–719.
18. Mautner, V. F., Lindenau, M., Baser, M. E., Kluwe, L., and Gottschalk, J., *Skin abnormalities in neurofibromatosis 2.* Arch Dermatol 1997. 133:1539–1543.
19. Jaffe, A. T., Heymann, W. R., and Schnur, R. E., *Clustered angiofibromas on the ear of a patient with neurofibromatosis type 2.* Arch Dermatol, 1998. 134:760–761.
20. Ettl, A., Marinkovic, M., and Koornneef, L., *Localized hypertrichosis associated with periorbital neurofibroma: Clinical findings and differential diagnosis.* Ophthalmology, 1996. 103:942–948.

21. Sawada, S., Honda, M., Kamide, R., and Niimura, M., *Three cases of subungual glomus tumors with von Recklinghausen neurofibromatosis.* J Am Acad Dermatol, 1995. 32:277–278.

22. Argenyz, Z. B., Thieberg, M. D., Hayes, C. M., and Whitaker, D. C., *Primary cutaneous meningioma associated with von Recklinghausen's disease.* J Cutan Pathol, 1994. 21:549–556.

23. Tommerup, N., Warburg, M., Gieselmann, V., Hansen, B. R., Koch, J., and Petersen, G. B., *Ring chromosome 22 and neurofibromatosis.* Clin Genet, 1992. 42:171–177.

24. Niimura, M., *Aspects in neurofibromatosis from the viewpoint of dermatology.* J Dermatol, 1992. 19:868–872.

25. Sahn, E. E., Dunlavey, E. S., and Parsons, J. L., *Multiple cutaneous granular cell tumors in a child with possible neurofibromatosis.* J Am Acad Dermatol, 1997. 36:327–330.

26. Riccardi, V. M., *Von Recklinghausen's neurofibromatosis.* N Eng J Med, 1981. 305:1617–1626.

27. Morier, P., Merot, Y., Paccaud, D., Beck, D., and Frenk, E., *Juvenile chronic granulocytic leukemia, juvenile xanthogranulomas, and neurofibromatosis. Case report and review of the literature.* J Am Acad Dermatol, 1990. 22:962–965.

28. Deb, G., Habertswallner, D., Helson, L., De Sio, L., Caniglia, M., and Donfrancesco, A., *Sporadic acute lymphocytic leukemia arising in a patient with neurofibromatosis and xanthogranulomatosis.* Cancer Invest, 1996. 14:109–111.

29. Rotte, J. J., de Vaan, G. A., and Koopman, R. J., *Juvenile xanthogranuloma and acute leukemia: A case report.* Med Pediatr Oncol, 1994. 23:57–59.

30. Ferner, R. E., Hughes, R. A., and Johnson, M. R., *Neurofibromatosis I and multiple sclerosis.* J Neurol Neurosurg Psychiatry, 1995. 58:582–585.

31. Angletti, G., Crispino, G., Bracaccia, M., Rosi, G., Caputo, N., Lupidi, G., and Sbordone, G. B., *Precocious puberty and neurofibromatosis of vonRecklinghausen. A clinical report.* Recent Prog Med, 1990. 81:806–808.

32. Wasserman, R., *Fibrosarcoma in a child with neurofibromatosis.* Med Pediatr Oncol, 1989. 17:271–273.

33. Ogawa, T., Mitsukawa, T., Ishikawa, T., and Tamura, K., *Familial pheochromocytoma associated with von Recklinghausen's disease.* Intern Med, 1994. 33:110–114.

34. Martuza, R. L., Philippe, I., Fitzpatrick, T. B., Zwaan, U., Seki, Y., and Lederman, J., *Melanin macroglobules as a cellular marker of neurofibromatosis: A quantitative study.* J Invest Dermatol, 1985. 85:347–350.

35. Slater, C., Hayes, M., Saxe, N., Temple-Camp, C., and Beighton, P., *Macromelanosomes in the early diagnosis of neurofibromatosis.* Am J Dermatopathol, 1986. 8:284–289.

36. Megahed, M., *Histopathologic variants of neurofibroma.* Am J Dermatopathol, 1994. 16:486–495.

37. Requena, L., and Sangueza, O. P., *Benign neoplasms with neural differntiation: A review.* Am J Dermatopathol, 1995. 17:75–96.

38. Fisher, D. A., Chu, P., and McCalmont, T., *Solitary neurofibroma is not pathognomonic of von Recklinghausen's neurofibromatosis: A report of a case.* Int J Dermatol, 1997. 36:439–442.

39. Fletcher, C. D. M., and Davies, S. E., *Benign plexiform (multinodular) schwannoma: A rare tumor unassociated with neurofibromatosis.* Histopathology, 1986. 10:971–980.

40. Woodruff, J. M., Godwin, T. A., Erlandson, R. A., Susin, M., and Martini, N., *Cellular schwannoma: A variety of schwannoma sometimes mistaken for a malignant tumor.* Am J Surg Pathol, 1981. 5:733–744.

41. Ducatman, B. S., Scheithauer, B. W., Piepgras, D. G., Reiman, H. M., and Ilstrup, D. M., *Malignant peripheral nerve sheath tumors. A clinicopathologic study of 120 cases.* Cancer, 1986. 57:215–226.

42. D'Agostino, A. N., Soule, E. H., and Miller, R. H., *Sarcomas of the peripheral nerves and somatic soft tissues associated with multiple neurofibromatosis (von Recklinghausen's disease).* Cancer, 1963. 16:1015–1027.

43. Sangueza, O. P., and Requena, L., *Neoplasms with neural differentiation: A review. Part II: Malignant neoplasms.* Am J Dermatopathol, 1998. 20:89–102.

44. Schmidt, M. A., Michels, V. V., and Dewald, G. W., *Cases of neurofibromatosis with rearrangements of chromosome 17 involving band 17q11.2.* Am J Med Genet, 1987. 28:771–777.

45. Webb, D. W., and Osborne, J. P., *New research in in tuberous sclerosis.* BMJ, 1992. 304:1647–1648.

46. Singer, K., *Genetic aspects of tuberous sclerosis in a Chinese population.* Am J Med Genet, 1971. 23:33–40.

47. Monaghan, H. P., Krafchik, B. R., MacGregor, D. L., and Fitz, C. R., *Tuberous sclerosis complex in children.* Am J Dis Child, 1981. 135:912–917.

48. Fryer, A. E., Chalmers, A., Connor, J. M., Fraser, I., Povey, S., Yates, A. D., Yates, J. R., and Osborne, J. P., *Evidence that the gene for tuberous sclerosis is on chromosome* Lancet 9. 1987. 1:659–661.

49. Kandt, R., Haines, J., Smith, M., Northrup, H., Gardner, R. J., Short, M. P., Dumars, K., Roach, E. S., et al., *Linkage of a major gene locus on tuberous sclerosis to a chromosome 16 marker for polycystic kidney disease.* Nat Genet, 1992. 2:37–41.

50. Webb, D. W., Clarke, A., Fryer, A., and Osborne, J. P., *The cutaneous features of tuberous sclerosis: A population study.* Br J Dermatol, 1996. 135:1–5.

51. Osborne, J. P., *Diagnosis of tuberous sclerosis.* Arch Dis child, 1988. 63:1423–1425.

52. Fryer, A. E., Osborne, J. P., and Schutt, W., *Forehead plaque: A presenting skin sign in tuberous sclerosis.* Arch Dis Child, 1987. 62:292–293.

53. Gil-Mateo, M. P., Miquel, F. J., Valasco, A. M., Pitarch, A., Fortea, J. M., and Aliaga, A., *Widespread angiokeratomas and tuberous sclerosis.* Br J Demratol, 1996. 135:280–282.

54. Riikonen, R., and Simell, O., *Tuberous sclerosis and infantile spasms.* Dev Med Child Neurol, 1990. 32:203–209.

55. Webb, D. W., Fryer, A. E., and Osborne, J. P., *On the incidence of fits and mental retardation in tuberous sclerosis.* J Med Genet, 1991. 28:395–397.

56. Fryer, A. E., Osborne, J. P., Tan, R., et al., *Tuberous sclerosis: A large family with no history of seizures or mental retardation.* J Med Genet, 1987. 24:547–548.

57. Stillwell, T. J., Gomez, M. R., and Kelalis, P. P., *Renal lesions in tuberous sclerosis.* J Urol, 1987. 138:477–481.

58. Chonko, A. M., Weiss, S. M., Stein, J. H., and Ferris, T. F., *Renal involvement in tuberous sclerosis.* Am J Med, 1974. 56:124–132.

59. Jozwiak, S., Pedich, M., Rajszys, P., and Michalowicz, R., *Incidence of hepatic hamartomas in tuberous sclerosis.* Arch Dis Child, 1992. 67:1363–1365.

60. Smith, H. C., Watson, G. H., Patel, R. G., and Super, M., *Cardiac rhabdomyomata in tuberous sclerosis: Their course.* Arch Dis Child, 1989. 64:196–200.

61. Mlynarczyk, G., *Enamel pitting: A common symptom of tuberous sclerosis.* Oral Surg Oral Med Oral Pathol, 1991. 71:63–67.

62. Hurwitz, S., and Braverman, L. M., *White spots in tuberous sclerosis.* J Pediatr, 1970. 77:587–594.

63. Jimbow, K., *Tuberous sclerosis and guttate leukodermas.* Semin Cutan Med Surg, 1997. 16:30–35.

64. Kousseff, B. G., *The phakomatoses as paracrine growth disorders (paracrinopathies).* Clin Genet, 1990. 37:97–105.

65. Braffman, B. H., Bilaniuk, L. T., Naidich, T., Altman, N. R., Post, M. J., Quencer, R. M., Zimmerman, R. A., and Brody, B. A., *MR imaging of tuberous sclerosis: Pathogenesis of this phakomatosis, use of gadopentetate dimeglumine, and literature review.* Radiology, 1992. 183:227–238.

66. Fahsold, R., Rott, H. D., and Lorenz, P., *A third gene locus for tuberous sclerosis is closely linked to the phenylalanine hydroxylase gene locus.* Hum Genet, 1991. 88:85–90.

67. Rand, R. E., and Baden, H. P., *The ichthyoses—a review.* J Am Acad Dermatol, 1983. 8:285–305.

68. Davies, M. G., Marks, R., Dykes, P. J., and Reynolds, D., *Epidermal abnormalities in Refsum's syndrome.* Br J Dermatol, 1997. 97:401–406.

69. Kuntzer, T., Ochsner, F., Schmid, F., and Regli, F., *Quantitative EMG analysis and longitudinal nerve conduction studies in a Refsum's disease patient.* Muscle Nerve, 1993. 16:857–863.

70. Blanchet-Bardon, C. I., Anton-Lamprecht, I., Puissant, A., and Schnyder, U. W., *Ultrastructural features of ichthyotic skin in Refsum's syndrome.* In *The Ichthoses,* R. Marks and P. J. Dykes, Eds. 1978, Spectrum Publications, Inc, New York, pp. 65–69.

71. Stokke, O., Skjeldal, O. H., and Hoie, K., *Disorders related to the matabolism of phytanic acid.* Scand J Clin Lab Invest Suppl, 1986. 184:3–10.

72. Singh, I., Pahan, K., Singh, A. K., and Barbosa, E., *Refsum disease: A defect in the alpha-oxidation of phytanic acid in peroxisomes.* J Lipid Res, 1993. 34:1755–1764.

73. Chahal, A., Khan, M., Pai, S. G., Barbosa, E., and Singh, I., *Restoration of phytanic acid oxidation in Refsum disease fibroblasts from patients with mutations in the phytanoyl-CoA hydroxylase gene.* FEBS Lett, 1998. 429:119–122.

74. Rizzo, W. B., Carney, G., and De Laurenzi, V., *A common deletion mutation in European patients with Sjögren-Larsson syndrome.* Biochem Mol Med, 1997. 62:178–181.

75. de Laurenzi, V., Rogers, G. R., Tarcsa, E., Carney, G., Marekov, L., Bale, S. J., Compton, J. G., Markova, N., et al., *Sjögren-Larsson syndrome is caused by a common mutation in northern European and Swedish patients.* J Invest Dermatol, 1997. 109:79–83.

76. Lacour, M., Middleton-Price, H. R., and Harper, J. I., *Confirmation of lineage of Sjögren-Larsson syndrome to chromosome 17 in families of different ethnic origins.* J Med Genet, 1996. 33:258–259.

77. Lacour, M., *Update on Sjögren-Larsson syndrome.* Dermatology, 1996. 193:77–82.

78. Jagell, S., and Heijbel, J., *Sjögren-Larsson syndrome: Physical and neurological features. A survey of 35 patients.* Helv Paediatr Acta, 1982. 37:519–530.

79. Jagell, S., and Liden, S., *Ichthyosis in the Sjögren-Larsson syndrome.* Clin Genet, 1982. 21:243–252.

80. Barnard, N. A., Patel, C., and Barnard, R. A., *Sjögren-Larsson syndrome: Case reports of two brothers.* Ophthalm Physiol Opt, 1991. 11:180–183.

81. Fivenson, D. P., Lucky, A. W., and Iannoccone, S., *Sjögren-Larsson syndrome associated with the Dandy-Walker malformation: Report of a case.* Pediatr Dermatol, 1989. 6:312–315.

82. Rizzo, W. B., *Sjögren-Larsson syndrome.* Semin Dermatol, 1993. 12:210–218.

83. Hofer, P. A., and Jagell, S., *Sjögren-Larsson syndrome: A dermato-histopathological study.* J Cutan Pathol, 1982. 9:360–376.

84. Ito, M., Oguro, K., and Sato, Y., *Ultrastructural study of the skin in Sjögren-Larsson syndrome.* Arch Dermatol Res, 1991. 283:141–148.

85. Paller, A. S., *Laboratory tests for ichthyosis.* Dermatol Clin, 1994. 12:99–107.

86. Scheimber, I., Harper, J. I., Malone, M., and Lake, B. D., *Inherited ichthyoses: A review of the histology of the skin.* Pediatr Pathol Lab Med, 1996. 16:359–378.

87. Paige, D. G., Morse-Fisher, N., and Harper, J. I., *Quantification of stratum corneum ceramides and lipid envelope ceramides in the hereditary ichthyoses.* Br J Dermatol, 1994. 131:23–27.

88. Kaufman, L. M., *A syndrome of retinitis pigmentosa, congenital ichthyosis, hypergonadotropic hypogonadism, small stature, mental retardation, crania dysmorphism, and abnormal electroencephalogram.* Ophthalmic Genet, 1998. 19:69–79.

89. Skinner, B. A., Greist, M. C., and Norins, A. L., *The dermatitis, ichthyosis, and deafness (KID) syndrome.* Arch Dermatol, 1981. 117:285–289.

90. Caceres-Rios, H., Tamayo-Sanchez, L., Duran-Mckinster, C., de la Luz Orozco, M., and Ruiz-Maldonado, R., *Keratitis, ichthyosis, and deafness (KID syndrome): Review of the literature and proposal of a new terminology.* Pediatr Dermatol, 1996. 13:105–113.

91. Nazzaro, V., Blanchet-Bardon, C., Lorette, G., and Civatte, J., *Familial occurrence of KID (keratitis, ichthyosis, deafness) syndrome. Case report of a mother and daughter.* J Am Acad Dermatol, 1990. 23:385–388.

92. Kone-Paut, I., Hesse, S., Palix, C., Rey, R., Remediani, K., Garnier, J. M., and Berbis, P., *Keratitis, ichthyosis, and deafness (KID) syndrome in half sibs.* Pediatr Dermatol, 1998. 15:219–221.

93. Wilson, G. N., Squires, R. H., Jr., and Weinberg, A. G., *Keratitis, hepatitis, ichthyosis, and deafness: Report and review of KID syndrome.* Am J Med Genet, 1991. 40:255–259.

94. Legrand, J., Litoux, P., Quere, M., Stalder, J. F., and Ertus, M., *Un syndrome rare oculoauritculo-cutané (syndrome de Burns).* J Fr Ophthalmol, 1982. 5:441–445.

95. Langer, K., Konrad, K., and Wolff, K., *Keratitis, ichthyosis, and deafness (KID)-syndrome: Report of three cases and a review of the literature.* Br J Dermatol, 1990. 122:689–697.

96. Grob, J. J., Breton, A., Bonafe, J. L., Sauvan-Ferdani, M., and Bonerandi, J. J., *Keratitis, ichthyosis, and deafness (KID) syndrome. Vertical transmission and death from multiple squamous cell carcinomas.* Arch Dermatol, 1987. 1987:777–782.

97. Harms, M., Gilardi, S., Levy, P. M., and Saurat, J. H., *KID syndrome (keratitis, ichthyosis, and deafness) and chronic mucocutaneous candidiasis: Case report and review of the literature.* Pediatr Dermatol, 1984. 2:1–7.

98. Helm, K., Lane, A. T., Orosz, J., and Metlay, L., *Systemic cytomegalovirus in a patient with the keratitis, ichthyosis, and deafness (KID) syndrome.* Pediatr Dermatol, 1990. 7:54–56.

99. Tsuzuku, T., Kaga, K., Kanematsu, S., Shibata, A., and Ohde, S., *Temporal bone findings in keratitis, ichthyosis, and deafness syndrome: Case report.* Ann Otol Rhinol Laryngol, 1992. 101:413–416.

100. McGrae, J. D., *Keratitis, ichthyosis, and deafness (KID) syndrome.* Int J Dermatol, 1990. 29:89–93.

101. Hsu, H. C., Lin, G. S., and Li, W. M., *Keratitis, ichthyosis, and deafness (KID) syndrome with cerebellar hypoplasia.* Int J Dermatol, 1988. 27:695–697.

102. Leventhal, L. J., Straka, P. C., and Schumacher, H. R., Jr., *Jaccoud arthropathy and acroosteolysis in KID syndrome.* J Rheumatol, 1989. 16:1274–1277.

103. Hazen, P. G., Carney, P., and Lynch, W. S., *Keratitis, ichthyosis and deafness syndrome with development of multiple cutaneous neoplasms.* Int J Dermatol, 1989. 28:190–191.

104. Reynolds, N. J., and Kennedy, C. T. C., *Keratitis, ichthyosis deafness (KID) syndrome.* Br J Dermatol, 1990. 123(Suppl):77–80.

105. Madariaga, J., Fromowitz, F., Phillips, M., and Hoover, H. C., Jr., *Squamous cell carcinoma in congenital ichthyosis with deafness and keratitis. A case report and review of the literature.* Cancer, 1986. 57:2026–2029.

106. Rycroft, R. J. G., Moynahan, E. J., and Wells, R. S., *Atypical ichthyosiform erythroderma, deafness and keratitis.* Br J Dermatol, 1976. 94:211–217.

107. de Berker, D., Branford, W. A., Soucek, S., and Michaels, L., *Fatal keratitis, ichthyosis and deafness syndrome (KIDS). Aural, ocular, and cutaneous histopathology.* Am J Dermatopathol, 1993. 15:64–69.

108. Weisz, J. M., Holland, G. N., Roer, L. N., Park, M. S., Yuge, A. J., Moorthy, R. S., Forster, D. J., Rao, N. A., et al., *Association between Vogt-Koyanagi-Harada syndrome and HLA-DR1 and -DR4 in Hispanic patients living in southern California.* Ophthalmology, 1995. 102:1012–1015.

109. Pivetti-Pezzi, P., Accorinti, M., Colabelli-Gisoldi, R. A., and Pirraglia, M. P., *Vogt-Koyanagi-Harada disease and HLA type in Italian patients.* Am J Ophthalmol, 1996. 122:889–891.

110. Goldberg, A. C., Yamamoto, J. H., Chiarella, J. M., Marin, M. L., Sibinelli, M., Neufeld, R., Hirata, C. E., Olivalves, E., et al., *HLA-DRB1*0405 is the predominant allele in Brazilian patients with Vogt-Koyanagi-Harada disease.* Hum Immunol, 1998. 59:183–188.

111. Ishikawa, A., Shiono, T., and Uchida, S., *Vogt-Koyanagi-Harada disease in identical twins.* Retina, 1994. 15:435–437.

112. Gruich, M. J., Evans, O. B., Story, J. M., Bradley, S. T., and Chen, C. J., *Vogt-Koyanagi-Harada syndrome in a 4 year-old child.* Pediatr Neurol, 1995. 13:50–51.

113. Barnes, L., *Vitiligo and the Vogt-Koyanagi-Harada syndrome.* Dermatol Clin, 1988. 6:229–239.

114. Kumakiri, M., Kimura, T., Miura, Y., and Tagawa, Y., *Vitiligo with an inflammatory erythema in Vogt-Koyanagi-Harada disease: Demonstration of filamentous masses and amyloid deposits.* J Cutan Pathol, 1982. 9:258–266.

115. Nordlund, J. J., Albert, D., Forget, B., and Lerner, A. B., *Halo nevi and the Vogt-Koyanagi-Harada syndrome. Manifestations of vitiligo.* Arch Dermatol, 1980. 116:690–692.

116. Moorthy, R. S., Inomata, H., and Rao, N. A., *Vogt-Koyanagi-Harada syndrome.* Surv Ophthalmol, 1995. 39:265–292.

117. Brouzas, D., Chatzoulis, D., Galina, E., Liaskou, A., and Koukoulomatis, P., *Corneal anesthesia in a case of Vogt-Koyanagi-Harada syndrome.* Acta Ophthalmol Scand, 1997. 75:4464–465.

118. Eibschitz-Tsimhoni, M., Gelfand, Y. A., Mezer, E., and Miller, B., *Bilateral angle closure glaucoma: An unusual presentation of Vogt-Koyanagi-Harada syndrome.* Br J Ophthalmol, 1997. 81:705–706.

119. Jaggarao, N., Voth, D., and Jacobsen, J., *The Vogt-Koyanagi-Harada syndrome: Association with hypothyroidism and diabetes mellitus.* Postgrad Med J, 1989. 65:587–588.

120. Jovic, N. S., Nesovic, M., Vranjesevic, D. N., Ciric, J., Marinkovic, D. M., and Bonaci, B., *The Vogt-Koyanagi-Harada syndrome: Association with autoimmune polyglandular syndrome type 1.* Postgrad Med J, 1996. 72:495–497.

121. Chi, H. I., Furue, M., and Ishibashi, Y., *Vogt-Koyanagi-Harada syndrome associated with Hashimoto's thyroiditis.* J Dermatol, 1994. 21:683–686.

122. Howsden, S. M., Herndon, J. H. Jr., and Freeman, R. G., *Vogt-Koyanagi-Harada syndrome and psoriasis.* Arch Dermatol, 1973. 108:395–398.

123. Watanabe, K., Kato, T., and Hayasaka, S., *Concurrent bilateral posterior scleritis and Vogt-Koyanagi-Harada disease in a patient with positive rheumatoid factor.* Ophthalmologica, 1997. 211:316–319.

124. Chuah, S. Y., Lyne, A. J., and Dronfield, M. W., *Vogt-Koyanagi-Harada syndrome, a rare association of Hodgkin's disease.* Postgrad Med J, 1991. 67:476–478.

125. Cipriani, D., Landonio, G., and Canepari, C., *A case of Vogt-Koyanagi-Harada syndrome in a patient affected by Hodgkin's disease.* J Neurol, 1989. 236:303–304.

126. Pettitt, A. R., Neoh, C., Wong, S. H., and Clark, R. E., *Vogt-Koyanagi-Harada syndrome complicating allogeneic bone marrow transplantation.* Bone Marrow Transplant, 1994. 13:225–227.

127. Walker, J., Ober, R. R., Khan, A., Yuen, D., and Rao, N. A., *Intraocular lymphoma developing in a patient with Vogt-Koyanagi-Harada syndrome.* Int Ophthalmol, 1993. 17:331–336.

128. Jimbow, M., and Jimbow, K., *Pigmentary disorders in Oriental skin.* Clin Dermatol, 1989. 7:11–27.

129. Okada, T., Sakamoto, T., Ishibashi, T., and Inomata, H., *Vitiligo in Vogt-Koyanagi-Harada disease: Immunohistochemical analysis of inflammatory infiltrate.* Graefes Arch Clin Exp Ophthalmol, 1996. 234:359–363.

130. Ohta, K., Norose, K., Wang, X. C., Ito, S., and Yoshimura, N., *Abnormal naive and memory T lymphocyte subsets in the peripheral blood of patients with uveitis.* Curr Eye Res, 1997. 16:650–655.

131. Ohta, K., and Yoshimura, N., *Expression of Fas antigen on helper T lymphocytes in Vogt-Koyanagi-Harada disease.* Graefes Arch Clin Exp Ophthalmol, 1998. 236:434–439.

132. Bassili, S. S., Peyman, G. A., Gebhardt, B. M., Daun, M., Ganiban, G. J., and Rifai, A., *Detection of Epstein-Barr virus DNA by polymerase chain reaction in the vitreous from a patient with Vogt-Koyanagi-Harada syndrome.* Retina, 1996. 16:160–161.

133. Baxter, G., and Beer, J., *Rubinstein-Taybi syndrome.* Psychol Rep, 1992. 70:451–456.

134. Marion, R. W., Garcia, D., and Karasik, J. B., *Apparent dominant transmission of the Rubinstein-Taybi syndrome.* Am J Med Genet, 1993. 46:284–287.

135. Hennekam, R. C., Stevens, C. A., and Van de Kamp, J. J., *Etiology and recurrence risk in Rubinstein-Taybi syndrome.* Am J Med Genet Suppl, 1990. 6:56–64.

136. Siraganian, P. A., Rubinstein, J. H., and Miller, R. W., *Keloids and neoplasms in the Rubinstein-Taybi syndrome.* Med Pediatr Oncol, 1989. 17:485–491.

137. Selmanowitz, V. J., and Stiller, M. J., *Rubinstein-Taybi syndrome. Cutaneous manifestations and colossal keloids.* Arch Dermatol, 1981. 117:504–506.

138. Kurwa, A. R., *Rubinstein-Taybi syndrome and spontaneous keloids.* Clin Exp Dermatol, 1979. 4:251–254.

139. Hendrix, J. D., Jr., and Greer, K. E., *Rubinstein-Taybi syndrome with multiple flamboyant keloids.* Cutis, 1996. 57:346–348.

140. Cambiaghi, S., Ermacora, E., Brusasco, A., Canzi, L., and Caupto, R., *Multiple pilomatricomas in Rubinstein-Taybi syndrome: A case report.* Pediatr Dermatol, 1994. 11:21–25.

141. Masuno, M., Imaizumi, K., Ishii, T., Kuroki, Y., Baba, N., and Tanaka, Y., *Pilomatrixomas in Rubinstein-Taybi syndrome.* Am J Med Genet, 1998. 77:81–82.

142. Herranz, P., Borbujo, J., Martinez, W., Vidaurrazaga, C., Diaz, R., and Casado, M., *Rubinstein-Taybi syndrome with piebaldism.* Clin Exp Dermatol, 1994. 19:170–172.

143. Atasu, M., *Dermatoglyphic findings in Rubinstein-Taybi syndrome.* J Ment Defic Res, 1979. 23:111–121.

144. Rubinstein, J. H., *Broad thumb-hallux (Rubinstein-Taybi) syndrome 1957–1988.* Am J Med Genet Suppl, 1990. 6:3–16.

145. Stevens, C. A., and Bhakta, M. G., *Cardiac abnormalities in the Rubinstein-Taybi syndrome.* Am J Med Genet, 1995. 59:346–348.

146. Skousen, G. J., Wardinsky, T., and Chenaille, P., *Medulloblastoma in patient with Rubinstein-Taybi syndrome.* Am J Med Genet, 1996. 66:367.

147. Burton, B. J., Kumar, V. G., and Bradford, R., *Granular cell tumour of the spinal cord in a patient with Rubinstein-Taybi syndrome.* Br J Neurosurg, 1997. 11:257–259.

148. Miller, R. W., and Rubinstein, J. H., *Tumors in Rubinstein-Taybi syndrome.* Am J Med Genet, 1995. 56:112–115.

149. Sobel, R. A., and Woerner, S., *Rubinstein-Taybi syndrome and nasopharyngeal rhabdomyosarcoma.* J Pediatr, 1981. 99:1000–1001.

150. Quaranta, L., and Quaranta, C. A., *Congenital glaucoma associated with Rubinstein-Taybi syndrome.* Acta Ophthalmol Scand, 1998. 76:112–113.

151. Kimura, H., Ito, Y., Koda, Y., and Hase, Y., *Rubinstein-Taybi syndrome with thymic hypoplasia.* Am J Med Genet, 1993. 46:293–296.

152. Jonas, D. M., Heilbron, D. C., and Ablin, A. R., *Rubinstein-Taybi syndrome and acute leukemia.* J Pediatr, 1978. 92:851–852.

153. Kanjilal, D., Basir, M. A., Verma, R. S., Rajegowda, B. K., Lala, R., and Nagaraj, A., *New dysmorphic features in Rubinstein-Taybi syndrome.* J Med Genet, 1992. 29:669–670.

154. Moran, R., Calthorpe, D., McGoldrick, F., Fogarty, E., and Dowling, F., *Congenital dislocation of the patella in Rubinstein Taybi syndrome.* Ir Med J, 1993. 86:34–35.

155. Taine, L., Goizet, C., Wen, Z. Q., Petrij, F., Breuning, M. H., Ayme, S., Saura, R., Arveiler, B., et al., *Submicroscopic deletion of chromosome 16p13.3 in patients with Rubinstein-Taybi syndrome.* Am J Med Genet, 1998. 78:267–270.

156. Reifer, H., and Sobel, E., *Contrasts in clinical presentation and genetic transmission of myotonic dystrophy.* J Am Podiatr Med Assoc, 1998. 88:313–322.

157. de Die-Smulers, C. E., Howeler, C. J., Thijs, C., Mirandolle, J. F., Anten, H. B., Smeets, H. J., Chandler, K. E., and Geraedts, J. P., *Age and causes of death in adult-onset myotonic dystrophy.* Brain, 1998. 121:1557–1563.

158. Delfino, M., Monfrecola, G., Ayala, F., Suppa, F., and Piccirillo, A., *Multiple familial pilomatricomas: A cutaneous marker for myotonic dystrophy.* Dermatologica, 1985. 170:128–132.

159. Filla, A., Perretti, A., Barbieri, F., Marolda, M., Pelosi,

L., Delfino, M., and Corona, M., *Myotonic dystrophy and pilomatricomas: An unusual assocation.* Acta Neurol (Napoli), 1982. 4:79–91.

160. Cantwell, A. R., Jr., and Reed, W. B., *Myotonia atypica and multiple calcifying epithelioma of Malherbe.* Acta Derm Venereol, 1965. 45:387–390.

161. Berberian, B. J., Colonna, T. M., Battaglia, M., and Sulica, V. I., *Multiple pilomatricomas in association with myotonic dystrophy and a family history of melanoma.* J Am Acad Dermatol, 1997. 37:268–269.

162. Graells, J., Servitje, O., Badell, A., Notario, J., and Peyri, J., *Multiple familial pilomatricomas associated with myotonic dystrophy.* Int J Dermatol, 1996. 35:732–733.

163. Farrell, A. M., Ross, J. S., Barton, S. E., and Bunker, C. B., *Multiple pilomatricomas and myotonic dystrophy in a patient with AIDS.* Clin Exp Dermatol, 1995. 20:423–424.

164. Runne, U., Chilf, G. N., and Zentner, J., *Multiple pilomatrixomas as symptoms of Curschmann-Steiner myotonia dystrophica.* Hauzarzt, 1982. 33:271–275.

165. Cusano, F., Feleppa, M., Capozzi, M., and Errico, G., *Cutis verticis gyrata and dystrophica myotonica.* G Ital Dermatol Venereol, 1987. 122:201.

166. Stieler, W., and Plewig, G., *Multiple basaliomas in Curschmann-Steinert myotonia atrophica.* Hautarzt, 1986. 37:226–229.

167. Ribera, M., Calderon, P., Barranco, C., and Ferrandiz, C., *Multiple pilomatrixomas associated with myotonic dystrophy and medullary carcinoma of the thyroid.* Med Cutan Ibero Lat Am, 1989. 17:395–398.

168. Friedenberg, W. R., Marx, J. J. Jr., Hansotia, P., and Gottschalk, P. G., *Granulocyte dysfunction and myotonic dystrophy.* J Neurol Sci, 1986. 73:1–10.

169. Kuroiwa, Y., Sugita, H., Toyokura, Y., Mizoguchi, M., Matsuo, H., and Nonaka, Y., *Immunologic derangement in myotonic dystrophy—Abnormal contact sensitization to dinitrochlorobenzene.* J Neurol Sci, 1980. 47:231–239.

170. Geifman-Holtzman, O., and Fay, K., *Prenatal diagnosis of congenital myotonic dystrophy and counseling of the pregnant mother: Case report and literature review.* Am J Med Genet, 1998. 78:250–253.

171. Lipsker, D., Piette, J. C., Laporte, J. L., Maunoury, L., and Frances, C., *Annular atrophic lichen planus and Sneddon's syndrome.* Dermatology, 1997. 195:402–403.

172. Richard, M. A., Grob, J. J., Durand, J. M., Noe, C., Basseres, N., and Bonerandi, J. J., *Sneddon syndrome.* Ann Dermatol Venereol, 1994. 121:331–337.

173. Kame, M., Imai, H., Motegi, M., Miura, A. B., and Namura, I., *Sneddon's syndrome (livedo racemosa and cerebral infarction) presenting psychiatric disturbance and shortening of fingers and toes.* Intern Med, 1996. 35:668–673.

174. Macario, F., Macario, M. C., Ferro, A., Goncalves, F., Campos, M., and Marques, A., *Sneddon's syndrome: A vascular systemic disease with kidney involvement?* Nephron, 1997. 75:94–97.

175. Schellong, S. M., Weissenborn, K., Niedermeyer, J.,

Wollenhaupt, J., Sosada, M., Ehrenheim, C., and Lubach, D., *Classification of Sneddon's syndrome.* Vasa, 1997. 26:215–221.

176. Michel, M., Bourquelot, P., and Hermine, O., *Essential thrombocythaemia: A cause of Sneddon's syndrome (letter).* Lancet, 1996. 347:395.

177. Alegre, V. A., Winkelmann, R. K., and Gastineau, D. A., *Cutaneous thrombosis, cerebrovascular thrombosis, and lupus anticoagulant—The Sneddon syndrome. Report of 10 cases.* Int J Dermatol, 1990. 29:45–49.

178. Daoud, M. S., Wilmoth, G. J., Su, W. P. D., and Pittelkow, M. R., *Sneddon syndrome.* Semin Dermatol, 1995. 14:166–172.

179. Pascual-Castroviejo, I., Lopez-Rodriguez, L., de la Cruz Medina, M., Salamanca-Maesso, C., and Roche Herrero, C., *Hypomelanosis of Ito. Neurological complications in 34 cases.* Can J Neurol Sci, 1988. 15:124–129.

180. Pascual-Castroviejo, I., Roche, C., Martinez-Bermejo, A., Arcas, J., Lopez-Martin, V., Tendero, A., Esquiroz, J. L., and Pascual-Pascual, S. I., *Hypomelanosis of Ito: A study of 76 infantile cases.* Brain Dev, 1998. 20:36–43.

181. Glover, M. T., Brett, E. M., and Atherton, D. J., *Hypomelanosis of Ito: Spectrum of the disease.* J Pediatr, 1989. 115:75–80.

182. Hatchwell, E., *Hypomelanosis of Ito and X;autosome translocations: A unifying hypothesis.* J Med Genet, 1996. 33:177–183.

183. Ruiz-Maldonado, R., Toussaint, S., Tamayo, L., Laterza, A., and del Castillo, V., *Hypomelanosis of Ito: Diagnostic criteria and report of 41 cases.* Pediatr Dermatol, 1992. 9:1–10.

184. Buzas, J. W., Sina, B., and Burnett, J. W., *Hypomelanosis of Ito: Report of a case and review of the literature.* J Am Acad Dermatol, 1981. 4:195–204.

185. Ballmer-Weber, B. K., Inaebnit, D., Brand, C. U., and Braathen, L. R., *Sporadic hypomelanosis of Ito with focal hypertrichosis in a 16–month-old girl.* Dermatology, 1996. 193:63–64.

186. Zemstrov, A., Boyd, A. S., and Giveon, T., *Hypomelanosis of Ito associated with palmoplantar keratoderma and normal magnetic resonance imaging findings.* Int J Dermatol, 1992. 31:284–285.

187. Urgelles, E., Pascual-Castroviejo, I., Roche, C., Moneo, J. L., Martinez, M. A., and Vega, A., *Arteriovenous malformation in hypomelanosis of Ito.* Brain Dev, 1996. 18:78–80.

188. Steiner, J., Adamsbaum, C., Desguerres, I., Lalande, G., Raynaud, F., Ponsot, G., and Kalifa, G., *Hypomelanosis of Ito and brain abnormalities: MRI findings and literature review.* Pediatr Radiol, 1996. 26:763–768.

189. Fryns, J. P., Dereymaeker, A. M., and Van Den Berghe, H., *Hypomelanosis of Ito and severe sensorineural deafness.* Genet Couns, 1992. 3:149–151.

190. Stewart, R. E., Funderbunk, S., and Setoguchi, Y., *A malformation complex of ectrodactyly, clefting and hypomelanosis of Ito (incontinentia pigmenti achromians).* Cleft Patale J, 1979. 16:358–362.

191. Tan, S. T., Slaney, S. F., Ashworth, G., and Poole,

M. D., *Hemifacial hypoplasia and hypomelanosis of Ito.* J Craniomaxillofac Surg, 1995. 23:274–279.

192. Daubeney, P. E., Pal, K., and Stanhope, R., *Hypomelanosis of Ito and precocious puberty.* Eur J Pediatr, 1993. 152:715–716.

193. Chevalier, C., Colon, S., Faraj, G., Bouvier, R., Pincon, J. A., and Cochat, P., *Glomerulopathy and hypomelanosis of Ito.* Nephrologie, 1997. 18:125–127.

194. Nordlund, J. J., Klaus, S. N., and Gino, J., *Hypomelanosis of Ito.* Acta Derm Venereol, 1977. 57:261–264.

195. Cavallari, V., Ussia, A. F., Siragusa, M., and Schepis, C., *Hypomelanosis of Ito: Electron microscopical observations on two new cases.* J Dermatol Sci, 1996. 13:87–92.

196. Cellini, A., Morroni, M., Simonetti, O., and Offidani, A., *Hypomelanosis of Ito: A case report with clinical and ultrastructural data.* J Eur Acad Dermatol Venereol, 1998. 10:73–76.

197. Sybert, V. P., *Hypomelanosis of Ito: A description, not a diagnosis.* J Invest Dermatol, 1994. 103(Suppl 5):141S–143S.

198. Gorski, J. L., and Burright, E. N., *The molecular genetics of incontinentia pigmenti.* Semin Dermatol, 1993. 12:255–265.

199. Scheuerle, A. E., *Male cases of incontinentia pigmenti: Case report and review.* Am J Med Genet, 1998. 18:201–218.

200. Kirchmann, T. T., Levy, M. L., Lewis, R. A., Kanzler, M. H., Nelson, D. L., and Scheuerle, A. E., *Gonadal mosaicism for incontinentia pigmenti in a healthy male.* J Med Genet, 1995. 32:887–890.

201. Fowell, S. M., Greenwald, M. J., Prendiville, J. S., and Jampol, L. M., *Ocular findings of incontinentia pigmenti in a male infant with Klinefelter's syndrome.* J Pediatr Ophthalmol Strabismus, 1992. 29:180–184.

202. Kunze, J., Frenzel, U. H., Huttig, E., Grosse, F.-R., and Wiedemann, H.-R., *Klinefelter's syndrome and incontinentia pigmenti Bolch-Sulzberger.* Hum Genet, 1977. 35:237–240.

203. O' Brien, J. E., and Feingold, M., *Incontinentia pigmenti: A longitudinal study.* Am J Dis Child, 1985. 139:711–712.

204. Carney, R. G., *Incontinentia pigmenti: A world statistical analysis.* Arch Dermatol, 1976. 112:535–542.

205. Dutheil, P., Vabres, C., Cayla, M. C., and Enjolras, O., *Incontinentia pigmenti: Late sequelae and genotypic diagnosis: A three-generation study of four patients.* Pediatr Dermatol, 1995. 12:107–111.

206. Abimelec, P., Rybojad, M., Cambiaghi, S., Moraillon, I., Cavelier-Balloy, B., Marx, C., and Morel, P., *Late, painful, subungual hyperkeratosis in incontinentia pigmenti.* Pediatr Dermatol, 1995. 12:340–342.

207. Adeniran, A., Townsend, P. L., and Peachey, R. D., *Incontinentia pigmenti (Bloch-Sulzberger syndrome) manifesting as painful periungual and subungual tumours.* J Hand Surg (Br), 1993. 18:667–669.

208. Simmons, D. A., Kegel, M. F., Scher, R. K., and Hines, Y. C., *Subungual tumors in incontinentia pigmenti.* Arch Dermatol, 1986. 122:1431–1434.

209. Yell, J. A., Walshe, M., and Desai, S. N., *Incontinentia pigmenti associated with bilateral cleft lip and palate.* Clin Exp Dermatol, 1991. 16:49–50.

210. Avrahami, E., Harel, S., Jurgenson, U., and Coh, D. F., *Computed tomographic demonstration of brain changes in incontinentia pigmenti.* Am J Dis Child, 1985. 139:372–374.

211. Yang, J. H., Ma, S. Y., and Tsai, C. H., *Destructive encephalopathy in incontinentia pigmenti: A case report.* J Dermatol, 1995. 22:340–343.

212. Aydingoz, U., and Midia, M., *Central nervous system involvement in incontinentia pigmenti: Cranial MRI of two siblings.* Neuroradiology, 1998. 40:364–366.

213. Goldberg, M. F., *The blinding mechanisms of incontinentia pigmenti.* Trans Am Ophthalmol Soc, 1994. 92:167–176.

214. Soltau, J. B., and Lueder, G. T., *Bilateral macular lesions in incontinentia pigmenti. Bloch-Sulzberger syndrome.* Retina, 1996. 16:38–41.

215. Ferreira, R. C., Ferreira, L. C., Forstot, L., and King, R., *Corneal abnormalities associated with incontinentia pigmenti.* Am J Ophthalmol, 1997. 123:549–551.

216. Manthey, R., Apple, D. J., and Kivlin, J. D., *Iris hypoplasia in incontinentia pigmenti.* J Pediatr Ophthalmol Strabismus, 1982. 19:279–280.

217. Smith, B., and Bedrossian, E. H. Jr., *Incontinentia pigmenti associated with nasolacrimal duct obstruction.* Ophthalmic Surg, 1984. 15:980–982.

218. Peltonen, L., *Incontinentia pigmenti in four generations.* Dermatologica, 1986. 172:201–204.

219. Rott, H. D., *Partial sweat gland aplasia in incontinentia pigmenti Bloch-Sulzberger. Implications for nosologic classification.* Clin Genet, 1984. 26:36–38.

220. Moss, C., and Inco, P., *Anhidrotic and achromians lesions in incontinentia pigmenti.* Br J Dermatol, 1987. 116:839–849.

221. Roberts, W. M., Jenkins, J. J., Moorhead, E. L. 2nd, and Douglass, E. C., *Incontinentia pigmenti, a chromosomal instability syndrome, is associated with childhood malignancy.* Cancer, 1988. 62:2370–2372.

222. Zillikens, D., Mehringer, A., Lechner, W., and Burg, G., *Hypo- and hyperpigmented areas in incontinentia pigmenti. Light and electron microscopic studies.* Am J Dermatopathol, 1991. 13:57–62.

223. Gorski, J. L., Bialecki, M. D., McDonald, M. T., Massa, H. F., Trask, B. J., and Burright, E. N., *Cosmids map to incontinentia pigmenti type I (IP1) translocation breakpoints to a 180-kb region within a 1.2-Mb YAC contig.* Genomics, 1996. 35:338–345.

224. Jouet, M., Stewart, H., Landy, S., Yates, J., Yong, S. L., Harris, A., Garret, C., Hatchwell, E., et al., *Linkage analysis in 16 families with incontinentia pigmenti.* Eur J Hum Genet, 1997. 5:168–170.

225. Takematsu, H., Terui, T., Torinuki, W., and Tagami, H., *Incontinentia pigmenti: Eosinophil chemotactic activity of the crusted scales in the vesiculobullous stage.* Br J Dermatol, 1986. 115:61–66.

226. Thyresson, N. H., Goldberg, N. C., Tye, M. J., and Leiferman, K. M., *Localization of oeosinophil granule major basic protein in incontinentia pigmenti.* Pediatr Dermatol, 1991. 8:102–106.

CHAPTER 10

Hematologic Malignancies and Skin Diseases

LYMPHOMAS

Hematopoietic diseases can present initially in the skin and remain localized or disseminate from there. Such cases are classified as "primary" cutaneous malignancies. Alternatively, the diseases can spread from lymph nodes or the bone marrow to involve the skin, in which case they are classified as "secondary" processes. This is an important distinction in terms of prognosis, although it may be a difficult, if not impossible, distinction to make on an isolated skin biopsy specimen. Only "secondary" lymphomas are discussed in this volume.

Large Cell Anaplastic Lymphoma

Epidemiology. The nomenclature regarding large cell anaplastic lymphoma is somewhat confusing. Primary cutaneous large cell anaplastic lymphoma arises in the skin and often has no underlying systemic involvement. The designation *secondary* cutaneous large cell anaplastic (Ki-1) lymphoma currently has two meanings. It can refer to lymphomas that develop as a result of a transformation from a primary cutaneous T-cell lymphoma such as mycosis fungoides or pleomorphic T-cell lymphoma [1, 2]. The same term can refer to lymphomas that develop from cutaneous involvement of a systemic large cell anaplastic lymphoma. It is impossible to make this distinction on histologic grounds, but it is an important distinction to make in terms of prognosis and

treatment options [3]. In general, the prognosis is believed to be quite poor for patients in whom large cell anaplastic lymphoma develops secondary to another type of primary cutaneous lymphoma, whereas it is excellent for patients with primary cutaneous large cell anaplastic lymphoma [1, 2]. Because these neoplasms are primarily cutaneous tumors without concurrent systemic disease, they are not addressed further in this volume. There are several excellent reviews of this type of lymphoma [3, 4]. The secondary cutaneous large cell lymphomas that occur in the setting of systemic lymphoma tend to occur in children and adolescents and have a bimodal age distribution [5, 6]. This age distribution is similar to that in Hodgkin's disease [5]. Most series suggest a male predominance [7, 8]. A t(2:5)(p23;q35) translocation has been associated with these secondary large cell lymphomas [9]. This association is not seen in patients with primary cutaneous large cell anaplastic lymphoma. The 2 year disease-free survival rate was 39% for all patients and 62% for patients presenting with stages I and II disease [8].

Cutaneous Features. Firm, erythematous to violaceous papules and nodules are the most common presentation of cutaneous involvement in secondary large cell anaplastic lymphoma. Often, the cutaneous lesions are relatively few in number and may be localized to a single anatomic location. Generalized lesions are not common. There is no apparent site predilection. Spontaneous regression of cutaneous lesions has been reported [10].

Associated Disorders. Secondary involvement of the skin by large cell anaplastic lymphoma occurs in the setting of marked extranodal disease. Up to 40% of patients with anaplastic large cell lymphoma will demonstrate extranodal disease [8]. Up to 90% of patients present with lymphadenopathy [11]. The extranodal organs most affected, in addition to the skin, include the lung, gastrointestinal tract, soft tissues, and bone [5, 6, 12]. Bone marrow involvement is uncommon in these patients [6, 8]. Anaplastic large cell lymphoma has been reported in patients with acquired immunodeficiency syndrome (AIDS) [13].

Histologic Features. Histologic features of primary and secondary cutaneous large cell anaplastic lymphomas are identical. The tumors are composed of a dense, diffuse dermal infiltrate of large, atypical cells (Fig. 10–1 *A*). The neoplastic cells are distributed throughout the dermis, and in most cases, epidermotropism is minimal [4]. A grenz zone may be present in the papillary dermis. The infiltrate often extends into the subcutaneous fat and may extend into cutaneous appendages. The cells can be multinucleated. Nuclei are vesicular and have one or more irregular and eccentrically placed nucleoli, which are often quite prominent. Cells resembling Reed-Sternberg cells may be present. Cytoplasm is abundant in these round to polygonal lymphocytes. Abundant mitotic figures, some of which may be atypical, and individual cell necrosis are present in most cases (Fig. 10–1 *B*). An infiltrate of reactive small lymphocytes is often present at the periphery of the tumor nodules.

There is some attempt in the literature to divide these large cell anaplastic lymphomas into those with pleomorphic nuclei and those with a more monomorphous-appearing infiltrate. Some argue that those with the monomorphic-type of anaplastic large cell lymphoma may have a worse prognosis [5]. Others, however, have suggested that those with the pleomorphic subtype of lymphoma have a more aggressive form of the disease [7].

Special Studies. The large cell anaplastic lymphoma is defined by its immunolabeling profile. CD30 (Ki-1) will label more than 75% of the atypical cells in the dermis [10, 14]. Although most cases represent T-cell lymphomas and will label with CD43, CD20-positive B-cell lymphomas can also be CD30 positive and may represent 10%–20% of all cases [8]. Indeterminate-lineage CD30-positive lymphomas may also occur [13]. CD25 is also positive in many cases. A Ki-67 stain will demonstrate a high proliferation index in these neoplasms [9]. CD15, which labels Reed-Sternberg cells in many cases of Hodgkin's disease, is not expressed by the atypical cells in anaplastic large cell lymphoma. This may be helpful in resolving a differential diagnosis. Gene rearrangement studies demonstrate clonal proliferations in most cases of anaplastic large cell lymphoma.

Pathogenesis. Epstein-Barr virus has been found in 33%–67% of patients with secondary cutaneous large cell anaplastic lymphoma [10, 15]. There is some evidence to suggest that CD30-positive lymphomas that are found to contain Epstein-Barr virus DNA have a more aggressive course [16]. It has been suggested that this viral infection plays some role in the pathogenesis of this neoplasm, but the exact role remains to be defined [13]. Human T-cell lymphotrophic virus type I has also been found in some patients with large cell anaplastic lymphoma, but this association is believed to be tenuous [10].

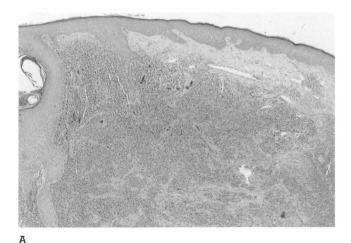

A

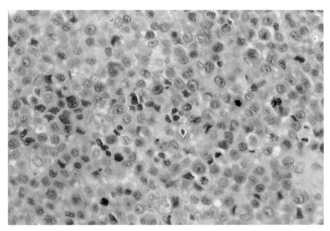

B

Fig. 10–1. *A,* A dense dermal infiltrate of atypical lymphocytes is seen in large cell anaplastic lymphoma. *B,* The cells are markedly atypical, with vesicular nuclei, prominent nucleoli, and abundant mitoses.

Angiocentric Lymphoma

Epidemiology. Angiocentric lymphoma is generally regarded as the malignant form of the spectrum of angiocentric immunoproliferative lesions [17]. Angiocentric lymphoma frequently involves extranodal sites, including the skin and the upper respiratory tract [18]. The most commonly affected region is the nasal cavity [19]. It remains controversial whether angiocentric lymphomas are identical to lymphomatoid granulomatosis or are distinct entities [20, 21] (see Chapter 6).

Cutaneous Features. Angiocentric lymphoma involves the skin with erythematous plaques and nodules that are frequently ulcerated.

Associated Disorders. A granulomatous panniculitis has been observed in some patients with angiocentric T-cell lymphoma [22]. It is unclear whether this observation may be one of overlap in diagnostic criteria between angiocentric T-cell lymphoma, subcutaneous T-cell lymphoma, and so-called cytophagic histiocytic panniculitis.

Angiocentric lymphomas frequently involve the gastrointestinal tract and upper respiratory tract. Pulmonary lesions are also common, especially in cases classified as lymphomatoid granulomatosis (see Chapter 6).

Histologic Features. Histologic features of angiocentric lymphoma involving the skin include a patchy and/or diffuse infiltrate of atypical lymphoid cells centered in the deeper dermis and subcutaneous fat. Extension into the superficial portions of the dermis may occur, but epidermotropism is uncommon. The atypical cells surround blood vessels and can be seen invading the vascular walls, leading to destruction and disruption of endothelial cells (Fig. 10–2 *A*). Throm-

bosis is commonly seen, with subsequent necrosis of the overlying epidermis and dermis (Fig. 10–2 *B*). The atypical lymphocytes are characterized by having large, indented nuclei and moderate amounts of cytoplasm. The neoplastic lymphocytes range in size from small to large cells [21]. Mitoses are common. Abundant cytoplasm within the neoplastic T cells gives the infiltrate a granulomatous appearance [22].

Special Studies. Immunolabeling of the neoplastic lymphocytes has revealed confusing data. In some cases, the tumor cells are purported to label as T cells [23]. More recent data have suggested that, while many T cells are present, the neoplastic lymphocytes are actually B cells. In some cases, the neoplastic cells label as natural killer cells [22]. Similarly, gene rearrangement studies have yielded conflicting results, suggesting that more than one type of neoplastic lymphoid proliferation may give rise to a similar pattern of clinical and histologic changes. Part of this confusion stems from definitions, with some authors differentiating between angiocentric lymphoma and lymphomatoid granulomatosis [20, 21] and others regarding the entities as identical [24, 25].

Pathogenesis. A high percentage of patients with angiocentric lymphoma are positive for the Epstein-Barr virus [18, 21]. Some patients with angiocentric lymphoma have been found to be infected with human T-cell lymphotrophic virus type I [23].

Subcutaneous T-Cell Lymphoma (Histiocytic Cytophagic Panniculitis)

Epidemiology. There is still some debate in the literature about whether histiocytic cytophagic panniculitis and subcutaneous T-cell lymphoma are synonymous or

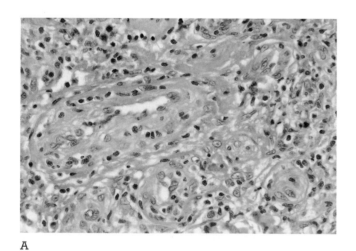

A

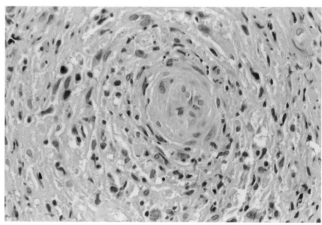

B

Fig. 10–2. Angiocentric T-cell lymphoma is characterized by infiltration of blood vessel walls by atypical lymphocytes *(A)*, leading to thrombosis and vascular occlusion *(B)*.

whether there is simply a large overlap between the two conditions. The disease occurs in middle-aged adults and appears to have a slight female predominance [26]. It is often fatal, with many patients dying within months of diagnosis [27]. Other patients, however, appear to have a better prognosis and recover without evidence of systemic lymphoma [28].

Cutaneous Features. Cutaneous lesions of subcutaneous T-cell lymphoma/histiocytic cytophagic panniculitis are those of a panniculitis. Tender, erythematous nodules and plaques are present, often on the lower extremities. Superficial ulceration with spontaneous drainage may be present. The trunk, extremities, and face can also be involved [26]. Purpura is also commonly seen [29].

Associated Disorders. Patients with subcutaneous T-cell lymphoma have constitutional symptoms that include chronic fever, mucosal ulceration, serositis, and hepatosplenomegaly. Liver failure occurs, and death is usually due to a hemorrhagic event [28]. Disseminated intravascular coagulation is present in almost half of these patients [26].

Some authors argue that not all patients with cytophagic histiocytic panniculitis have subcutaneous T-cell lymphoma and that the same symptom complex is associated with a wide range of viral illnesses, most commonly Epstein-Barr virus, cytomegalovirus, and human immunodeficiency virus type 1 (HIV-1) [30]. Others argue that while there are considerable similarities between the two entities, there are subtle differences that suggest that they are distinct entities [31]. A patient has been reported who had both a T-cell lymphoma and active Epstein-Barr virus infection [32]. Patients with similar symptoms and histologic changes were found to have B-cell lymphomas [33].

Histologic Features. Subcutaneous T-cell lymphoma/histiocytic cytophagic panniculitis usually spares the epidermis and upper portions of the dermis. The upper dermis may demonstrate a mild lymphohistiocytic infiltrate. Located in the deep reticular dermis and in the subcutaneous fat, there are benign-appearing large, foamy histiocytes, edema, and hemorrhage [28] (Fig. 10–3 A). The infiltrate is predominantly lobular, but also involves the septa, and there is abundant fat necrosis (Fig. 10–3 B). The characteristic diagnostic cells are large, atypical lymphocytes with abundant cytoplasm in which multiple lymphocytes, platelets, and erythrocytes can be seen. These cells have been called "bean bag" cells [27] (Fig. 10–3 C). Karyorrhectic debris may be present.

Special Studies. Clonal proliferations of T cells have been demonstrated [31, 34].

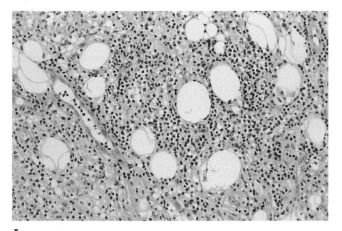

A

B

C

Fig. 10–3. *A, B,* Subcutaneous T-cell lymphoma is characterized by a dense infiltrate of lymphocytes within the deep reticular dermis and subcutaneous fat. *C,* Emperipolesis is a common finding.

Pathogenesis. The pathogenesis of subcutaneous T-cell lymphoma remains unknown. It is still not resolved whether this it even a single entity or if this clinicopathologic disease pattern is seen in patients with lymphomas and also in patients with viral illnesses.

Intravascular Lymphoma (Malignant Angioendotheliomatosis)

Epidemiology. Intravascular lymphoma is a very rare entity. The tumor was initially believed to be a proliferation of endothelial cells, giving rise to its initial designation of malignant angioendotheliomatosis. Subsequent work has, however, demonstrated this neoplasm to be an intravascular lymphoma [35]. The disease is usually found in middle-aged to elderly adults, with no gender predilection [36]. The median survival time is approximately 13 months after diagnosis [36]. It is important to differentiate between the "malignant" variant, that is, a true lymphoma, and the "reactive" variant, which represents a reactive proliferation of endothelial cells.

Cutaneous Features. Most patients with intravascular lymphoma present with cutaneous or neurologic changes caused by vascular occlusion [37]. Cutaneous involvement is quite varied and may manifest with generalized telangiectasias [38], asymptomatic purpuric patches [39], a vasculitic appearance [40], or tender, indurated nodules resembling panniculitis [41].

Associated Disorders. Patients frequently present with mild anemia, an elevated sedimentation rate, and elevated lactate dehydrogenase levels [42]. Fevers and myalgias may be present.

    Visceral involvement is present in approximately 65% of patients [43]. The central nervous system is another frequent site of involvement. Described symptoms include mental status changes, pyramidal tract signs, and peripheral neuropathy [44]. Tumor infiltrating muscles and peripheral nerves has also been reported [45]. Adrenal glands may be infiltrated by intravascular lymphoma [46].

    Intravascular lymphoma has been reported in a patient with rheumatoid arthritis and Sjögren's syndrome [47]. Symmetric polyarthritis was the presenting sign in another patient [48].

    Involvement of the lungs has led to the clinical presentation of adult respiratory distress syndrome in a patient with intravascular lymphoma [49]. Epstein-Barr virus has been detected in the neoplastic cells of a patient with intravascular lymphoma, raising the possibility of a causal association [50].

Histologic Features. Intravascular lymphoma is characterized by widely ectatic vessels in the dermis and subcutaneous fat that are filled by large, atypical cells that are noncohesive (Fig. 10–4 *A*). These cells have hyperchromatic, irregular nuclei and little cytoplasm. Nucleoli may be present and quite conspicuous, and mitotic activity is often brisk [46] (Fig. 10–4 *B*).

Special Studies. Most cases of intravascular lymphoma have been shown to be B-cell lymphomas [51,

52]. This histologic pattern in others has been labeled as T-lymphocyte proliferation [46] or has demonstrated a T-cell lineage with polymerase chain reaction analyses [49].

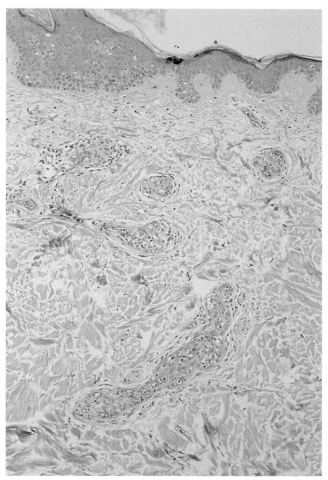

A

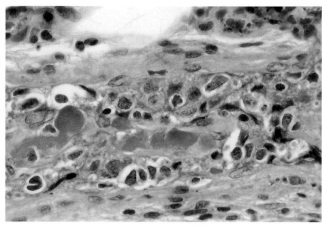

B

Fig. 10–4. *A,* Dermal blood vessels are distended with atypical lymphocytes in intravascular lymphoma. *B,* These markedly atypical lymphocytes are largely confined to vascular lumina.

Pathogenesis. The pathogenesis of intravascular lymphoma remains unknown.

Secondary B-Cell Lymphoma

Epidemiology. B-cell lymphomas may arise primarily in the skin or appear in the skin as a manifestation of systemic disease. The primary cutaneous B cell lymphomas fall outside the purview of this volume and are not discussed further. Moreover, the systemic manifestations of B-cell lymphoma are better addressed in other contexts. The remainder of this discussion focuses on the cutaneous presentation of systemic B-cell lymphomas as they affect the skin. Secondary involvement of the skin is found in approximately 10% of patients with nodal-based B-cell lymphomas [53]. Except in medium-grade lymphomas, cutaneous involvement conveys a poor prognosis [53]. Lymphoblastic and diffuse small cleaved types of lymphoma are most likely to secondarily affect the skin, while immunoblastic and small lymphocytic are least likely [54].

Cutaneous Features. The usual cutaneous presentation of B-cell lymphoma secondarily involving the skin is that of erythematous to violaceous, firm dermal nodules. The head and neck are the most common sites of involvement, but lymphoma nodules have been described on the trunk, buttocks, and virtually all other body sites. The papules and nodules may be grouped or disseminated.

Associated Disorders. Although systemic lymphomas are associated with myriad other clinical disorders, including immunosuppression, viral infections, and heritable chromosomal abnormalities, there are no associations that are specifically related to cutaneous involvement.

Histologic Features. Histologic features of secondary cutaneous lymphoma replicate the primary nodal-based lymphoma in most cases. It has been shown that a correct histologic diagnosis of follicular lymphoma is possible based on skin biopsy results in about 60% of cases

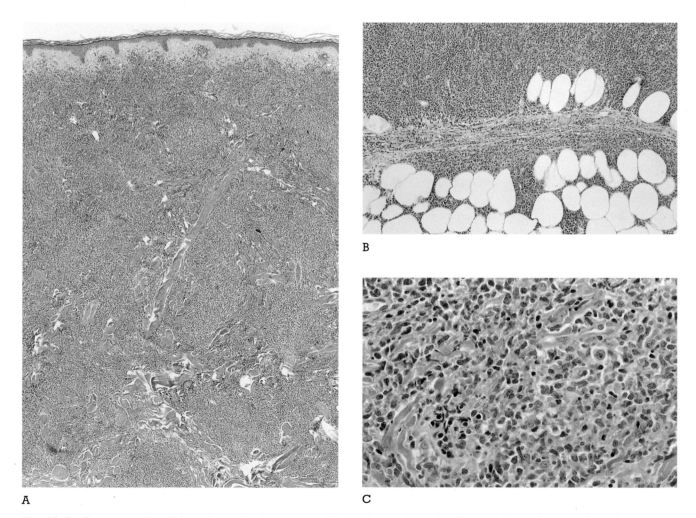

A

B

C

Fig. 10–5. Cutaneous B-cell lymphoma is characterized by a dense dermal infiltrate of lymphocytes that often spares the epidermis *(A)* and can extend into the subcutaneous fat *(B)*. A uniform population of irregular lymphocytes is seen throughout the infiltrate *(C)*.

Table 10–1. Lymphocyte Surface Markers Useful in the Classification of Lymphoma

Marker	Targets Labeled
CD2	Pan T cells
CD3	Pan T cells
CD4	Helper T cells
CD5	Pan T cells
CD7	Pan T cells
CD8	Cytotoxic/suppressor T cells
CD10	Follicular center cells, pre-B cells, some T cells
CD11c	Myelomonocytic antigen
CD15	Reed-Sternberg cells
CD19	Pan B cells
CD20	Pan B cells
CD22	Pan B cells
CD25	Interleukin-2 receptors
CD30	Activated T and B cells, lymphomatoid papulosis, Hodgkin's disease, large cell anaplastic lymphoma
CD43	Pan T cells
CD45RO	OPD4− subset of memory T cells
CD56	Natural killer cells, angiocentric lymphoma
CD57	Natural killer cells, angiocentric lymphoma
MIB-1	Proliferating cells
Ki-67	Proliferating cells
kappa	Subset of B cells
lambda	Subset of B cells
IgM	Subset of B cells
bcl-2	Malignant follicular center cells, reactive T cells

[55]. In general, the histologic features depend on the subtype of lymphoma that has spread to involve the skin. B-cell lymphomas tend to be centered in the dermis, with minimal epidermotropism. A Grenz zone is often, but not always, present [56] (Fig. 10–5 A). The infiltrate of lymphocytes can be either diffuse or nodular. In some, but not all, cases a "bottom-heavy" pattern may be present, and extension into the subcutaneous fat is common (Fig. 10–5 B). In some cases, tumor cells infiltrate and destroy the cutaneous appendages. The characteristics of the neoplastic cells depend on the particular subtype of lymphoma involving the skin. Absence of admixed histiocytes and eosinophils is helpful in distinguishing neoplastic B-cell proliferations from reactive infiltrates (Fig. 10–5 C).

Special Studies. Immunolabeling is very helpful in establishing or confirming a diagnosis of B-cell lymphoma involving the skin. Most benign, reactive cutaneous infiltrates have relatively few B cells, and in these settings they are centered in reactive germinal centers containing tingible-body macrophages and other features of benignity. A pan-B-cell marker, such as CD20, is helpful in demonstrating sheets of B cells, a finding that is very suggestive of B-cell lymphoma. Antibodies directed against kappa and lambda light chains can also be use-

ful in detecting clonality of a population of B cells, but these markers can be difficult to use when examining mature B cells. A wide panel of other immunomarkers has been described that are helpful in subclassifying the type of lymphoma (Table 10–1) [57]. Gene rearrangement studies have also been shown to be very sensitive for detecting early lesions of lymphoma. This is not often, however, necessary in patients with known node-based lymphoma in whom skin lesions appear.

Pathogenesis. It is not currently understood what permits some lymphomas to extend into the skin while others do not. Epstein-Barr virus has been implicated in the pathogenesis of some types of B-cell lymphomas [58].

Hodgkin's Disease Involving the Skin

Epidemiology. Cutaneous involvement with Hodgkin's disease is very uncommon, occurring in 1%–3.4% of cases [59, 60]. In most cases, it appears late in the course of the disease, when the process is widely disseminated and patients have stage IVB disease. In these cases, the prognosis is very poor, with most patients dying within several months of developing skin lesions [60]. Some patients do well, however, even after secondary cutaneous involvement [61].

Cutaneous Features. Patients with Hodgkin's disease may have specific lesions or nonspecific lesions. Nonspecific lesions are more common and include ichthyosis, lichenification, and herpes zoster infection. Only specific lesions are described in more detail in this section. The most common types of cutaneous presentations include single or multiple dermal or subcutaneous papules and nodules [60]. The chest is the most commonly affected site [62]. These nodules are often located in the skin distal to affected lymph nodes [62]. Several other types of lesions have been described in these patients, including poikiloderma atrophicans vasculare [63] and ulcers [64]. Direct extension into the skin from underlying tumor nodules has also been described.

Lymphomatoid papulosis rarely occurs in patients with Hodgkin's disease and may appear at any time during the course of their disease. Approximately 10%–20% of patients with lymphomatoid papulosis will also have systemic lymphoma at some time during their lives [65]. It is assumed by many authors that these entities are closely related [65, 66]. Lymphomatoid papulosis is characterized by multiple erythematous papules and nodules at different stages of development. They are usually relatively asymptomatic [67]. The papules are often hemorrhagic and necrotic within days to weeks [68]. They heal with hyperpigmentation or varioliform scars over weeks to months. The true nosology of lymphomatoid papulosis occurring with Hodgkin's disease is uncertain.

Associated Disorders. Patients with Hodgkin's disease may present with many types of nonspecific cutaneous lesions including generalized pruritus, erythema annulare centrifugum [69], granulomatous panniculitis [70],

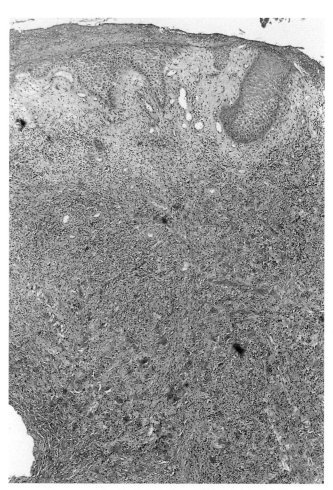

A

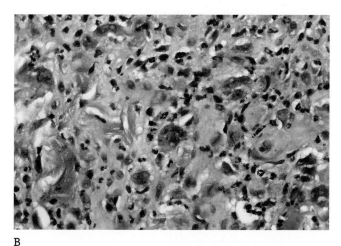

B

Fig. 10–6. Cutaneous Hodgkin's disease is characterized by a dense dermal infiltrate of lymphocytes *(A)*, scattered eosinophils, and occasionally Reed-Sternberg cells *(B)*.

symmetric peripheral gangrene secondary to disseminated intravascular coagulation [71], prurigo nodularis [72], vasculitis [73], urticarial vasculitis [74], and pyoderma gangrenosum [75].

Involvement of the skin by Hodgkin's disease has been reported in patients with AIDS [76]. Infection with Epstein-Barr virus has also been reported in about half of patients with Hodgkin's disease [77]. The significance of this finding remains unknown.

There is a complex relationship between Hodgkin's disease, lymphomatoid papulosis, and mycosis fungoides [65]. The waxing and waning papules and nodules of lymphomatoid papulosis may antedate [65], coincide with, or postdate [66] the appearance of Hodgkin's disease and/or mycosis fungoides. Similarly, many patients have been reported in whom there coexists mycosis fungoides and Hodgkin's disease and lymphomatoid papulosis [78].

Granulomatous slack skin is a rare cutaneous disorder that has been associated with Hodgkin's disease and/or mycosis fungoides in many cases [79]. Approximately 50% of patients with granulomatous slack skin (believed to be a variant of cutaneous T-cell lymphoma) have Hodgkin's disease [79, 80]. There is a marked male predominance, and the disease tends to affect younger adults [79]. Patients develop erythematous patches within flexures, which gradually develop into pendulous, lax folds of skin.

Histologic Features. The histologic features of Hodgkin's disease involving the skin resemble those seen in affected lymph nodes. Each of the subtypes, including nodular sclerosing, lymphocyte predominant, mixed cellularity, and lymphocyte–depleted Hodgkin's disease, can give rise to cutaneous lesions that resemble their nodal counterparts. In some cases, it is possible to subtype the disease based on the cutaneous histologic findings. In all cases, there is a dense dermal infiltrate of lymphocytes, which largely spares the epidermis and papillary dermis (Fig. 10–6 A). The infiltrate is diffuse, and an admixture of cell types, including eosinophils, may be present. Most of the cells are small lymphocytes that are admixed with macrophages. Reed-Sternberg cells and lacunar cells are found in most cases [81] (Fig. 10–6 B). In some forms of the disease, bands of fibrosis are present, dividing the infiltrating lymphocytes into nodules.

Granulomatous slack skin is characterized by a granulomatous infiltrate present within the dermis. Epidermotropism may be seen. Admixed with the granulomas are atypical lymphocytes that may be hyperconvoluted. Elastolysis is present [79]. Degenerated elastic tissue fibers can be found within giant cells.

Histologic features of *lymphomatoid papulosis* have been well described [82]. The epidermis may be slightly spongiotic with an overlying parakeratotic scale. Ero-

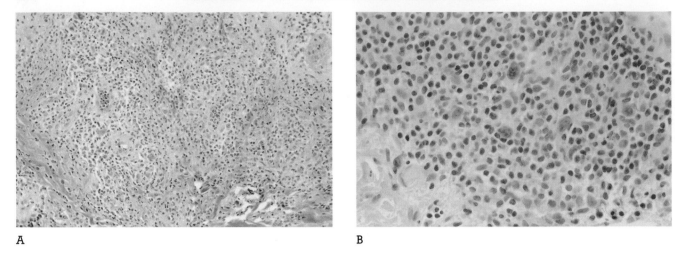

A   B

Fig. 10–7. *A*, Lymphomatoid papulosis is characterized by a dense dermal infiltrate of lymphocytes with scattered eosinophils and perivascular neutrophils. *B*, Scattered atypical cells are interspersed within the infiltrate.

sions or ulcerations may be seen. Dermal infiltrates are polymorphous and dense and show focal epidermotropism. A wedge shape to the infiltrate may be apparent (Fig. 10–7 *A*). Most of the infiltrating lymphocytes are small, reactive T cells. There is a variable admixture of larger, more atypical-appearing cells. These may appear similar to Reed-Sternberg cells (type A) or Sézary cells (type B) [83] (Fig. 10–7 *B*). Eosinophils and neutrophils are often present around vessels and may result in endothelial cell and fibrin deposition [84].

Special Studies. Immunolabeling is useful in establishing a diagnosis of Hodgkin's disease. The Reed-Sternberg cells are positive for CD30 and negative for CD45 (leukocyte common antigen). Most of these cells also express CD15, unlike similar-appearing cells found in large cell anaplastic (Ki-1 lymphoma) and lymphomatoid papulosis [81].

Pathogenesis. Cutaneous involvement with Hodgkin's disease appears to occur by retrograde lymphatic spread, direct extension from an underlying nodal focus of involvement or from hematogenous dissemination [60]. For cases with coexisting lymphomatoid papulosis and Hodgkin's disease, it has been suggested that a t(8;9) genetic translocation may be involved in the pathogenesis of lymphomatoid papulosis and its progression to Hodgkin's disease [65]. Alternatively, lymphomatoid papulosis may represent a lymphoma from the outset. Clonal T-cell gene rearrangements have been found in patients with lymphomatoid papulosis, giving support to this contention [85].

Nonlymphoid hematopoietic processes can present initially in the skin and disseminate from there, in which case they are classified as "primary" cutaneous malignancies. Alternatively, they can spread from lymph nodes or the bone marrow to involve the skin, in which case they are classified as "secondary" processes. This is an important distinction in terms of prognosis, although it may be a difficult, if not impossible, distinction to make with an isolated skin biopsy specimen.

LANGERHANS' CELL PROLIFERATIONS

Histiocytosis X. Langerhans' cell proliferations, previously known as histiocytosis X, encompass the entities of Letterer-Siwe disease, Hand-Schuller-Christian disease, and eosinophilic granuloma. It has been suggested that these forms can be respectively regarded as the acute disseminated, the chronic progressive, and the benign localized forms of Langerhans' cell histiocytosis [86]. It is also now generally believed that congenital self-healing reticulohistiocytosis is also within the spectrum of Langerhans' cell histiocytosis [87, 88]. Because the cell types implicated in the disease processes are identical, the entities are discussed together, making note of differences in clinical presentation.

Epidemiology. Biologic behavior varies from a highly aggressive, fatal disease leading to death to a benign, self-limited course. Presence of organ dysfunction, age, and extent of disease are the best predictors of the disease course [89]. Children older than 2 years of age tend to fare better than younger ones. Others believe that young age and multisystem involvement do not necessarily imply a bad prognosis [90]. The overall mortality rate in children less than 2 years is about 40% [89]. Langerhans' cell histiocytosis occurs rarely in adults [91, 92].

Cutaneous Features. The cutaneous features of Langerhans' cell histiocytosis are quite varied. The most common presentation is that of rose-yellow, and often petechial, 1–2 mm macules and papules in a seborrheic type of distribution involve the face, neck, upper chest, and back. This pattern is seen in more than half of affected infants with the Letterer-Siwe variant of the disease [86]. Pustules have been reported, often on the scalp [91]. Xanthoma-like papules are also observed, often on the eyelids [93]. Less commonly, nodules and ulcers may be seen. A granuloma annulare-like eruption has been reported in adult patients [94].

Cutaneous manifestations occur in about one-third of patients with the Hand-Schuller-Christian variant. These are identical to the cutaneous findings described in patients with the Letterer-Siwe variant, although they may be fewer in number.

Patients with the eosinophilic granuloma form of Langerhans' cell histiocytosis rarely display skin findings. When there is skin involvement, ulcerated nodules may be present. A periorificial location has been reported [95, 96].

Congenital self-healing reticulohistiocytosis usually presents at birth, but may become clinically apparent during the first few months of life [97]. The cutaneous findings are often indistinguishable from those of the Letterer-Siwe form of the disease at the time of presentation and diagnosis. Only the rapid clearing of the lesions with minimal intervention allows the correct diagnosis to be made. The clinical presentation is usually that of widespread papules and nodules in a seborrheic distribution. Vesicles have also been reported [98]. The lesions resolve spontaneously, usually within 3–4 years; however, subsequent relapse has also been reported in these patients [99]. Mucous membranes are usually not affected [100]. In contrast to those with the Letterer-Siwe form of the disease, children with the benign, localized form are not clinically ill.

A purely genital form of the disease has been reported in adults. In these cases, the cutaneous macules and papules are limited to the genital region at the time of presentation and in some cases disseminate [101, 102].

Associated Disorders. Table 10–2 summarizes the organ systems involved in each type of Langerhans' cell histiocytosis. Pulmonary involvement, which may be asymptomatic, is present in more than half of patients with the Letterer-Siwe form of the disease [86]. Hepatosplenomegaly is a major finding in patients with systemic Langerhans' cell histiocytosis. Liver dysfunction adversely affects survival more than any other affected organ [90]. Less than one-third of patients with splenomegaly survive [103]. Bone lesions are present in about 60% of patients with this form of the disease. Thrombocytopenia and anemia may be seen in very severe cases.

Patients with the Hand-Schuller-Christian variant are

Table 10–2. Langerhans' Cell Histiocytoses: Involvement of Internal Organs

Variant of Langerhans' Cell Histiocytosis	Organs Involved and Symptoms
Letterer-Siwe disease	Lungs (>50%)
	Hepatosplenomegaly (majority)
	Bone lesions (>60%)
	Thrombocytopenia (uncommon)
	Anemia (uncommon)
Hand-Schuller-Christian disease	Pituitary
	Exophthalmos
	Bone lesions (>80%)
Eosinophilic granuloma	Bone lesions
	Lymph nodes (rare)
	Lungs (rare)
Congenital self-healing reticulohistiocytosis	None

usually between the ages of 2 and 6 years and have involvement of the pituitary gland, resulting in diabetes insipidus. Exophthalmos may also be present in these patients. Overall, approximately 20% of children with Langerhans' cell histiocytosis experience diabetes insipidus [90, 104]. Bone lesions are found in up to 80% of patients with this form of the disease [91]. Pulmonary infiltrates are present in about 20% of these patients. Hepatomegaly and lymphadenopathy are rare [91].

Lytic bone lesions are the most common finding in patients with eosinophilic granuloma. The lymph nodes and lungs may also be involved [86].

Mucocutaneous involvement with Langerhans' cell histiocytosis is uncommon and may be more prevalent in adults [91, 92]. Involvement of the thymus has also been reported in a series of patients [105]. Acute leukemia has been associated with Langerhans' cell histiocytosis in several patients [90, 106].

Histologic Features. Langerhans' cell histiocytosis demonstrates a dense infiltrate of Langerhans' cells within the dermis. Ulceration may be present. The dermal infiltrate is patchy in most cases and has a per-ivascular distribution. A band-like infiltrate along the dermal–epidermal junction is commonly seen, and epidermotropism into the overlying epidermis is common, occurring in 70% of cases [91] (Fig. 10–8 *A*). The epidermis can be unaffected, but is usually either atrophic or acanthotic. Papillary dermal edema is present in most early lesions [86]. A peri-appendageal infiltrate has been reported in some cases [93]. An admixture of lymphocytes, neutrophils, and abundant eosinophils is usually present. The Langerhans' cells display slight pleomorphism and nuclear hyperchromatism. They have large amounts of eosinophilic cytoplasm and a grooved, or reniform, nucleus (Fig. 10–8 *B*). Small nucleoli may be seen. In the Letterer-Siwe form

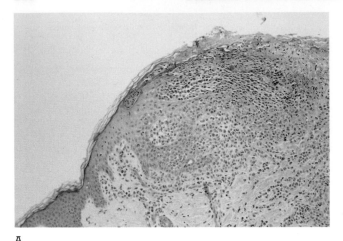
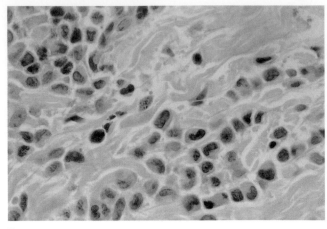

A   B

Fig. 10–8. Langerhans' cell histiocytoses are characterized by a dense infiltrate within the dermis and epidermis *(A)* of Langerhans' cells and eosinophils *(B)*.

of the disease, the Langerhans' cells may demonstrate more pleomorphism and nuclear atypia. Some cells within the infiltrate of older lesions may demonstrate cytoplasmic lipid [86]. In rare cases, this feature is prominent.

Special Studies. Langerhans' cells are easily identified with immunolabeling with S100 protein and CD1a. CD1a expression is more specific than S100 expression. The antibody is commercially available and works in routinely processed tissue. These tests are sometimes necessary to confirm the cell type responsible for the infiltrate. These cells also express HLA-DR and the Fc receptor. Birbeck's granules can be identified within the cytoplasm of a minority of the tumor cells using electron microscopy. The need for this technique has largely been replaced with immunohistochemistry.

Pathogenesis. It remains very controversial whether Langerhans' cell histiocytosis represents a neoplastic clonal transformation or is a reactive process. Several studies have demonstrated a nonrandom skewing pattern of X-chromosome inactivation to argue in favor of a neoplastic transformation [107, 108]. As expected, T-cell gene rearrangement studies failed to reveal a clonal rearrangement [108]. Others maintain that Langerhans' cell histiocytosis is a reactive disorder [109]. Herpesvirus-6 has been detected in lesional tissue of a significant percentage of these patients in one study [110]. The significance of this observation remains unknown.

Indeterminate Cell Disorder

Epidemiology. Indeterminate cell disorder is a rare proliferation of antigen-presenting cells initially described in 1985 [111], and fewer than 50 cases have been recognized and reported since then [112]. The disease occurs equally in men and women and is most common in adults. One congenital case has been reported [113]. Although malignant behavior has been reported [114], spontaneous remission of the lesions has been seen in several patients [111, 115].

Cutaneous Features. Indeterminate cell disorder most commonly presents as a solitary cutaneous nodule. Other patients have presented with widespread papules and papulonodules. Extracutaneous lesions have also been reported as the initial presentation [116].

Associated Disorders. Indeterminate cell disorder has been associated with B-cell chronic lymphocytic leukemia [114] and with mast cell leukemia [117].

Histologic Features. The histologic features of indeterminate cell disorder include a diffuse dermal infiltrate of nonlipidized histiocytes (Fig. 10–9 *A*). These cells have pale cytoplasm and bland, grooved nuclei and are indistinguishable from those of histiocytosis X on routine histologic sections. Nucleoli, when present, are inconspicuous. Mitotic figures are rare. There may be scattered lymphocytes and multinucleated giant cells (Fig. 10–9 *B*). In the rare cases that have a malignant clinical course, the histiocytes display marked cytologic atypia, and mitoses are abundant [111].

Special Studies. Immunolabeling studies are essential to discriminate the cells in indeterminate cell disorder from those in Langerhans' cell histiocytoses. Indeterminate cells are defined as expressing S100 protein but not CD1a. They also lack the Birbeck's granules characteristic of Langerhans' cells.

Pathogenesis. It is unknown what triggers the proliferation of this population of indeterminate, poorly defined mononuclear cells.

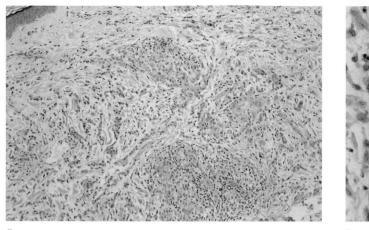
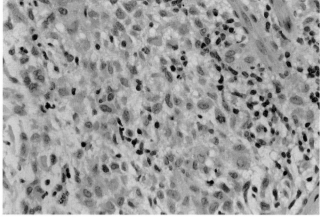

A

B

Fig. 10–9. Indeterminate cell disorder has a dense dermal infiltrate of histiocytic cells *(A)* admixed with smaller lymphocytes *(B)*.

LEUKEMIAS AND THE SKIN

Primary Leukemia Cutis

Epidemiology. Although uncommon, there are many reports in the literature of patients in whom the initial presentation of leukemia is in the skin [118–121]. This includes patients in whom there is no evidence of bone marrow involvement for weeks to months after the initial presentation [122]. Leukemia cutis at the time of birth has heralded the later onset of marrow involvement [122]. Although there are insufficient cases to arrive at a valid statistical analysis about which subtypes of leukemia are most likely to initially present in the skin, it appears as though it may be more likely in the nonlymphocytic leukemias.

Cutaneous Features. The most common appearance of primary leukemia cutis is of one or several red-purple papules or nodules [121, 122]. Erythematous, urticarial macules and papules on the face and extremities have also been reported [120], as has an indurated plaque on the scalp, followed by similar lesions on the trunk [119]. A "seborrheic dermatitis"–like eruption was ultimately diagnosed as leukemia in a single patient [118].

Associated Disorders. Patients who present with "aleukemic" leukemia invariably progress to leukemia over weeks to months. Patients with myelodysplastic syndrome often progress to develop extramedullary myeloid tumors [123].

Histologic Features. The histologic features of primary leukemia cutis are indistinguishable from leukemia cutis originating elsewhere. The epidermis

is usually uninvolved, but epidermotropism has been described in some lymphocytic leukemias. The dermis is filled with sheets of atypical hematopoietic cells that course individually between collagen bundles. There is some predilection for accumulation of these cells around blood vessels and eccrine apparatus [123]. The cells have a high mitotic rate, and individual cell necrosis is prominent. The cells features dependent on the type of leukemia that is present in the skin. These differences are described later in Secondary Leukemia cutis.

Special Studies. A chloroacetate esterase (Leder) stain is often helpful in establishing a diagnosis of myeloid lineage leukemias. Immunolabeling is also helpful in determining the malignant nature of the cells. Table 10–3 summarizes some markers useful for making a diagnosis of leukemia in the skin.

Pathogenesis. It remains unknown why leukemic infiltrates appear in the skin before any evidence of marrow involvement.

Table 10–3. Immunomarkers for Diagnosing Cutaneous Leukemia

Marker	Cells Labeled
CD3	T lymphocytes
CD20	B lymphocytes
CD34	Immature hematopoietic precursors
CD43	T lymphocytes
CD68	Histiocytes
CD99	Lymphoblasts, myeloblasts
Ki-67	Proliferation marker

From references 255 and 256.

Secondary Leukemia Cutis

Epidemiology. Any of the subtypes of leukemia can involve the skin secondarily. In one series of 40 patients with leukemia and cutaneous involvement, most patients had myeloid leukemias (especially subtypes M2 and M4). Only three patients in this series had specific cutaneous infiltrates with chronic lymphocytic leukemia [123]; however, it is well known that chronic lymphocytic leukemia may be present within the skin without giving rise to specific lesions [124]. In another series, chronic forms of leukemia were more likely than acute forms to involve the skin in an adult population [125]. This may reflect the incidence of leukemia subtypes in this population group. Other investigators have also documented higher incidences of cutaneous involvement with monocytic and myelomonocytic leukemias [126]. Cutaneous involvement with leukemia occurs in 25%–30% of children with leukemia [127]. In one series, cutaneous lesions were the presenting sign of leukemia in 17% of patients with chronic lymphocytic leukemia [128]. The prognosis is generally poor for patients with leukemia that spreads to involve the skin [126]. Complete remission has been difficult to attain in many of these patients [129].

Cutaneous Features. In most cases, leukemia cutis presents as erythematous to violaceous papules or nodules. They can be single or multiple and can occur on any site. In widely disseminated cases occurring in newborns, the infants display what has been termed a "blueberry muffin" appearance [130]. This appearance is not specific for leukemia cutis, however, and various other disorders can give rise to a similar clinical appearance. Gingival infiltration with leukemic cells occurs in about 7% of patients with leukemia [131]. This is most commonly seen with acute monocytic leukemia, followed by acute myelomonocytic leukemia.

A wide spectrum of other clinical appearances for leukemic involvement of the skin has been described. Leukemia cutis has been described as mimicking guttate psoriasis [132], urticaria [133], circinate plaques [134], erythema chronicum migrans [135], stasis dermatitis [136], and primary syphilis [137]. A positive Darier's sign (urtication with gentle stroking typical of mastocytosis) has been described in an infant with lymphoblastic leukemia [127].

Several nonspecific cutaneous disorders have also been described in association with leukemia cutis. These include cutis verticis gyrata [138], porphyria cutanea tarda [139], acral erythema [140], atrophie blanche [141], neutrophilic eccrine hidradenitis [142], pyoderma gangrenosum [143], pruritus [144], vasculitis [145], and follicular mucinosis[146].

Multiple secondary cutaneous neoplasms have been reported to occur in patients with leukemia cutis [147]. These include squamous cell carcinomas, basal cell carcinomas, and keratoacanthomas [124, 148]. It has been suggested that this might be related to alterations in immunosurveillance. Rare cases of Merkel cell carcinoma have also been reported in patients with leukemia [149].

Pityriasis rubra pilaris has been described as the initial cutaneous manifestation in a patient with acute leukemia [150]. Rare patients with myeloid leukemias have demonstrated xanthomas as their initial cutaneous manifestations [151]. An unusual pustulovesicular eruption has also been described as the presenting cutaneous lesions in a child with Down's syndrome and chronic myelogenous leukemia [152]. A patient presented with dermatomyositis 3 years before acute myelomonocytic leukemia developed [153].

Associated Disorders. The association of Down's syndrome and leukemia has been well documented [154, 155]. A 10–20-fold increased risk for developing leukemia has been described for patients with Down's syndrome [156]. Acute lymphocytic leukemia, acute megalokaryocytic leukemia, and chronic myelogenous leukemias have all occurred with increased frequency in patients with Down's syndrome. A "transient megakaryocytic leukemia," a true clonal proliferation, develops in some patients, and up to 25% of these patients will fully recover [157]. Monosomy 7 syndrome is associated with juvenile chronic myelogenous leukemia [155].

Patients with leukemia experience secondary cutaneous infections with fungi, (including *Candida* [158] and *Fusarium* [159]), bacteria, and actinomycosis [160]. Countless less common organisms have also been described to cause cutaneous infections in these patients [161]. Demodicidosis has also been described as causing an opportunistic skin infection in patients with leukemia that resembles folliculitis or acne vulgaris [162].

Sweet's disease (acute febrile neutrophilic dermatosis) and pyoderma gangrenosum are both associated with leukemia (see Chapter 30). They are both covered more extensively in Chapter 5.

Histologic Features

Leukemia cutis. Histologic features of secondary leukemia cutis are identical to those seen in patients with primary involvement. Atypical hematopoietic cells are present throughout the dermis (Fig. 10–10 A). This infiltrate usually spares the epidermis and papillary dermis, although epidermotropic infiltrates have been described. The atypical cells course individually between collagen bundles, and there may be a tendency to aggregate around dermal blood vessels and eccrine structures [123]. Cytologic characteristics of the neoplastic cells are related to the subtype of leukemia present. Myeloid leukemias are characterized by the presence of immature myeloid forms, including myeloblasts, promyelocytes, metamyelocytes, band forms, and mature neutrophils (Fig. 10–10 B). The less differentiated forms characterize the acute myeloid leukemias, whereas later forms are more common in chronic myelocytic leukemia. Cytoplasmic granularity can be seen in routine sections in many cases of chronic myelocytic and monomyelocytic leukemia. Lymphocytic leukemias are characterized by the presence of either immature lymphoblasts with a high mitotic rate and abundant individual cell necrosis in the acute forms or a monomorphous population of small, well-differentiated lymphocytes that are identifiable as atypical, primarily on the basis of their monotony, in the chronic form (Fig. 10–10 C).

Several interesting patterns of leukemic infiltration within the skin have been described. A dense aggregation of leukemic cells has been reported in patients with herpes zoster [128], varicella [163], and the inflammatory infiltrate underlying primary keratinocytic neoplasms [124]. The inflammatory infiltrate in psoriasis has been shown to be entirely leukemic [164]. An exaggerated response to arthropod bites has been demonstrated in patients with cutaneous lymphocytic leukemia [165].

Special studies. Chloroacetate esterase is sometimes helpful in accentuating the cytoplasmic granules, thereby establishing a diagnosis of myeloid lineage leukemia. Immunostaining with myeloperoxidase and CD34 can also be helpful for this purpose. CD99 has been shown to be expressed by lymphoblasts in all cases of acute lymphoblastic leukemia and by immature myeloid precursors in up to 80% of cases of acute myelogenous leukemia [166]. As this marker is not usually expressed by mature hematopoietic cells, it may be a sensitive but not a specific marker for a leukemic infiltrate.

NOTE: Neutrophilic eccrine hidradenitis is considered in Chapter 25.

PLASMA CELL DYSCRASIAS AND RELATED CUTANEOUS DISORDERS

Multiple Myeloma. Patients with multiple myeloma experience a range of cutaneous problems. Most of these are rare associations and are addressed briefly at the end of this section.

Extramedullary Plasmacytoma

Epidemiology. Extramedullary plasmacytomas are almost always associated with underlying late-stage mul-

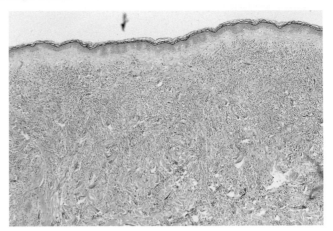

A

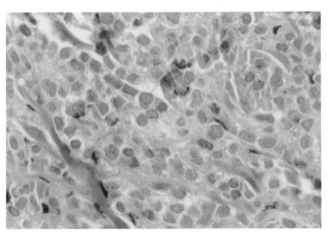

B

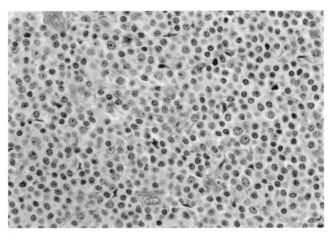

C

Fig. 10–10. Leukemia cutis involves the skin with a diffuse, dense dermal infiltrate (A). Immature blast forms are present in acute myelogenous leukemia (B), and a monomorphous appearance of relatively mature-appearing lymphocytes is seen in chronic lymphocytic leukemia (C).

tiple myeloma [167]. Rare examples have been reported in which no systemic disease has been present [168]; however, it should be noted that up to one-fourth of patients with no apparent systemic disease will develop multiple myeloma within 2 years [169]. The prognosis is dismal for patients with multiple myeloma and extramedullary plasmacytosis within the skin [170]. It is not possible to determine the presence or absence of systemic involvement based on skin biopsy results [171].

Cutaneous Features. Plasmacytomas appear as firm, single or multiple dermal nodules. They are usually red-brown in color and have no overlying surface changes unless they are ulcerated [168]. The trunk is the most commonly affected skin site, followed by the legs and the face [172]. Plasmacytoma was reported to occur in a single patient at the site of previous herpes zoster [171].

Associated Disorders. The disorders associated with extramedullary plasmacytomas are those associated with multiple myeloma and include amyloidosis, cryoglobulinemia, anemia, leukopenia and thrombocytopenia, Raynaud's syndrome, xanthomatosis, and purpura [173].

Histologic Features. The histologic appearance of an extramedullary plasmacytoma is that of a dense, diffuse dermal collection of plasma cells. Typically, the malignant infiltrate spares the epidermis and papillary dermis (Fig. 10–11 *A*). These cells may resemble normal plasma cells or may display varying amounts of cytologic atypia [174]. Nucleoli may be multiple and prominent (Fig. 10–11 *B*). Mitoses are sometimes abundant. The cellular infiltrate tends to cluster around dermal blood vessels and appendages but does not cause destruction of these structures [171]. The malignant infiltrate can extend into the subcutaneous fat [175].

Some authors have suggested that the presence of immature cells resembling B immunoblasts may convey a worse prognosis [176].

Special Studies. Immunolabeling is helpful in determining the monoclonal nature of the cells in extramedullary plasmacytoma. Plasma cells are typically negative when stained with CD20, but show light chain restriction for either kappa or lambda light chains. In some cases, no light chain expression is detected, and staining with antibodies directed against heavy chains can be helpful [169].

Pathogenesis. The pathogenesis of multiple myeloma and extramedullary plasmacytoma remains unknown.

Scleromyxedema

Epidemiology. Scleromyxedema is a disease of middle-aged people with no gender predilection [177]. It has a chronic, progressive course and with little tendency for spontaneous regression [178]. Scleromyxedema may be fatal. Most authors consider scleromyxedema either to be synonymous with lichen myxedematosus or to be a more indurated variant.

Cutaneous Features. Scleromyxedema is characterized by the appearance of multiple waxy 2–3 mm papules and variably distributed induration of the skin. The hands and feet are often the initial site of involvement, but lesions rapidly spread to the head and neck, trunk, and upper extremities [179]. With severe disease, a mask-like face or a leonine face may be apparent.

Associated Disorders. Scleromyxedema is often associated with paraproteinemia. Most patients have circulating IgG lambda paraproteins [180]. The associa-

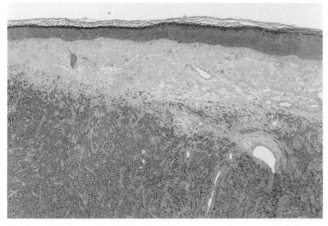

A

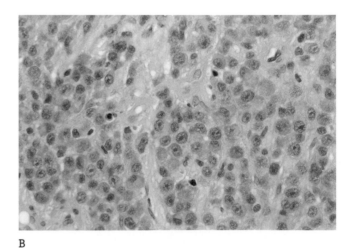

B

Fig. 10–11. *A*, Plasmacytoma is characterized by a dense dermal infiltrate of plasma cells that spares the epidermis and papillary dermis. *B*, Cytologic atypia is often present.

tion with fully developed multiple myeloma is much less common, but does occur more commonly than a random association [179]. Scleromyxedema has also been reported in a patient with non-Hodgkin's lymphoma [181] and in a patient with angioimmunoblastic lymphadenopathy [182].

Systemic involvement with scleromyxedema is uncommon. Gastrointestinal involvement is the most common extracutaneous site of change in patients with scleromyxedema [183]. Scleromyxedematous involvement of the small bowel has been reported in a patient with multiple myeloma [184]. Involvement of the esophagus has also been reported [177].

Severe myopathy has been reported in several patients with scleromyxedema [177, 185, 186]. This has been described as an atypical necrotizing vacuolar myopathy with no increase in acid mucopolysaccharides and minimal inflammation within the muscle [185]. Elevated creatine kinase and aldolase may be present in these patients [186].

Ophthalmologic abnormalities, including corneal opacities and ectropion, have been reported in a series of patients with scleromyxedema. Hyaluronic acid deposits have been demonstrated within the cornea of affected individuals [187, 188]. Other neurologic complications include progressive degenerative changes, median neuropathy [189, 190], and coma [191].

Patients with cor pulmonale, decreased pulmonary diffusion capacity, and "scleroderma kidney" and coexisting scleromyxedema have been reported [177]. A patient with arthritis and scleromyxedema has also been reported [192].

Scleromyxedema occurred in one patient with a long-standing history of psoriasis [193]. An association has also been made between scleromyxedema and adenocarcinomas of the stomach and pancreas [194].

Histologic Features. The histologic features of scleromyxedema include an increase in fibroblasts within the upper half of the reticular dermis (Fig. 10–12 *A*). The overlying epidermis is usually unremarkable and the papillary dermis and deep reticular dermis are unaffected by the process. There may be hyperkeratosis or parakeratosis in some cases. Within the superficial reticular dermis, there is an increase in acid mucopolysaccharides, giving a blue-gray appearance to the ground substance. Early lesions have abundant, round or stellate-shaped fibroblasts, and a mild lymphocytic inflammatory infiltrate is present around vessels [195]. Increased numbers of mast cells may be present [194]. Later lesions are less cellular and have less mucin, and the dermis appears more fibrotic.

Special Studies. Colloidal iron and Alcian blue stains performed at pH 2.5 demonstrate increased acid mucopolysaccharides (Fig. 10–12 *B*). This staining can be eliminated with pretreatment by hyaluronidase, identifying the ground substance as hyaluronic acid. In most cases, these stains are not necessary because the increased ground substance is readily apparent on routine sections.

Pathogenesis. In vitro studies have demonstrated that sera from patients with scleromyxedema cause increased production of hyaluronic acid and prostaglandin E by fibroblasts, without increasing cellular proliferation rates [196]. Other studies, however, have suggested exactly the opposite, that is, an increase in fibroblast proliferation without an increase in glycosaminoglycan production [197]. Additional studies demonstrated increased amounts of type I collagen and decreased amounts of type III collagen in the superficial dermis in a patient with scleromyxedema [198]. The exact relationship between increased serum im-

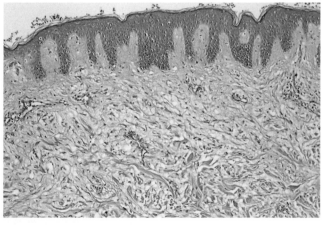

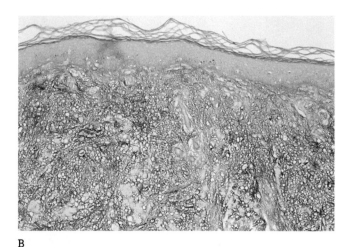

A   B

Fig. 10–12. *A,* Scleromyxedema is characterized by increased numbers of fibroblasts within the superficial dermis. *B,* and increased dermal mucin is detected with colloidal iron stain.

munoglobulins and dermal hyaluronic acid remains unclear.

Other Mucocutaneous Conditions Associated with Multiple Myeloma.

Cutis laxa acquisita has been reported to occur in several patients with multiple myeloma. Destruction of elastic tissue affects the skin, as well as lungs, heart, gastrointestinal tract, and urogenital tract. It has been postulated that immune complex–mediated elastin destruction is responsible for the destruction of the elastic tissue that results in the laxity of the skin in the axilla. McCarty et al. [199] suggest that cutis laxa acquisita be regarded as a paraneoplastic process of multiple myeloma.

Follicular spicules of the nose are described in several patients with multiple myeloma [200, 201]. These small cutaneous horns are present mainly on the face and centered on the nose. Histologic evaluation demonstrated the presence of IgG paraprotein deposits between keratinocytes in the upper layers of the follicular infundibula and in the surrounding epidermis [200]. Follicular cavities were filled with parakeratotic cells and paraprotein giving rise to a horny spicule [201]. Bork et al. [201] suggest that the predilection for the nose is related to cryoprecipitation of the paraprotein. In a related condition, parakeratotic horns, again with strong deposits of epidermal immunoglobulin, were found in a generalized distribution in a patient with multiple myeloma [202].

A bullous lichenoid eruption in the oral cavity has been reported in a patient with multiple myeloma [203] as has a case of acquired hyalinosis cutis et mucosae [204]. Subcorneal pustular dermatosis is also seen in patients with IgA myeloma [205].

Necrobiotic xanthogranuloma with paraproteinemia [206] and normolipemic planar xanthomas [207] have been associated with multiple myeloma and are discussed more fully in Chapter 29. Pityriasis rotunda has been associated with multiple myeloma [208] and is discussed in Chapter 30. Systemic amyloidosis occurs in patients with multiple myeloma and is discussed in Chapter 7, and pyoderma gangrenosum and Sweet's syndrome [209] have both been associated with multiple myeloma and are addressed in Chapter 5 and Chapter 30.

Waldenström's Macroglobulinemia

Epidemiology. Waldenström's macroglobulinemia is a monoclonal proliferation of plasma cells in the spleen, marrow, and lymph nodes. Affected individuals usually have increased levels of circulating monoclonal IgM. It occurs in middle-aged to elderly individuals and has a slight male predominance. The classic triad involves a lymphoplasmacytic lymphoma, an IgM M spike of greater than 3 g, and the hyperviscosity syndrome. Skin involvement is quite unusual in this disease [210].

Cutaneous Features. Nonspecific cutaneous signs of Waldenström's macroglobulinemia include erythematous to violaceous papulonodules, ulcers, leukocytoclastic vasculitis, and livedo reticularis [211]. The papules have been described as being "infiltrated" or firm, and they are painful in some patients [210]. A more common association is with urticaria, a constellation of findings known as Schnitzler's syndrome [212, 213]. In addition, translucent small papules filled with IgM, called "storage papules," have been observed in some patients [214, 215]. It is unclear if these cases are similar to one patient who was described as having Waldenström's macroglobulinemia and xanthoma disseminatum [216]. A bullous eruption has also been reported in several of these patients [211].

Associated Disorders. Patients with Waldenström's macroglobulinemia suffer from weakness, fatigue, increased bleeding, weight loss, and neurologic disturbances [217]. Other symptoms include cryoglobulinemia, hyperviscosity, and cold agglutinin-positive hemolytic anemia.

Glomerular disease, amyloidosis, and neuropathy may be seen in patients with Waldenström's macroglobulinemia secondary to deposits of IgM in the tissues [218]. Lupus erythematosus has been reported to occur in several patients with Waldenström's macroglobulinemia [219, 220].

Histologic Features. The macules and papules of Waldenström's macroglobulinemia are characterized by dense lymphoplasmacytoid cell infiltrates within the dermis [221]. They are perivascular or diffuse and typically spare the papillary dermis. Some of the infiltrating cells can be immature forms [222].

Histologic features of the bullae associated with Waldenström's macroglobulinemia include a subepidermal blister and occlusion of small and large vessels within the dermis and subcutaneous fat by periodic acid–Schiff positive eosinophilic material. There is no inflammation [211] (Fig. 10–13).

Urticaria, in cases of Waldenström's macroglobulinemia, demonstrates a perivascular mixed inflammatory infiltrate with neutrophils and nuclear dust [223]. Biopsy material from ulcers in these patients have demonstrated IgM paraproteins within dermal vessel walls, causing luminal obstruction [224]. The "storage papules" associated with Waldenström's macroglobulinemia contain abundant eosinophilic material in the

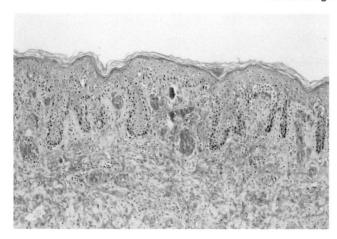

Fig. 10–13. Waldenström's macroglobulinemia is characterized by occlusion of small and large vessels with minimal inflammation.

dermis (probably representing immunoglobulins), in addition to a dense lymphoplasmacytic infiltrate [225].

Special Studies. Immunostained sections of skin demonstrate monoclonal IgM deposits within occluded vessels. Similar deposits have been described along the basement membrane zone [211]. In other studies, the immunoglobulin depositions have been localized to the roof [226] and to the base [210] of the blister in different patients. Immunolabeling of the lymphoplasmacytoid infiltrate reveals monoclonality in these cases based on light chain restriction [222].

Pathogenesis. The pathogenesis of this plasmacellular malignancy remains unknown.

MISCELLANEOUS SYSTEMIC HEMATOPOIETIC PROLIFERATIONS IN THE SKIN

Angioimmunoblastic Lymphadenopathy

Epidemiology. Angioimmunoblastic lymphadenopathy (AILD) is a very rare immunoproliferative disorder that transforms into T-cell lymphoma in a subset of patients [227]. Patients with AILD, independent of whether transformation to lymphoma occurs or not, tend to have a poor prognosis.

Cutaneous Features. Cutaneous involvement occurs in approximately 40% of patients with AILD. The most common manifestation is that of pruritic, generalized macules and papules [228]. Less commonly, plaques

and nodules have been described in these patients. Urticaria and exfoliative erythroderma are also reported [227]. In many patients, the cutaneous eruption may precede any other signs of systemic disease [229]. It has been suggested that patients with cutaneous involvement may have a worse prognosis [230].

Associated Disorders. Most patients with AILD present with constitutional symptoms including fever, weight loss, and malaise. Generalized lymphadenopathy is present in most patients. Hepatosplenomegaly can also be present. Occasional patients with AILD present with polyarthritis [231]. Common laboratory abnormalities include hemolytic anemia and polyclonal hypergammaglobulinemia [232].

There are numerous reports of patients with coexisting Kaposi's sarcoma and AILD [233].

Histologic Features. Histologic features of AILD include an extensive superficial and deep perivascular and periappendageal infiltrate of lymphocytes admixed with a vascular proliferation (Fig. 10–14 A). A mixture of small and large lymphocytes is present. A high mitotic index is seen within these cells. Extravasation of erythrocytes is also seen commonly [234]. Scattered plasma cells are present within the infiltrate [235] (Fig. 10–14 B). A lymphocytic vasculitis has been described in some patients with AILD [236].

Special Studies. Special studies with skin biopsy tissue are not helpful in making a diagnosis of AILD. Gene rearrangement studies, however, are essential in determining the presence of an evolving T-cell lymphoma.

Pathogenesis. The exact pathogenesis of AILD is unknown. It has been suggested that the process develops due to an excessive proliferation of transformed lymphocytes due to chronic antigen stimulation. Human herpesvirus-6 has been implicated in some cases [237] and Epstein-Barr virus in others [238].

Sinus Histiocytosis with Massive Lymphadenopathy (Rosai-Dorfman Disease)

Epidemiology. Sinus histiocytosis with massive lymphadenopathy (SHML) occurs in patients of any age, but has a mean age of onset of about 21 years [239]. There is a slight male predominance. In most cases, the disease is self-limited and spontaneously regresses [240].

Cutaneous Features. Extranodal SHML occurs in up to 43% of patients with the disease. The skin is the most common extranodal site of involvement and can

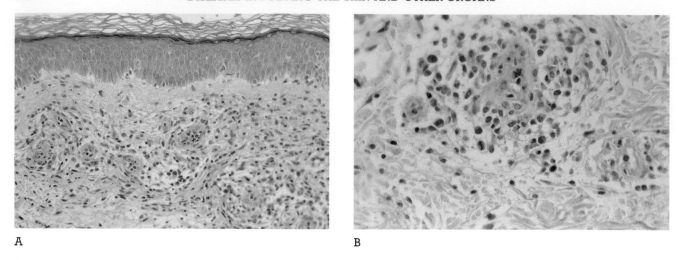

A   B

Fig. 10–14. Angioimmunoblastic lymphadenopathy demonstrates a superficial and deep perivascular lymphocytic infiltrate *(A)* with admixed plasma cells. Mitoses are often prominent *(B)*.

be affected in the absence of associated lymph node involvement. Yellow papules, similar in appearance to xanthomas, have been described most frequently; however, papules, dermal nodules, scaly patches, diffuse erythema, indurated plaques, and subcutaneous nodules have also been reported [239].

Associated Disorders. Constitutional symptoms in patients with SHML include fever, weight loss, and malaise. Night sweats occur infrequently.

Lymphadenopathy is the most common clinical finding in patients with SHML. The cervical nodes are involved in 87% of cases, but any lymph nodes can be affected. Mild hepatomegaly is seen in about 20% of patients with SHML [239]. Osteolytic bone lesions have been reported. The nasal cavity is a common ex-

tranodal site of involvement for SHML. Ocular and central nervous systems have also been involved.

Several types of neoplasia, including non-Hodgkin's lymphoma, Langerhans' cell histiocytosis, multiple myeloma, melanoma, and papillary thyroid carcinoma have been reported in patients with SHML. As these are all individual case reports, it is not clear that they represent true associations.

Histologic Features. The histologic features of SHML involving the skin are quite similar to the changes reported in affected lymph nodes. Within the dermis, there is a dense nodule of pale-staining histiocytes along with lymphocytes and neutrophils (Fig. 10–15 *A*). The histiocytes are frequently present within the lumen of dilated lymphatic channels [241]. Emperipolesis, or

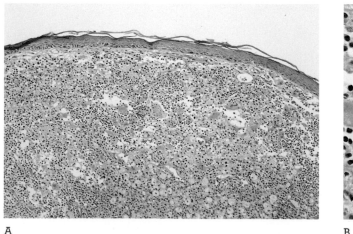

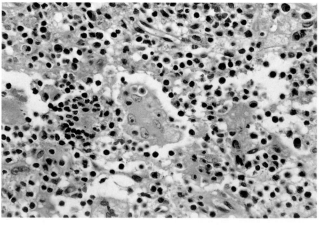

A   B

Fig. 10–15. *A,* Sinus histiocytosis with massive lymphadenopathy is characterized by sheets of histiocytes and perivascular aggregates of plasma cells. *B,* Emperipolesis is evident in large histiocytes.

phagocytosis of lymphocytes and erythrocytes, is commonly seen and is helpful in making a diagnosis of SHML (Fig. 10–15 *B*). Abundant plasma cells are present along the dilated lymphatics [239]. Lymphoid aggregates and germinal centers are frequently present at the periphery of the infiltrates [241].

Special Studies. Antibodies directed against S100 protein and pan-macrophage markers such as CD68 stain the histiocytes in SHML. These cells do not stain with antibodies directed against CD1a [242].

Pathogenesis. The pathogenesis of SHML is currently not known. The disease is best regarded as a proliferation of functionally active macrophages derived from circulating monocytes [242]. Several series have implicated human herpesvirus-6 in the cases of SHML [243, 244].

Cutaneous Eruptions of Lymphocyte Recovery

Epidemiology. The cutaneous eruption of lymphocyte recovery occurs in 50%–75% of patients receiving cytoreductive therapy without marrow support [245]. The concept of eruption of lymphocyte recovery includes allogeneic and autologous graft-versus-host reactions (GVHRs). Allogeneic GVHRs occur in 50%–95% of patients depending on type of transplant, age of the recipient, prophylactic regimen, and manipulation of the marrow, among other factors. The development of allogeneic graft-versus-host disease confers protection against tumor relapse [246]. Autologous GVHR evolves in roughly 10% of patients when the transplant is unmodified [247]. The addition of low-dose cyclosporin results in a cutaneous eruption resembling a GVHR in 50%–70% of patients, thereby hopefully inducing a graft-versus-tumor effect [245]. Further modification of the transplant through the addition of interferon-γ and interleukin-2 increases the incidence and severity of cutaneous eruptions developing after autologous marrow transplantation. Chronic graft-versus-host disease occurs as lichenoid and sclerodermoid forms, generally after 60 days post-transplant in 10%–20% of patients.

Cutaneous Features. Erythematous macules and papules arise in any distribution in the cutaneous eruption of lymphocyte recovery and an acute GVHR. Both eruptions usually occur after 14–21 days of hospitalization. A GVHR often first appears on acral surfaces, especially the palms, soles, and pinnae, but may begin on the trunk. As the distribution of the eruption increases, bullae may arise within the erythematous macules, imparting close resemblance to toxic epidermal necrolysis (Table 10–4).

Table 10–4. Clinical Stages of Graft-Versus-Host Reactions	
Stage	*Involvement*
1	<25% of body surface
2	25%–50% of body surface
3	Erythroderma
4	Bullae

The lichenoid GVHR greatly resembles lichen planus with erythematous to violaceous papules in variable distribution. Further similarity exists with oral findings of white lacy patches resembling changes seen in idiopathic lichen planus [248]. The sclerodermatoid GVHR presents with progressive induration of the skin in varying distribution and intensity. Whole-body involvement may ensue. Loss of hair, chronic erosion, ulceration, and joint contracture develop in long-standing cases.

Associated Disorders. Graft-versus-host reactions are associated with any diseases that are treated wtih bone marrow transplantation. Less commonly, GVHR may be seen after solid organ transplantations [249] and blood transfusions [250].

Histologic Features. Samples of the cutaneous eruption of lymphocyte recovery display a mild upper dermal perivascular infiltrate composed of lymphocytes with mild overlying exocytosis and spongiosis with occasional necrotic keratinocytes [251]. In an acute GVHR the lymphocytes assume a perivascular and interstitial array with basal layer vacuolization, exocytosis, and necrosis of keratinocytes [246] (Fig. 10–16). Melanophages accumulate in the upper dermis. After

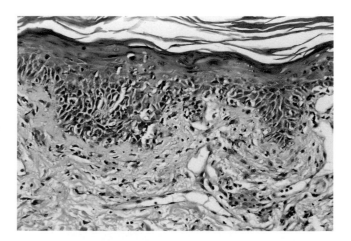

Fig. 10–16. Graft-versus-host disease is demonstrated in a superficial lymphocytic infiltrate that extends into the epidermis. Dying keratinocytes are present.

Table 10–5. Grading Scheme for Histologic Findings in Acute Graft-Versus-Host Reactions

Grade	Features
0	Normal skin or diagnosis unrelated to the marrow transplant
1	Basal vacuolization and mild spongiosis
2	Grade 1 plus keratinocyte necrosis and dermal lymphocytes
3	Cleft formation at the dermal–epidermal junction
4	Separation of epidermis from dermis

liver transplantation and transfusions, GVHRs display similar findings. Table 10–5 provides the grading scheme for the histologic diagnosis of an acute GVHR. By convention, grade 2 changes comprise the diagnostic findings of a GVHR.

After unmodified autologous marrow transplants, samples of cutaneous eruptions display findings of the eruption of lymphocyte recovery. Administration of cyclosporin results in changes resembling an acute allogeneic GVHR, whereas the addition of interferon-γ and interleukin-2 results in greater numbers of lymphocytes in the dermal infiltrate and more pronounced exocytosis and spongiosis.

The histologic findings of lichenoid and sclerodermoid GVHRs greatly resemble their idiopathic counterparts. In sclerodermatous disease, basal vacuolization accompanies the collagen alteration [252]. Unlike

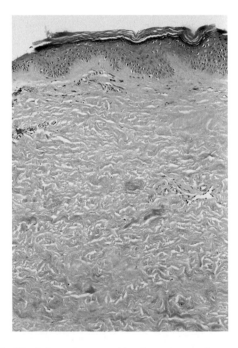

Fig. 10–17. Sclerodermatoid chronic graft-versus-host disease demonstrates marked thickening and sclerosis of the reticular dermis.

morphea and progressive systemic sclerosis, a superficial panniculitis is generally absent (Fig. 10–17).

Special Studies. No special studies aid the diagnosis of any cutaneous eruption of lymphocyte recovery.

Pathogenesis. Mechanisms of disease for the entities considered here are poorly understood. After allogeneic marrow transplant between MHC-matched individuals who are related or unrelated, minor antigen mismatch presumably drives the immunologic reaction [253]. In the autologous setting, unregulated effector activity and homing of recovery lymphocytes to the skin may underlie the frequent development of cutaneous eruptions. The addition of low-dose cyclosporin to autologous transplantation regimens may promote autoreactive cells by abrogating processes that normally delete T lymphocytes with self-recognition receptors [254]. The autoimmune mechanisms responsible for chronic GVHRs remain highly speculative.

NOTE: Post-transplant lymphoproliferative disease is described in Chapter 8.

References

1. Sterry, W., Korte, B., and Schubert, C., *Pleomorphic T-cell lymphoma and large cell anaplastic lymphoma of the skin.* Am J Dermatopathol, 1989. 11:112–123.
2. Kaudewitz, P., Stein, H., and Dallenbach, F., *Primary and secondary cutaneous Ki-1+ (CD30+) anaplastic large cell lymphomas.* Am J Pathol, 1989. 135:359–367.
3. Willemze, R., and Beljaards, R. C., *Spectrum of primary cutaneous CD30 (Ki-1)-positive lymphoproliferative disorders.* J Am Acad Dermatol, 1993. 28:973–980.
4. Krishnan, J., Tomaszewski, M.-M., and Kao, G. F., *Primary cutaneous CD30-positive anaplastic large cell lymphoma. Report of 27 cases.* J Cutan Pathol, 1993. 20:193–202.
5. Chott, A., Kaserer, K., Augustin, I., Vesely, M., Heniz, R., Oehlinger, W., Hanak, H., and Radaszkiewicz, T., *Ki-1–positive large cell lymphoma: A clinicopathologic study of 41 cases.* Am J Surg Pathol, 1990. 14:439–448.
6. Kadin, M. E., Sako, D., and Berliner, N., *Childhood Ki-1 lymphoma presenting with skin lesions and peripheral lymphadenopathy.* Blood, 1986. 68:1042–1049.
7. Chan, J. K. C., Ng, C. S., Hui, P. K., Leung, T. W., Los, E. S., Lau, W. H., and McGuire, L. J., *Anaplastic large cell Ki-1 lymphoma. Delineation of two morphologic types.* Histopathology, 1989. 15:11–34.
8. Greer, J. P., Kinney, M. C., Collins, R. D., Salhany, K. E., Wolff, S. N., Hainsworth, J. D., Flexner, J. M., and Stein, R. S., *Clinical features of 31 patients with Ki-1 anaplastic large cell lymphoma.* J Clin Oncol, 1991. 9:539–547.
9. Bitter, M. A., Franklin, W. A., and Larson, R. A., *Morphology in Ki-1 (CD30) positive non-Hodgkin's lym-*

phomas is correlated with clinical features and the presence of a unique chromosomal abnormality, t(2;5) (p23;q35). Am J Surg Pathol, 1990. 14:305–316.

10. Kaudewitz, P., Kind, P., and Sander, C. A., *CD30+ anaplastic large cell lymphoma.* Semin Dermatol, 1994. 13:180–186.

11. Rodriguez, J., Pugh, W., Romaguera, J., and Cabanillas, F., *Anaplastic Ki-1+ large-cell lymphoma.* Cancer Invest, 1993. 11:554–558.

12. Agnarsson, B. A., and Kadin, M. E., *Ki-1 positive large cell lymphoma: A morphologic and immunologic study of 19 cases.* Am J Surg Pathol, 1988. 21:264–274.

13. Chadburn, A., Cesarman, E., Jagirdar, J., Subar, M., Mir, R. N., and Knowles, D. M., *CD30 (Ki-1) positive anaplastic large cell lymphoma in individuals infected with the human immunodeficiency virus.* Cancer, 1993. 72:3078–3090.

14. Stein, H., Mason, D. Y., Gerdes, J., O'Connor, N., Wainscoat, J., Pallesen, G., Gratter, K., Fallini, B., et al., *The expression of Hodgkin's disease–associated antigen Ki-1 in reactive and neoplastic lymphoid tissue: evidence that Reed-Sternberg cells and histiocytic malignancies are derived from activated lymphoid tissue.* Blood, 1985. 66:848–858.

15. Kanavaros, P., Jiwa, N. M., De Bruin, P. C., Van Der Valk, P., Noordyn, L. A., Van Heerde, P., Gordijn, R., Horstman, A., et al., *High incidence of EBV genome in CD30-positive non-Hodgkin's lymphomas.* J Pathol, 1992. 168:307–315.

16. Su, I. J., Hseih, H. C., Lin, K. H., Uen, W. C., Kao, C. L., Chen, C. J., Cheng, A. L., Kadin, M. E., et al., *Aggressive peripheral T-cell lymphomas containing Epstein-Barr viral DNA: A clinicopathologic and molecular analysis.* Blood, 1991. 77:799–808.

17. Jaffe, E. S., *Pathology of the Lymph Nodes and Related Organs.* 1985, W B Saunders Company, Philadelphia.

18. Chan, J. K. C., Ng, C. S., Ngan, K. C., Hui, P. K., Lo, S. T., and Lau, W. H., *Angiocentric T-cell lymphoma of the skin.* Am J Surg Pathol, 1988. 12:861–876.

19. Sander, C. A., Kind, P., Kaudewitz, P., Raffeld, M., and Jaffe, E. S., *The revised European-American classification of lymphoid neoplasms (REAL): A new perspective for the classification of cutaneous lymphomas.* J Cutan Pathol, 1997. 24:329–341.

20. Guinee, D., Jaffe, E., Kingma, J. D., Fishback, N., Wallberg, K., Krishnan, J., Fizzera, G., Travis, W., et al., *Pulmonary lymphomatoid granulomatosis: evidence for a proliferation of Epstein-Barr virus infected B-lymphocytes with a prominent T-cell component and vasculitis.* Am J Surg Pathol, 1994. 18:753–764.

21. Jaffe, E. S., Chan, J. K. C., Su, I. J., Frizzera, G., Morri, S., Feller, A. C., and Ho, F. C., *Report of the workshop on nasal and related extranodal angiocentric T/NK lymphomas: Definitions, differential diagnosis, and epidemiology.* Am J Surg Pathol, 1996. 20:103–111.

22. Takeshita, M., Kimura, N., Suzumiya, J., Ohshima, K., Kikuchi, M., Watanabe, R., Okamura, T., and Goto, H., *Angiocentric lymphoma with granulomatous panniculitis in the skin expressing natural killer cell and large granular T-cell phenotypes.* Virchows Archiv, 1994. 425:499–504.

23. McNutt, N. S., Smoller, B. R., Kline, M., Choen, S. R., Hsu, A., Saltz, L., Cash, K., and Safai, B., *Angiocentric T-cell lymphoma associated with human T-cell lymphotropic virus type I.* Arch Pathol Lab Med, 1990. 114:170–175.

24. Nicholson, A. G., Wotherspoon, A. C., Diss, T. C., Singh, N., Butcher, D. N., Pan, L. X., Isaacson, P. G., and Corrin, B., *Lymphomatoid granulomatosis: Evidence that some cases represent Epstein-Barr virus–associated B-cell lymphoma.* Histopathology, 1996. 29:317–324.

25. Madison McNiff, J., Cooper, D., Howe, G., Crotty, P. L., Tallini, G., Crouch, J., and Eisen, R. N., *Lymphomatoid granulomatosis of the skin and lung. An angiocentric T-cell–rich B-cell lymphoproliferative disorder.* Arch Dermatol, 1996. 132:1464–1470.

26. Alegre, V. A., and Winkelmann, R. K., *Histiocytic cytophagic panniculitis.* J Am Acad Dermatol, 1989. 20:177–185.

27. Crotty, C. P., and Winkelmann, R. K., *Cytophagic histiocytic panniculitis with fever, cytopenia, liver failure and terminal hemorrhagic diathesis.* J Am Acad Dermatol, 1981. 4:181–194.

28. Pettersson, T., Kariniemi, A.-L., Tervonen, S., and Franssila, K., *Cytophagic histiocytic panniculitis: A report of four cases.* Br J Dermatol, 1992. 127:635–640.

29. Smith, K. J., Skelton, H. G. I., Yeager, J., Angritt, P., Wagner, K., James, W. D., Giblin, W. J., and Lupton, G. P., *Cutaneous histopathologic, immunohistochemical, and clinical manifestations in patients with hemophagocytic syndrome.* Arch Dermatol, 1992. 128:193–200.

30. Perniciaro, C., Winkelmann, R. K., and Erhardt, D. R., *Fatal systemic cytophagic histiocytic panniculitis: A histopathologic and immunohistochemical study of multiple organ sites.* J Am Acad Dermatol, 1994. 31:901–905.

31. Mehregan, D. A., Su, W. P. D., and Kurtin, P. J., *Subcutaneous T-cell lymphoma: A clinical, histopathologic, and immunohistochemical study of six cases.* J Cutan Pathol, 1994. 21:110–117.

32. Smith, K. J., Skelton, H. G. I., Giblin, W. L., and James, W. D., *Cutaneous lesions of hemophagocytic syndrome in a patient with T-cell lymphoma and active Epstein-Barr virus.* J Am Acad Dermatol, 1991. 25:919–924.

33. Peters, M. S., and Winkelmann, R. K., *Cytophagic panniculitis and B cell lymphoma.* J Am Acad Dermatol, 1985. 13:882–885.

34. Coupe, M., Foroni, L., Stamp, G., Lovatt, D., Barnard, M., Krausz, T., Kalofonos, H., Epenetos, A., et al., *Conal rearrangement of the T-cell receptor γ gene associated with a bizarre lymphoproliferative syndrome.* Eur J Hematol, 1988. 41:289–294.

35. Wick, M. R., Mills, S. E., Scheithaur, B. W., Cooper, P. H., Davitz, M. A., and Parkinson, K., *Reassessment of malignant "angioendotheliomatosis." Evidence in favor of its reclassification as "intravascular lymphomatosis."* Am J Surg Pathol, 1986. 10:112–123.

36. Remberger, K., Nawrath-Koll, I., Gokel, J. M., and Haider, M., *Systemic angioendotheliomatosis of the lung.* Pathol Res Pract, 1987. 182:265–274.

37. Dubas, F., Saint-Andre, J. P., Pouplard-Barthelaix, A., Delestre, F., and Emile, J., *Intravascular malignant lymphomatosis (so-called malignant angioendotheliomatosis): A case confined to the lumbosacral spinal cord and roots*. Clin Neuropathol, 1990. 9:115–120.

38. Ozguroglu, E., Buyulbabani, N., Ozguroglu, M., and Baykal, C., *Generalized telangiectasia as the major manifestation of (intravascular) lymphoma*. Br J Dermatol, 1997. 137:422–425.

39. Chang, A., Zic, J. A., and Boyd, A. S., *Intravascular large cell lymphoma: A patient with asymptomatic purpuric patches and a chronic clinical course*. J Am Acad Dermatol, 1998. 39:318–321.

40. Walker, U. A., Herbst, E. W., Ansorge, O., and Peter, H. H., *Intravascular lymphoma simulating vasculitis*. Rheumatol Int, 1994. 14:131–133.

41. Perniciaro, C., Winkelmann, R. K., Daoud, M. S., and Su, W. P. D., *Malignant angioendotheliomatosis is an angiotropic intravascular lymphoma. Immunohistochemical, ultrastructural, and molecular genetics studies*. Am J Dermatopathol, 1995. 17:242–248.

42. Sleater, J. P., Segal, G. H., Scott, M. D., and Masih, A. S., *Intravascular (angiotropic) large cell lymphoma: Determination of monoclonality by polymerase chain reaction on paraffin-embedded tissues*. Mod Pathol, 1994. 7:593–598.

43. Wick, M. R., Banks, P. M., and McDonald, T. J., *Angioendotheliomatosis of the nose with fatal systemic dissemination*. Cancer, 1981. 48:2510–2517.

44. Devlin, T., Moll, S., Hulette, C., and Morgenlander, J. C., *Intravascular malignant lymphomatosis with neurologic presentation: Factors facilitating antemortem diagnosis*. South Med J, 1998. 91:672–676.

45. Levin, K. H., and Lutz, G., *Angiotropic large-cell lymphoma with peripheral nerve and skeletal muscle involvement: Early diagnosis and treatment*. Neurology, 1996. 47:1009–1011.

46. Lopez-Gil, F., Roura, M., Umbert, I., and Umbert, P., *Malignant proliferative angioendotheliomatosis or angiotropic lymphoma associated with soft-tissue lymphoma*. J Am Acad Dermatol, 1992. 26:101–104.

47. Chakravarty, K., Goyal, M., Scott, D. G., and McCann, B. G., *Malignant "angioendotheliomatosis" (intravascular lymphomatosis)—an unusual cutaneous lymphoma in rheumatoid arthritis*. Br J Rheumatol, 1993. 32:932–934.

48. von Kempis, J., Kohler, G., Herbst, E. W., and Peter, H. H., *Intravascular lymphoma presenting as symmetric polyarthritis*. Arthritis Rheum, 1998. 41:1126–1130.

49. Gabor, E. P., Sherwood, T., and Mercola, K. E., *Intravascular lymphomatosis presenting as adult respiratory distress syndrome*. Am J Hematol, 1997. 56:155–160.

50. Au, W. Y., Shek, W. H., Nicholls, J. T., Tse, K. M., Todd, D., and Kwong, Y. L., *T-cell intravascular lymphomatosis (angiotropic large cell lymphoma): Association with Epstein-Barr viral infection*. Histopathology, 1997. 31:563–567.

51. Cuter, T. P., and Wiltshire, C. R., *Malignant proliferating angioendotheliomatosis*. Br J Dermatol, 1989. 121:76–77.

52. Willemze, R., Kruyswijk, M. R. J., de Bruin, C. D., Meijer, C. J., and Von Berkel, W., *Angiotropic (intravascular) large-cell lymphoma of the skin previously classified as malignant angioendotheliomatosis*. Br J Dermatol, 1987. 116:393–399.

53. Sterry, W., Kruger, G. R., and Steigleder, G. K., *Skin involvement of malignant B-cell lymphomas*. J Dermatol Surg Oncol, 1984. 10:276–277.

54. Patterson, J. W., *Lymphomas*. Dermatol Clin, 1992. 10:235–251.

55. Dabski, K., Banks, P. M., and Winkelmann, R. K., *Clinicopathologic spectrum of cutaneous manifestations in systemic follicular lymphoma. A study of 11 patients*. Cancer, 1989. 64:1480–1485.

56. Glusac, E. J., Kindel, S. E., Soslow, R. A., and Smoller, B. R., *Evaluation of classic architectural criteria in nonmycosis fungoides cutaneous lymphomas*. Am J Dermatopathol, 1998. 19:557–561.

57. Smoller, B. R., *The role of immunohistochemistry in the diagnosis of cutaneous lymphoma*. In *Advances in Dermatology*, C. J. Cockerell, Ed. 1998, Mosby, St. Louis, pp. 207–234.

58. Kulwichit, W., Edwards, R. H., Davenport, E. M., Basker, J. F., Godfrey, V., and Raab-Traub, N., *Expression of the Epstein-Barr virus latent membrane protein 1 induces B cell lymphoma in transgeneic mice*. Proc Natl Acad Sci USA, 1998. 95:11963–11968.

59. Tassies, D., Sierra, J., Montserrat, E., Marti, R., Estrach, T., and Rozman, C., *Specific cutaneous involvement in Hodgkin's disease*. Hematol Oncol, 1992. 10:75–79.

60. White, R. M., and Patterson, J. W., *Cutaneous involvement in Hodgkin's disease*. Cancer, 1985. 55:1136–1145.

61. Morman, M. R., and Petrozzi, J. W., *Cutaneous Hodgkin's disease*. Cutis, 1980. 26:483–484.

62. Smith, J. L., and Butler, J. J., *Skin involvement in Hodgkin's disease*. Cancer, 1980. 45:354–361.

63. Bardach, H., and Kuhbock, J., *Localized poikiloderma vascularis atrophicans as an early manifestation of Hodgkin's disease of the nodular-sclerosing type*. Hautarzt, 1981. 32:126–129.

64. Misra, R. S., Mukherjee, A., Ramesh, V., Jain, R. K., and Sharma, A. K., *Specific skin ulcers in Hodgkin's disease*. Cutis, 1987. 39:247–248.

65. Davis, T. H., Morton, C. C., Miller-Cassman, R., Balk, S. P., and Kadin, M. E., *Hodgkin's disease, lymphomatoid papulosis, and cutaneous T-cell lymphoma derived from a common T-cell clone*. N Engl J Med, 1992. 326:1115–1122.

66. Kaudewitz, P., Stein, H., Plewig, G., Schwarting, R., Gerdes, J., Burg, G., Kind, P., Eckert, F., et al., *Hodgkin's disease followed by lymphomatoid papulosis. Immunophenotypic evidence for a close relationship between lymphomatoid papulosis and Hodgkin's disease*. J Am Acad Dermatol, 1990. 22:999–1006.

67. Willemze, R., *Lymphomatoid papulosis*. Dermatol Clin, 1985. 3:735–747.

68. Weinman, V. F., and Ackerman, A. B., *Lymphomatoid papulosis: A critical review and new findings*. Am J Dermatopathol, 1981. 3:129–163.

69. Leimert, J. T., Corder, M. P., Skibba, C. A., and Gingrich, R. D., *Erythema annulare centrifugum and Hodgkin's disease: Association with disease activity.* Arch Intern Med, 1979. 139:486–487.

70. Sina, B., Goldner, R., and Burnett, J. W., *Granulomatous panniculitis and Hodgkin's disease.* Cutis, 1984. 33:403–404.

71. Molos, M. A., and Hall, J. C., *Symmetrical peripheral gangrene and disseminated intravascular coagulation.* Arch Dermatol, 1985. 121:1057–1061.

72. Shelnitz, L. S., and Paller, A. S., *Hodgkin's disease manifesting as prurigo nodularis.* Pediatr Dermatol, 1990. 7:136–139.

73. Wooten, M. D., and Jasin, H. E., *Vasculitis and lymphoproliferative diseases.* Semin Arthritis Rheum, 1996. 26:564–574.

74. Strickland, D. K., and Ware, R. E., *Urticarial vaculitis: An autoimmune disorder following therapy for Hodgkin's disease.* Med Pediatr Oncol, 1995. 25:208–212.

75. Flipo, R. M., Hardoin, P., Walter, M. P., Thomas, P., Bauters, F., and Duquesnoy, B., *Pyoderma gangrenosum and paraneoplastic chronic polyarthritis disclosing Hodgkin's lymphoma.* Rev Med Interne, 1990. 11:149–150.

76. Shaw, M. T., and Jacobs, S. R., *Cutaneous Hodgkin's disease in a patient with human immunodeficiency virus infection.* Cancer, 1989. 64:2585–2587.

77. Vassef, M. A., Kamel, O. W., Chen, Y.-Y., Medeiros, L. J., and Weiss, L. M., *Detection of Epstein-Barr virus in multiple sites involved by Hodgkin's disease.* Am J Pathol, 1995. 147:1408–1415.

78. Simrell, C. R., Boccia, R. V., Longo, D. L., and Jaffe, E. S., *Coexisting Hodgkin's disease and mycosis fungoides. Immunohistochemical proof of its existence.* Arch Pathol Lab Med, 1986. 110:1029–1034.

79. Noto, G., Pravata, G., Miceli, S., and Arico, M., *Granulomatous slack skin: Report of a case associated with Hodgkin's disease and a review of the literature.* Br J Dermatol, 1994. 131:275–279.

80. van Haselen, C. W., Toonstra, J., van der Putte, S. J., van Dongen, J. J., van Hees, C. L., and can Vloten, W. A., *Granulomatous slack skin. Report of three patients with an updated review of the literature.* Dermatology, 1998. 196:382–391.

81. Cerroni, L., Beham-Schmidt, C., and Kerl, H., *Cutaneous Hodgkin's disease: An immunohistochemical analysis.* J Cutan Pathol, 1995. 22:229–235.

82. Karp, D. L., and Horn, T. D., *Lymphomatoid papulosis.* J Am Acad Dermatol, 1994. 30:379–395.

83. Willemze, R., Meyer, C. J., van Vloten, W. A., and Scheffer, E., *The clinical and histological spectrum of lymphomatoid papulosis.* Br J Dermatol, 1982. 107:131–144.

84. Macaulay, W. L., *Lymphomatoid papulosis. A continuing self-healing eruption, clinically benign-histologically malignant.* Arch Dermatol, 1968. 97:23–30.

85. Kadin, M. E., Vonderheid, E. C., Sako, D., Clayton, L. K., and Olbricht, S., *Clonal composition of T cells in lymphomatoid papulosis.* Am J Pathol, 1987. 126:13–17.

86. Gianotti, F., and Caputo, R., *Histiocytic syndromes: A review.* J Am Acad Dermatol, 1985. 13:383–404.

87. Favara, B. E., *Histocytosis syndromes: Classification, diagnostic features and current concepts.* Leuk Lymphoma, 1990. 2:141–150.

88. Favara, B. E., *Langerhans cell histiocytosis: Pathobiology and pathogenesis.* Semin Oncol, 1991. 18:3–7.

89. Lahey, M. E., *Histiocytosis X. An analysis of prognostic factors.* J Pediatr, 1975. 87:184–189.

90. Ceci, A., de Terlizzi, M., Colella, R., Loiacono, G., Balducci, D., Surico, G., Castello, M., Testi, A. M., et al., *Langerhans cell histiocytosis in childhood: Results from the Italian Cooperative AIEOP-CNR-H.X '83 study.* Med Pediatr Oncol, 1993. 21:259–264.

91. Caputo, R., Grimalut, R., Laterza, A., Bencini, P. L., and Veraldi, S., *Mucocutaneous expressions of Langerhans cell histiocytosis in adults.* Eur J Dermatol, 1994. 4:528–531.

92. Sheehan, M. G., Condemi, J. J., and Rosenfeld, S. I., *Position dependent livedo reticularis in cholesterol emboli syndrome.* J Rheumatol, 1993. 20:1973–1974.

93. Helm, K. F., Lookingbill, D. P., and Marks, J. G. Jr., *A clinical and pathologic study of histiocytosis X in adults.* J Am Acad Dermatol, 1993. 29:166–170.

94. Lichtenwald, D. J., Jakubovic, H. R., and Rosenthal, D., *Primary cutaneous Langerhans cell histiocytosis in an adult.* Arch Dermatol, 1991. 127:1545–1548.

95. Fitzpatrick, R., Rapaport, M. J., and Silva, D. G., *Histiocytosis X.* Arch Dermatol, 1980. 117:253–257.

96. Winkelmann, R. K., *The skin in histiocytosis X.* Mayo Clin Proc, 1968. 44:535–549.

97. Schaumburg-Lever, G., Rechowicz, E., Fehrenbacher, B., Moller, H., and Nau, P., *Congenital self-healing reticulohistiocytosis—a benign Langerhans cell disease.* J Cutan Pathol, 1993. 21:59–66.

98. Alexis, J. B., Poppiti, R. J., and Turbat-Herrera, E., *Congenital self-healing reticulohistiocytosis. Report of a case with 7 year follow-up and a review of the literature.* Am J Dermatopathol, 1991. 13:189–194.

99. Longaker, M. A., Frieden, I. J., LeBoit, P. E., and Shertz, E. F., *Congenital "self-healing" Langerhans cell histiocytosis. The need for long-term follow-up.* J Am Acad Dermatol, 1994. 31:910–916.

100. Divaris, D. X. G., Ling, F. C. K., and Prentice, R. S. A., *Congenital self-healing histiocytosis. Report of two cases with histochemical and ultrastructural studies.* Am J Dermatopathol, 1991. 13:481–487.

101. Axiotis, C. A., Merino, M. J., and Duray, P. H., *Langerhans cell histiocytosis of the female genital tract.* Cancer, 1991. 67:1650–1660.

102. Meehan, S., and Smoller, B. R., *Langerhans cell histiocytosis of the genitalia in the elderly: A unique clinical pathologic presentation.* J Cutan Pathol, 1998. 25:370–374.

103. Lycaya, J., *Histiocytosis X.* Am J Dis Child, 1971. 121:289–295.

104. Dunger, D. B., Broadbent, V., Yeoman, E., Seckl, J. R., Lightman, S. L., Grant, D. B., and Pritchard, J., *The frequency and natural history of diabetes insipidus in children with Langerhans-cell histiocytosis.* N Engl J Med, 1989. 321:1157–1162.

105. Siegal, G. P., Dehner, L. P., and Rosai, J., *Histiocytosis X (Langerhans' cell granulomatosis) of the thymus. A clinicopathologic study of four childhood cases.* Am J Surg Pathol, 1985. 9:117–124.

106. Arico, M., Comelli, A., Bossi, G., Raiteri, E., Piombo, M., and Maarten Egeler, R., *Langerhans cell histiocytosis and acute leukemia: Unusual association in two cases.* Med Pediatr Oncol, 1993. 21:271–273.

107. Yu, R. C., Chu, C., Buluwela, L., and Chu, A. C., *Clonal proliferation of Langerhans cells in Langerhans cell histiocytosis.* Lancet, 1994. 343:767–768.

108. Willman, C. L., Busque, L., Griffith, B. B., Favara, B. E., McClain, K. L., Duncan, M. H., and Gilliland, G., *Langerhans-cell histiocytoses (histiocytosis x)—a clonal proliferative disease.* N Engl J Med, 1994. 331:154–160.

109. Komp, D. M., *Langerhans cell histiocytosis.* N Engl J Med, 1987. 316:747–748.

110. Leahy, M. A., Krejci, S. M., Friednash, M., Stockert, S. S., Wilson, H., Huff, J. C., Weston, W. L., and Brice, S. L., *Human herpesvirus 6 is present in lesions of Langerhans cell histiocytosis.* J Invest Dermatol, 1993. 101:642–645.

111. Wood, G. S., Hu, C.-H., Beckstead, J. H., Turner, R. R., and Winkelmann, R. K., *The indeterminate cell proliferative disorder: Report of a case manifesting as an unusual cutaneous histiocytosis.* J Derm Surg Oncol, 1985. 11:1111–1119.

112. Wood, G. S., and Haber, R. S., *Novel histiocytoses considered in the context of histiocyte subset differentiation.* Arch Dermatol, 1992. 129:210–214.

113. Levisohn, D., Seidel, D., Phelps, A., and Burgdorf, W., *Solitary congenital indeterminate cell histiocytoma.* Arch Dermatol, 1993. 129:81–85.

114. Bonetti, F., Knowles, D. M., Chilosi, M., Pisa, R., Fiaccavento, S., Rizzuto, N., Zamboni, G., Menestrina, F., et al., *A distinctive cutaneous malignant neoplasm expressing the Langerhans cell phenotype: Synchronous occurrence with B-chronic lymphocytic leukemia.* Cancer, 1985. 55:2417–2425.

115. Contreras, F., Fonseca, E., Gamallo, C., and Burgos, E., *Multiple self-healing indeterminate cell lesions of the skin in an adult.* Am J Dermatopathol, 1990. 12:396–401.

116. Chan, W. C., and Zaatari, G., *Lymph node interdigitating cell sarcoma.* Am J Clin Pathol, 1986. 85:739–744.

117. Kolde, G., and Brocker, E. B., *Multiple skin tumors of indeterminate cells in an adult.* J Am Acad Dermatol, 1986. 15:591–597.

118. Friedlander, S. F., West, A., and Eichenfield, L. F., *Isolated leukemia cutis presenting as "seborrheic dermatitis."* Clin Pediatr (Phila), 1996. 35:531–534.

119. Konstantopoulos, K., Kanellopoulou, G., Angelopoulou, M. K., Androulaki, A., Hatzidimitriou, D., Patsouris, S., Yataganas, X., and Pangalis, G. A., *Leukemia cutis preceding acute myelomonocytic leukaemia.* Haematologica (Budap), 1997. 28:169–172.

120. Chen, M. J., Huang, M. L., Hung, I. J., and Kuo, T. T., *Leukemia cutis as the initial manifestation of acute nonlymphocytic leukemia in a young child.* Cutis, 1997. 60:263–264.

121. Tomasini, C., Quaglino, P., Novelli, M., and Fierro, M. T., *"Aleukemic" granulomatous leukemia cutis.* Am J Dermatopathol, 1998. 20:417–421.

122. Monpoux, F., Lacour, J. P., Hatchuel, Y., Hofman, P., Raynaud, S., Sudaka, I., Ortonne, J. P., and Mariani, R., *Congenital leukemia cutis preceding monoblastic leukemia by 3 months.* Pediatr Dermatol, 1996. 13:472–476.

123. Longacre, T. A., and Smoller, B. R., *Leukemia cutis. Analysis of 50 biopsy-proven cases with an emphasis on occurrence in myelodysplastic syndromes.* Am J Clin Pathol, 1993. 100:276–284.

124. Smoller, B. R., and Warnke, R. A., *Cutaneous infiltrate of chronic lymphocytic leukemia and relationship to primary cutaneous epithelial neoplasms.* J Cutan Pathol, 1997. 25:160–164.

125. Desch, J. K., and Smoller, B. R., *The spectrum of cutaneous disease in leukemias.* J Cutan Pathol, 1993. 20:407–410.

126. Ratnam, K. V., Khor, C. J., and Su, W. P., *Leukemia cutis.* Dermatol Clin, 1994. 12:419–431.

127. Yen, A., Sanchez, R., Oblender, M., and Raimer, S., *Leukemia cutis: Darier's sign in a neonate with acute lymphoblastic leukemia.* J Am Acad Dermatol, 1996. 34:375–378.

128. Cerroni, L., Zenahlik, P., Hofler, G., Kaddu, S., Smolle, J., and Kerl, H., *Specific cutaneous infiltrates of B-cell chronic lymphocytic leukemia: A clinicopathologic and prognostic study of 42 patients.* Am J Surg Pathol, 1996. 20:1000–1010.

129. Byrd, J. C., Weiss, R. B., Arthur, D. C., Lawrence, D., Baer, M. R., Davey, F., Trikha, E. S., Carroll, A. J., et al., *Extramedullary leukemia adversely affects hematologic complete remission rate and overall survival in patients with t(8;21)(q22;q22): Results from Cancer and Leukemia Group B 8461.* J Clin Oncol, 1997. 15:466–475.

130. Gottesfeld, E., Silverman, R. A., Coccia, P. F., Jacobs, G., and Zaim, M. T., *Transient blueberry muffin appearance of a newborn with congenital monoblastic leukemia.* J Am Acad Dermatol, 1989. 21:347–351.

131. Dreizen, S., McCredie, K. B., Keating, M. J., and Luna, M. A., *Malignant gingival and skin "infiltrate" in adult leukemia.* Oral Surg Oral Med Oral Pathol, 1983. 55:572–579.

132. Berger, B. J., Gross, P. R., Daniels, R. B., and Lankton, B. B., *Leukemia cutis masquerading as guttate psoriasis.* Arch Dermatol, 1973. 108:416–418.

133. McCune, A., and Cohen, B. A., *Urticarial skin eruption in a child. Leukemia cutis.* Arch Dermatol, 1990. 126:1499.

134. Buescher, L., and Anderson, P. C., *Circinate plaques heralding juvenile chronic myelogenous leukemia.* Pediatr Dermatol, 1990. 7:122–125.

135. Inoue, S., Gordon, R., and Berner, G., *Erythema chronicum migrans as the presenting manifestation of juvenile chronic myelocytic leukemia.* Cutis, 1989. 43:333–337.

136. Butler, D. F., Berger, T. G., and Rodman, O. G., *Leukemia cutis mimicking stasis dermatitis.* Cutis, 1985. 35:47–48.

137. Czarnecki, D. B., O'Brien, T. J., Rotstein, H., and Brenan, J., *Leukaemia cutis mimicking primary syphilis.* Acta Derm Venereol, 1981. 61:368–369.

138. Passarini, B. N., Patrizi, A., and Masina, M., *Cutis verticis gyrata secondary to acute monoblastic leukemia.* Acta Derm Venereol, 1993. 73:148–149.

139. Hacker, S. M., Berkwitz, M., and Cody, R., *Porphyria cutanea tarda in a patient with hairy cell leukemia.* Cutis, 1993. 51:251–252.

140. Cohen, P. R., *Acral erythema: A clinical review.* Cutis, 1993. 51:175–179.

141. Sadick, N. S., and Allen, S. L., *Atrophie blanche in chronic myelogenous leukemia.* Cutis, 1988. 42:206–209.

142. Flynn, T. C., Harrist, T. J., Murphy, G. F., Loss, R. W., and Moschella, S. L., *Neutrophilic eccrine hidradenitis: A distinctive rash associated with cytarabine therapy and acute leukemia.* J Am Acad Dermatol, 1984. 11:584–590.

143. Lewis, J. R., *Bullous pyoderma gangrenosum with chronic myelogenous leukemia: Report of a case.* Cutis, 1980. 25:82–83.

144. Botero, F., *Pruritis as a manifestation of systemic disorders.* Cutis, 1978. 21:873–880.

145. Jones, D., Dorfman, D. M., Barnhill, R. L., and Granter, S. R., *Leukemic vasculitis: A feature of leukemia cutis in some patients.* Am J Clin Pathol, 1997. 107:637–642.

146. Sumner, W. T., Grichnik, J. M., Shea, C. R., Moore, J. O., Miller, W. S., and Burton, C. S., *Follicular mucinosis as a presenting sign of acute myeloblastic leukemia.* J Am Acad Dermatol, 1998. 38:803–805.

147. Levi, F., Randimbison, L., Te, V. C., and La Vecchia, C., *Non-Hodgkin's lymphomas, chronic lymphocytic leukaemias and skin cancers.* Br J Cancer, 1996. 74:1847–1850.

148. Fowler, J. F. Jr., and Knuckles, M. L., *Multiple cutaneous squamous cell carcinomas in a patient with chronic lymphocytic leukemia.* Cutis, 1985. 36:467–469.

149. Quaglino, D., Di Leonardo, G., Lalli, G., Pasqualoni, E., Di Simone, S., Vecchio, L., and Ventura, T., *Association between chronic lymphocytic leukaemia and secondary tumours: Unusual occurrence of a neuroendocrine (Merkel cell) carinoma.* Eur Rev Pharmacol Sci, 1997. 1:11–16.

150. Reinhardt, L. A., and Rosen, T., *Pityriasis rubra pilaris as the initial manifestation of leukemia.* Cutis, 1983. 31:100–102.

151. Miralles, E. S., Escribano, L., Bellas, C., Nunez, M., and Ledo, A., *Cutaneous xanthomatous tumors as an expression of chronic myelomonocytic leukemia?* Clin Exp Dermatol, 1996. 21:145–147.

152. Lerner, L. H., Wiss, K., Gellis, S., and Barnhill, R., *An unusual pustular eruption in an infant with Down syndrome and a congenital leukemoid reaction.* J Am Acad Dermatol, 1996. 35:330–333.

153. Tzavara, V., Stamoulis, K., Aroni, K. G., Kordossis, T., and Boki, K. A., *Facial heliotrope rash as the initial manifestation of acute myelomonocytic leukemia.* Leuk Lymphoma, 1997. 25:393–398.

154. Drabkin, H. A., and Erickson, P., *Down syndrome and leukemia, an update.* Prog Clin Biol Res, 1995. 393:169–176.

155. Hess, J. L., Zutter, M. M., Castleberry, R. P., and Emanuel, P. D., *Juvenile chronic myelogenous leukemia.* Am J Clin Pathol, 1996. 105:238–248.

156. Fong, C. T., and Brodeur, G. M., *Down's syndrome and leukemia: Epidemiology, genetics, cytogenetics and mechanisms of leukogenesis.* Cancer Genet Cytogenet, 1987. 28:55–76.

157. Zipursky, A., Brown, E., Christensen, H., Sutherland, R., and Doyle, J., *Leukemia and/or myeloproliferative syndrome in neonates with Down syndrome.* Semin Perinatol, 1997. 21:97–101.

158. Klingspor, L., Stintzing, G., and Tollemar, J., *Deep Candida infection in children with leukaemia: Clinical presentations, diagnosis and outcome.* Acta Pediatr, 1997. 86:30–36.

159. Kumar, R. R., Kumar, B. R., Shafiulla, M., Lakshmaiah, K. C., and Sridhar, H., *Fusarium solani infection in a patient with acute myelogenous leukemia—a case report.* Indian J Pathol Microbiol, 1997. 40:555–557.

160. Takeda, H., Mitsuhashi, Y., and Kondo, S., *Cutaneous disseminated actinomycosis in a patient with acute lymphocytic leukemia.* J Dermatol, 1998. 25:37–40.

161. Torok, L., Simon, G., Csorani, A., Tapai, M., and Torok, I., *Scedosporium apiospermum infection imitating lymphocutaneous sporotrichosis in a patient with myeloblastic-monocytic leukemia.* Br J Dermatol, 1995. 133:805–809.

162. Ivy, S. P., Mackall, C. L., Gore, L., Gress, R. E., and Hartley, A. H., *Demodicidosis in childhood acute lymphoblastic leukemia: An opportunistic infection occurring with immunosuppression.* J Pediatr, 1995. 127:751–754.

163. Doutre, M. S., Beylot-Barry, M., Beylot, C., Dubus, P., LaFont, M. E., Belleannee, G., Broustet, A., and Merlio, J. P., *Cutaneous localization of chronic lymphocytic leukemia at the site of chickenpox.* J Am Acad Dermatol, 1997. 36:98–99.

164. Metzler, G., Cerroni, L., Schmidt, H., Soyer, H. P., Sill, H., and Kerl, H., *Leukemic cells within skin lesions of psoriasis in a patient with acute myelogenous leukemia.* J Cutan Pathol, 1997. 24:445–448.

165. Davis, M. D., Perniciaro, C., Dahl, P. R., Randle, H. W., McEvoy, M. T., and Leiferman, K. M., *Exaggerated arthropod-bite lesions in patients with chronic lymphocytic leukemia: A clinical, histopathologic, and immunopathologic study of eight patients.* J Am Acad Dermatol, 1998. 39:27–35.

166. Dorfman, D. M., Kraus, M., Perez-Atayde, A. R., Barnhill, R. L., Pinkus, G. S., and Granter, S. R., *CD99 (p30/32MIC2) immunoreactivity in the diagnosis of leukemia cutis.* Mod Pathol, 1997. 10:283–288.

167. Green, T., Grant, J., Pye, R., and Marcus, R., *Multiple primary cutaneous plasmacytomas.* Arch Dermatol, 1992. 128:962–965.

168. Nakamura, S., Hoshi, K., Onda, S., and Kamiya, S., *Primary cutaneous IgA plasmacytoma.* J Dermatol, 1984. 11:482–486.

169. Meis, J. M., Butler, J. J., Osborne, B. M., and Ordonez, N. G., *Solitary plasmacytomas of bone and extramedullary plasmacytomas.* Cancer, 1987. 59:1475–1485.

170. Wiltshaw, E., *The natural history of extramedullary plasmacytoma and its relation to solitary myeloma of bone and myelomatosis.* Medicine, 1976. 55:217–238.

171. Torne, R., Su, W. P. D., Winkelmann, R. K., Smolle, J., and Kerl, H., *Clinicopathologic study of cutaneous plasmacytoma.* Int J Dermatol, 1990. 29:562–566.

172. Alberts, D. S., and Lynch, P., *Cutaneous plasmacytoma in myeloma: Relationship to tumor cell burden.* Arch Dermatol, 1978. 114:1784–1787.

173. Bluefarb, S. M., *Cutaneous manifestations of multiple myeloma.* Arch Dermatol, 1955. 72:506–522.

174. Wong, K. F., Chan, J. K. C., Li, L. P. K., and Yau, T. K., *Primary cutaneous plasmacytoma—report of two cases and review of the literature.* Am J Dermatopathol, 1994. 16:392–397.

175. Edwards, G. A., and Zawadzki, Z. A., *Extraosseous lesions in plasma cell myeloma: A report of six cases.* Am J Med, 1967. 43:194–205.

176. Durie, B. G. M., and Salmon, S. E., *A clinical staging system for multiple myeloma: Correlation of measured myeloma cell mass with presenting clinical features, response to treatment and survival.* Cancer, A1975. 36:842–854.

177. Gabriel, S. E., Perry, H. O., Oleson, G. B., and Bowles, C. A., *Scleromyxedema: A sclerodermal-like disorder with systemic manifestations.* Medicine (Baltimore), 1988. 67:58–65.

178. Krasagakis, K., Zouboulis, C. C., Owsianowski, M., Ramaker, J., Trautman, C., Tebbe, B., and Orfanos, C. E., *Remission of scleromyxedema following treatment with extracorporeal photopheresis.* Br J Dermatol, 1996. 135:463–466.

179. Kantor, G. B., Bergfeld, W. F., Katzin, W. E., Reynolds, O. D., Biscardi, A. P., Lobour, D. M., Box, T. A., Schreiber, M. J., et al., *Scleromyxedema associated with scleroderma renal disease and acute psychosis.* J Am Acad Dermatol, 1986. 14:879–888.

180. Kitamura, W., Matsuoka, Y., Miyagawa, S., and Sakamoto, K., *Immunochemical analysis of the monoclonal paraprotein in scleromyxedema.* J Invest Dermatol, 1978. 70:305–308.

181. Gimenez Garcia, R., Garcia, S. G., D., S. V., and Moro Sanchez, M. J., *Scleromyxedema associated with non-Hodgkin's lymphoma.* Int J Dermatol, 1989. 28:670–671.

182. Rahmani, R., Brenner, S., Krakowski, A., Lipitz, R., Ilie, B., and Behar, A. J., *Angioimmunoblastic lymphadenopathy with scleromyxedema-like lesions and serum monoclonal protein.* Isr J Med Sci, 1983. 19:235–239.

183. Dineen, A. M., and Dicken, C. H., *Scleromyxedema.* J Am Acad Dermatol, 1995. 33:37–43.

184. Dowling, J. P., Griffiths, J. D., and McLeish, J. A., *Myeloma associated scleromyxedema with extensive involvement of small bowel.* Pathology, 1991. 23:244–247.

185. Verity, M. A., Toop, J., McAdam, L. P., and Pearson, C. M., *Scleromyxedema myopathy. Histochemical and electron microscopic observations.* Am J Clin Pathol, 1978. 69:446–451.

186. Helfrich, D. J., Walker, E. R., Martinez, A. J., and Medsger, T. A. Jr., *Scleromyxedema myopathy: Case report and review of the literature.* Arthritis Rheum, 1988. 31:1437–1441.

187. Davis, M. L., Bartley, G. B., Gibson, L. E., and Maguire, L. J., *Ophthalmic findings in scleromyxedema.* Ophthalmology, 1994. 101:252–255.

188. Goldin, H. M., Axelrod, A. J., Bronson, D. M., Torczynski, E., Arroyave, C. M., and Barsky, S., *Scleromyxedema with corneal deposits.* Ophthalmology, 1987. 94:1334–1338.

189. Frayha, R. A., *Papular mucinosis, destructive arthropathy, median neuropathy, and sicca complex.* Clin Rheumatol, 1983. 2:277–284.

190. Webster, G. F., Matsuoka, L. Y., and Burchmore, D., *The association of potentially lethal neurologic syndromes with scleromyxedema (papular mucinosis).* J Am Acad Dermatol, 1993. 28:105–108.

191. Verier, A., Jouet, J. P., Muller, J. P., Destee, A., Thomas, P., and Warot, P., *Recurrent coma, papular mucinosis and benign dysglobulinemia.* Rev Neurol (Paris), 1987. 143:791–797.

192. Espinosa, A., De Miguel, E., Morales, C., Fonseca, E., and Gijon-Banos, J., *Scleromyxedema associated with arthritis and myopathy: A case report.* Clin Exp Rheumatol, 1993. 11:545–547.

193. Wright, R. C., Franco, R. S., Denton, D., and Blaney, D. J., *Scleromyxedema.* Arch Dermatol, 1976. 112:63–66.

194. Farmer, E. R., Hambrick, G. W. Jr., and Shulman, L. E., *Papular mucinosis. A clinicopathologic study of four patients.* Arch Dermatol, 1982. 118:9–13.

195. Truhan, A. P., and Roegnik, H. H., *The cutaneous mucinoses.* J Am Acad Dermatol, 1986. 14:1–18.

196. Yaron, M., Yaron, I., Yust, I., and Brenner, S., *Lichen myxedematosus (scleromyxedema) serum stimulates hyaluronic acid and prostaglandin E production by human fibroblasts.* J Rheumatol, 1985. 12:171–175.

197. Ferrarini, M., Helfrich, D. J., Wlker, E. R., Medsger, T. A. Jr., and Whiteside, T. L., *Scleromyxedema serum increases proliferation but not the glycosaminoglycan synthesis of dermal fibroblasts.* J rheumatol, 1989. 16:837–841.

198. Alves, M. F., Filgueria, A. L., Lorena, D. E., and Porto, L. C., *Type I and type III collagens in cutaneous mucinosis.* Am J Dermatopathol, 1998. 20:41–47.

199. McCarty, M. J., Davidson, J. M., Cardone, J. S., and Anderson, L. L., *Cutis laxa acquisita associated with multiple myeloma: A case report and review of the literature.* Cutis, 1996. 57:267–270.

200. Requena, L., Sarasa, J. L., Ortiz Masllorens, F., Martin, L., Pique, E., Olivares, M., Farina, M. C., Prieto, E., et al., *Follicular spicules of the nose: A peculiar cutaneous manifestation of multiple myeloma with cryoglobulinemia.* J Am Acad Dermatol, 1995. 32:834–839.

201. Bork, K., Bockers, M., and Pfeifle, J., *Pathogenesis of paraneoplastic follicular hyperkeratotic spicules in multiple myeloma. Follicular and epidermal accumulation*

of IgG dysprotein and cryoglobulin. Arch Dermatol, 1990. 126:509–513.

202. Kuokkanen, K., Niemi, K. M., and Reunala, T., *Parakeratotic horns in a patient with myeloma.* J Cutan Pathol, 1987. 14:54–58.

203. Bowden, J. R., Scully, C., Eveson, J. W., Flint, S., Harman, R. R., and Jones, S. K., *Multiple myeloma and bullous lichenoid lesions: An unusual associaton.* Oral Surg Oral Med Oral Pathol, 1990. 70:587–589.

204. von der Helm, D., Ring, J., Schmoeckel, C., and Braun-Falco, O., *Acquired hyalinosis cutis et mucosae in plasmacytoma with monoclonal IgG-lambda gammopathy.* Hautarzt, 1989. 40:153–157.

205. Takata, M., Inaoki, M., Shodo, M., Hirone, T., and Kaya, H., *Subcorneal pustular dermatosis associated with IgA myeloma and intraepidermal IgA deposits.* Dermatology, 1994. 189 (Suppl. 1):111–114.

206. Plotnik, H., Taniguchi, Y., Hashimoto, K., Negendank, W., and Tranchida, L., *Periorbital necrobiotic xanthogranuloma and stage I multiple myeloma. Ultrastructure and response to pulsed dexamethasone documented by magnetic resonance imaging.* J Am Acad Dermatol, 1991. 25:373–377.

207. Feingold, K. R., Castro, G. R., Ishikawa, Y., Fielding, P. E., and Fielding, C. J., *Cutaneous xanthoma in association with paraproteinemia in the absence of hyperlipidemia.* J Clin Invest, 1989. 83:796–802.

208. Etoh, T., Nagakawa, H., and Ishibashi, Y., *Pityriasis rotunda associated with multiple myeloma.* J Am Acad Dermatol, 1991. 24:303–304.

209. Breier, F., Hobisch, G., and Groz, S., *Sweet syndrome. Acute neutrophilic dermatosis in multiple myeloma.* Hautarzt, 1993. 44:229–231.

210. Pech, J. H., Moreau-Cabarrot, A., Oksman, F., Bedane, C., Bernard, P., and Bazex, J., *Waldenström's macroglobulinemia with antibasement membrane activity of monoclonal immunoglobulin.* Ann Dermatol Venereol, 1997. 124:325–328.

211. West, J. Y., Fitzpatrick, J. E., David-Bajar, K. M., and Bennion, S. D., *Waldenström macroglobulinemia-induced bullous dermatosis.* Arch Dermatol, 1998. 134:1127–1131.

212. Torok, L., Borka, I., and Szabo, G., *Waldenström's macroglobulinemia presenting with cold urticaria and cold purpura.* JClin Exp Dermatol, 1993. 18:277–279.

213. Janier, M., Bonvalet, D., Blanc, M. F., Lemarchand, F., Cavelier, B., Ribrioux, A., Aguenier, B., and Civatte, J., *Chronic urticaria and macroglobulinemia (Schnitzler's syndrome): Report of two cases.* J Am Acad Dermatol, 1989. 20:206–211.

214. Green, T., *Cutaneous manifestations of Waldonström's macroglobulinaemia.* Br J Dermatol, 1989. 121(Suppl 34):55.

215. Lowe, L., Fitzpatrick, J. E., Huff, J. C., Shanley, P. F., and Golitz, L. E., *Cutaneous macroglobulinosis.* Arch Dermatol, 1992. 128:377–380.

216. Goodenberger, M. E., Piette, W. W., Macfarlane, D. E., and Argenyi, Z. B., *Xanthoma disseminatum and Waldenström's macroglobulinemia.* J Am Acad Dermatol, 1990. 23:1015–1018.

217. Kyle, R. A., *The monoclonal gammopathies.* Clin Chem, 1994. 40:2154–2161.

218. Dimopoulos, M. A., and Alexian, R., *Waldenström's macroglobulinemia.* Blood, 1994. 83:1452–1459.

219. Abdou, N. L., and Abdou, N. I., *Discoid lupus erythematosus with macroglobulinemia. Correlations between autoimmunity and B cell malignancy with hyperimmunoglobulinemia.* Am J Med, 1974. 57:631–637.

220. Habib, G. S., Stimmer, M. M., and Quismorio, F. P. Jr., *Hypergammaglobulinemic purpura of Waldenström associated with systemic lupus erythematosus: Report of a case and review of the literature.* Lupus, 1995. 4:19–22.

221. Mozzanica, N., Finzi, A. F., Facchetti, G., and Villa, M. L., *Macular skin lesion and monoclonal lymphoplasmacytoid infilrates. Occurrence in primary Waldenström's macroglobulinemia.* Arch Dermatol, 1984. 120:778–781.

222. Bergroth, V., Reitamo, S., Konttinen, Y. T., and Wegelius, O., *Skin lesions in Waldenström's macroglobulinaemia. Characterization of the cellular infiltrate.* Acta Med Scand, 1981. 209:129–131.

223. Morita, A., Sakakibara, S., Yokota, M., and Tsuji, T., *A case of urticarial vasculitis associated with macroglobulinemai (Schnitzler's syndrome).* J Dermatol, 1995. 22:32–35.

224. Wagner, D. R., Eckert, F., Gresser, U., Landthaler, M., Middeke, M., and Zollner, N., *Deposits of paraprotein in small vessels as a cause of skin ulcers in Waldenström's macroglobulinemia.* Clin Invest, 1993. 72:46–49.

225. Mascaro, J. M., Montserrat, E., Estrach, T., Feliu, E., Ferrando, J., Castel, T., Mallolas, J., and Rozman, C., *Specific cutaneous manifestations of Waldenström's macroglobulinemia. A report of two cases.* Br J Dermatol, 1982. 106:217–222.

226. Whittaker, S. J., Bhogal, B. S., and Black, M. M., *Acquired immunobullous disease: A cutaneous manifestation of IgM macroglobulinemia.* Br J Dermatol, 1996. 135:283–286.

227. Su, W. P. D., *Angioimmunoblastic lymphadenopathy.* Dermatol Clin, 1985. 3:759–768.

228. Matlof, R. B., and Neiman, R. S., *Angioimmunoblastic lymphadenopathy. A generalized lymphoproliferative disorder with cutaneous manifestations.* Arch Dermatol, 1978. 114:92–94.

229. Bernstein, J. E., Soltani, I., and Lorincz, A. L., *Cutaneous manifestations of angioimmunoblastic lymphodenopathy.* J Am Acad Dermatol, 1979. 1:227–232.

230. Archimbaud, E., Coiffier, B., Bryon, P. A., Brizard, C. P., and Viala, J. J., *Rash implies poor prognosis in angioimmunoblastic lymphadenopathy.* Lancet, 1983. 1(8331):998–999.

231. Layton, M. A., Musgrove, C., and Dawes, P. T., *Polyarthritis, rash and lymphadenopathy: Case reports of two patients with angioimmunoblastic lymphadenopathy presenting to a rheumatology clinic.* Clin Rheumatol, 1998. 17:148–151.

232. Schauer, P. K., Staus, D. J., Bagley, C. M. Jr., Rudolph, R. H., McCracken, J. D., Huff, J., Glucksburg, H., Bauermeister, D. E., et al., *Angioimmunoblastic lymphadenopathy: Clinical spectrum of disease.* Cancer, 1981. 48:2493–2498.

233. Varsano, S., Manor, Y., Steiner, Z., Griffel, B., and Klajman, A., *Kaposi's sarcoma and angioimmunoblastic lymphadenopathy.* Cancer, 1984. 54:1582–1585.

234. Schmuth, M., Ramaker, J., Trautmann, C., Hummel, M., Schmitt-Graff, A., Stein, H., and Goerdt, S., *Cutaneous involvement in prelymphomatous angioimmunoblastic lymphadenopathy.* J Am Acad Dermatol, 1997. 36:290–295.

235. Seehafer, J. R., Goldberg, N. C., Dicken, C. H., and Su, W. P. D., *Cutaneous manifestations of angioimmunoblastic lymphadenopathy.* Arch Dermatol, 1980. 116:41–45.

236. Pavlidis, N. A., Klouvas, G., Tsokos, M., Bai, M., and Moutsopoulos, H. M., *Cutaneous lymphocytic vasculopathy in lymphoproliferative disorders—a paraneoplastic lymphocytic vasculitis of the skin.* Leuk Lymphoma, 1995. 16:477–482.

237. Daibata, M., Ido, E., Murakami, K., Kuzume, T., Kubonishi, I., Taguchi, H., and Miyoshi, I., *Angioimmunoblastic lymphadenopathy with disseminated human herpesvirus 6 infection in a patient with acute myeloblastic leukemia.* Leukemia, 1997. 11:882–885.

238. Su, I. J., and Hseih, H. C., *Clinicopathological spectrum of Epstein-Barr virus-associated T cell malignancies.* Leuk Lymphoma, 1992. 7:47–53.

239. Foucar, E., Rosai, J., and Dorfman, R., *Sinus histiocytosis with massive lymphadenopathy (Rosai-Dorfman disease): Review of the entity.* Semin Diagn Pathol, 1990. 7:19–73.

240. Komp, D. M., *The treatment of sinus histiocytosis with massive lymphadenopathy (Rosai-Dorfman disease).* Semin Diagn Pathol, 1990. 7:83–86.

241. Chu, P., and LeBoit, P. E., *Histologic features of cutaneous sinus histiocytosis (Rosai-Dorfman disease): Study of cases both with and without systemic involvement.* J Cutan Pathol, 1992. 19:201–206.

242. Eisen, R. N., Buckley, P. J., and Rosai, J., *Immunophenotypic characterization of sinus histiocytosis with massive lymphadenopathy (Rosai-Dorman disease).* Semin Diagn Pathol, 1990. 7:74–82.

243. Levine, P. H., Jahan, N., Murari, P., Manak, M., and Jaffe, E. S., *Detection of human herpesvirus 6 in tissues involved by sinus histiocytosis with massive lymphadenopathy (Rosai-Dorfman disease).* J Infect Dis, 1992. 166:291–295.

244. Luppi, M., Barozzi, P., Garber, R., Maiorana, A., Bonacorsi, G., Artusi, T., Trovato, R., Marasca, R., et al., *Expression of human herpesvirus-6 antigen in benign and malignant lymphoproliferative diseases.* Am J Pathol, 1998. 153:815–823.

245. Jones, R. J., Vogelsang, G. B., Hess, A. D., Farmer, E. R., Mann, R. B., Geller, R. B., Piantadosi, S., and Santos, G. W., *Induction of graft-versus-host reaction and cutaneous eruption of lymphocyte recovery.* Lancet, 1989. 8641:754–757.

246. Horn, T. D., Altomonte, V., Vogelsang, G., and Kennedy, M. J., *Erythroderma after autologous bone marrow transplantation modified by administration of cyclosporine and interferon gamma for breast cancer.* J Am Acad Dermatol, 1996. 34:413–417.

247. Hood, A. F., Vogelsang, G. B., Black, L. P., Famer, E. R., and Santos, G. W., *Acute graft-versus-host disease: Development following autologous and syngeneic bone marrow transplantation.* Arch Dermatol, 1987. 123:745–750.

248. Freemer, C. S., Farmer, E. R., Corio, R. L., Altomonte, V. L., Wagner, J. E., Vogelsang, G. B., and Santos, G. W., *Lichenoid chronic graft-vs-host disease occurring in a dermatomal distribution.* Arch Dermatol, 1994. 130:70–72.

249. Redondo, P., Espana, A., Herrero, I., Quiroga, J., Cienfuegos, J. A., Azanza, J. R., and Prieot, J., *Graft-versus-host disease after liver transplantation.* J Am Acad Dermatol, 1993. 29:314–317.

250. Sola, M. A., Espana, A., redondo, P., Idoate, M. A., Fernandez, A. L., Llorens, R., and Quintanilla, E., *Transfusion-associated acute graft-versus-host disease in a heart transplant recipient.* Br J Dermatol, 1994. 132:626–630.

251. Bauer, D. J., Hood, A. F., and Horn, T. D., *Histologic comparison of autologous graft-versus-host reaction and cutaneous eruption of lymphocyte recovery.* Arch Dermatol, 1993. 129:855–858.

252. Chosidow, O., Bagot, M., Vernant, J.-P., Roujeau, J.-C., Cordonnier, C., Kuentz, M., Weschler, J., Andre, C., et al., *Sclerodermatous chronic graft-versus-host disease: Analysis of seven cases.* J Am Acad Dermatol, 1992. 26:49–55.

253. Ferrara, J. L. M., and Deeg, H. J., *Graft-versus-host disease.* N Engl J Med, 1991. 324:667–674.

254. Jenkins, M. K., Schwartz, R. H., and Pardoll, D. M., *Effects of cyclosporine A on T cell development and clonal detection.* Science, 1989. 241:252–259.

255. Dorfman, D. M., Kraus, M., Perez-Atayde, A. R., Barnhill, R. L., Pinkus, G. S., and Granter, S. R., *CD99 (p30/32^{MIC2}) immunoreactivity in the diagnosis of leukemia cutis.* Mod Pathol, 1997. 10:283–288.

256. Kaiserling, E., Horny, H.-P., Geerts, M.-L., and Schmid, U., *Skin involvement in myelogenous leukemia: Morphologic and immunophenotypic heterogeneity of skin infiltrates.* Mod Pathol, 1995. 7:771–774.

CHAPTER 11

Musculoskeletal and Skin Diseases

Klippel-Trénaunay-Weber Syndrome

Epidemiology. Klippel-Trénaunay-Weber syndrome is a rare, sporadic congenital vascular disease of unknown etiology [1]. The syndrome is defined as the triad of capillary malformations, varicosities or venous malformations, and bony or soft tissue hypertrophy usually affecting extremities [2]. Approximately 98% of patients with Klippel-Trénaunay-Weber syndrome have port-wine stains, 72% display venous malformations, and limb hypertrophy was present in 67% [2]. Sixty-three percent of patients demonstrated all three features, and 37% had two of the three [2]. Rare cases of autosomal dominant inheritance have been described [3]. In some series, there is a 2:1 female to male predominance [4]. In one patient, a 5:11 balanced chromosomal translocation was detected, suggesting a genetic defect in some cases [5].

Cutaneous Features. Port-wine stain, or nevus flammeus, is the most common cutaneous manifestation of Klippel-Trénaunay-Weber syndrome, being present in up to 98% of affected patients [2]. These appear initially as lightly erythematous macules of varying sizes that continue to grow and darken throughout life. They can eventually become nodular. Arteriovenous malformations have also been described in patients with Klippel-Trénaunay-Weber syndrome, as have rare cases of spindle cell hemangioma. The cutaneous vascular processes associated with the Klippel-Trénaunay-Weber syndrome do not appear different from those unasso-ciated with underlying soft tissue and bony anomalies. A dermatomal distribution of the vascular anomalies is often noted [6].

Associated Disorders. The most common extracutaneous manifestation of Klippel-Trénaunay-Weber syndrome is elongation of the affected limb [7]. There is hypertrophy of the soft tissues in the affected limbs [8] and overgrowth of the bones [9]. Varicose veins are also present in about one-third of patients [7]. The face is also commonly affected, which may lead to dental anomalies [10]. Facial hemihypertrophy may occur in concert with the limb hypertrophy [11].

Macrodactyly, syndactyly, and various other malformations of the fingers and toes have been described in patients with Klippel-Trénaunay-Weber syndrome [4].

The vascular malformations that occur in patients with the syndrome can affect many organ systems (Table 11–1). Lymphatic involvement of the lungs has been reported, leading to plexiform hyperplasia of the lymphatic channels [1]. Gastrointestinal involvement, which can be associated with significant bleeding [12], and splenic involvement [13] have also been described. Central nervous system defects, including brain stem infarction, occur when vascular malformations affect this region [14], and similar arteriovenous malformations may affect the spinal cord [15]. Retinal and renal vascular malformations have also been described in patients with Klippel-Trénaunay-Weber syndrome [16]. Maternal angiomatosis has led to fetal growth re-

Table 11-1. Klippel-Trénaunay-Weber Syndrome	
Organ Involved	*Clinical Manifestations*
Lung lymphatics	Respiratory defects
Gastrointestinal tract	Bleeding
Spleen	
Central nervous system	Infarction
Eye	Blindness
Kidney	Renal vascular malformations

striction [17]. A patient in whom multiple cutaneous squamous cell carcinomas and basal cell carcinomas developed overlying the site of a vascular malformation has been described [18]. The significance of this observation remains unknown.

Histologic Features. The histologic findings of the cutaneous vascular anomalies observed within Klippel-Trénaunay-Weber syndrome resemble those of cutaneous vascular anomalies that are unassociated with the syndrome. Port-wine stains appear as an increased number of thin-walled, ectatic blood vessels located primarily within the reticular dermis. Vessels are progressively ectatic and congested as lesions become older [19] (see Chapter 12, Figs. 12–10 and 12–11). Arteriovenous fistulas display an increase in both thin-walled and thick-walled vessels within the dermis.

Kaposi's sarcoma-like proliferations are sometimes found in patients with Klippel-Trénaunay-Weber syndrome [20]. These probably develop secondary to increased blood flow through altered vascular beds in a manner analogous to acral angiodermatitis.

Special Studies. Special studies are not required to establish a diagnosis of the cutaneous vascular anomalies associated with Klippel-Trénaunay-Weber syndrome.

Pathogenesis. The pathogenesis of Klippel-Trénaunay-Weber syndrome remains unknown. It is generally believed that the increased blood flow from the vascular malformations probably plays some role in inducing soft tissue and bony hypertrophy in the underlying tissues. The pathogenesis of the cutaneous vascular malformations is not known. A decrease in cutaneous innervation has been demonstrated in port-wine stains. It has been suggested that the lack of neural modulation of blood vessels accounts for the progressive vascular ectasia seen in port-wine stains [21]. Similar observations have not been made in arteriovenous malformations, nor have the port-wine stains specifically associated with Klippel-Trénaunay-Weber syndrome been studied.

Maffucci's Syndrome and Ollier's Disease

Epidemiology. Ollier's disease and Maffucci's syndrome are two congenital conditions that are characterized by the presence of cutaneous vascular malformations and multiple enchondromas. There is no evidence for genetic transmission of the conditions. There is no gender preference. Maffucci's syndrome has been associated with a high rate of malignancy. Ollier's disease does not have this association, except for sarcomatous change within enchondromas. There is, however, some overlap between the two conditions, and some authors believe them to represent a spectrum of a single disease [22]. Some authors suggest that unilateral predominance favors a diagnosis of Ollier's disease [23]. The two conditions are discussed together in this section.

Cutaneous Features. Cutaneous and soft tissue hemangiomas are the most common features seen in patients with Maffucci's syndrome and Ollier's disease. The hands are the most commonly affected site, but the hemangiomas can occur at any location. Lymphangiomas and arteriovenous malformations have also been reported in these patients. Some of these malformations appear to be true anomalies with venous and arterial components. Others appear to be entirely venous, with compensatory hyperplasia and arterialization of vascular walls.

Another vascular neoplasm associated with Maffucci's syndrome is spindle cell hemangioma. These tumors usually arise on the distal extremities of young patients with a mean age in the fourth decade [24]. Multiple discrete nodules may be present [25]. These are thought to be vascular tumors of low malignant potential, with local recurrence occurring in about half of patients [24], but with a low risk for metastatic spread. Approximately 5% of patients with spindle cell hemangioma have Maffucci's syndrome [24]. Malignant degeneration of the vascular neoplasms in Maffucci's syndrome is quite rare, with cases of angiosarcoma and lymphangiosarcoma reported [26, 27].

Associated Disorders. Multiple enchondromas are the characteristic tumor associated with Ollier's disease and Maffucci's syndrome. These tumors can arise in any location, but the hands are particularly affected. The cartilaginous involvement of the disease is often self-limited, as the disease stops spontaneously, with tumors even regressing, as the patient grows [23]. In some patients, unequal leg length has been attributed to varus angulation of the lower femur [28].

Sarcomatous change has been reported to develop within enchondromas in 15%–30% of patients with

Maffucci's syndrome [27, 29]. These can occur in any location, including intracranial [30].

Central nervous system tumors, including malignant astrocytomas [22, 31], have been described in patients with Maffucci's syndrome. Ovarian neoplasms, including fibrosarcoma [32], Sertoli-Leydig cell tumor [33], and granulosa cell tumors [34] have been reported in patients with Maffucci's syndrome. Breast tumors, including adenomas [33] and carcinomas [35], have also been reported in patients with Maffucci's syndrome. Less commonly, pituitary adenomas have been described in patients with Maffucci's syndrome [35], as has a case of multicentric paraganglioma [36] and one of epidermoid carcinoma of the nasopharynx [37]. A case of acute lymphoid leukemia has been reported in a patient with Maffucci's syndrome [38].

Histologic Features. The hemangiomas and arteriovenous malformations present in Maffucci's syndrome are histologically identical to those seen independent of the syndrome. Well-developed vessels lined by unremarkable endothelial cells are present throughout the affected dermis and subcutaneous tissue. In the malformations, some of the vessels may display thickening of the vascular walls (see Chapter 12, Fig. 12–6).

Spindle cell hemangioendothelioma is a dermal tumor with areas of well-formed dilated vessels admixed with areas of spindle cell proliferation. The areas with dilated vessels histologically resemble cavernous hemangiomas. The other zones are characterized by more solid sheets of spindle-shaped cells with thin slit-like vascular spaces and extravasated erythrocytes. The endothelial cells may appear epithelioid. Scattered mitotic figures may be seen, but there is not significant cytologic atypia. These areas are histologically similar to Kaposi's sarcoma [25]. Many of these neoplasms are partly or entirely intravascular. The following entities must be considered in the differential diagnosis of spindle cell hemangioendothelioma:

- Acquired tufted angioma
- Angiosarcoma
- Kaposi's sarcoma
- Pyogenic granuloma

Special Studies. Special studies are not helpful in diagnosing the cutaneous lesions in patients with Maffucci's syndrome.

Pathogenesis. The pathogenesis of Maffucci's syndrome is not known. Because of the findings of increased nerves within hemangiomas and enchondromas, it has been suggested that upregulation of the neuropeptidergic nervous system may be related to the development of the cartilaginous and vascular tumors seen in the syndrome [39].

Goltz's Syndrome (Focal Dermal Hypoplasia)

Epidemiology. Goltz's syndrome is an X-linked dominant syndrome that is usually lethal to affected male patients. It is characterized by a wide range of defects involving components of both mesodermal and ectodermal tissues. There is marked variability in the expression of the syndrome, with some patients displaying only mild changes such as aplasia cutis congenita and dental anomalies [40]. Rare cases have been documented in men [41] and attributed to half chromatid mutations [42].

Cutaneous Features. The most common cutaneous defects observed in patients with Goltz's syndrome include aplasia cutis congenita, multiple atrophic patches, linear striae, papillomatosis of the skin, and lipomatous growths [43].

Atrophic hyper- and hypopigmented macules characteristically demonstrate a linear arrangement. They may be erythematous. Multiple focal atrophic patches are commonly found randomly distributed and may be extensive, involving virtually the entire skin surface. These lesions are often oval or elongated.

Multiple 1–2 mm verrucous papules have been described commonly in patients with Goltz's syndrome. These are often located on the face, especially on the eyelids and around the mouth [44]. Mucosal papillomatosis has also been described [43]. The verrucous papules have a smooth surface and may be pedunculated or sessile. Common acrochordons are also seen frequently in these patients.

The striae described in Goltz's syndrome spread from early oval macules to erythematous, atrophic streaks that are most common along the extremities.

Aplasia cutis congenita, appearing as a scar-like or ulcerated linear plaque, is usually located in the midline on the scalp. It has been reported in patients with Goltz's syndrome. It is clinically identical to similar lesions occurring in patients without the syndrome.

Herniations of subcutaneous fat into the overlying skin are commonly seen in patients with Goltz's syndrome. Perianal herniations are especially common. Multiple hidrocystomas have been reported in patients with Goltz's syndrome [41, 45].

Associated Disorders. Skeletal anomalies are common in patients with Goltz's syndrome. These include syndactyly that resembles a lobster claw, short stature, scoliosis, and clinodactyly [44]. In rare patients, osteochondromas [46] and aneurysmal bone cysts [47] may develop. Osteopathia striata is also found [44].

Dental anomalies are frequent in these patients and include caries, hypodontia, and malocclusion [44]. Congenital papillomatosis in locations other than the skin, including the esophagus, has been reported in patients with Goltz's syndrome, as has hiatal herniation [45, 48]. Central nervous system anomalies have also been described in patients with Goltz's syndrome. These include myelomeningocele, Arnold-Chiari anomaly, and hydrocephalus [49], as well as porencephalic cysts [42]. Cortical and cerebellar atrophy have been reported [44].

Ocular defects described in patients with Goltz's syndrome include corneal abnormalities, microphthalmos, anophthalmos, and colobomas [50], as well as hypoplasia of the optic nerve [44]. Urinary tract anomalies, including bifid ureters and renal pelvices, are found in patients with Goltz's syndrome [44]. Horseshoe kidney is an unusual finding in these patients [51]. Herniations of the ventral wall have been observed in patients with Goltz's syndrome [52]. Malrotation of the intestine and mediastinum have also been reported [53].

Histologic Features. Histologic features of the earliest changes seen in Goltz's syndrome have not been completely described. In one study, a lymphocytic inflammatory infiltrate and marked papillary dermal edema were found admixed with fibroblasts and clusters of adipocytes within the dermis of red, linear atrophic lesions [54]. Dermal collagen is reported to still be present in the earliest lesions [43]. It is not known if these changes are commonly found before the development of the classic changes of focal dermal hypoplasia.

The histologic findings of the areas of focal dermal hypoplasia and striae include an atrophic epidermis, with flattening of the rete ridge pattern. The dermis is markedly attenuated to absent, and adipose tissue is present almost adjacent to the epidermis [44] (Fig. 11–1). Increased small blood vessels are present in the papillary dermis and are surrounded by adipose tissue. No inflammation is seen in well-developed lesions. The following entities must be considered in the histologic differential diagnosis of focal dermal hypoplasia:

- Aplasia cutis congenita
- Fibrolipoma
- Fibrous hamartoma of infancy
- Nevus lipomatosis superficialis

Lipomatous tumors appear histologically as proliferations of mature adipose tissue that overgrow the dermis and produce nodules underlying an intact, flattened epidermis. They differ from ordinary lipomas solely by their very superficial anatomic location. Papillomas

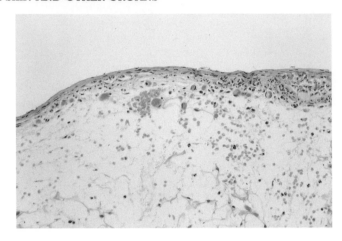

Fig. 11–1. Focal dermal hypoplasia is characterized by adipose tissue and increased vascularity in the place of dermal collagen.

found in Goltz's syndrome are characterized by epidermal papillomatosis and acanthosis. They contain a thin stalk of collagen and a slight inflammatory infiltrate.

Special Studies. Special studies are not required to make a diagnosis of focal dermal hypoplasia.

Pathogenesis. Although the exact pathogenesis of Goltz's syndrome is not known, a defect in the X chromosome is known to cause the observed anomalies. It has been suggested that random inactivation of the X chromosome bearing the mutant gene may be responsible for the variable degrees of expression demonstrated by patients with the syndrome [40].

Based on data from sequential biopsies performed on patients for up to 30 years, it has been suggested that the lipomatous lesions seen in patients with Goltz's syndrome represent lipomatous hamartomas rather than dermal hypoplasia [43]. Other investigators have arrived at a similar conclusion [55], although the hypothesis has not yet been definitively proved. Other groups have, however, hypothesized that the absence of dermal collagen can be attributed to a defect in the ability of fibroblasts to produce collagen [41, 56].

Congenital Hemidysplasia with Ichthyosiform Erythroderma and Limb Defects (CHILD) Syndrome

Epidemiology. CHILD syndrome occurs almost exclusively in girls. It is a congenital syndrome [57]. It has been suggested that CHILD syndrome is caused by an X-linked dominant mutation and is lethal for affected male embryos [58]. A woman with an isolated CHILD nevus (see later) may be at increased risk of transmitting the full-blown CHILD syndrome to a daughter [59].

Cutaneous Features. The most common cutaneous finding in patients with CHILD syndrome is unilateral ichthyosiform erythroderma, which usually develops shortly after birth. In some patients, there is a tendency for greater involvement of skin folds (ptychotropism) [57]. Unilateral epidermal nevi have been described in patients with CHILD syndrome [60]. Verruciform xanthomas have been noted in multiple patients with the syndrome [60]. It has been proposed that each of the above designations is inappropriate and that patients with this syndrome have a characteristic cutaneous finding that is best designated a CHILD nevus [59]. This nevus is unique in its waxy yellow scaling and its diffuse and linear pattern of unilateral involvement, in addition to its characteristic histologic features (see later) [59]. Cutaneous abnormalities also include widespread areas of hypotrichosis and onychodystrophy [58].

Associated Disorders. CHILD syndrome has been associated with fused vertebrae, hemivertebrae, and renal agenesis [58]. Hexadactyly has also been described in these patients [61]. Chondrodysplasia punctata occurs in patients with CHILD syndrome [62]. Absence of facial muscles, ventricular septal defects, and shortening of limbs have been described [63]. The skeletal and visceral anomalies usually occur ipsilateral to the cutaneous findings.

Histologic Features. It has been suggested that the usual histologic changes in cutaneous lesions of patients with CHILD syndrome (i.e., a CHILD nevus) are those of a verruciform xanthoma, which distinguishes this syndrome from others in which epidermal nevi are found [57]. Histologic features of verruciform xanthoma are indistinguishable from those occurring in other settings. They include verrucous epidermal hyperplasia with overlying hyperkeratosis and parakeratosis (Fig. 11–2). The papillary dermis is filled with lipid-laden histiocytes that abut the epidermis but do not invade (Fig. 11–3). There is a minimal associated inflammatory infiltrate.

Special Studies. No special studies are necessary to make a diagnosis of a CHILD nevus.

Pathogenesis. It has been proposed that inactivation of the X chromosome prevents development of a clone of cells that control a large developmental field [63]. Abnormalities in fibroblast proliferation rates and rate of production of prostaglandin E_2 have been found in affected skin compared with uninvolved skin from patients with CHILD syndrome [64]. It has also been

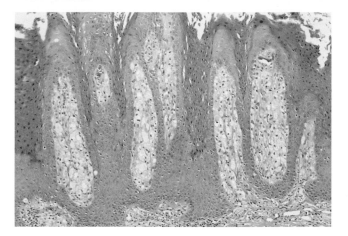

Fig. 11–2. Verruciform xanthoma displaying hyperkeratosis, parakeratosis, and epidermal hyperplasia.

shown that fibroblasts from these individuals have peroxisomal defects [62]. It has been suggested that dermal factors, such as fibroblasts, may have a role in influencing the abnormal protein expression seen in lesional keratinocytes in this syndrome [65].

Papillon-Lefèvre Syndrome

Epidemiology. Papillon-Lefèvre syndrome is an autosomal recessive condition characterized by keratoderma, severe periodontitis, and recurrent pyogenic infections. The syndrome appears to be related to a locus in the region of chromosome 11q14–11q21[66, 67]. An autosomal recessive inheritance pattern has been established [68].

Cutaneous Features. Pronounced hyperkeratotic plaques overlying the knees, elbows, and interphalangeal joints characterize the keratoderma of Papillon-Lefèvre syn-

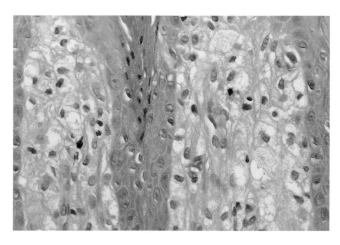

Fig. 11–3. The papillary dermis is distended with lipid-laden histiocytes in verruciform xanthoma.

drome. Marked hyperkeratosis of the palms and soles occurs in all of these patients, as well.

Associated Disorders. Periodontitis is the most common extracutaneous finding in patients with Papillon-Lefèvre syndrome. The diagnosis of periodontitis marginalis profunda is highly specific for Papillon-Lefèvre syndrome [69]. Periodontal disease results in the premature loss of teeth in many affected patients [70].

Recurrent cutaneous infections are also a problem in some patients with Papillon-Lefèvre syndrome [71, 72]. Rare cases of ocular nystagmus have been reported in patients with the syndrome [73], as has acro-osteolysis [74]. Calcification of the falx has also been reported in some patients with Papillon-Lefèvre syndrome [68].

Histologic Features. The histologic findings in Papillon-Lefèvre syndrome are nonspecific. Affected skin has marked hyperkeratosis. Parakeratosis is not generally seen. The epidermis has a thickened granular layer and is often slightly acanthotic. The underlying dermis is unremarkable (Fig. 11–4). These features occur in a number of syndromes associated with keratoderma.

Special Studies. Special studies are not helpful in making the diagnosis of Papillon-Lefèvre syndrome. Electron microscopic studies demonstrated lipid-like vacuoles in keratinocytes within the stratum corneum and stratum granulosum. These cells had decreased numbers of tonofilaments and irregularly shaped keratohyaline granules [75].

Pathogenesis. Studies have demonstrated several immunologic anomalies in patients with Papillon-Lefèvre syndrome. Some patients have impaired reactivity to both T- and B-cell mitogens, but this finding did not correlate with increased susceptibility to infection in affected patients [76]. Neutrophil chemotaxis was depressed in another group of patients with the syndrome [77]. The relationship between increased infections and the observed cutaneous hyperkeratosis is not understood.

Epidermal Nevus Syndrome

Epidemiology. Epidermal nevus syndrome is a congenital syndrome that affects the skin and multiple other organ systems. The age of clinical onset ranges from birth to 14 years [78]. In about one third of patients, the epidermal nevi will extend beyond the original distribution. Its mode of inheritance is not known, but chromosomal mosaicisms have been detected in some patients [79]. In rare cases, a familial association has been documented, suggesting the possibility of autosomal dominant inheritance with decreased penetrance [80]. Given the rarity of familial clustering, this is thought to be unlikely by most investigators.

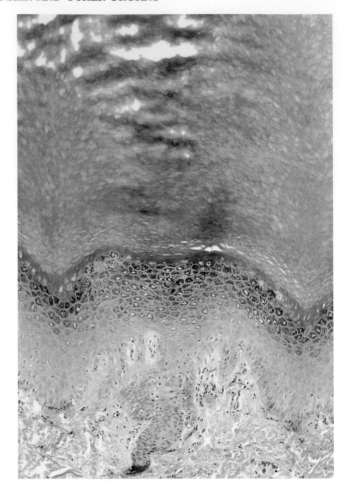

Fig. 11–4. Papillon-Lefèvre syndrome is characterized by marked orthokeratotic hyperkeratosis, acanthosis, and hypergranulosis.

The term *epidermal nevus syndrome* has been called into question by some authors, who argue that there are several different syndromes that fall into this category, including Proteus syndrome, sebaceous nevus syndrome, and CHILD syndrome, leaving few cases that remain unclassified [81].

Cutaneous Features. The epidermal nevus syndrome is characterized by linear, hyperkeratotic verrucous papules. The most common sites of involvement are the head and neck. Lesions are widespread in up to 13% of patients [78].

Giant woolly hair nevi [82] and inflammatory linear verrucous epidermal nevi (ILVEN) [83] have been described in patients with the epidermal nevus syndrome.

Cutaneous vascular lesions such as hemangiomas and hemangioendotheliomas have been reported in some patients with the epidermal nevus syndrome [80]. Trichilemmal cysts have been described in several patients [84].

Associated Disorders. Epidermal nevus syndrome is associated with malformations in multiple organ systems, including the central nervous system (frequently), the musculoskeletal system, eyes, and cardiovascular system. Up to one-third of patients demonstrate extracutaneous anomalies, and about 5% have five or more such problems [78]. Reported anomalies include mental retardation, hemiparesis, epilepsy, cortical atrophy [85], and megalencephaly and vascular malformations [86].

The epidermal nevus syndrome is also frequently associated with abnormalities of the musculoskeletal system, including vitamin D–resistant rickets [87], macrodactyly [88], scoliosis [89], osteolysis of the skull, multiple fractures [90], and hemihypertrophy [91].

Precocious puberty has been described in patients with the epidermal nevus syndrome [82, 87].

Early onset of neoplasms, including several malignancies, has also been reported in these patients [82], with an overall incidence of less than 5% [78]. Some of the associated neoplasms include chondroblastoma [92], gliomatosis cerebri [93], rhabdomyosarcoma [94], and transitional cell carcinoma of the bladder [89].

Histologic Features. Multiple histologic patterns of epidermal nevi have been described [95]. The most common pattern demonstrates hyperkeratosis with focal parakeratosis overlying a hyperplastic epidermis (Fig. 11–5 and 11–6). The granular layer is thickened, and there is a papillomatous architecture that may resemble "church spires." Increased melanin within basal keratinocytes is sometimes present. Foci of acantholysis and cornoid lamellae are present in some cases. The following entities must be considered in the histologic differential diagnosis of an epidermal nevus:

- Acanthosis nigricans
- Acrokeratosis verruciformis of Hopf

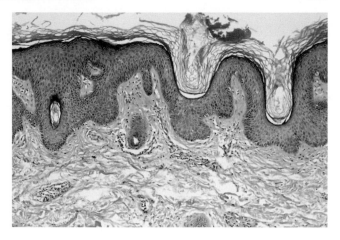

Fig. 11–6. Epidermal nevus with acanthosis and increased pigmentation in basal keratinocytes.

- Confluent and reticulated papillomatosis of Gougerot and Carteaud
- Dowling-Degos syndrome
- Nevus sebaceus of Jadassohn
- Seborrheic keratosis
- Verruca vulgaris

Less commonly, epidermal nevi may demonstrate epidermolytic hyperkeratosis. In these cases, there is perinuclear vacuolization within the superficial portions of the epidermis. Increased numbers of irregularly shaped and enlarged keratohyalin granules are present within the upper spinous layers. There is prominent overlying hyperkeratosis (Fig. 11–7). These patients may have a forme fruste of nonbullous congenital ichthyosiform erythroderma, as focal genetic defects in keratins 1 and 10 have been reported.

In a subset of patients with classic epidermal nevi, inflammatory linear verrucous epidermal nevi may also

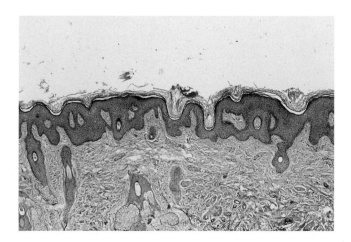

Fig. 11–5. Epidermal nevus demonstrates epidermal hyperplasia and papillomatosis.

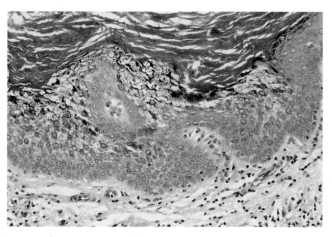

Fig. 11–7. Epidermolytic hyperkeratosis in an epidermal nevus demonstrates dissolution of the keratinocytes in the upper portions of the epidermis.

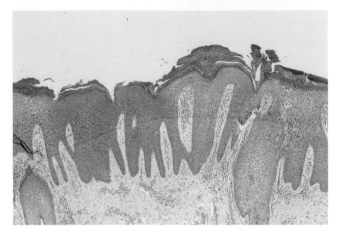

Fig. 11–8. Inflammatory verrucous epidermal nevus (ILVEN) demonstrates psoriasiform hyperplasia and overlying parakeratosis and hyperkeratosis.

be present. These hamartomas are characterized by psoriasiform hyperplasia of the epidermis with overlying alternating zones of hyperkeratosis and parakeratosis (Fig. 11–8). There is suprapapillary thinning, tortuosity and ectasia of thin-walled capillaries within the dermal papillae, and a lymphohistiocytic inflammatory cell infiltrate in the dermis (Fig. 11–9).

Special Studies. Special studies are not necessary to make a diagnosis of epidermal nevus.

Pathogenesis. Some authors have hypothesized a gene mosaicism theory of pathogenesis [86]. A somatic mutation occurring during fetal life is believed to be the cause of the hamartomatous changes seen in epidermal nevus syndrome [84]. Neuronal migratory abnormalities during development may play a

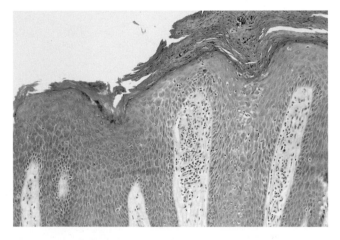

Fig. 11–9. Inflammatory verrucous epidermal nevus (ILVEN) demonstrates alternating orthokeratosis and parakeratosis, psoriasiform epidermal hyperplasia, and ectatic papillary dermal blood vessels.

significant role in causing the epidermal nevus syndrome [93].

Buschke-Ollendorff Syndrome

Epidemiology. Buschke-Ollendorff syndrome, also known as *dermatofibrosis lenticularis disseminata*, is an autosomal dominant syndrome that affects the skin and bones.

Cutaneous Features. Connective tissue hamartomas are found in virtually all patients with Buschke-Ollendorff syndrome. Patients develop disseminated white to skin-colored papules that are often grouped. The papules are asymmetrically distributed and appear at any early age [96]. They can be scattered and few or widespread and abundant.

Associated Disorders. Osteopoikilosis is found in two-thirds of affected patients [96]. The osteopoikilosis can affect any bones, including the pelvis and lumbosacral spine. There is no bone weakness or any other clinical manifestation associated with the radiographic changes [97].

A rare case of Buschke-Ollendorff syndrome associated with protein C deficiency has been reported. The authors suggest that the association may not be fortuitous, as the genes for elastin and protein C are both located on chromosome 2q [98].

Histologic Features. The cutaneous papules known as *dermatofibrosis lenticularis disseminata* have the histologic changes of connective tissue hamartomas. Biopsy specimens demonstrate skin with unremarkable epidermis. The dermis appears thickened by an overgrowth of disordered, thickened interlacing elastic fibers. Electron microscopy reveals markedly branched elastic fibers [99]. The following entities must be considered in the histologic differential diagnosis of a connective tissue nevus:

- Normal back skin
- Scar
- Scleroderma/ morphea
- Sclerotic fibroma

Special Studies. An elastic tissue stain (Verhoeff–van Gieson) is helpful in demonstrating the altered quantity and quality of the dermal elastic fibers in cutaneous lesions of the Buschke-Ollendorff syndrome.

Pathogenesis. Alterations of calcium and phosphorous metabolism have been described in a series of patients with Buschke-Ollendorff syndrome [100]; however, this finding does not appear to be widespread among patients with the syndrome. Cultured fibroblasts from affected patients have been shown to produce increased amounts of elastin than those from people without the disease [101].

Ehlers-Danlos Syndrome

Epidemiology. Ehlers-Danlos syndrome is composed of a group of conditions that share various combinations of joint hyperextensibility, skin fragility, and easy bruising and bleeding. Each subtype is associated with its own pattern of inheritance. Table 11–2 summarizes the subtypes of Ehlers-Danlos syndrome.

Cutaneous Features. Cutaneous changes in Ehlers-Danlos syndrome vary depending on the syndrome subtype. In general, the changes include hyperelastic skin with a dough-like consistency, easy bruisibility that

Table 11–2. Subtypes of Ehlers-Danlos Syndrome				
Subtype	Mode of Inheritance	Cutaneous Abnormalities	Biochemical Deficiency	Histologic Abnormality
I	AD	Herniations of fat into dermis; scarring; tumors	COL5A1 mutation	
II	AD	Mild cutaneous changes	COL5A1 mutation	
III	AD	Joint hypermobility, minimal skin changes	Unknown	Loss of type III collagen
IV	AD/AR variants	Rupture of large arteries and internal viscera; translucent face skin	Mutation in COL3A1 gene leads to decreased collagen III production	Increased solar elastosis; thinning of dermis
V	X-linked	Cutaneous hyperextensibility; other cutaneous changes resembling type I	?Lysyl oxidase defect	
VI	AR	Ocular fragility; kyphoscoliosis; prominent joint and skin changes; muscular hypotonia; arterial rupture; retinal detachment	Peptidyl lysyl hydroxylase deficiency causes abnormal cross links in types I and III collagen	Thinning of dermis
VII	Unknown	Joint instability; multiple dislocations at birth	Defect in conversion of type I procollagen to collagen	
VIII	AD	Easy bruising; Pretibial hyperpigmentation; periodontal disease; hyperextensible joints	Unknown	
IX*	X-linked	Occipital horn syndrome*		
X	Unknown	Defect in platelet aggregation; moderately severe skin and joint changes	Related to fibronectin	
XI*	AD	Familial benign joint hypermobility syndrome*		

AD = Autosomal dominant; AR = autosomal recessive.

*No longer currently recognized as a subtype of Ehlers-Danlos syndrome in this classification scheme.

From references 106–108.

heals with atrophic scars, and connective tissue fragility. Trauma may result in the formation of "molluscoid" pseudotumors. Characteristic "fish mouth" scars develop over the knees and elbows in many patients. Calcified, firm, subcutaneous nodules are found in some patients. Premature aging of the face may be observed.

Associated Disorders. Skeletal, vascular, and visceral anomalies have been described in the various subtypes of Ehlers-Danlos syndrome. These findings are summarized in Table 11–2. Elastosis perforans serpiginosum has been described in patients with type IV Ehlers-Danlos syndrome [102].

Histologic Features. Routine histologic sections of tissue from patients with Ehlers Danlos syndrome usually do not demonstrate any abnormalities and thus are not helpful in making the diagnosis. In some patients with type VI, thinning of the dermis has been described [103]. Investigators have also reported increased solar elastosis in patients with type IV disease [103]. Others have reported thinning of the dermis in some patients with type IV Ehlers-Danlos syndrome [104]. Loss of type III collagen has been shown, with immunohistochemistry, in some biopsy specimens from patients with type IV Ehlers-Danlos syndrome [105]. These findings are included in Table 11–2.

Special Studies. Electron microscopic studies of dermal collagen have demonstrated altered collagen fibers in some types of Ehlers-Danlos syndrome. Histologic examination of skin is not, however, the preferred method of making a diagnosis of Ehlers-Danlos syndrome, as the changes are often minimal and not well described.

Pathogenesis. Each of the subtypes of Ehlers-Danlos syndrome has its own genetic defect. In some types, the specific biochemical or genetic defect has been isolated, whereas in other types it remains unknown. These are summarized in Table 11–2.

References

1. Joshi, M., Cole, S., Knibbs, D., and Diana, D., *Pulmonary abnormalities in Klippel-Trénaunay syndrome. A histologic, ultrastructural, and immunocytochemical study.* Chest, 1992. 102:1274–1277.
2. Jacob, A. G., Driscoll, D. J., Shaughnessy, W. J., Stanson, A. W., Clap, R. P., and Gloviczki, P., *Klippel-Trénaunay syndrome: Spectrum and management.* Mayo Clin Proc, 1998. 73:28–36.
3. Ceballos-Quintal, J. M., Pinto-Escalante, D., and Castillo-Zapata, I., *A new case of Klippel-Trénaunay-Weber (KTW) syndrome: Evidence of autosomal dominant inheritance.* Am J Med Genet, 1996. 14:426–427.
4. McCrory, B. J., Amadio, P. C., Dobyns, J. H., Stickler, G. B., and Unni, K. K., *Anomalies of the fingers and toes associated with Klippel-Trénaunay syndrome.* J Bone Joint Surg (Am), 1991. 73:1537–1546.
5. Whelan, A. J., Watson, M. S., Porter, F. D., and Steiner, R. D., *Klippel-Trénaunay-Weber syndrome associated with a 5:11 balanced translocation.* Am J Med Genet, 1995. 59:492–494.
6. Robinson, D., Tieder, M., Halperin, N., Burshtein, D., and Nevo, Z., *Maffucci's syndrome—the result of neural abnormalities.* Cancer, 1994. 74:949–957.
7. Servelle, M., *Klippel and Trénaunay's syndrome. 768 operated cases.* Ann Surg, 1985. 201:365–373.
8. Meine, J. G., Schwartz, R. A., and Janniger, C. K., *Klippel-Trénaunay-Weber syndrome.* Cutis, 1997. 60:127–132.
9. Atiyeh, B. S., and Musharrafieh, R. S., *Klippel-Trénaunay-type syndrome: An eponym for various expressions of the same entity.* J Med, 1995. 26:253–260.
10. Steiner, M., Gould, A. R., Graves, S. M., and Kuerschner, T. W., *Klippel-Trénaunay-Weber syndrome.* Oral Surg Oral Med Oral Pathol, 1987. 63:208–215.
11. Burke, J. P., West, N. F., and Strachan, I. M., *Congenital nystagmus, anisomyopia, and hemimegalencephaly in the Klippel-Trénaunay-Weber syndrome.* J Pediatr Ophthalmol Strabismus, 1991. 28:41–44.
12. Myers, B. M., *Treatment of colonic bleeding in Klippel-Trénaunay syndrome with combined partial colectomy and endoscopic laser.* Dig Dis Sci, 1993. 38:1351–1353.
13. Nusser, C. A., Tuggle, D. W., McLanahan, K. B., and Leonard, J. C., *Splenic lymphangioma. An unusual manifestation of the Klippel-Trénaunay-Weber syndrome.* Clin Nucl Med, 1995. 20:844–845.
14. Alberti, E., *Ischaemic infarct of the brain stem combined with bisymptomatic Klippel-Trénaunay-Weber syndrome and cutis laxa.* J Neurol Neurosurg Psychiatry, 1976. 39:581–585.
15. Djindjian, M., Djindjian, R., Hurth, M., Rey, A., and Houdart, R., *Spinal cord arteriovenous malformations and the Klippel-Trénaunay-Weber syndrome.* Surg Neurol, 1977. 8:229–237.
16. Brod, R. D., Shields, J. A., Shields, C. L., Oberkircher, O. R., and Sabol, I. J., *Unusual retinal and renal vacular lesions in the Klippel-Trénaunay-Weber syndrome.* Retina, 1992. 12:355–358.
17. Fait, G., Daniel, Y., Kupferminc, M. J., Gull, I., Peyser, M. R., and Lessing, J. B., *Klippel-Trénaunay-Weber syndrome associated with fetal growth restriction.* Hum Reprod, 1996. 11:2544–2545.
18. Salman, S. M., Phillips, T., and Rogers, G. M., *Klippel-Trénaunay syndrome and cutaneous carcinomas.* J Dermatol Surg Oncol, 1993. 19:582–584.
19. Finley, J. L., Noe, J. M., Arndt, K. A., and Rosen, S., *Port wine stains: Morphologic variations and developmental lesions.* Arch Dermatol, 1984. 120:1453–1455.
20. Del-Rio, E., Aguilar, A., Amrojo, P., Velez, A., and

Sanchez Yus, E., *Pseudo-Kaposi sarcoma induced by minor trauma in a patient with Klippel-Trénaunay-Weber syndrome*. Clin Exp Dermatol, 1993. 18:151–153.

21. Smoller, B. R., and Rosen, S., *Port wine stains: An alteration of neural modulation of blood vessels*. Arch Dermatol, 1986. 122:177–179.

22. Mellon, C. D., Carter, J. D., and Owen, D. B., *Ollier's disease and Maffucci's syndrome: Distinct entities or a continuum. Case report: Enchondromatosis complicated by an intracranial glioma*. J Neurol, 1988. 235:376–378.

23. Miyawaki, T., Kinoshita, Y., and Iizuka, T., *A case of Ollier's disease of the hand*. Ann Plast Surg, 1997. 38:77–80.

24. Perkins, P., and Weiss, S. W., *Spindle cell hemangioendothelioma: An analysis of 78 cases with reassessment of its pathogenesis and biologic behavior*. Am J Surg Pathol, 1996q. 20:1196–1204.

25. Fanburg, J. C., Meis-Kindblom, J. M., and Rosenberg, A. E., *Multiple enchondromas associated with spindle-cell hemangioendotheliomas. An overlooked variant of Maffucci's syndrome*. Am J Surg Pathol, 1995. 19:1029–1038.

26. Kerr, H. D., Keep, J. C., and Chiu, S., *Lymphangiosarcoma associated with lymphedema in a man with Maffucci's syndrome*. South Med J, 1991. 84:1039–1041.

27. Davidson, T. I., Kissin, M. W., Bradish, C. F., and Westbury, G., *Angiosarcoma arising in a patient with Maffucci syndrome*. Eur J Surg Oncol, 1985. 11:381–384.

28. Chew, D. K., Menelaus, M. B., and Richardson, M. D., *Ollier's disease: Varus angulation at the lower femur and its management*. J Pediatr Orthop, 1998. 18:202–208.

29. Albregts, A. E., and Rapini, R. P., *Malignancy in Maffucci's syndrome*. Dermatol Clin, 1995. 13:73–78.

30. Ramina, R., Coelho Neto, M., Meneses, M. S., and Pedrozo, A. A., *Maffucci's syndrome associated with a cranial base chondrosarcoma: Case report and literature review*. Neurosurgery, 1997. 41:269–272.

31. Bendel, C. J., and Gelmers, H. J., *Multiple enchondromatosis (Ollier's disease) complicated by malignant astrocytoma*. Eur J Radiol, 1991. 12:135–137.

32. Christman, J. E., and Ballon, S. C., *Ovarian fibrosarcoma associated with Maffucci's syndrome*. Gynecol Oncol, 1990. 37:290–291.

33. Weyl-Ben Arush, M., and Olander, L., *Ollier's disease associated with Sertoli-Leydig cell tumor and breast adenoma*. Am J Pediatr Hematol Oncol, 1991. 13:49–51.

34. Plantaz, D., Flamant, F., Vassal, G., Chappius, J. P., Baranzelli, M. C., Bouffet, E., Dyon, J. F., Armari, C., et al., *Granulosa cell tumors of the ovary in children and adolescents. Multicenter retrospective study in 40 patients aged 7 months to 22 years*. Arch Fr Pediatr, 1992. 49:793–798.

35. Marymount, J. V., Fisher, R. F., Emde, G. E., and Limbird, T. J., *Maffucci's syndrome complicated by carcinoma of the breast, pituitary adenoma and mediastinal hemangioma*. South Med J, 1987. 80:1429–1431.

36. Lamovec, J., Frkovic-Grazio, S., and Bracko, M., *Non-sporadic cases and unusual morphological features in pheochromocytoma and paraganglioma*. Arch Pathol Lab Med, 1998. 122:63–68.

37. Yazidi, A., Benzekri, L., Senouci, K., Bennouna-Biaz, F., and Hassam, B., *Maffucci syndrome associated with epidermoid carcinoma of the nasopharynx*. Ann Dermatol Venereol, 1998. 125:50–51.

38. Rector, J. T., Gray, C. L., Sharpe, R. W., Hall, F. W., Thomas, W., and Jones, W., *Acute lymphoid leukemia associated with Maffucci's syndrome*. Am J Pediatr Hematol Oncol, 1993. 15:427–429.

39. Robinson, D., Tieder, M., Halperin, N., Burshtein, D., and Nevo, Z., *Maffucci's syndrome—the result of neural abnormalities? Evidence of mitogenic neurotransmitters present in enchondroma and soft tissue hemangiomas*. Cancer, 1994. 74:949–957.

40. Weschler, M. A., Papa, C. M., Haberman, F., and Marion, R. W., *Variable expression in focal dermal hypoplasia. An example of differential X-chromosome inactivation*. Am J Dis Child, 1988. 142:297–300.

41. Buchner, S. A., and Itin, P., *Focal dermal hypoplasia syndrome in a male patient. Report of a case and histologic and immunological studies*. Arch Dermatol, 1992. 128:1078–1082.

42. Sule, R. R., Dhumawat, D. J., and Gharpuray, M. B., *Focal dermal hypoplasia*. Cutis, 1994. 53:309–312.

43. Howell, J. B., and Freeman, R. G., *Cutaneous defects of focal dermal hypoplasia: An ectomesodermal dysplasia syndrome*. J Cutan Pathol, 1989. 16:237–258.

44. Gunduz, K., Gunalp, I., and Erden, I., *Focal dermal hypoplasia (Goltz's syndrome)*. Ophthalmic Genet, 1997. 18:143–149.

45. Zala, L., Elltin, C., and Krebs, A., *Focal dermal hypoplasia with keratoconus, papillomatosis of esophagus and hidrocystomas*. Dermatologica, 1975. 150:176–185.

46. Cox, N. H., and Paterson, W. D., *Osteochondroma of humerus in focal dermal hypoplasia (Goltz) syndrome*. Clin Exp Dermatol, 1991. 16:283–284.

47. D'Alise, M. D., Timmons, C. F., and Swift, D. M., *Focal dermal hypoplasia (Goltz syndrome) with vertebral solid aneurysmal bone cyst variant. A case report*. Pediatr Neurosurg, 1996. 24:151–154.

48. Brinson, R. R., Schuman, B. M., Mills, L. R., Thigpen, S., and Freedman, S., *Multiple squamous papillomas of the esophagus associated with Goltz syndrome*. Am J Gastroenterol, 1987. 82:1177–1179.

49. Almeida, L., Anyane-Yeboa, K., Grossman, M., and Rosen, T., *Myelomeningocele, Arnold-Chiari anomaly and hydrocephalus in focal dermal hypoplasia*. Am J Med Genet, 1988. 30:917–923.

50. Lueder, G. T., and Steiner, R. D., *Corneal abnormalities in a mother and daughter with focal dermal hypoplasia (Goltz-Gorlin syndrome)*. Am J Ophthalmol, 1995. 120:256–258.

51. Suskan, E., Kurkcuoglu, N., and Uluoglu, O., *Focal dermal hypoplasia (Goltz syndrome) with horseshoe kidney abnormality*. Pediatr Dermatol, 1990. 7:283–286.

52. Bhatia, A. M., Clericuzio, C. L., and Musemeche,

C. A., *Congenital ventral hernia in association with focal dermal hypoplasia.* Pediatr Dermatol, 1995. 12:336–339.

53. Irvine, A. D., Stewart, F. J., Bingham, E. A., Nevin, N. C., and Boston, V. E., *Focal dermal hypoplasia (Goltz syndrome) associated with intestinal malrotation and mediastinal dextroposition.* Am J Med Genet, 1996. 62:213–215.

54. Mann, M., Weintrabu, R., and Hashimoto, K., *Focal dermal hypoplasia with an initial inflammatory phase.* Pediatr Dermatol, 1990. 7:278–282.

55. Ishii, N., Baba, N., Kanaizuka, I., Nakajima, H., Ono, S., and Amemiya, F., *Histopathological study of focal dermal hypoplasia (Goltz syndrome).* 1992. 17:24–26.

56. Sato, M., Ishikawa, O., Yokoyama, Y., Kondo, A., and Miyachi, Y., *Focal dermal hypoplasia (Goltz syndrome): A decreased accumulation of hyaluronic acid in three-dimensional culture.* Acta Derm Venereol, 1996. 76:365–367.

57. Happle, R., *Epidermal nevus syndromes.* Semin Dermatol, 1995. 14:111–121.

58. Happle, R., Karlic, D., and Steijlen, P. M., *CHILD syndrome in a mother and daughter.* Hautarzt, 1990. 41:105–108.

59. Happle, R., Mittag, H., and Kuster, W., *The CHILD nevus: A distinct skin disorder.* Dermatology, 1995. 191:210–216.

60. Zamora-Martinez, E., Martin-Moreno, L., Barat-Cascante, A., and Castro-Torres, A., *Another CHILD syndrome with xanthomatous pattern.* Dermatologica, 1990. 180:263–266.

61. Peter, C., and Meinecke, P., *CHILD syndrome. Case report of a rare genetic dermatosis.* Hautarzt, 1993. 44:590–593.

62. Emami, S., Rizzo, W. B., Hanley, K. P., Taylor, J. M., Goldyne, M. E., and Williams, M. L., *Peroxisomal abnormality in fibroblasts from involved skin of CHILD syndrome. Case study and review of peroxisomal disorders in relation to skin disease.* Arch Dermatol, 1992. 128:1213–1222.

63. Fink-Puches, R., Soyer, H. P., Pierer, G., Kerl, H., and Happle, R., *Systematized inflammatory epidermal nevus with symmetrical involvement: An unusual case of CHILD syndrome?* J Am Acad Dermatol, 1997. 36:823–826.

64. Goldyne, M. E., and Williams, M. L., *CHILD syndrome. Phenotypic dichotomy in eicosanoid metabolism and proliferative rates among cultured dermal fibroblasts.* J Clin Invest, 1989. 84:357–360.

65. Dale, B. A., Kimball, J. R., Fleckman, P., Herbert, A. A., and Holbrook, K. A., *CHILD syndrome: Lack of expression of epidermal differentiation markers in lesional ichthyotic skin.* J Invest Dermatol, 1992. 98:442–449.

66. Hart, T. C., Bowden, D. W., Ghaffar, K. A., Wang, W., Cutler, C. W., Cebeci, I., Efeoglu, A., and Firatli, E., *Sublocalization of the Papillon-Lefèvre syndrome locus on 11q14–q21.* Am J Med Genet, 1998. 79:134–139.

67. Laass, M. W., Hennies, H. C., Preis, S., Stevens, H. P., Jung, M., Leigh, I. M., Wienker, T. F., and Reis, A., *Localisation of a gene for Papillon-Lefèvre syndrome to chromosome 11q14–q21 by homozygosity mapping.* Hum Genet, 1997. 101:376–382.

68. Landow, R. K., Cheung, H., and Bauer, M., *Papillon-Lefèvre syndrome.* Int J Dermatol, 1983. 22:177–179.

69. Bork, K., and Lost, C., *Extrapalmoplantar skin symptoms and additional clinical, etiological and immunological aspects in particular, in Papillon-Lefèvre syndrome.* Hautarzt, 1980. 31:179–183.

70. Hattab, F. N., Rawashdeh, M. A., Yassin, O. M., al-Momani, A. S., and al-Ubosi, M. M., *Papillon-Lefèvre syndrome: A review of the literature and review of 4 cases.* J Periodontol, 1995. 66:413–420.

71. Verma, K. C., Chaddha, M. K., and Joshi, R. K., *Papillon-Lefèvre syndrome.* Int J Dermatol, 1979. 18:146–149.

72. Borroni, G., Pagani, A., Carcaterra, A., Pericoli, R., Gabba, P., and Marconi, M., *Immunologic alterations in a case of Papillon-Lefèvre syndrome with recurrent cutaneous infections.* Dermatologica, 1985. 170:27–30.

73. Mhaiskar, U., Kulkarni, S., and Shah, M. D., *Papillon-Lefèvre syndrome with ocular nystagmus: A case report.* J Postgrad Med, 1980. 26:267–268.

74. Trattner, A., David, M., and Sandbank, M., *Papillon-Lefèvre syndrome with acroosteolysis.* J Am Acad Dermatol, 1991. 24:835–838.

75. Nazzaro, V., Blanchet-Bardon, C., Mimoz, C., Revuz, J., and Puissant, A., *Papillon-Lefèvre syndrome. Ultrastructural study and successful treatment with acitretin.* Arch Dermatol, 1988. 124:533–539.

76. Levo, Y., Wollner, S., and Hacham-Zadeh, S., *Immunologic study of patients with the Papillon-Lefèvre syndrome.* Clin Exp Immunol, 1980. 40:407–410.

77. Firatli, E., Tuzun, B., and Efeoglu, A., *Papillon-Lefèvre syndrome. Analysis of neutrophil chemotaxis.* J Periodontol, 1996. 67:617–620.

78. Rogers, M., McCrossin, I., and Commens, C., *Epidermal nevi and the epidermal nevus syndrome. A review of 131 cases.* J Am Acad Dermatol, 1989. 20:476–488.

79. Stosiek, N., Ulmer, R., von den Driesch, P., Claussen, U., Hornstein, O. P., and Rott, H. D., *Chromosomal mosaicism in two patients with epidermal verrucous nevus. Demonstration of chromosomal breakpoint.* J Am Acad Dermatol, 1994. 30:622–625.

80. Mesechia, J. F., Junkins, E., and Hofman, K. J., *Familial systematized epidermal nevus syndrome.* Am J Med Genet, 1992. 44:664–667.

81. Happle, R., *How many epidermal nevus syndromes exist?* J Am Acad Dermatol, 1991. 25:550–556.

82. Tay, Y. K., Weston, W. L., Ganong, C. A., and Klingensmith, G. J., *Epidermal nevus syndrome: Association with central precocious puberty and woolly hair nevus.* J Am Acad Dermatol, 1996. 35:839–842.

83. Golitz, L. E., and Weston, W. L., *Inflammatory linear verrucous epidermal nevus. Association with epidermal nevus syndrome.* Arch Dermatol, 1979. 115:1208–1209.

84. Iglesias Zamora, M. E., and Vazquez-Doval, F. J., *Epidermal naevi associated with trichilemmal cysts and chromosomal mosaicism.* Br J Dermatol, 1997. 137:821–824.

85. Sasaki, M., Matsuda, H., Arai, Y., and Hashimoto, T.,

Startle-induced epilepsy in a patient with epidermal nevus syndrome. Pediatr Neurol, 1998. 18:346–349.

86. Gurecki, P. J., Holden, K. R., Sahn, E. E., Dyer, D. S., and Cure, J. K., *Developmental neural abnormalities and seizures in epidermal nevus syndrome.* Dev Med Child Neurol, 1996. 38:716–723.

87. Ivker, R., Resnick, S. D., and Skidmore, R. A., *Hypophosphatemic vitamin D–resistant rickets, precocious puberty, and the epidermal nevus syndrome.* Arch Dermatol, 1997. 133:1557–1561.

88. Greenberg, B. M., Pess, G. M., and May, J. W. Jr., *Macrodactyly and the epidermal nevus syndrome.* J Hand Surg (Am), 1987. 12:730–733.

89. Rosenthal, D., and Fretzin, D. F., *Epidermal nevus syndrome: Report of association with transitional cell carcinoma of the bladder.* Pediatr Dermatol, 1986. 3:455–458.

90. Camacho Martinez, F., and Moreno Gimenez, J. C., *Epidermal nevus syndrome.* Ann Dermatol Venereol, 1985. 112:143–147.

91. Pavone, L., Curatolo, P., Rizzo, P., Micali, G., Incorpora, G., Garg, B. P., Dunn, D. W., and Dobyns, W. B., *Epidermal nevus syndrome: A neurologic variant with hemimegalencephaly, gyral malformation, mental retardation, seizures, and facial hemihypertrophy.* Neurology, 1991. 41:266–271.

92. Chow, M. J., and Fretzin, D. F., *Epidermal nevus syndrome: Report of association with chondroblastoma of bone.* Pediatr Dermatol, 1989. 6:358.

93. Choi, B. H., and Kudo, M., *Abnormal neuronal migration and gliomatosis cerebri in epidermal nevus syndrome.* Acta Neuropathol (Berl), 1981. 53:319–325.

94. Dimond, R. L., and Amon, R. B., *Epidermal nevus and rhabdomyosarcoma.* Arch Dermatol, 1976. 112:1424–1426.

95. Su, W. P. D., *Histopathologic varieties of epidermal nevus. A study of 160 cases.* Am J Dermatopathol, 1982. 4:161–170.

96. Morrison, J. G., Jones, E. W., and MacDonald, D. M., *Juvenile elastoma and osteopoikilosis (the Buschke-Ollendorff syndrome).* Br J Dermatol, 1977. 97:417–422.

97. Al Attia, H. M., and Sherif, A. M., *Buschke-Ollendorff syndrome in a grande multipara: A case report and short review of the literature.* Clin Rheumatol, 1998. 17:172–175.

98. de la Salmoniere, P., Janier, M., Chemlal, K., Lazareth, I., Carlotti, A., Charasson, I., Priollet, P., and Daniel, F., *Buschke-Ollendorff syndrome.* Am Dermatol Venereol, 1994. 121:718–720.

99. Uitto, J., Santa Cruz, D. J., Starcher, B. C., Whyte, M. P., and Murphy, W. A., *Biochemical and ultrastructural demonstration of elastin accumulation in the skin lesions of the Buschke-Ollendorff syndrome.* J Invest Dermatol, 1981. 76:284–287.

100. Llado Blanch, A., Covas Planells, I., and Estrach Planella, T., *Changes in phosphorous-calcium metabolism in osteopoikilosis (Buschke-Ollendorff syndrome).* An Esp Pediatr, 1989. 31:139–141.

101. Giro, M. G., Duvic, M., Smith, L. T., Kennedy, R., Rapini, R., Arnett, F. C., and Davidson, J. M., *Buschke-Ollendorff syndrome associated with elevated elastin production by affected skin fibroblasts in culture.* J Invest Dermatol, 1992. 99:129–137.

102. Woo, T. Y., and Rasmussen, J. E., *Disorders of transepidermal elimination.* Int J Dermatol, 1985. 24:267–279.

103. Sulica, V. I., Cooper, P. H., Pope, F. M., Hambrick, G. W., Jr., Gerson, B. M., and McKusick, V. A., *Cutaneous histologic features in Ehlers-Danlos syndrome.* Arch Dermatol, 1979. 115:40–42.

104. Holbrook, K. A., and Byers, P. H., *Structural abnormalities in the dermal collagen and elastic matrix from the skin of patients with inherited connective tissue disorders.* J Invest Dermatol, 1982. 79:7s–16s.

105. Shishkina, L. V., Lazarev, V. A., Meshcheriakova, A. V., and Printseva, O. I., *Connective tissue pathology in patients with aneurysms of the cerebral arteries (Ehlers Danlos syndrome).* Ark Patol, 1993. 55:16–20.

106. Smith, L. T., Schwarze, U., Goldstein, J., and Byers, P. H., *Mutations in the COL3A1 gene result in the Ehlers-Danlos syndrome type IV and alterations in the size and distribution of the major collagen fibrils of the dermis.* J Invest Dermatol, 1997. 108:241–247.

107. Pope, F. M., *Ehlers-Danlos syndrome: Subtypes.* In *Balliere's Clinical Rheumatology.* 1991, Harcourt Brace and Co., New York, pp. 321–349.

108. De Paepe, A., Nuytinck, L., Hausser, I., Anton-Lamprecht, I., and Naeyaert, J. M., *Mutations in the COL5A1 gene are causal in the Ehlers-Danlos syndromes I and II.* Am J Hum Genet, 1997. 60:547–554.

Vascular Anomalies and Skin Diseases

Pseudoxanthoma Elasticum

Epidemiology. Pseudoxanthoma elasticum is a disease that displays multiple inheritance patterns. It is characterized by fragmentation and subsequent calcification of elastic fibers in the skin and other organs. It occurs in about 1 person per 100,000 and is twice as common in women as in men [1]. Two forms of autosomal dominant inheritance and two forms of autosomal recessive inheritance have been described [2], but 90% of affected people in the United States have an autosomal recessive form of the disease [1]. These four variants of the disease differ mainly in extent of symptoms.

Cutaneous Features. The most common cutaneous manifestations of pseudoxanthoma elasticum are multiple grouped, yellow papules and plaques on the skin overlying flexural areas [3]. The skin often takes on a "plucked chicken skin" appearance around the neck and in the axillae [4]. Redundant skin folds develop in flexural regions.

A rare, acquired form of pseudoxanthoma elasticum occurs in a periumbilical distribution in obese, middle-aged multiparous women [5]. Periumbilical, well-demarcated plaques with keratotic papules at the periphery are present. These lesions frequently perforate [5, 6].

Associated Disorders. Destruction of the elastic lamina within vessels throughout the body leads to complications for some patients with pseudoxanthoma elas-

ticum. Within the eyes, angioid streaks occur within the fundi oculi, often in young children [7]. Angioid streaks are linear cracks in Bruch's membrane that are accompanied by changes in the retinal pigment epithelium. Severe chorioretinitis is also seen in these patients [2]. Blindness is a consequence in some patients [1].

In the gastrointestinal tract, vascular disruption may cause bleeding in the stomach [8] in up to 13% of cases [9] or in the lower gastrointestinal tract. Bleeding affecting the uterus, bladder, nasal cavities, and joint spaces has also been reported [10].

Cardiovascular complications including myocardial infarction [11, 12], mitral valve prolapse [3], intimal fibroelastotic thickening, atherosclerosis [13], and restrictive cardiomyopathy [14] have been attributed to vascular damage in patients with pseudoxanthoma elasticum. Aortic insufficiency may occur in these patients [15]. Pseudoxanthoma elasticum is associated with hypertension that may be refractory to treatment and appears early in childhood [16].

Neurologic complications occur in patients with pseudoxanthoma elasticum. These include cerebrovascular insufficiency, lacunar infarcts, aneurysms, subarachnoid and intracerebral hemorrhage, decreased mentation, seizures, and possible cortical atrophy. These changes are attributed to alteration of cerebral blood vessels. [17].

Pulmonary complications are unusual in pseudoxanthoma elasticum, but calcification and loss of parenchymal elastic tissue have been described [18]. Pregnancy-related complications including increased risk of early miscarriage, increased placental calcifications, and increased risks for developing abdominal striae [19] have been reported in patients with pseudoxanthoma elasticum. These risks are small and may be overstated [20]. Pregnancy has been associated with increased severity of the disease [1].

Calcification of renal parenchyma occurs in patients with pseudoxanthoma elasticum and can result in renal disease [21]. Late-onset pseudoxanthoma elasticum has also been reported in patients with chronic renal failure undergoing hemodialysis [22].

The periumbilical form of the disease is often associated with idiopathic hypertension [5]. Other extracutaneous manifestations are unusual with this variant, but chronic renal failure and angioid streaks in the eyes have been described [5].

Pseudoxanthoma elasticum has been reported in patients taking long-term, high-dose penicillamine [4], but in these patients the elastic tissue fibers fail to calcify [1]. Similar changes have been reported in patients ingesting saltpeter [23]. Pseudoxanthoma elasticum may also be seen in association with Schnitzler's syndrome (urticaria and macroglobulinemia) [24].

Histologic Features. Histologic features of pseudoxanthoma elasticum include marked fragmentation and clumping of elastic tissue fibers within the reticular dermis (Fig. 12–1). The fibers are very basophilic and are readily apparent on routine sections (Fig. 12–2). In well-developed lesions, the elastic fiber fragments are coated with calcium phosphate, which is also easily visualized on routine sections. The epidermis is unremarkable, and elastic tissue fibers within the papillary dermis are relatively spared.

Histologic features of pseudoxanthoma elasticum may be present in clinically normal skin in patients with

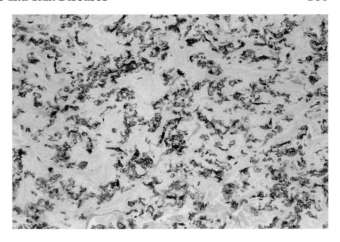

Fig. 12–2. High-power of pseudoxanthoma elasticum shows basophilia of the clumped elastic tissue fibers.

pseudoxanthoma elasticum [10]. The following entities must be considered in the differential diagnosis of pseudoxanthoma elasticum:

- Elastosis perforans serpiginosum
- Nodular elastosis
- Perforating calcific elastosis

Special Studies. A von Kossa stain is helpful in highlighting the calcium phosphate deposition on elastic tissue fibers, but is rarely necessary to establish the diagnosis. A Verhoeff-van Gieson stain demonstrates fragmentation and clumping of elastic tissue fibers (Fig. 12–3), but also is rarely necessary to make a diagnosis of pseudoxanthoma elasticum.

Scanning electron microscopic studies of the dermal elastic fibers from patients with pseudoxanthoma elasticum demonstrate characteristic changes. There is a

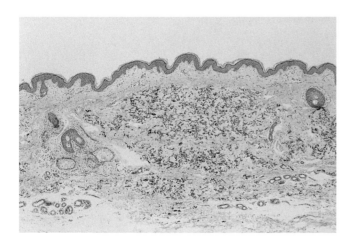

Fig. 12–1. Pseudoxanthoma elasticum demonstrates marked clumping of elastic tissue fibers in the reticular dermis.

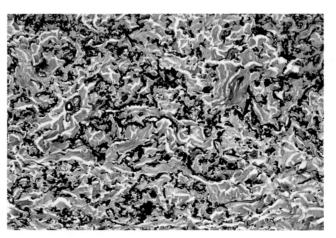

Fig. 12–3. Verhoeff-van Gieson stain demonstrates clumping and increase in elastic tissue fibers in pseudoxanthoma elasticum.

normal-appearing portion of the fiber that is composed of thin fibrils, a thickened tortuous portion covered with amorphous material, and a markedly damaged portion that is calcified [25]. It is not necessary to perform electron microscopic examination on skin biopsy specimens to make the diagnosis of pseudoxanthoma elasticum.

Pathogenesis. The primary pathologic change that underlies many of the processes in pseudoxanthoma elasticum is that of degeneration of elastic tissue fibers with subsequent calcification of the degenerated fibers. The mutated gene responsible for this process has not yet been identified [26]. It has been speculated that polyionic deposits such as glycoproteins attract calcium that leads to damage of elastin [27]. Fibroblasts from patients with pseudoxanthoma elasticum have been shown to produce stronger polyanion properties than do normal fibroblasts [28].

Fabry's Disease

Epidemiology. Fabry's disease is an X-linked recessive disorder that is seen predominantly in male patients and is thought to be a lethal mutation in girls.

Cutaneous Features. Most patients with Fabry's disease develop multiple papular, erythematous, vascular proliferations. In some patients, a hyperkeratotic collarette can be seen surrounding the vascular tumor. Rare patients may have the disease and lack the characteristic angiokeratomas [29]. Other cutaneous findings in patients with Fabry's disease include generalized anhidrosis and painful fingers, although these are uncommon findings [30].

Associated Disorders. About 50% of patients with Fabry's disease experience mild, vague gastrointestinal symptoms [31]. In some patients, decreased intestinal motility is present, perhaps related to affected autonomic innervation [32].

About half of patients with Fabry's disease also have cardiovascular involvement. Many of these patients suffer from mitral valve prolapse [33] and complete atrioventricular block [34]. Hypertrophic cardiomyopathies have been reported, as has renovascular hypertension [33]. Cerebrovascular accidents occur in as many as one-fourth of patients with Fabry's disease and may occur at a young age [35].

Autonomic nervous system function is impaired in many patients with Fabry's disease. This manifests with orthostatic hypotension, decreased sweating, impaired pupillary constriction, and reduced tear and saliva formation [32]. A child with priapism has also been described [36]. Other neural deficits including decreased

thermal sensation and cold sensitivity have been reported, even in asymptomatic carriers [37]. Vascular dementia has also been attributed to vascular involvement within the brain [38]. Eye involvement including corneal dystrophy occurs in patients with Fabry's disease [39].

Testicular and epididymal involvement has been reported in patients with Fabry's disease, but no associated infertility has been reported [40]. A possible case of primary hypothyroidism due to Fabry's disease has also been reported [41]. Rare patients demonstrate sensorineural hearing loss due to ear involvement [42]. Airway obstruction due to fixed narrowing by glycosphingolipids is a common finding in patients with Fabry's disease [43]. Uremia and renal failure is the ultimate cause of death in many patients with Fabry's disease.

Histologic Features. Histologic sections of the angiokeratomas associated with Fabry's disease are similar to sporadically occurring angiokeratomas. Dilated capillaries are present within the dermal papillae [44]. These may be widely ectatic and thrombosed. There is overlying epidermal hyperplasia, which may give rise to the deceptive appearance that the dilated vessels are actually within the epidermis (Fig. 12–4). The vascular proliferation is usually confined to the superficial vessels within the superficial vascular plexus and the papillary dermal capillaries, but involvement of vessels within the deeper reticular dermis can occur. The following entities must be considered in the differential diagnosis of angiokeratoma:

- Bacillary angiomatosis
- Capillary hemangioma
- Lymphangioma circumscriptum
- Pyogenic granuloma
- Venous lake

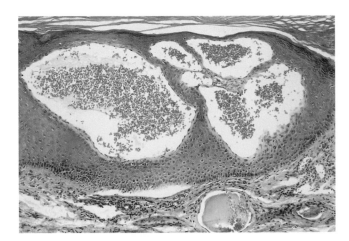

Fig. 12–4. Angiokeratoma demonstrates ectatic vessels high in dermal papillae with surrounding hyperplastic epidermis.

Special Studies. Electron microscopic examination of the skin from patients with Fabry's disease reveals electron-dense deposits within the cytoplasm of endothelial cells, pericytes, myocytes, fibroblasts, and adipocytes [45]. Secretory cells of the eccrine glands can also contain inclusions [29]. The inclusions are composed of parallel stacks of lipid-containing membranes that have been called "zebra bodies" or "myeloid bodies." Clinically unaffected skin will demonstrate similar findings. In many patients, electron microscopic examination of a skin biopsy specimen is the preferred morphologic method for establishing the diagnosis. Assays for leukocyte α-galactosidase activity are also helpful in establishing the diagnosis [46].

Pathogenesis. Lack of lysosomal α-galactosidase results in the accumulation of glycosphingolipids in endothelial, perithelial, and smooth muscle cells of blood vessels, ganglion cells within the autonomic nervous system, and renal tubules [42]. Multiple mutations in the Xq22.1 gene have been described in these patients and are responsible for the decreased enzyme activity [47].

Osler-Weber-Rendu Disease (Hereditary Hemorrhagic Telangiectasia)

Epidemiology. Osler-Weber-Rendu syndrome, also known as hereditary hemorrhagic telangiectasia syndrome (HHT), is inherited in an autosomal dominant manner. It is characterized by cutaneous, mucosal, and visceral vascular ectasias. In one large series, 62% of affected patients were symptomatic by age 16 years and all of them by age 40 years [48]. Epistaxis was the presenting sign in 90% of patients. Two forms of the disease, HHT1 and HHT2, have been described. The genetic defect in HHT1 has been localized to chromosome 9q3 [49] and the HHT2 defect to chromosome 12q13 [50]. Familial occurrence is seen in 94% of cases [51].

Cutaneous Features. Cutaneous telangiectasias are present in up to 75% of patients with HHT. These are present in up to 50% of patients before age 30 years. Telangiectasias occurred on the hands and wrists in about 40% of patients and on the face in up to one-third [51]. The individual vascular ectasias range from one to several millimeters in diameter, and most patients with HHT will have hundreds of these telangiectasias widely scattered over their entire skin surface. Epistaxis occurs in 96% of patients with HHT, starting before age 20 years in 50% of them [51].

Associated Disorders. Visceral involvement is present in up to one-fourth of patients with HHT [51]. Gastrointestinal bleeding secondary to vascular ectasias is the most common manifestation of visceral involvement in patients with HHT [52]. The vascular anomalies can occur at any location within the gastrointestinal tract, including the ampulla of Vater [53], stomach, duodenum, and jejunum [54].

Cerebrovascular malformations are present in about 20% of patients with HHT [55]. These consist of arteriovenous malformations and purely venous malformations. These anomalies are more common in younger patients with HHT [51].

Multiple coronary arteriovenous malformations leading to anginal chest pain has been described in a patient with HHT [56]. High-output congestive heart failure has also been reported in patients with HHT [57].

Pulmonary arteriovenous fistulas may be seen in patients with HHT, leading to dyspnea and hemoptysis [58]. It has been suggested that this finding is more prevalent in patients with HHT1 than in those with HHT2 [59] and appears to be a more frequent complication in younger patients with HHT [51].

Conjunctival telangiectasias may be present [60]. Hepatic vascular malformations occur in patients with HHT and when severe lead to cholestasis [61] and hepatolithiasis [62]. Urinary tract involvement has been reported but is quite exceptional [51].

Histologic Features. Histologic features of HHT demonstrate ectatic dermal postcapillary venules (Fig. 12–5). As the vascular telangiectasias progress, the postcapillary venules continue to enlarge and connect with dilated arterioles via the capillary network. Over time, the capillary network disappears, giving rise to direct arteriovenous malformations (Fig. 12–6). A slight lymphohistiocytic inflammatory infiltrate is seen surrounding the vessels of the superficial vascular plexus [63].

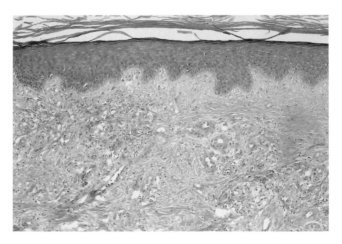

Fig. 12–5. Hereditary hemorrhagic telangiectasia with multiple ectatic venules in superficial vascular plexus. Some of the vessels have thickened walls.

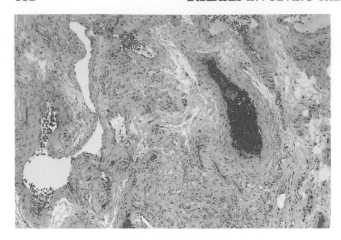

Fig. 12–6. Arteriovenous-type hemangioma demonstrates thickening of some of the vessel walls, while other vessel walls remain relatively thin.

Special Studies. Electron microscopic examination of dermal blood vessels in HHT reveals dilated vessels with thickened walls. Dehiscence of the vessel walls is seen, giving rise to the hemorrhage observed in these patients [64].

Pathogenesis. The chromosomal anomalies seen in patients with HHT1 produce insufficiency of endoglin (CD105), a tumor growth factor-β (TGF-β) binding protein [65]. It is believed that endoglin deficiency is involved in the formation of the arteriovenous malformations and telangiectasias. Patients with HHT2 have been shown to have a deficiency in activin receptor-like kinase I [50]. This gene has also been related to the TGF-β family of proteins and suggests a central role for TGF-β ligand–receptor interactions in vascular homeostasis [66].

Blue Rubber Bleb Nevus Syndrome

Epidemiology. Blue rubber bleb nevus syndrome (BRBNS) is a rare autosomal dominant disorder characterized by multiple vascular malformations of the skin and internal organ systems. Signs and symptoms appear at or soon after birth. Occasional cases have apparent sporadic occurrence [67]. Very rare cases have been reported with adult onset [68].

Cutaneous Features. Multiple red-blue tumors are present on virtually any cutaneous sites in patients with BRBNS. Oral [69] and genital [70] vascular lesions have also been reported. These tumors are exophytic and occasionally have a rubbery consistency [71]. They may thrombose, giving rise to rapidly enlarging, darker colored tumors. The tumors vary greatly in size, ranging from several millimeters to multiple centimeters in diameter.

Associated Disorders. The gastrointestinal tract is frequently involved in patients with BRBNS and may lead to occult blood loss and subsequent anemia [72]. Vascular neoplasms may be present in the esophagus, stomach, and small and large intestine [73]. Similar lesions have been reported in the liver and retroperitoneum [73]. Gastrointestinal vascular malformations rarely can occur in the absence of cutaneous lesions.

Virtually all other organ systems can develop vascular malformations in patients with BRBNS, leading to a wide range of complications. These include paraparesis [74], urinary bladder complications [75], sudden cardiac death [76], microcephaly, deficient motor coordination, decreased visual acuity [77], progressive ataxia [71], and suffocation [78]. Multiple ocular hemangiomas [79] and coagulopathies [74] have also been reported in patients with BRBNS.

Histologic Features. Histologic features of the tumors seen in BRBNS are similar to those of tumors unassociated with the syndrome. In most patients, the vascular tumors are capillary and cavernous hemangiomas

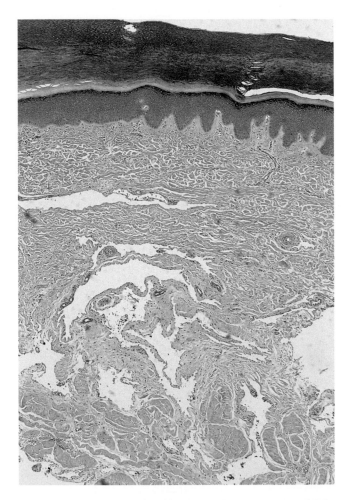

Fig. 12–7. Cavernous hemangioma demonstrates widely ectatic blood vessels throughout the dermis.

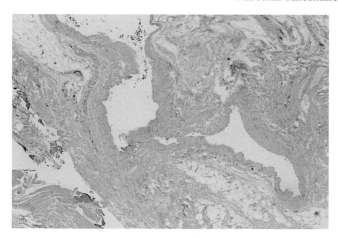

Fig. 12–8. Cavernous hemangioma demonstrates widely ectatic vessels with thin vascular walls.

[76]. In some series, cavernous hemangiomas are the most common histologic neoplasm found [68]. In some patients, the vascular neoplasms are angiokeratomas [80]. Arteriovenous malformations have also been reported [76].

Cavernous hemangiomas are characterized by the presence of widely ectatic, thin-walled vessels present throughout the dermis and frequently extending into the subcutaneous fat (Fig. 12–7). The epidermis is unremarkable. The endothelial cells are usually flattened and unremarkable (Fig. 12–8). Thrombi and foci of recanalization are common findings in these types of lesions.

Capillary hemangiomas are also characterized by the presence of ectatic vessels coursing throughout the dermis. The vessel walls are, however, usually of a smaller caliber diameter and extend less deeply into the subcutaneous fat than those seen in cavernous hemangiomas. The epidermis is usually unremarkable to slightly attenuated overlying these vascular neoplasms (Fig. 12–9).

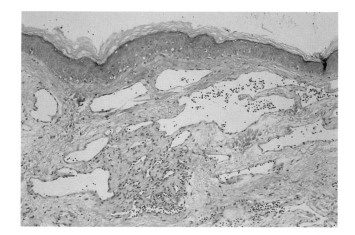

Fig. 12–9. Capillary hemangioma demonstrates a more superficial proliferation of ectatic vessels.

Angiokeratomas are characterized by the presence of widely ectatic, thin-walled vessels located very superficially within the papillary dermal tips, sometimes extending deeper into the dermis (Fig. 12–2). The overlying epidermis is acanthotic, with elongated rete ridges extending downward and surrounding the superficially located dermal vessels. This makes the vessels appear intraepidermal, which is not the case. Thrombi are frequently seen in these superficial, dilated vessels.

Special Studies. No special studies are necessary to make a diagnosis of BRBNS.

Pathogenesis. Evidence suggests that BRBNS may be linked to a defect in chromosome 9p [67, 81].

Cobb's Syndrome

Epidemiology. Cobb's syndrome is a very rare syndrome that is characterized by the presence of a nevus flammeus (port-wine stain) or angiokeratoma occurring in a dermatomal distribution associated with an underlying spinal hemangioma [82]. The syndrome is believed by some to be a mesodermal phakomatosis [83].

Cutaneous Features. Port-wine stains are the most common vascular malformation observed in patients with Cobb's syndrome. These vascular ectasias appear as erythematous macules or plaques that over time can become more verrucous. They are often distributed in a dermatomal pattern and are clinically indistinguishable from sporadically occurring port-wine stains. Rarely, lymphangioma circumscriptum may be the cutaneous vascular abnormality associated with the underlying spinal angioma [82]. Café-au-lait spots have been reported in rare patients [84].

Associated Disorders. Occasional patients with Cobb's syndrome may demonstrate ipsilateral hypertrophy of the extremities [84]. In these cases, there is some overlap with the Klippel-Trénaunay-Weber syndrome.

Histologic Features. Nevus flammeus, or port-wine stain, associated with Cobb's syndrome is histologically identical to the sporadic vascular anomaly. In early lesions, the epidermis is unremarkable, and there is a very slight increase in number of dermal blood vessels. In some cases the vessels are congested and ectatic, but in many cases they appear essentially normal (Fig. 12–10). In more developed lesions, the dermal vascularity is more prominent and the ectatic vessels are often congested. In some cases, overlying epidermal hyperplasia may develop (Fig. 12–11).

Special Studies. No special studies are necessary to make a diagnosis of port-wine stain.

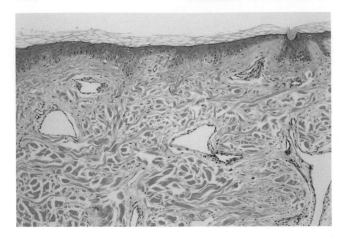

Fig. 12–10. Early port-wine stain demonstrates ectatic blood vessels in superficial vascular plexus. Many of the vessels are not congested.

Pathogenesis. The pathogenesis of Cobb's syndrome is not known. It has been postulated that port-wine stains represent progressive vascular ectasias and not true vascular proliferations. The progressive ectasia has been attributed to decreased autonomic innervation of the dermal blood vessels within a given dermatome [85]. How this observation relates to the spinal angiomas is not yet understood.

Sturge-Weber Syndrome

Epidemiology. Sturge-Weber syndrome is a rare genodermatosis characterized by a combination of facial port-wine stains and associated intracranial venous malformations. Exceptional patients with the Sturge-Weber syndrome may not have any cutaneous manifestations of their disease [86].

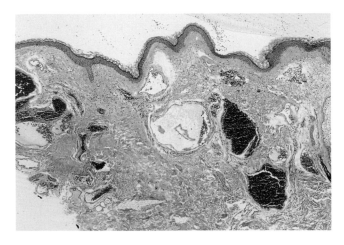

Fig. 12–11. Well-developed port-wine stain demonstrates ectatic, congested blood vessels throughout the dermis.

Cutaneous Features. Port-wine stains are present along the ophthalmic branch of the trigeminal nerve in virtually all patients with Sturge-Weber syndrome [87]. The upper eyelid and forehead are involved in all patients reported in several series [87, 88]. As many as half the patients may have additional port-wine stains on the trunk or extremities. These vascular ectasias are initially macular, but may become papular and even verrucous in older, well-developed lesions.

Associated Disorders. Approximately 80% of patients with Sturge-Weber syndrome suffer from seizures [87]. Seizures are more common in patients with bilateral port-wine stains than in those with unilateral lesions. About 75% of patients with bilateral port-wine stains will have seizures during their first year of life. The seizures are caused by intracranial and leptomeningeal vascular malformations. Intracerebral calcifications with a characteristic "railway line" appearance are seen in most afflicted patients [89]. More than half of patients with the syndrome display developmental delay. Glaucoma is present in up to half of affected patients and is found in the first year of life in most [87]. Other findings include hemiparesis and mental retardation, which may be seen to some degree in up to half of people with Sturge-Weber syndrome [90]. Choroidal hemangiomas have also been reported in patients with Sturge-Weber syndrome [91].

Patients with Sturge-Weber syndrome and concomitant nevus of Ota have been reported [92]. Rare patients with phakomatosis pigmentovascularis present with clinically overlapping symptoms of Sturge-Weber syndrome. The relationship between these entities is not fully established [93]. Some authors suggest that abnormal vessels in Sturge-Weber syndrome differ from the vessels in patients with phakomatosis pigmentovascularis and that the syndromes are clearly distinguishable [94].

Histologic Features. Port-wine stains associated with Sturge-Weber syndrome are histologically indistinguishable from similar lesions occurring sporadically or as part of the Klippel-Trenaunay-Weber syndrome as described in Chapter 11.

Special Studies. No special studies are necessary to make a diagnosis of port-wine stain associated with Sturge-Weber syndrome.

Pathogenesis. The pathogenesis of the Sturge-Weber syndrome remains unknown. Abnormal autonomic innervation of intracranial vessels has been described within the vascular lesions in some patients with Sturge-Weber syndrome [95].

von Hippel-Lindau Disease

Epidemiology. von Hippel-Lindau disease (VHL) is inherited in an autosomal dominant manner [96]. One in 36,000 people are affected, and renal neoplasms are one of the main causes of death in these patients [97].

Cutaneous Features. Vascular tumors may be present in any location on the skin, in addition to within the central nervous system and other internal organ systems. The cutaneous vascular lesions can vary widely in size and configuration and have no particular distinguishing clinical characteristics. They are similar in appearance to sporadically occurring port-wine stains and those associated with Sturge-Weber syndrome, Cobb's syndrome, and Klippel-Trénaunay Weber syndrome (see Chapter 11).

Associated Disorders. The most common extracutaneous findings in patients with VHL include hemangioblastomas of the central nervous system and retina. Retinal angiomatosis may give rise to glaucoma [98]. Other anomalies found in these patients include pheochromocytomas and renal cysts and renal cell carcinomas [96]. The presence of clear cell renal cell carcinomas, especially when they occur sporadically, in young patients, or are bilateral, is very suggestive of VHL disease [97].

von Hippel-Lindau disease involves the pancreas in 16%–29% of patients. Serous cystadenomas are the most common types of tumors, and polycystic pancreas has also been reported [96]. Islet cell tumors also occur in some patients with VHL, as do endolymphatic sac tumors [99]. Epididymal cystadenomas are also found in patients with VHL [97].

Histologic Features. The usual cutaneous findings in patients with VHL include port-wine stains (Figs. 12–10 and 12–11) and café-au-lait macules. Port-wine stains have been described fully in the discussion of Klippel-Trénaunay-Weber syndrome (Chapter 11). Café-au-lait macules are discussed in the section concerning neurofibromatosis (Chapter 9).

The histologic features of hemangioblastoma are well described in the neuropathology literature, but cutaneous counterparts have not been similarly described. Hemangioblastomas are well circumscribed but not encapsulated tumors. The neoplasms consist of large numbers of closely packed, well-formed blood vessels. The vascular walls are lined by plump endothelial cells and a separate population of large, polygonal cells with abundant foamy cytoplasm. The exact nature of these cells is not known.

Special Studies. Special studies are not required to make a diagnosis of hemangioblastoma; however, genetic testing may be helpful in arriving at a diagnosis of VHL.

Pathogenesis. The VHL gene has been located at 3p25–3p26 and is known to be a tumor suppressor gene [100]. When the gene is inactivated, the affected person is predisposed to development of neoplasms. The germ cell mutation is found in 70% of patients with VHL [97].

NOTE: Cholesterol emboli are discussed in Chapter 7.

References

1. Nelder, K. H., *Pseuduoxanthoma elasticum.* Int J Dermatol, 1988. 27:98–100.
2. Pope, F. M., *Historical evidence for the genetic heterogeneity of pseudoxanthoma elasticum.* Br J Dermatol, 1975. 92:493–509.
3. Lebwohl, M. G., Distefano, D., Prioleau, P. G., Uram, M., Yannuzzi, L. A., and Fleischmajer, R., *Pseudoxanthoma elasticum and mitral-valve prolapse.* N Engl J Med, 1982. 307:228–231.
4. Bolognia, J. L., and Braverman, I., *Pseudoxanthoma elasticum-like changes induced by penicillamine.* Dermatology, 1992. 184:12–18.
5. Sapadin, A. N., Lebwohl, M. G., Teich, S. A., Phelps, R. G., DiCostanzo, D., and Cohen, S. R., *Periumbilical pseudoxanthoma elasticum.* J Am Acad Dermatol, 1998. 39:338–344.
6. Hicks, J., Carpenter, C. L. Jr., and Reed, R. J., *Periumbilical perforating pseudoxanthoma elasticum.* Arch Dermatol, 1979. 115:300–303.
7. Gomolin, J. E., *Development of angioid streaks in association with pseudoxanthoma elasticum.* Can J Ophthalmol, 1992. 27:30–31.
8. Spinzi, G., Strocchi, E., Imperiali, G., Sangiovanni, A., Terruzzi, V., and Minoli, G., *Pseudoxanthoma elasticum: A rare cause of gastrointestinal bleeding.* Am J Gastroenterol, 1996. 91:1631–1634.
9. Bonotto, G., Tonetto, F., Baraglia, E., Battistioli, M., Fabi, F., Arrigoni, M., and Spolaore, R., *Pseudoxanthoma elasticum. A rare cause of upper digestive hemorrhage.* Minerva Chir, 1992. 47:1641–1645.
10. McKusick, V. A., *Pseudoxanthoma elasticum.* In *Heritable Disorders of Connective tissue*, P. Baghton, Ed., 1972, Mosby, St. Louis, pp. 475–520.
11. Slade, A. K., John, R. M., and Swanton, R. H., *Pseudoxanthoma elasticum presenting with myocardial infarction.* Br Heart J, 1990. 63:372–373.
12. Klingel, R., Poralla, T., Dippold, W., and Meyer zum Buschenfelde, K. H., *Pseudoxanthoma elasticum (Gronblad-Strandberg syndrome) and rheumatoid arthritis.* Deutsche Med Wochenschr, 1990. 115:1911–1916.
13. Mendelsoh, G., Bulkley, B. H., and Hutchins, G. M., *Cardiovascular manifestations of pseudoxanthoma elasticum.* Arch Pathol Lab Med, 1978. 102:298–302.

14. Navarro-Lopez, F., Llorian, A., Ferrer-Roca, O., Betriu, A., and Sanz, G., *Restrictive cardiomyopathy in pseudoxanthoma elasticum.* Chest, 1980. 78:113–115.

15. Irani, C., Dagonet, Y., Casasoprana, A., and Ribierre, M., *Pseudoxanthoma elasticum with aortic insufficiency and arterial hypertension in a 12-year-old boy.* Arch Fr Pediatr, 1984. 41:337–339.

16. Ekim, M., Turner, N., Atmaca, L., Anadolu, R., Salih, M., Donmez, O., and Ozkaya, N., *Pseudoxanthoma elasticum: A rare cause of hypertension in children.* Pediatr Nephrol, 1998. 12:183–185.

17. Iqbal, A., Alter, M., and Lee, S. H., *Pseudoxanthoma elasticum: A review of neurological complications.* Ann Neurol, 1978. 4:18–20.

18. Jackson, A., and Loh, C. L., *Pulmonary calcification and elastic tissue damage in pseudoxanthoma elasticum.* Histopathology, 1980. 4:607–611.

19. Viljoen, D. L., Beatty, S., and Beighton, P., *The obstetric and gynaecological implications of pseudoxanthoma elasticum.* Br J Obstet Gynaecol, 1987. 94:884–888.

20. Yoles, A., Phelps, R., and Lebwohl, M., *Pseudoxanthoma elasticum and pregnancy.* Cutis, 1996. 58:161–164.

21. Gresser, U., Stautner-Bruckman, C., and Zoller, W. G., *Kidney involvement in pseudoxanthoma elasticum—sonography shows early calcinosis of the kidney parenchyma.* Bildgebung, 1987–89. 56:179–180.

22. Nickoloff, B. J., Noodleman, F. R., and Abel, E. A., *Perforating pseudoxanthoma elasticum associated with chronic renal failure and hemodialysis.* Arch Dermatol, 1985. 121:1321–1322.

23. Nielsen, A. O., Christensen, O. B., Hentzer, B., Johnson, E., and Kobayasi, T., *Saltpeter-induced dermal changes electron-microscopically indistinguishable from pseudoxanthoma elasticum.* Acta Derm Venereol, 1978. 58:323–327.

24. Machet, L., Vaillant, L., Machet, M. C., Esteve, E., De Muret, A., Khallour, R., Arbeille, B., Muller, C., et al., *Schnitzler's syndrome (urticaria and macroglobulinemia) associated with pseudoxanthoma elasticum.* Acta Derm Venereol, 1992. 72:22–24.

25. Tsuji, T., *Three-dimensional architecture of altered dermal elastic fibers in pseduoxanthoma elasticum: Scanning electron microscopic studies.* J Invest Dermatol, 1984. 82:518–521.

26. Christiano, A. M., Lebwohl, M. G., Boyd, C. D., and Uitoo, J., *Workshop on pseudoxanthoma elasticum: Molecular biology and pathology of the elastic fibers. Jefferson Medical Collete, Philadelphia, Pennsylvania, June 10, 1992.* J Invest Dermatol, 1992. 99:660–663.

27. Martinez-Hernandez, A., and Huffer, W. E., *Pseudoxanthoma elasticum: Dermal polyanions and the mineralization of elastic fibers.* Lab Invest, 1974. 31:181–186.

28. Passi, A., Albertini, R., Baccarani Contri, M., de Luca, G., de Paepe, A., Pallavicini, G., Pasquali Ronchetti, I., and Tiozzo, R., *Proteoglycan alterations in skin fibroblast cultures from patients affected with pseudoxanthoma elasticum.* Cell Biol Funct, 1996. 14:111–120.

29. Kang, W. H., Chun, S. I., and Lee, S., *Generalized anhidrosis associated with Fabry's disease.* J Am Acad Dermatol, 1987. 17:883–887.

30. Shelley, E. D., Shelley, W. B., and Kurczynski, T. W., *Painful fingers, heat intolerance, and telangiectasias of the ear: Easily ignored childhood signs of Fabry's disease.* Pediatr Dermatol, 1995. 12:215–219.

31. Sheth, K. J., Werlin, S. L., Freeman, M. E., and Hodach, A. E., *Gastrointestinal structure and function in Fabry's disease.* Am J Gastroenterol, 1981. 76:246–251.

32. Cable, W. J., Kolodny, E. H., and Adams, R. D., *Fabry's disease: Impaired autonomic function.* Neurology, 1982. 32:498–502.

33. Sakuraba, H., Yanagawa, Y., Igarashi, T., Suzuki, Y., Suzuki, T., Watanabe, K., Ieki, K., Shimoda, K., et al., *Cardiovascular manifestations in Fabry's disease. A high incidence of mitral valve prolapse in hemizygotes and heterozygotes.* Clin Genet, 1986. 29:276–283.

34. Ikari, Y., Kuwako, K., and Yamaguchi, T., *Fabry's disease with complete atrioventricular block: Histological evidence of involvement of the conduction system.* Br Heart J, 1992. 68:323–325.

35. Grewal, R. P., *Stroke in Fabry's disease.* J Neurol, 1994. 241:153–156.

36. Jaureguizar Monreo, E., Lopez Pereira, P., Cabo, J., Gutierrez, J. M., Garcia-Consuegra, J., Martinez Olivas, J., and Lopez Santamaria, M., *Priapism associated with Fabry's disease.* Cir Pediatr, 1990. 3:138–140.

37. Morgan, S. H., Rudge, P., Smith, S. J., Bronstein, A. M., Kendall, B. E., Holly, E., Young, E. P., Crawford, M. D., et al., *The neurological complications of Anderson-Fabry's disease (alpha-galactosidase A deficiency)—investigation of symptomatic and presymptomatic patients.* Q J Med, 1990. 75:491–507.

38. Mendez, M. F., Stanley, T. M., Medel, N. M., Li, Z., and Tedesco, D. T., *The vascular dementia of Fabry's disease.* Dementia Geriatr Cogn Disord, 1997. 8:252–257.

39. Klein, P., *Ocular manifestations of Fabry's disease.* J Am Optom Assoc, 1986. 57:672–674.

40. Nistal, M., Paniagua, R., and Picazo, M. L., *Testicular and epididymal involvement in Fabry's disease.* J Pathol, 1983. 1983:113–124.

41. Tojo, K., Oota, M., Honda, H., Shibasaki, T., and Sakai, O., *Possible thyroidal involvement in a case of Fabry's disease.* Intern Med, 1994. 33:172–176.

42. Schachern, P. A., Shea, D. A., Paparella, M. M., and Yoon, T. H., *Otologic histopathology of Fabry's disease.* Ann Otol Rhinol Laryngol, 1989. 98:359–363.

43. Brown, L. K., Miller, A., Bhuptani, A., Sloane, M. F., Zimmerman, M. I., Schilero, G., Eng, C. M., and Desnick, R. J., *Pulmonary involvement in Fabry's disease.* Am J Respir Crit Care Med, 1997. 155:1004–1010.

44. Braverman, I. M., and Ken-Yen, A., *Ultrastructural and three-dimensional reconstruction of several macular and papular telangiectasias.* J Invest Dermatol, 1983. 81:489–497.

45. Le Charpentier, Y., Crouzet, J., Le Charpentier, M., Lessana-Leibowitch, M., Di Crescenzo, M. C., Bennet, B., and Abelanet, R., *Fabry's disease without cutaneous angiokeratoma: Diagnosis by electron microscope study of skin biopsy.* Sem Hop, 1981. 57:78–82.

46. Peters, F. P., Sommer, A., Vermeulen, A., Cheriex, E. C., and Kho, T. L., *Fabry's disease: A multidisciplinary disorder.* Postgrad Med J, 1997. 73:710–712.

47. Eng, C. M., and Desnick, R. J., *Molecular basis of Fabry disease: Mutations and polymorphisms in the human alpha-galactosidase A gene.* Hum Mutat, 1994. 3:103–111.

48. Porteous, M. E., Burn, J., and Proctor, S. J., *Hereditary haemorrhagic telangiectasia: A clinical analysis.* J Med Genet, 1992. 29:527–530.

49. Gallione, C. J., Klaus, D. J., Yeh, E. Y., Stenzel, T. T., Xue, Y., Anthony, K. B., McAllister, K. A., Baldwin, M. A., et al., *Mutation and expression analysis of the endoglin gene in hereditatry hemorrhagic telangiectasia reveals null alleles.* Hum Mutat, 1998. 11:286–294.

50. Berg, J. N., Gallione, C. J., Stenzel, T. T., Johnson, D. W., Allen, W. P., Schwartz, C. E., Jackson, C. E., Porteus, M. E., et al., *The activin receptor-like kinase i gene: Genomic structure and mutations in herediatry hemorrhagic telangiectasia type 2.* Am J Hum Genet, 1997. 61:60–67.

51. Plauchu, H., de Chadarevian, J. P., Bideau, A., and Robert, J. M., *Age-related clinical profile of hereditary hemorrhagic telangiectasia in an epidemiologically recruited population.* Am J Med Genet, 1989. 32:291–297.

52. Vase, P., and Grove, O., *Gastrointestinal lesions in hereditary hemorrhagic telangiectasia.* Gastroenterology, 1986. 91:1079–1083.

53. Chu, K. M., Lai, E. C., and Ng, I. O., *Hereditary hemorrhagic telangiectasias involving the ampulla of Vater presented wtih recurrent gastrointestinal bleeding.* Am J Gastroenterol, 1993. 88:1116–1119.

54. Zolotarevskii, V. B., and Nekrasova, T. P., *A case of hereditary hemorrhagic telangiectasia with predominant involvement of the small intestine.* Ark Patol, 1998. 60:56–58.

55. Fullbright, R. K., Chaloupka, J. C., Putnam, C. M., Sze, G. K., Merriam, M. M., Lee, G. K., Fayad, P. B., Awad, I. A., et al., *MR of hereditary hemorrhagic telangiectasia: Prevalence and spectrum of cerebrovascular malformations.* Am J Neuroradiol, 1998. 19:477–484.

56. Gurevitch, Y., Hasin, Y., Gotsman, M. S., and Rozenman, Y., *Coronary arteriovenous malformations in a patient with hereditary hemorrhagic telangiectasia—a case report.* Angiology, 1998. 49:577–580.

57. Peery, W. H., *Clinical spectrum of hereditary hemorrhagic telangiectasia (Osler-Weber-Rendu disease).* Am J Med, 1987. 82:989–997.

58. Marchesani, F., Cecarini, L., Pela, R., Catalini, G., Sabbatini, A., Fianchini, A., and Sanguinetti, C. M., *Pulmonary arteriovenous fistula in a patient with Renda-Osler-Weber syndrome.* Respiration, 1997. 64:367–370.

59. Porteous, M. E., Curtis, A., Williams, O., Marchuk, D., Bhattacharya, S. S., and Burn, J., *Genetic heterogeneity in hereditary haemorrhagic telangiectasia.* J Med Genet, 1994. 31:925–926.

60. Swensson, B., Swensson, O., and Haring, G., *Progressive disseminated essential telangiectasia with conjunctival involvement.* Klin Monatsblat Augenheilkd, 1998. 212:116–119.

61. Buscarini, E., Buscarini, L., Danesino, C., Piantanida, M., Civardi, G., Quaretti, P., Rossi, S., Di Stasi, M., et al., *Hepatic vascular malformations in hereditary hemorrhagic telangiectasia: Doppler sonographic screening in a large family.* J Hepatol, 1997. 26:111–118.

62. Ball, N. J., and Duggan, M. A., *Hepatolithiasis in hereditary hemorrhagic telangiectasia.* Arch Pathol Lab Med, 1990. 114:423–425.

63. Braverman, I. M., Keh, A., and Jacobson, B. S., *Ultrastructural and three-dimensional organization of the telangiectasias of hereditary hemorrhagic telangiectasia.* J Invest Dermatol, 1990. 95:422–427.

64. Tsianakas, P., Teillac-Hamel, D., Fraitag, S., De Prost, Y., and Prost, C., *Ultrastructural study of hereditary benign telangiectasia. Differential diagnosis from Osler-Rendu disease.* Ann Dermatol Venereol, 1995. 122:517–520.

65. Shovlin, C. L., *Glaxo/MRS Young Investigator Medal. Molecular studies on adenosine deaminase deficiency and hereditary haemorrhagic telangiectasia.* Clin Sci, 1998. 94:207–218.

66. Shovlin, C. L., *Molecular defects in rare bleeding disorders: Hereditary haemorrhagic telangiectasia.* Thomb Haemost, 1997. 78:145–150.

67. Gallione, C. J., Pasyk, K. A., Boon, L. M., Lennon, F., Johnson, D. W., Helmbold, E. A., Markel, D. S., Vikkula, M., et al., *A gene for familial venous malformations maps to chromosome 9p in a second large kindred.* J Med Genet, 1995. 32:197–199.

68. Oranje, A. P., *Blue rubber bleb nevus syndrome.* Pediatr Dermatol, 1986. 3:304–310.

69. Sumi, Y., Taguchi, N., and Kaneda, T., *Blue rubber bleb nevus syndrome with oral hemangiomas.* Oral Surg Oral Med Oral Pathol, 1991. 71:84–86.

70. Busund, B., Stray-Pedersen, S., Iversen, O. H., and Austad, J., *Blue rubber bleb nevus syndrome with manifestations in the vulva.* Acta Obstet Gynecol Scand, 1993. 72:310–313.

71. Satya-Murti, S., Navada, S., and Eames, F., *Central nervous system involvement in blue-rubber-bleb-nevus syndrome.* Arch Neurol, 1986. 43:1184–1186.

72. MacKinlay, J. R., Kaiser, J., Barrett, T. L., and Graham, B., *Blue rubber bleb nevus syndrome.* Cutis, 1998. 62:97–98.

73. Kisu, T., Yamaoka, K., Uchida, Y., Mori, H., Nakama, T., Hisatsugu, T., Miyaji, H., and Motooka, M., *A case of blue rubber bleb nevus syndrome with familial onset.* Gastroenterol Jpn, 1986. 21:262–266.

74. Wong, Y. C., Li, Y. W., and Chang, M. H., *Gastrointestinal bleeding and paraparesis in blue rubber bleb nevus syndrome.* Pediatr Radiol, 1994. 24:600–601.

75. Radke, M., Waldschmidt, J., Stolpe, H. J., Mix, M., and Richter, I., *Blue rubber-bleb-nevus syndrome with predominant urinary bladder hemangiomatosis.* Eur J Pediatr Surg, 1993. 3:313–316.

76. Ishii, T., Asuwa, N., Suzuki, S., Suwa, H., and Shimada, K., *Blue rubber bleb naevus syndrome.* Virchows Arch A Pathol Anat Histopathol, 1988. 413:485–490.

77. Gallman, T., and Boltshauser, E., *Blue rubber bleb nevus syndrome with CNS involvement.* Klin Padiatr, 1987. 199:382–384.

78. Crepeau, J., and Poliquin, J., *The blue rubber bleb nevus syndrome.* J Otolaryngol, 1981. 10:387–390.

79. Crompton, J. L., and Taylor, D., *Ocular lesions in the blue rubber bleb naevus syndrome.* Br J Ophthalmol, 1981. 65:133–137.

80. Trattner, A., Krichely, D., and David, M., *Blue rubber bleb nevus syndrome associated with diffuse angiokeratoma.* Cutis, 1997. 59:264–266.

81. Bonde, C. T., Jacobsen, E., and Hasselcalch, H. C., *"Blue rubber bleb nevus syndrome"—or Bean's syndrome.* Ugeskr Laeger, 1997. 159:4274–4275.

82. Shim, J. H., Lee, D. W., and Cho, B. K., *A case of Cobb syndrome associated with lymphangioma circumscriptum.* Dermatology, 1996. 193:45–47.

83. Gordon-Firing, S., Purriel, J. A., Pereyra, D., and Brodbek, I., *Report of a new case of Cobb syndrome. Meningo-spinal cutaneous angiomatosis.* Acta Neurol Latinoam, 1981. 27:99–111.

84. Zala, L., and Mumenthaler, M., *Cobb syndrome: Association with verrucous angioma, ipsilateral hypertrophy of the extremities and café-au-lait spots.* Dermatologica, 1981. 163:417–425.

85. Smoller, B. R., and Rosen, S., *Port wine stains: An alteration of neural modulation of blood vessels.* Arch Dermatol, 1986. 122:177–179.

86. Pascual-Castroviejo, I., Pascual-Pascual, S. I., Viano, J., Martinez, V., and Coya, J., *Sturge-Weber syndrome without facial nevus.* Neuropediatrics, 1995. 26:220–222.

87. Sujansky, E., and Conradi, S., *Sturge-Weber syndrome: Age of onset of seizures and glaucoma and the prognosis for affected children.* J Child Neurol, 1995. 10:49–58.

88. Uram, M., and Zubillaga, C., *The cutaneous manifestations of Sturge-Weber syndrome.* J Clin Neuroophthalmol, 1982. 2:245–248.

89. Prieto, M. L., de Juan, J., Anton, M., Roiz, C., and Crespo, M., *Sturge-Weber syndrome with atypical calcifications.* Rev Neurol, 1997. 25:1411–1413.

90. Pascual-Castroviejo, I., Diaz-Gonzalez, C., Garcia-Melian, R. M., Gonzalez-Casado, I., and Munoz-Hiraldo, E., *Sturge-Weber syndrome: Study of 40 patients.* Pediatr Neurol, 1993. 9:283–288.

91. Enjolras, O., Riche, M. C., and Merland, J. J., *Facial port-wine stains and Sturge-Weber syndrome.* Pediatrics, 1985. 76:48–51.

92. Recupero, S. M., Abdolrahimzadeh, S., De Dominicis, M., and Mollo, R., *Sturge-Weber syndrome associated with naevus of Ota.* Eye, 1998. 12:212–213.

93. Gilliam, A. C., Ragge, N. K., Perez, M. I., and Bolognia, J. L., *Phakomatosis pigmentovascularis type IIb with iris mammillations.* Arch Dermatol, 1993. 129:340–342.

94. Ruiz-Maldonado, R., Tamayo, L., Laterza, A. M., Brawn, G., and Lopez, A., *Phacomatosis pigmentovascularis: A new syndrome? Report of four cases.* Pediatr Dermatol, 1987. 4:189–196.

95. Cunha e Sa, M., Barroso, C. P., Caldaas, M. C., Edvinsson, L., and Gulbenkian, S., *Innervation pattern of malformative cortical vessels in Sturge-Weber disease: An histochemical, immunohistochemical, and ultrastructural study.* Neurosurg, 1997. 41:872–876.

96. Girelli, R., Bassi, C., Falconi, M., De Santis, L., Bonora, A., Caldiron, E., Sartori, N., Salvia, R., et al., *Pancreatic cystic manifestations in von Hippel-Lindau disease.* Int J Pancreatol, 1997. 22:101–109.

97. Richard, S., Beroud, C., Joly, D., Chretien, Y., and Benoit, G., *Von Hippel-Lindau disease and renal cancer: 10 years of genetic progress. GEFVHL (French-Speaking Study Group on von Hippel-Lindau disease).* Prog Urol, 1998. 8:330–339.

98. Janotka, H., and Laskowski, A., *Secondary glaucoma in retinal angiomatosis (Hippel-Lindau disease).* Klin Oczna, 1980. 82:165–166.

99. Richards, F. M., Webster, A. R., McMahon, R., Woodward, E. R., Rose, S., and Maher, E. R., *Molecular genetic analysis of von Hippel-Lindau disease.* J Intern Med, 1998. 243:527–533.

100. Sobottka, S. B., Frank, S., Hampl, M., Schackert, H. K., and Schackert, G., *Multiple intracerebral hemangioblastomas in identical twins with von Hippel-Lindau disease—a clinical and molecular study.* Acta Neurochir, 1998. 140:281–285.

CHAPTER 13

Endocrine Abnormalities and Skin Diseases

Pretibial Myxedema

Epidemiology. Pretibial myxedema is an uncommon manifestation of hyperthyroidism. It usually is seen in patients after treatment for Graves' disease. Less commonly it is associated with Hashimoto's thyroiditis and can occur in the absence of known thyroid disease. It tends to occur late in the course of the disease, but has been reported as a presenting sign [1]. It has also been reported in patients who were euthyroid or even hypothyroid [1–3]. Spontaneous regression occurs in some but not all cases [4].

Cutaneous Features. Pretibial myxedema almost invariably affects the anterior aspect of the shins, presenting as nonpitting edema. Other locations such as the upper extremities and thighs may rarely be involved [5]. Nodules and waxy, indurated plaques with a peau d'orange appearance develop in more florid cases [1]. The follicular ostia become prominent. Localized hyperhidrosis is reported in rare cases [6, 7].

Hyperthyroid-associated acropachy with hypertrophic osteoarthropathy is associated with pretibial myxedema in about 7% of cases [1, 6]. Hyperpigmentation of the lower extremities may also be encountered rarely in patients with hyperthyroidism [8].

Associated Disorders. In one series, 88% of patients with pretibial myxedema also demonstrated significant proptosis, and only one patient failed to have an opthalmopathy [1]. The triad of bilateral exophthalmus, pretibial myxedema, and acropachyderma of the fingers and toes is known as Diamond's syndrome.

Most patients with pretibial myxedema have elevated levels of long-acting thyroid stimulator in their sera, but this protein does not appear to be pathogenetic in the development of the cutaneous changes [9].

Histologic Features. Pretibial myxedema is characterized by deposits of mucin in the superficial portion of the reticular dermis, leading to thickening of the dermis. Fibroblasts are normal in number to slightly increased and have a stellate appearance (Fig. 13–1). In most cases, a zone of sparing is present within the papillary dermis [10]. Splitting of collagen and elastic tissue fibers may be appreciated on routine histologic sections or with the aid of special stains. The following entities must be considered in the histologic differential diagnosis of pretibial myxedema:

- Dermatomyositis
- Generalized myxedema
- Papular mucinosis
- Reticular erythematous mucinosis
- Scleromyxedema/lichen myxedematosus

Special Studies. Colloidal iron or Alcian blue stains performed at pH 4.5 demonstrate a marked increase in nonsulfated acid mucopolysaccharides within the superficial reticular dermis (Fig. 13–2). Predigestion with hyaluronidase eliminates the material. Elastic tissue

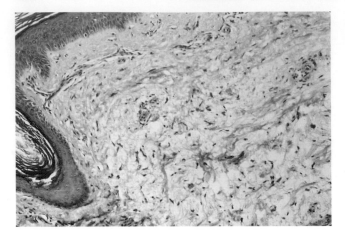

Fig. 13–1. Pretibial myxedema has increased mucin in the superficial reticular dermis, and scattered stellate fibroblasts are also present.

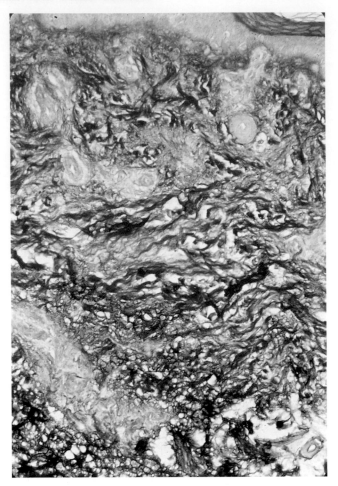

Fig. 13–2. Colloidal iron stains performed at pH 4.5 demonstrate markedly increased amounts of acid mucopolysaccharides.

stains demonstrate splitting and decreased numbers of elastic tissue fibers within the reticular dermis [11].

Pathogenesis. It has been suggested that cutaneous fibroblasts are stimulated to produce increased amounts of hyaluronic acid by cross-reactivity with antibodies directed against thyroid antigens [4]. Fibroblasts in unaffected regions of the skin do not appear to be similarly affected [12]. Patients with pretibial myxedema have also been shown to have increased levels of thyroid-stimulating hormone receptor antibodies in their sera, as well as on the plasma membranes of fibroblasts from lesional skin [13].

Generalized Myxedema

Epidemiology. Generalized myxedema is a condition that is associated with hypothyroidism.

Cutaneous Features. Hypothyroidism is only occasionally associated with cutaneous changes. In these patients, a generalized myxedema is seen. They typically also have dry skin. Localized myxedematous areas have been described in rare patients [14]. Trichorrhexis nodosa is another change associated with hypothyroidism and thus may be seen in patients with generalized myxedema [15].

Associated Disorders. Myxedematous skin is also associated with weakness, cold intolerance, mental and physical slowness, and a hoarse voice. Affected patients may demonstrate a characteristic facies [16]. Constipation, sustained reflexes, and alopecia are also present in some patients.

A case of myxedema related to hypothyroidism has been associated with cutis verticis gyrata [17]. Palmo-

plantar keratoderma has also been reported in this setting [18]. Vitiligo is associated with autoimmune thyroid disease (hyperthyroidism and hypothyroidism) and thus may be seen in patients who also have myxedema [19].

Histologic Features. Accumulation of acid mucopolysaccharides within the dermis account for the histologic appearance of generalized myxedema. The amount of dermal mucin is much less than that seen in pretibial myxedema, often making it difficult to detect on routine sections and even with special stains. There is no increase in numbers of dermal fibroblasts in this entity.

Special Studies. In some cases, colloidal iron or Alcian blue stains performed at pH 4.5 or 2.5 may be helpful in detecting increased levels of acid mucopolysaccharides within the dermis. The degree of mucin is hard to detect over baseline levels, however, often precluding a definitive histologic diagnosis. Decreased numbers of elastic tissue fibers, with increased splitting of these fibers, has been demonstrated in patients with generalized myxedema [11].

Pathogenesis. Increased amounts of hyaluronic acid accumulate in the skin of patients with myxedema. Hyaluronic acid has a strong water-binding capacity, which may contribute to the nonpitting edema observed in these patients [20]. Inadequate lymphatic draining may also play a role in the accumulation of dermal fluids [21].

Vitiligo

Epidemiology. Vitiligo may occur as part of one of several syndromes (see Chapter 9) or as an isolated cutaneous process. It affects from 1% to 3% of the world's population [22, 23] and appears to be slightly more common in women [24]. About half of those affected acquire the disease before age 20 years, and new onset is uncommon in the elderly [25]. Large epidemiologic studies have failed to confirm an association between vitiligo and any major histocompatibility antigen [26].

Cutaneous Features. Vitiligo has several different clinical presentations. It may appear as depigmented patches confined to a single dermatome or may be disseminated. Disseminated disease is the most common presentation. In these patients, the depigmentation is symmetric and bilateral and is most pronounced in a periorificial distribution. Unilateral disease is also encountered and tends to occur in a younger age group than in those with disseminated disease [27]. Universal vitiligo is uncommon and refers to loss of pigment throughout the entire body surface. Koebnerization occurs in some patients with vitiliginous areas [28]. Disease progression occurs in up to 89% of patients and is more frequent in patients with nonsegmental disease, Koebner's phenomenon, and mucosal involvement [29]. Vitiligo may occur concurrently with other cutaneous eruptions, including psoriasis [30] and lichen planus [31].

Associated Disorders. Vitiligo has been associated with multiple autoimmune disorders, including thyroid disease, diabetes, pernicious anemia, rheumatoid arthritis, and alopecia areata [23, 32–34]. Up to 25% of patients with vitiligo have some evidence of thyroid disease [35]. Less commonly, vitiligo has been associated with autoimmune chronic active hepatitis [36, 37] and primary biliary cirrhosis [38]. An uncommon association is with dermatitis herpetiformis [39]. A case of inherited acanthosis nigricans coexisting with vitiligo has been reported [40]. A statistical association has been established for vitiligo and the presence of thyroid disease, while the other associations have not been as firmly demonstrated [24]. The association between vitiligo and autoimmune disease is strongest for patients with disseminated, bilateral vitiligo [27] and is very weak for those with segmental disease [41].

Vitiligo has been reported in patients with halo nevi [28]. Congenital nevi are also three times as prevalent in patients with vitiligo as in normal population controls [24]. Nevus depigmentosus has been reported to coexist in a patient with vitiligo [42].

Vitiligo may be present in patients with metastatic melanoma. It has been suggested that it may serve as a marker for a relatively good prognosis in this group of patients [43, 44].

Multiple cutaneous neoplasms including actinic keratoses and squamous cell carcinomas have been reported in patients with vitiligo, usually after prolonged treatment with psoralen ultraviolet actinotherapy [45, 46]. The cutaneous neoplasms are more likely related to treatment than to the vitiligo, although the loss of protection from ultraviolet light certainly plays a role in this process. Vitiligo has been associated with oral medications including chloroquine and clofazamine [47, 48] (see also Vogt- Koyanagi-Harada Syndrome in Chapter 9).

Histologic Features. The histologic changes of vitiligo are described in detail in Chapter 9. In brief, well-developed lesions are devoid of melanocytes and intraepidermal melanin pigment. Minimal inflammation is present (Fig. 13–3). In earlier, actively inflamed vitiliginous patches, a mild lymphohistiocytic infiltrate is present around vessels of the superficial vascular plexus, with scattered exocytosis [49]. Melanocytes with degenerative changes may be observed. Pigment incontinence is minimal.

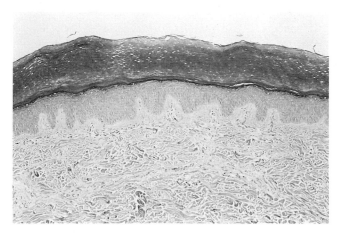

Fig. 13–3. Vitiligo is characterized by loss of melanocytes with only minimal dermal inflammation.

It is difficult to make a histologic diagnosis of vitiligo. In some cases, comparison of affected and unaffected adjacent skin is very helpful. The following entities must be considered in the histologic differential diagnosis of vitiligo:

- Nevus depigmentosus
- Normal skin
- Postinflammatory pigmentary alteration

Special Studies. Immunostaining with antibodies directed against S100 protein demonstrates a complete loss of melanocytes in well-developed lesions. Care should be taken with the interpretation of an S100 stain, as Langerhans' cell hyperplasia has been reported in patients with vitiligo. A CD1a stain may be helpful in determining if the S100-positive cells are Langerhans' cell or melanocytes. A MART-1 stain may also be helpful, as it will stain melanocytes but not Langerhans' cells. A Fontana stain for melanin will accentuate the loss of epidermal pigment (Fig. 13–4). Dopa stains performed on fresh tissue will also demonstrate the loss of melanocytes.

Ultrastructural studies reveal a complete loss of melanocytes within vitiliginous skin in long-standing lesions. Biopsies from earlier affected skin demonstrate melanocytes with various cellular abnormalities [50].

Absence of Merkel cells has also been reported in lesional skin [51]. The significance of this finding remains unknown.

Pathogenesis. The pathogenesis of vitiligo remains unknown. Some investigators believe that lesional T cells rather than circulating antimelanocyte antibodies are responsible for the patchy destruction of melanocytes [52–54]. Serum interleukin-2 receptors are elevated in patients with vitiligo [55]. Others argue that both cellular and humoral immunities play a role in the pathogenesis of this disease [56]. Still others argue for a defect in humoral immunity as the primary cause of vitiligo [57]. Inherent melanocyte defects, such as defective c-kit receptors, have also been reported in lesional melanocytes [58]. Free radical–mediated melanocyte damage has been suggested as the primary process in the observed melanocyte degeneration seen in vitiligo [59]. Primary neural defects have been implicated in the pathogenesis by some authors [25].

Mucosal Neuroma Syndrome

Epidemiology. Mucosal neuroma syndrome (MEN) is a rare, autosomal dominant syndrome that is characterized by multiple mucosal neuromas, a marfanoid habitus, medullary thryoid carcinoma, and pheochromocytomas [60]. It has also been referred to as MEN type III [60]. Nonfamilial, sporadic cases have also been described.

Cutaneous Features. Patients with MEN type IIB have characteristic unusual facial manifestations including multiple pedunculated nodules on the lips, cheeks, buccal mucosa, and tongue [61]. The lips and upper eyelids are characteristically thickened [62]. The nasal bridge may be broadened and the corneal nerves thickened. Increased cutaneous pigmentation has been reported but is not a common feature of the syndrome [63].

Associated Disorders. Medullary carcinoma of the thyroid develops in virtually all affected patients. More than half of patients develop pheochromocytomas [60]. The majority of neoplasms arise about the time of the onset of puberty. Medullary carcinoma has a high likelihood of metastasizing early when it develops in patients with MEN type IIb [64].

Neurogangliomas are present within the gastrointestinal tract [65] and may give rise to megacolon and almost continuous diarrhea and/or constipation. Dysphagia due to eosphageal ganglioneuromatosis has also been reported [66]. Hypertension is also found in many affected patients [62].

Anomalies of dentition, including premature eruption of permanent teeth, malocclusion, and facial asymmetry have been described [61]. The lower incisor teeth have shortened roots [62]. Hypotonia and developmental delay may be present when presentation occurs during the neonatal period [67].

Histologic Features. Independent of location, the mucosal nodules have a similar histologic appearance. Numerous hypertrophic, enlarged axons are admixed with Schwann cells and new collagen fibers. The histologic

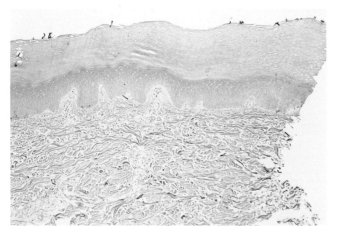

Fig. 13–4. A Fontana stain demonstrates only minimal melanin pigment within the basal layer of the epidermis.

changes are similar to those in traumatic neuromas and have no distinguishing features [68].

Special Studies. Serum calcitonin levels are important in screening for the development of medullary carcinoma of the thyroid in these patients [60].

Pathogenesis. Germline mutations in the RET proto-oncogene are responsible for the MEN IIB syndrome [69].

Necrolytic Migratory Erythema

Epidemiology. Necrolytic migratory erythema is an uncommon eruption that occurs most frequently in patients with α-cell, glucagon-secreting pancreatic neoplasms. Cutaneous lesions are often the presenting symptoms in these patients and may antedate the recognition of a neoplasm by years.

Cutaneous Findings. Lesions appear as annular, erythematous, scaling patches. Flaccid, superficial blisters may be present, especially after mild trauma. The lesions tend to be periorificial, but have been observed in all cutaneous locations. The inguinal region is also a commonly affected site. Cutaneous lesions may be associated with glossitis, angular stomatitis, and mucositis in some cases.

Associated Disorders. In the vast majority of cases, necrolytic migratory erythema is associated with glucagon-secreting pancreatic neoplasms. The cutaneous eruption most commonly precedes discovery of the tumor, and removal of the tumor often results in complete, rapid resolution of the cutaneous manifestations. Similar eruptions have been described in patients with zinc deficiency and amino acid deficiencies. Rare cases have been reported in patients with cirrhosis [70]. Clinical and histologic similarities with acrodermatitis enteropathica may lead to some confusion in diagnostic classification. A similar entity called *necrolytic acral erythema* has recently been described in patients with viral hepatitis C [71]. This entity differs only in sites affected.

Histologic Features. The histologic features of necrolytic migratory erythema depend in part on the type of lesion biopsied. The characteristic changes are those of pallor and necrosis of the upper portion of the epidermis (Fig. 13–5). The necrosis may result in superficial blister formation. Pyknotic nuclei are present. Diffuse parakeratosis is present overlying the affected epidermis. Acanthosis may be present. Vacuolar degeneration of basal keratinocytes may be seen. A modest perivascular lymphocytic infiltrate may be seen in

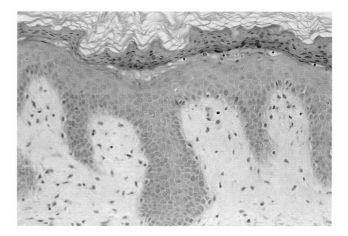

Fig. 13–5. Necrolytic migratory erythema, with abrupt pallor and necrosis of the epidermis, psoriasiform epidermal hyperplasia, and scant lymphohistiocytic inflammatory infiltrate.

the superficial dermis. Neutrophilic abscesses are occasionally present within the necrotic epidermis. The following entities must be considered in the histologic differential diagnosis:

- Acrodermatitis enteropathica
- Cystic fibrosis–related nutritional deficiency
- Pellagra

Special Studies. Special studies are not required to make a diagnosis of necrolytic migratory erythema.

Pathogenesis. Almost all patients with necrolytic migratory erythema have aminoaciduria and decreased serum levels of amino acids. This may also be an explanation for the similar clinical and histologic changes seen in acrodermatitis enteropathica. Authors have speculated that zinc deficiency or essential fatty acid deficiency may play a central role in the pathogenesis of this condition [72, 73].

Alopecia Areata

Epidemiology. Approximately 1% of the population will have had alopecia areata by the age of 50 years [74]. The peak incidence is in children and young adults. A single case of congenital alopecia areata has been described [75].

Cutaneous Features. Alopecia areata is an asymptomatic, nonscarring, noninflammatory alopecia. Sharply demarcated patches of hair loss characterize it. Follicular ostia are preserved, and there is minimal scaling or erythema on clinical examination. "Exclamation mark" hairs are present. These are tapered anagen hair shafts that have broken. The disease has an abrupt on-set and undergoes spontaneous remissions and exacer-bations. More extensive variants include alopecia to-talis, with loss of all scalp hair but with preservation of eyelids and eyebrows, and alopecia universalis, char-acterized by loss of all body hair. Red lunula and dys-trophic nails have been described in patients with alope-cia areata [76, 77].

Associated Disorders. Alopecia areata has been asso-ciated with atopic dermatitis, vitiligo, Down's syn-drome, pernicious anemia, and endocrine diseases such as Hashimoto's disease and myasthenia gravis [32, 74, 78–80]. Up to 17% of patients with myasthenia gravis and an associated thymoma will develop alopecia areata [79]. It has also been reported in a child with common variable immunodeficiency [81]. Coexistent human immunodeficiency virus infection and alopecia areata has been reported [82].

A small series of patients with Ullrich-Turner syn-

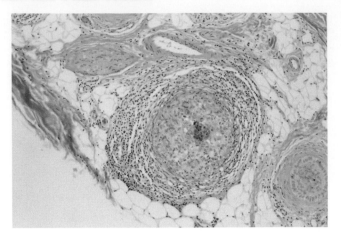

Fig. 13–7. Horizontally sectioned biopsy specimen of alopecia areata demonstrates "swarm of bees" appear-ance of lymphocytes at the level of the follicular bulb.

drome has been reported to have alopecia areata, along with other autoimmune diseases [83]. Alopecia areata has been demonstrated to co-localize with papules of lichen planus [84]. Alopecia universalis has developed in a patient with psoriasis [85]. Rare cases of alopecia areata have been associated with various medications including cyclosporine and lithium, although cy-closporine has also been used as an effective treatment for alopecia areata [86, 87].

Histologic Features. Alopecia areata is characterized by a sparse, peribulbar lymphocytic infiltrate that has been said to resemble a "swarm of bees" (Fig. 13–6). Lymphocytes are present within the follicular epithe-lium with accompanying mild spongiosis (Figure 13–7). In other cases, the infiltrate may be less concentrated around the follicular bulb, making the diagnosis more difficult. Increased catagen and telogen phase hairs may be present, as can pigment casts. Vellus hairs are present in increased numbers [88]. In horizontal sections, affected miniaturized follicles lack a competent keratinized hair shaft, unlike in adrogenic alopecia. Eosinophils are often present within the inflammatory infiltrate and may be a useful diagnostic sign [89].

A proliferation of eccrine ducts, resembling a sy-ringoma, has been described in biopsy specimens of alopecia areata, but is not thought to be part of the primary pathology [90, 91]. The nail changes seen in alopecia areata demonstrate parakeratosis [92]. The following entities must be considered in the histologic differential diagnosis of alopecia areata:

- Androgenetic alopecia
- Hair shaft abnormality
- Telogen effluvium
- Traction alopecia

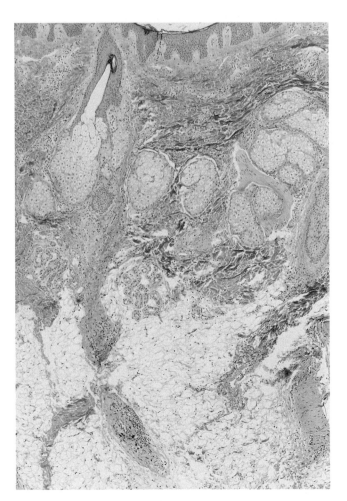

Fig. 13–6. Traditionally sectioned biopsy specimen of alopecia areata demonstrates a scant peribulbar lym-phocytic infiltrate.

Special Studies. Although not technically a "special study," transverse sectioning of routine histologic sections is especially helpful in making a diagnosis of alopecia areata. It enables the pathologist to examine many more hairs at many levels through the tissue, maximizing the chances of detecting scant foci of peribulbar inflammation. Electron microscopic examination demonstrates cytoplasmic vacuoles within keratinocytes and loss of keratin fibers [92].

Pathogenesis. The pathogenesis of alopecia areata remains unknown. It is generally believed to be an immunologically mediated process driven by CD4-positive lymphocytes [93]. Some investigators believe the disease to be autoimmune [82, 94]. It has been suggested that vascular hyperreactivity secondary to altered local cutaneous neuropeptides may play a role in the development of patches of alopecia [95].

Addison's Disease

Epidemiology. More than 80% of cases of Addison's disease are autoimmune in nature [96]. The disease can also be acquired by any inflammatory or neoplastic process that destroys the adrenal cortices, including sarcoidosis, tuberculosis, and non-Hodgkin's lymphoma [97].

Cutaneous Features. Addison's disease is characterized by diffuse hyperpigmentation without a preceeding inflammatory dermatosis [98]. Mucosal hyperpigmentation is also present in most patients with Addison's disease. Eruptive nevi have been reported in a patient with Addison's disease [99].

Associated Disorders. Primary adrenal insufficiency leads to weight loss, asthenia, weakness, and hypoglycemia [96]. Myalgias and muscle contractures may be present in patients with Addison's disease [100].

Addison's disease is often associated with other autoimmune processes such as pernicious anemia [101]. It has been assoicated with dermatitis herpetiformis and celiac disease in a small series of patients [102]. It has also been reported in a patient with Wiskott-Aldrich syndrome [103] and in another with Rothmund-Thomson syndrome [104].

Histologic Features. Histologic features of skin in Addison's disease include increased melanin within basal keratinocytes. There is no increase in number of melanocytes. There is no inflammatory infiltrate in most cases. In cases with excessive melanin, pigment incontinence may be recognized, with melanophages present within the papillary dermis and surrounding the superficial vascular plexus.

Special Studies. Special studies on skin biopsy specimens are not necessary to make a diagnosis of Addison's disease. The diagnosis is usually based on clinical findings and serologic laboratory data.

Pathogenesis. Prolonged periods of increased levels of adrenocorticotropic hormone lead to increased production of melanin by melanocytes. This results in increased melanin within basal layer keratinocytes and diffuse hyperpigmentation.

NOTE: Calciphylaxis is discussed in Chapter 8. Pancreatic panniculitis is discussed in Chapter 5. Multiple lentigines syndrome is discussed in Chapter 7.

References

1. Fatourechi, V., Pahouhi, M., and Fransway, A. F., *Dermopathy of Graves' disease (pretibial myxedema). Review of 150 cases.* Medicine (Baltimore), 1994. 73:1–7.
2. Chen, J. J., and Ladenson, P. W., *Euthyroid pretibial myxedema.* Am J Med, 1987. 82:318–320.
3. Kind, R., and Hornstein, O. P., *Clinical picture of pretibial myxedema and new aspects of diagnosis and pathogenesis.* Hautarzt, 1976. 27:375–381.
4. Kriss, J. P., *Pathogenesis and treatment of pretibial myxedema.* Endrocrinol Metab Clin North Am, 1987. 16:409–415.
5. Missner, S. C., Ramsay, E. W., Houck, H. E., and Kauffman, C. L., *Graves' disease presenting as localized myxedema in a thigh donor graft site.* J Am Acad Dermatol, 1998. 39:846–849.
6. Kato, N., Ueno, H., and Matsubara, M., *A case report of EMO syndrome showing localized hyperhidrosis in pretibial myxedema.* J Dermatol, 1991. 18:598–604.
7. Gitter, D. G., and Sato, K., *Localized hyperhidrosis in pretibial myxedema.* J Am Acad Dermatol, 1990. 23:250–254.
8. Banba, K., Tanaka, N., Fujioka, A., and Tajima, S., *Hyperpigmentation caused by hyperthyroidism: Differences from the pigmentation of Addison's disease.* Clin Exp Dermatol, 1999. 24:196–198.
9. Truhan, A. P., *Pretibial myxedema.* Am Fam Physician, 1985. 31:135–138.
10. Somach, S. C., Helm, T. N., Lawlor, K. B., Bergfeld, W. F., and Bass, J., *Pretibial mucin. Histologic patterns and clinical correlation.* Arch Dermatol, 1993. 129: 1152–1156.
11. Matsouka, L. Y., Wortsman, J., Uitto, J., Hashimoto, K., Kupchella, C. E., Eng, A. M., and Dietrich, J. E., *Altered skin elastic fibers in hypothyroid myxedema and pretibial myxedema.* Arch Intern Med, 1985. 145:117–121.
12. Pearcey, S. R., Flemming, L., Messenger, A., and Weetman, A. P., *Is Graves' dermopathy a generalized disorder?* Thyroid, 1996. 6:41–45.

13. Chang, T. C., Wu, S. L., Hsaio, Y. L., Kuo, S. T., Chien, L. F., Kuo, Y. F., Change, C. G., et al., *TSH and TSH receptor antibody-binding sites in fibroblasts of pretibial myxedema are related to the extracellular domain of entire TSH receptor.* Clin Immunol Immunopathol, 1994. 71:113–120.

14. Forgie, J. C., Highet, A. S., and Kelly, S. A., *Myxoedematous infiltrate of the forehead in treated hypothyroidism.* Clin Exp Dermatol, 1994. 19:168–169.

15. Lurie, R., Hodak, E., Ginzburg, A., and David, M., *Trichorrhexis nodosa: A manifestation of hypothyroidism.* Cutis, 1996. 57:358–359.

16. McConahey, W. M., *Diagnosing and treating myxedema and myxedema coma.* Geriatrics, 1089. 33:61–66.

17. Corbalan-Velez, R., Perez-Ferriols, A., and Aliaga-Bouiche, A., *Cutis verticis gyrata secondary to hypothyroid myxedema.* Int J Dermatol, 1999. 38:781–783.

18. Hodak, E., David, M., and Feuerman, E. J., *Palmoplantar keratoderma in association with myxedema.* Acta Derm Venereol, 1986. 66:354–357.

19. Mullin, G. E., and Eastern, J. S., *Cutaneous signs of thyroid disease.* Am Fam Physician, 1986. 34:93–98.

20. Lund, P., Horslev-Petersen, K., Helin, P., and Parving, H. H., *The effect of l-thyroxine treatment on skin accumulation of acid glycosaminoglycans in primary myxoedema.* Acta Endocrinol (Copenh), 1986. 113:56–58.

21. Parving, H. H., Hansen, J. M., Nielsen, S. L., Rossing, N., Munck, O., and Lassen, N. A., *Mechanisms of edema formation in myedema—increased protein extravasation and relatively slow lymphatic drainage.* N Engl J Med, 1979. 301:460–465.

22. Hann, S. K., and Lee, H. J., *Segmental vitiligo: Clinical findings in 208 patients.* J Am Acad Dermatol, 1996. 35:671–674.

23. Kennedy, J. A. Jr., *Vitiligo.* Dermatol Clin, 1988. 6:425–434.

24. Schallreuter, K. U., Lemke, R., Brandt, O., Schwartz, R., Westhofen, M., Montz, R., and Berger, J., *Vitiligo and other diseases: Coexistence or true assocation? Hamburg study on 321 patients.* Dermatology, 1994. 188:269–275.

25. Kovacs, S. O., *Vitiligo.* J Am Acad Dermatol, 1998. 38:647–666.

26. Schallreuter, K. U., Levenig, C., Kuhnl, P., Loliger, C., Hohl-Tehari, M., and Berger, J., *Histocompatibility antigens in vitiligo: Hamburg study on 102 patients from northern Germany.* Dermatology, 1993. 187:186–192.

27. Barona, M. I., Arrunateui, A., Falabella, R., and Alzate, A., *An epidemiologic case–control study in a population with vitiligo.* J Am Acad Dermatol, 1995. 33:621–625.

28. Koga, M., and Tango, T., *Clinical features and course of type A and type B vitiligo.* Br J Dermatol, 1988. 118:223–228.

29. Hann, S. K., Chun, W. J., and Park, Y. K., *Clinical characteristics of progressive vitiligo.* Int J Dermatol, 1997. 36:353–355.

30. Dhar, S., Malakar, S., and Dhar, S., *Colocalization of vitiligo and psoriasis in a 9-year-old boy.* Pediatr Dermatol, 1998. 15:242–243.

31. Antsey, A., and Marks, R., *Colocalization of lichen planus and vitiligo.* Br J Dermatol, 1993. 128:103–104.

32. Adams, B. B., and Lucky, A. W., *Colocalization of alopecia areata and vitiligo.* Pediatr Dermatol, 1999. 16:364–366.

33. Abraham, Z., Rozenbaum, M., Gluck, Z., Feuerman, E. J., Lahat, N., and Kinarty, A., *Vitiligo, rheumatoid arthritis and pernicious anemia.* J Dermatol, 1993. 20:418–423.

34. Dhar, S., and Kanwar, A. J., *Colocalization of vitiligo and alopecia areata.* Pediatr Dermatol, 1994. 11:85–86.

35. Frati, R., Frati, C., Sassano, P. P., and Antonaci, A., *Vitiligo, autoimmune thyroiditis: A rare thyroid cancer arising with bone metastases on maxillofacial area.* J Exp Clin Cancer Res, 1999. 18:85–87.

36. Dippel, E., Hass, N., and Czarnetzki, B. M., *Porokeratosis of Mibelli associated with active chronic hepatitis and vitiligo.* Acta Derm Venereol, 1994. 74:463–464.

37. Sacher, M., Blumel, P., Thaler, H., and Manns, M., *Chronic active hepatitis associated with vitiligo, nail dystrophy, alopecia and a new variant of LKM antibodies.* J Hepatol, 1990. 10:364–369.

38. Zauli, D., Crespi, C., Miserocchi, F., Bianchi, F. B., Tosti, A., Lama, L., and Veronesi, S., *Primary biliary cirrhosis and vitiligo.* J Am Acad Dermatol, 1986. 15:105–107.

39. Hogan, D. J., and Lane, P. R., *Dermatitis herpetiformis and vitiligo.* Cutis, 1986. 38:195–197.

40. Blume-Peytavi, U., Spieker, T., Reupke, H., and Orfanos, C. E., *Generalised acanthosis nigrans with vitiligo.* Acta Derm Venereol, 1996. 76:377–380.

41. Schwartz, R. A., and Janniger, C. K., *Vitiligo.* Cutis, 1997. 60:239–244.

42. Kang, I. K., and Hann, S., K., *Vitiligo coexistent with nevus depigmentosus.* J Dermatol, 1996. 23:187–190.

43. Cavallari, V., Cannavo, S. P., Ussia, A. F., Moretti, G., and Albanese, A., *Vitiligo associated with metastatic malignant melanoma.* Int J Dermatol, 1996. 35:738–740.

44. Nordlund, J. J., Kirkwood, J. M., Forget, B. M., Milton, G., Albert, D. M., and Lerner, A. B., *Vitiligo in patients with metastatic melanoma: A good prognostic sign.* J Am Acad Dermatol, 1983. 9:689–696.

45. Buckley, D. A., and Rogers, S., *Multiple keratoses and squamous cell carcinoma after PUVA treatment of vitiligo.* Clin Exp Dermatol, 1996. 21:43–45.

46. Takeda, H., Mitsuhashi, Y., and Kondo, S., *Multiple squamous cell carcinomas in situ in vitiligo lesions after long-term PUVA therapy.* J Am Acad Dermatol, 1998. 38:268–270.

47. Selvaag, E., *Chloroquine-induced vitiligo.* Acta Derm Venereol (Stockh), 1996. 76:166–167.

48. Brown-Harrell, V., Nitta, A. T., and Goble, M., *Apparent exacerbation of vitiligo syndrome in a patient with pulmonary Mycobacterium avium complex disease who received clofazamine therapy.* Clin Infect Dis, 1996. 22:581–582.

49. Horn, T. D., and Abanmi, A., *Analysis of the lympho-*

cytic infiltrate in a case of vitiligo. Am J Dermatopathol, 1997. 19:400–402.

50. Galadari, E., Mehregan, A. H., and Hashimoto, K., *Ultrastructural study of vitiligo.* Int J Dermatol, 1993. 32:269–271.

51. Bose, S. K., *Absence of Merkel cells in lesional skin of vitiligo.* Int J Dermatol, 1994. 33:481–483.

52. Badri, A. M., Todd, P. M., Garioch, J. J., Gudgeon, J. E., Stewart, D. G., and Goudie, R. B., *An immunohistochemical study of cutaneous lymphocytes in vitiligo.* J Pathol, 1993. 170:149–155.

53. Le Poole, I. C., van den Wijngaard, R. M., Westerhof, W., and Das, P. K., *Presence of T cells and macrophages in inflammatory vitiligo skin parallels melanocyte disappearance.* Am J Pathol, 1996. 148:1219–1228.

54. Mahmoud, F., Q. al-Saleh, A. H., Haines, D., Burleson, J., and Morgan, G., *Peripheral T-cell activation in nonsegmental vitiligo.* J Dermatol, 1998. 25:637–640.

55. Yeo, U. C., Yang, Y. S., Park, K. B., Sung, H. T., Jung, S. Y., Lee, E. S., and Shin, M. H., *Serum concentration of the soluble interleukin-2 receptor in vitiligo patients.* J Dermatol Sci, 1999. 19:182–188.

56. Abdel-Naser, M. B., Kruger-Krasagakes, S., Krasagakis, K., Gollnick, H., Abdel-Fattah, A., and Orfanos, C. E., *Further evidence for involvement of both cell mediated and humoral immunity in generalized vitiligo.* Pigmented Cell Res. 7:108, 1994.

57. Gilhar, A., Zelickson, B., Ulman, Y., and Etzioni, A., *In vivo destruction of melanocytes by the IgG fraction of serum from patients with vitiligo.* J Invest Dermatol, 1995. 105:683–686.

58. Norris, A., Todd, C., Graham, A., Quinn, A. G., and Thody, A. J., *The expression of the c-kit receptor by epidermal melanocytes may be reduced in vitiligo.* Br J Dermatol, 1996. 134:299–306.

59. Maresca, V., Roccella, M., Roccella, F., Camera, E., Del Porto, G., Passi, S., Grammatico, P., et al., *Increased sensitivity to peroxidative agents as a possible pathogenic factor of melanocyte damage in vitiligo.* J Invest Dermatol, 1997. 109:310–313.

60. Khairi, M. R., Dexter, R. N., Burzynski, N. J., and Johnston, C. C. Jr., *Mucosal neuroma, pheochromocytoma and medullary thyroid carcinoma: Multiple endocrine neoplasia type 3.* Medicine (Baltimore), 1975. 54:89–112.

61. Edwards, M., and Reid, J. S., *Multiple endocrine neoplasia syndrome type IIb: A case report.* Int J Paediatr Dent, 1998. 8:55–60.

62. Schenberg, M. E., Zajec, J. D., Lim-Tio, S., Collier, N. A., Brooks, A. M., and Reade, P. C., *Multiple endocrine neoplasia syndrome—type 2b. Case report and review.* Int J Oral Maxillofac Surg, 1992. 21:110–114.

63. Cunliffe, W. J., Hudgson, P., Fulthorpe, J. J., Black, M. M., Hall, R., Johnston, I. D., and Shuster, S., *A calcitonin-secreting medullary thyroid carcinoma associated with mucosal neuromas, marfanoid features, myopathy and pigmentation.* Am J Med, 1970. 48:120–126.

64. Kaufman, F. R., Roe, T. F., Isaacs, H. Jr., and Weitzman, J. J., *Metastatic medullary thyroid carcinoma in young children with mucosal neuroma syndrome.* Pediatrics, 1982. 70:263–267.

65. Netzloff, M. L., Garnica, A. D., Rodgers, B. M., and Frias, J. L., *Medullary carcinoma of the thyroid in the multiple mucosal neuromas syndrome.* Ann Clin Lab Sci, 1979. 9:368–373.

66. Cuthbert, J. A., Gallagher, N. D., and Turtle, J. R., *Colonic and oesophageal disturbance in a patient with multiple endocrine neoplasia, type 2b.* Aust NZ J Med, 1978. 8:518–520.

67. Moyes, C. D., and Alexander, F. W., *Mucosal neuroma syndrome presenting in a neonate.* Dev Med Child Neurol, 1977. 19:518–534.

68. Miller, R. L., Burzynski, N. J., and Giammara, N. L., *The ultrastructure of oral neuromas in multiple mucosal neuromas, pheochromocytoma, medullary thyroid carcinoma syndrome.* J Oral Pathol, 1977. 6:253–263.

69. Uchino, S., Noguchi, S., Yamashita, H., Sato, M., Adachi, M., Yamashita, H., Watanabe, S., et al., *Somatic mutations in RET exons 12 and 15 in sporadic medullary thyroid carcinomas: Different spectrum of mutations in sporadic type from hereditary type.* Jpn J Cancer Res, 1999. 90:1231–1237.

70. Doyle, J. A., Schoeter, A. L., and Rogers, R. S., *Hyperglucagonaemia and necrolytic migratory erythema in cirrhosis-possible pseudoglucagonoma syndrome.* Br J Dermatol, 1979. 101:581–587.

71. Darouti, M. E., and Ela, M. A. E., *Necrolytic acral erythema: A cutaneous marker of viral hepatitis C.* Int J Dermatol, 1996. 35:252–256.

72. Blackford, S., Wright, S., and Roberts, D. I., *Necrolytic migratory erythema without glucagonoma: The role of dietary essential fatty acids.* Br J Dermatol, 1991. 125:460–462.

73. Sinclair, S. A., and Reynolds, N. J., *Necrolytic migratory erythema and zinc deficiency.* Br J Dermatol, 1997. 136:783–785.

74. Sahn, E. E., *Alopecia areata in childhood.* Semin Dermatol, 1995. 14:9–14.

75. de Viragh, P. A., Gianadda, B., and Levy, M. L., *Congenital alopecia areata.* Dermatology, 1997. 195:96–98.

76. Wilkerson, M. G., and Wilkin, J. K., *Red lunulae revisited: A clinical and histopathologic examination.* J Am Acad Dermatol, 1989. 20:453–457.

77. Fanti, P. A., and Tosti, A., *Histologic aspects of dystrophy of the 20 nails associated with alopecia areata.* G Ital Dermatol Venereol, 1988. 123:533–534.

78. Kocak Altintas, A. G., Gul, U., and Duman, S., *Bilateral keratoconus associated with Hashimoto's disease, alopecia areata and atopic keratoconjunctivitis.* Eur J Ophthalmol, 1999. 9:130–133.

79. Kubota, A., Komiyama, A., and Hasegawa, O., *Myasthenia gravis and alopecia areata.* Neurology, 1997. 48:774–775.

80. Weitzner, J. M., *Alopecia areata.* Am Fam Physician, 1990. 41:1197–1201.

81. Kilic, S., Ersoy, F., Sanal, O., Turkbay, D., and Tezcan, I., *Alopecia universalis in a patient with common variable immunodeficiency.* Pediatr Dermatol, 1999. 16:305–307.

82. Stewart, M. I., and Smoller, B. R., *Alopecia universalis in an HIV-positive patient: Possible insight into pathogenesis.* J Cutan Pathol, 1993. 20:180–183.

83. Tebbe, B., H. Gollnick, Muller, R., Reupke, H. J., and Orfanos, C. E., *Alopecia areata and diffuse hypotrichosis associated with Ullrich-Turner syndrome. Presentation of 4 patients.* Hautarzt, 1993. 44:647–652.

84. Dhar, S., and Dhar, S., *Colocalization of alopecia areata and lichen planus.* Pediatr Dermatol, 1996. 13:258–259.

85. Yamamoto, T., Watanabe, K., Katayama, I., and Nishioka, K., *Alopecia universalis in a patient with psoriasis vulgaris.* J Dermatol, 1995. 22:623–624.

86. Cerottini, J. P., Panizzon, R. G., and de Viragh, P. A., *Multifocal alopecia areata during systemic cyclosporine A therapy.* Dermatology, 1999. 198:415–417.

87. Silvestri, A., Santonastaso, P., and Paggiarin, D., *Alopecia areata during lithium therapy. A case report.* Gen Hosp Psychiatry, 1988. 10:46–48.

88. Kim, I. H., Jo, H. Y., Cho, C. G., Choi, H. C., and Oh, C. H., *Quantitative image analysis of hair follicles in alopecia areata.* Acta Derm Venereol, 1999. 79:214–216.

89. Elston, D. M., McCollough, M. L., Bergfeld, W. F., Liranzo, M. O., and Heibel, M., *Eosinophils in fibrous tracts and near hair bulbs: A helpful diagnostic feature of alopecia areata.* J Am Acad Dermatol, 1997. 37:101–106.

90. Mehregan, A. H., and Mehregan, D. A., *Syringoma-like sweat duct proliferation in scalp alopecias.* J Cutan Pathol, 1990. 17:355–357.

91. Barnhill, R. L., Goldberg, S., and Stenn, K. S., *Proliferation of eccrine sweat ducts associated with alopecia areata.* J Cutan Pathol, 1988. 15:36–39.

92. Laporte, M., Andre, J., Stouffs-Vanhoof, F., and Achten, G., *Nail changes in alopecia areata: Light and electron microscopy.* Arch Dermatol Res, 1988. 280: S85–89.

93. Ghersetich, I., Campanile, G., and Lotti, T., *Alopecia areata: Immunohistochemistry and ultrastructure of infiltrate and identification of adhesion molecule receptors.* Int J Dermatol, 1996. 35:28–33.

94. Kalish, R. S., Johnson, K. L., and Hordinsky, M. K., *Alopecia areata. Autoreactive T cells are variably enriched in scalp lesions relative to peripheral blood.* Arch Dermatol, 1992. 128:1072–1077.

95. Rossi, R., Del Biano, E., Isolani, D., Baccari, M. C., and Cappugi, P., *Possible involvement of neuropeptidergic sensory nerves in alopecia areata.* Neuroreport, 1997. 8:1135–1138.

96. Burke, C. W., *Adrenocortical insufficiency.* Clin Endocrinol Metab, 1985. 14:947–976.

97. Takahashi, T., Ishii, S., Atsumi, S., Mita, H., Hayashi, T., Adachi, A., Hinoda, Y., et al., *Bilateral non-Hodgkin's lymphoma of the adrenal glands with adrenal insufficiency.* Rinsho Ketsueki, 1996. 37:867–869.

98. Schurer, N., Zumdick, M., and Goerz, G., *Hyperpigmentation in primary adrenal cortex insufficiency: Addison's disease.* Hautzart, 1993. 44:300–305.

99. Ibsen, H. H., and Clemmensen, O., *Eruptive nevi in Addison's disease.* Arch Dermatol, 1990. 126:1239–1240.

100. Shapiro, M. S., Trebich, C., Shilo, L., and Shenkman, L., *Myalgias and muscle contractures as the presenting signs of Addison's disease.* Postgrad Med J, 1988. 64:222–223.

101. Graner, J. L., *Addison, pernicious anemia and adrenal insufficiency.* CMAJ, 1985. 133:855–857.

102. Reunala, T., Salmi, J., and Karvonen, J., *Dermatitis herpetiformis and celiac disease associated with Addison's disease.* Arch Dermatol, 1987. 123:930–932.

103. Latal Hajnal, B., Lops, U., Friedrich, W., Zachmann, M., and Berthet, F., *Addison disease 10 years after bone marrow transplant for Wiskott-Alrich syndrome.* Eur J Pediatr, 1995. 154:729–731.

104. Lapunzina, P., Fonseca, E., Gracia, R., and Delicado, A., *Rothmund-Thomson syndrome and Addison's disease.* Pediatr Dermatol, 1995. 12:164–169.

PART III

Metabolic and Storage Diseases

Storage Diseases

Tangier Disease

Epidemiology. Tangier disease is caused by a deficiency of high-density plasma lipoproteins. It is inherited in an autosomal codominant manner. The genetic defect has been localized to chromosome 9q31 [1]. The disease is largely limited to inhabitants of Tangier Island, located in the Chesapeake Bay.

Cutaneous Features. Cutaneous manifestations of Tangier disease are very uncommon. The skin does, however, demonstrate lipid deposits within cells of the reticuloendothelial system (see later).

Associated Diseases. Enlarged, orange-yellow or gray tonsils are seen in most patients with Tangier disease [2]. Hepatosplenomegaly may be present as an early manifestation. Lymphadenopathy is also seen. [3]. Polyneuropathy is seen in most patients with Tangier disease [4, 5]. Cardiovascular disease affects approximately 20% of patients with Tangier disease [4]. Membranous phospholipid and cholesterol inclusions within the stroma of the cornea may be present in patients with Tangier disease and lead to corneal opacification [6]. The gastrointestinal tract may demonstrate tiny flat orange lesions throughout the mucosal surfaces [3, 7]. Hemolytic anemia has also been described in patients with Tangier disease [8].

Histologic Features. Skin biopsy specimens from patients with Tangier disease demonstrate deposits of cholesteryl esters within cells of the reticuloendothelial system. These deposits are birefringent and can be spherical or crystalline in shape [2]. Similar deposits can be seen in jejunal submucosa, bone marrow, Schwann cells within peripheral nerves, and nonvascular smooth muscle cells [2].

Special Studies. Electron microscopic examination reveals extensive nonmembrane-bound vacuoles in Schwann cells, endoneurial fibroblasts, perineurial cells, and macrophages [5]. Melanocytic nevus cells have also demonstrated similar vacuoles [5].

Pathogenesis. Patients affected by Tangier disease have markedly decreased levels of plasma high-density lipoprotein (HDL) and apolipoprotein A-1 (apo A-1). It is believed that these patients synthesize apo A-1, but have increased fractional catabolism of these proteins, thought to be, at least in part, due to a structural defect in the apo A-1 protein [9].

Niemann-Pick Disease

Epidemiology. Niemann-Pick disease is an autosomal recessive lysosomal storage disorder caused by the absence of sphingomyelinase. There are several subtypes described and designated types A through E. Type A disease is the most common and almost invariably follows a course leading to death during childhood. It is characterized by massive enlargement of the liver and spleen and involvement of the central nervous system leading to mental deterioration. Type B disease has similar visceral involvement, but does not involve the central nervous system. These patients often survive into adulthood because the nervous system is spared. Type

C disease is similar to type A disease but has a later onset, and patients succumb to disease usually by the age of 20 years. Niemann-Pick disease types D and E are quite rare [10].

Cutaneous Features. Most patients with Niemann-Pick disease do not display cutaneous manifestations. In rare patients, however, a papular eruption has been reported [11]. In other patients, indurated, brown plaques are described [12]. Juvenile xanthogranuloma has also been described in a patient with Niemann-Pick disease [13], as have cutaneous xanthomas [14]. Nummular dermatitis has been attributed to the disease process in a patient with type B Niemann-Pick disease [15].

Associated Diseases. Patients with Niemann-Pick disease have involvement of various viscera, depending on the subtype of the disease. Psychiatric disorders and low levels of HDL cholesterol have been described in patients with type B disease [16]. Delayed puberty, lung involvement, and stunted physical development have also been reported in these patients [15]. Progressive dementia, ataxia, and dysarthrias have been described in patients with type C disease [17]. Mental retardation may be severe and may be accompanied by involuntary movements and poor coordination [18]. Xanthomas of the gastrointestinal tract may be present. Splenomegaly and hepatomegaly are present in most patients with type C disease [19]. Bony infarcts and hyperlipidemia may also be present [19].

Histologic Features. Foam cells are present within the reticuloendothelial system throughout the body in patients affected by Niemann-Pick disease. Foamy histiocytes are present throughout the dermis, admixed with scattered lymphocytes (Fig. 14–1).

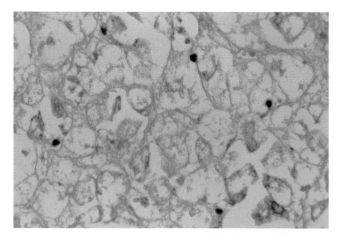

Fig. 14–1. Cells of the reticuloendothelial system are distended with accumulated syphingomyelin in this kidney from a patient with Niemann-Pick disease.

Special Studies. Lysosomal inclusions are present to varying degrees in patients with Niemann-Pick disease [20]. Ultrastructural analysis of skin biopsy specimens from patients with type C Niemann-Pick disease demonstrates lysosomes containing dark, lamellated structures within a clear matrix sometimes referred to as "zebra bodies" [21]. These inclusions are present within macrophages, axons, pericytes, Schwann cells, smooth cells, and fibroblasts. Melanocytes and endothelial cells are relatively spared [22]. Intracytoplasmic inclusions have also been described in clear cells of the eccrine coils and in follicular epithelium and basal keratinocytes [18].

Oil red O and Sudan black stain the foamy histiocytes within the dermis [14], and they will label metachromatically with toluidine blue [11].

Pathogenesis. Sphingomyelinase deficiency, resulting in increased levels of sphingomyelin, is the primary lesion in patients with Niemann-Pick disease. A number of genetic defects have been described in patients with Niemann-Pick disease, but no clear pattern has emerged.

Gaucher's Disease

Epidemiology. Gaucher's disease is an autosomal recessive disorder caused by a defect in acid β-glucocerebrosidase. It is the most common lysosomal storage disease [23]. Three subtypes of patients with Gaucher's disease have been described. Patients with type I disease do not experience neurologic symptoms. The acute neuoronopathic form is type II, and the subacute neuronopathic form is type III Gaucher's disease [24].

Cutaneous Features. Patients with type I Gaucher's disease demonstrate diffuse pigmentation, transient brown macules, and easy tanning [25]. Patients with type II Gaucher's disease frequently present with ichthyosiform changes [26, 27]. Coexistence with a restrictive dermopathy has been described in a single patient [28]. A collodian membrane characterized by lamellar desquamation may be present at birth in some infants with Gaucher's disease [29].

Associated Diseases. Immune thrombocytopenic purpura has been reported in patients with Gaucher's disease [30]. Hypersplenism can lead to severe cytopenia in these patients. Hepatomegaly is also present and is caused by accumulation of Gaucher's disease cells and fibrosis [31]. Gaucher's disease cells are cells that range in size from 20 to 100 μm in diameter. They have one or few small nuclei and abundant material positive for periodic acid–Schiff in the wrinkled-appearing cytoplasm.

Histologic Features. Clinically normal skin from patients with Gaucher's disease does not demonstrate any abnormalities on routine histologic examination. Skin biopsy specimens from patients with ichthyoses and Gaucher's disease have not been adequately described.

Special Studies. Unlike many of the other storage diseases, no specific abnormalities could be detected on ultrastructural analysis of skin biopsy material taken from patients with Gaucher's disease [32, 33]. In patients with ichthyosis and Gaucher's disease, persistence of incompletely processed lamellar bodies throughout the stratum corneum has been described [27].

Pathogenesis. Progressive accumulation of glucosylceramide within cells of the reticuloendothelial cell system leads to the physical changes seen in patients with Gaucher's disease [23]. The ichthyosiform changes seen in patients with type II Gaucher's disease are attributed to lack of glucocerebrosidase necessary to generate functionally competent cellular membranes for effective epidermal barrier function [27, 34]. In some patients, a mutation has been demonstrated in sphingolipid activator proteins necessary for lysosomal hydrolysis of glucosylceramide [35].

Fucosidosis

Epidemiology. Fucosidosis is a rare, autosomal recessive inborn error of metabolism caused by a loss of α-L-fucosidase. This leads to a lysosomal storage disorder.

Cutaneous Features. Fucosidosis is characterized by diffuse angiokeratomas. These appear as erythematous, nonblanchable papules that are up to 1 cm in diameter and are identical in appearance to those seen in Fabry's disease or as isolated, sporadic occurrences [36]. The oral mucosa may be involved [37].

Other cutaneous manifestations of fucosidosis include distal transverse purple nail bands associated with acrocyanosis. A nevus anemicus has also be described in a patient with fucosidosis [38].

Associated Diseases. Patients with fucosidosis develop mental retardation, cardiomegaly, progressive neurologic deterioration, and premature death [39]. Death is frequently related to recurrent upper respiratory tract infections [37]. Dyostosis multiplex is seen on x-ray examination of some patients with fucosidosis [38]. Coarse facial features and spondyloepiphyseal dysplasia are often present [37].

Histologic Features. Angiokeratomas associated with fucosidosis are histologically identical to those seen in

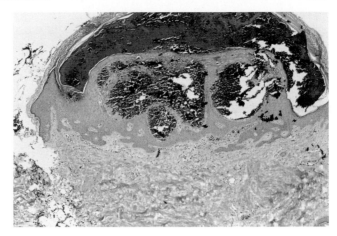

Fig. 14–2. Angiokeratoma in fucosidosis demonstrates collarette of hyperplastic epidermis surrounding thin-walled vessels located high in the papillary dermal tips.

association with Fabry's disease (see Chapter 12) and to the sporadically occurring vascular tumors. A hyperplastic epidermis is present surrounding ectatic papillary dermal blood vessels (Fig. 14–2). Hyperkeratosis and hypergranulosis are variably present, and the epidermis is irregularly acanthotic. Thin-walled vessels are widely dilated within papillary dermal tips and are increased in number (Fig. 14–3). Similarly ectatic vessels may be seen in the superficial reticular dermis, but do not ordinarily extend into the deeper dermis. Endothelial cells are flattened and unremarkable.

Special Studies. Electron microscopic examination of clinically normal-appearing skin reveals empty-appearing storage vesicles in melanocytes, endothelial cells, sweat glands, and fibroblasts [40]. Dense inclusion bodies with an internal lamellar structure may also be present. Similar findings may be present within Schwann cells [41].

Pathogenesis. Deficiency of α-L-fucosidase affects the way in which fucose-containing lipids are processed, resulting in the increase of glycoproteins and oligo- and polysaccharides in tissue [40]. Removal of a single N-linked oligosaccharide from the α-L-fucosidase appears to be responsible for the loss of function [42].

It has been suggested that the progressive storage of material within endothelial cells leads to occlusion of some dermal blood vessels, resulting in progressive angiectasis [43].

Farber's Lipogranulomatosis

Epidemiology. Farber's lipogranulomatosis is a lipid storage disease characterized by the deposition of excessive ceramide within cells of the reticuloendothelial

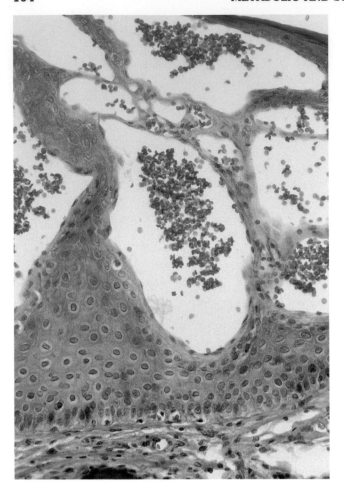

Fig. 14–3. Thin-walled vessels give the appearance of being intraepidermal in angiokeratomas associated with fucosidosis.

system. Three subtypes, varying in degree of severity, have been described [44]. Disease severity does not, however, appear to correlate with levels of acid ceramidase. Siblings affected by Farber's lipogranulomatosis have been reported [45, 46].

Cutaneous Features. Periarticular subcutaneous nodules are a common finding in patients with Farber's lipogranulomatosis [44]. In some cases, erythematous plaques are seen [45].

Associated Diseases. Hepatosplenomgealy is present in most affected patients [46]. Widespread erosions within the gastrointestinal tract have been reported [47]. Lymphadenopathy may also be seen.

Hoarseness, difficulty swallowing, and painful, swollen joints and progressive arthropathies are common features of Farber's lipogranulomatosis. Limb swelling and contractures may be present [45]. Coarse facial features and cloudy corneas are present in some affected infants [48].

Frequent respiratory infections are described in patients with Farber's lipogranulomatosis and may contribute to the mortality in these patients [49]. Nystagmus and mental and developmental growth retardation occur in patients with Farber's lipogranulomatosis [50]. Rare reports of renal involvement are present in the literature [46]. Hydrops fetalis has been described in a series of patients with Farber's lipogranulomatosis [51].

Histologic Features. Routine histologic sections from clinically normal skin are essentially nonspecific. In biopsy specimens from erythematous plaques, lipid-laden histiocytes are found in the dermis [45]. Biopsy material from subcutaneous nodules in patients with Farber's lipogranulomatosis demonstrate granulomatous foci composed of spindle- and oval-shaped lipid-laden histiocytes admixed with fibroblasts. Foamy-appearing histiocytes are present in some cases. Fibrosis is present [47].

Special Studies. Ultrastructural examination reveals curvilinear bodies within the cytoplasm of histiocytes, fibroblasts, and endothelial cells, known as "Farber bodies" [47, 52]. Zebra body–like structures and needle-like lysosomal inclusions have been described within keratinocytes in some affected individuals [44]. Similar zebra bodies have been demonstrated within endothelial cells [52]. Spindle-shaped inclusions, known by some as "banana bodies" [53], are present in Schwann cells in some cases [52]. Concentric lamellar bodies have also been described [48].

Pathogenesis. Farber's lipogranulomatosis is due to a deficiency of lysosomal acid ceramidase [48]. This results in markedly delayed degradation of ceramide [54].

References

1. Rust, S., Walter, M., Funke, H., von Eckardstein, A., Cullen, P., Kroes, H. Y., Hordijk, R., Geisel, J., et al., *Assignment of Tangier disease to chromosome 9q31 by a graphical linkage exclusion strategy.* Nat Genet, 1998. 20:96–98.
2. Ferrans, V. J., and Frederickson, D. S., *The pathology of Tangier disease. A light and electron microscopic study.* Am J Pathol, 1975. 78:101–158.
3. Lachaux, A., Sassolas, A., Bouvier, R., Le Gall, C., Loras, I., Regnier, F., Plauchu, H., Froelich, P., et al., *Early manifestations of Tangier disease.* Arch Pediatr, 1995. 2:447–451.
4. Serfaty-Lacrosniere, C., Civeira, F., Lanzberg, A., Isaia, P., Berg, J., Janus, E. D., Smith, M. P., Jr., Pritchard, P. H., et al., *Homozygous Tangier disease and cardiovascular disease.* Atherosclerosis, 1994. 107:85–98.

5. Gibbels, E., Schaefer, H. E., Runne, U., Schroder, J. M., Haupt, W. F., and Assmann, G., *Severe polyneuropathy in Tangier disease mimicking syringomyelia or leprosy. Clinical, biochemical, electrophysiological, and morphological evaluation, including electron microscopy of nerve, muscle, and skin biopsies.* J Neurol, 1985. 232: 283–294.

6. Winder, A. F., Alexander, R., Garner, A., Johnston, D., Vallance, D., McCreanor, G., and Frohlich, J., *The pathology of cornea in Tangier disease (familial high density lipoprotein deficiency).* J Clin Pathol, 1996. 49: 407–410.

7. Frosini, G., Marini, M., Galgani, P., Carnicelli, N., Farnetani, L., and Pettorali, M., *Tangier disease: An unusual diagnosis for the endoscopist.* Endoscopy, 1994. 26:373.

8. Reinhart, W. H., Gossi, U., Butikofer, P., Ott, P., Sigrist, H., Schatzmann, H. J., Lutz, H. U., and Straub, P. W., *Haemolytic anaemia in an alpha-lipoproteinaemia (Tangier disease): Morphological, biochemical, and biophysical properties of the red blood cell.* Br J Haematol, 1989. 72:272–277.

9. Kay, L. L., Ronan, R., Schaefer, E. J., and Brewer, H. B. Jr., *Tangier disease: a structural defect in apolipoprotein A-1 (apoA-1 Tangier).* Proc Natl Acad Sci USA, 1982. 79:2485–2489.

10. Brady, R. O., *Niemann-Pick disease.* In *The Metabolic Basis of Inherited Disease*, J. B. Stanbury, J. B. Wyngaarden, and D. S. Fredrickson, Eds. 1983, McGraw-Hill, New York, pp. 831–841.

11. Toussaint, M., Worret, W. I., Drosner, M., and Marquardt, K. H., *Specific skin lesions in a patient with Niemann-Pick disease.* Br J Dermatol, 1994. 131:895–897.

12. Mardini, M. K., Gergen, P., Akhtar, M., and Ghandour, M., *Niemann-Pick disease: Report of a case with skin involvement.* Am J Dis Child, 1982. 136:650–651.

13. Sibulkin, D., and Olichney, J. J., *Juvenile xanthogranuloma in a patient with Niemann-Pick disease.* Arch Dermatol, 1973. 108:829–831.

14. Crocker, A. C., and Farber, S., *Niemann-Pick disease: A review of eighteen patients.* Medicine (Baltimore), 1958. 37:1–95.

15. Pavone, L. F., Fiumara, A., and LaRosa, M., *Niemann-Pick disease type B: Clinical signs and follow-up of a new case.* J Inherit Metab Dis, 1986. 9:73–78.

16. Dubois, G., Mussini, J. M., Auclair, M., Battesti, J., Boutry, J. M., Kemeny, J. L., Maziere, J. C., Turpin, J. C., et al., *Adult sphingomyelinase deficiency: Report of two patients who initially presented with psychiatric disorders.* Neurology, 1990. 40:132–136.

17. Hulette, C. M., Earl, N. L., Anthony, D. C., and Crain, B. J., *Adult onset Niemann-Pick disease type C presenting with dementia and absent organomegaly.* Clin Neuropathol, 1992. 11:293–297.

18. Arsenio-Nunes, M. L., and Goutieres, F., *Morphological diagnosis of Niemann-Pick disease type C by skin and conjunctival biopsies.* Acta Neuropathol Suppl (Berl), 1981. 7:204–207.

19. Filling-Katz, M. R., Miller, S. P., Merrick, H. F., Travis, W. D., Greeg, R. E., Tsokos, M., Comly, M., Kaneski, C. R., et al., *Clinical, pathologic, and biochemical fea-tures of a cholesterol lipidosis accompanied by hyperlipidemia and xanthomas.* Neurology, 1992. 42:1768–1774.

20. Natowicz, M. R., Stoler, J. M., Prence, E. M., and Liscum, L., *Marked heterogeneity in Niemann-Pick disease, type C. Clinical and ultrastructural findings.* Clin Pediatr (Phila), 1995. 34:190–197.

21. Wood, W. S., Dimmick, J. E., and Dolman, C. L., *Niemann-Pick disease and juvenile xanthogranuloma. Are they related?* Am J Dermatopathol, 1987. 9:433–437.

22. Boutsany, R. N., Kaye, E., and Alroy, J., *Ultrastructural findings in skin from patients with Niemann-Pick disease, type C.* Pediatr Neurol, 1990. 6:177–183.

23. Pastores, G. M., *Gaucher's disease: Pathological features.* Baillieres Clin Haematol, 1997. 10:739–749.

24. Willemsen, R., van Dongen, J. M., Ginns, E. I., Sips, H. J., Schram, A. W., Tager, J. M., Barranger, J. A., and Reuser, A. J., *Ultrastructural localization of glucocerebrosidase in cultured Gaucher disease fibroblasts by immunocytochemistry.* J Neurol, 1987. 234:44–51.

25. Goldblatt, J., and Beighton, P., *Cutaneous manifestations of Gaucher disease.* Br J Dermatol, 1984. 111:331–334.

26. Fujimoto, A., Tayebi, N., and Sidransky, E., *Congenital ichthyosis preceding neurologic symptoms in two sibs with type 2 Gaucher disease.* Am J Med Genet, 1995. 20:356–358.

27. Sidransky, E., Fartasch, M., Lee, R. E., Metlay, L. A., Abella, S., Zimran, A., Gao, W., Elias, P. M., et al., *Epidermal abnormalities may distinguish type 2 from type 1 and type 3 of Gaucher disease.* Pediatr Res, 1996. 39:134–141.

28. Sherer, D. M., Metlay, L. A., Sinkin, R. A., Mongeon, C., Lee, R. E., and Woods, J. R. Jr., *Congenital ichthyosis with restrictive dermopathy and Gaucher disease: A new syndrome wqith associated prenatal diagnostic and pathology findings.* Obstet Gynecol, 1993. 81:842–844.

29. Lui, K., Commens, C., Choong, R., and Jaworski, R., *Collodion babies with Gaucher's disease.* Arch Dis Child, 1988. 63:854–856.

30. Lester, T. J., Grabowski, G. A., Goldblatt, J., Leiderman, I. Z., and Zaroulis, C. G., *Immune thrombocytopenia and Gaucher's disease.* Am J Med, 1984. 77:569–571.

31. Giraldo, P., Perez-Calvo, J., Cortes, T., Civeira, F., and Rubio-Felix, D., *Type I Gaucher's disease: Clinical, evolutive, and therapeutic features in 8 cases.* Sangre (Barc), 1994. 39:3–7.

32. Dolman, C. L., MacLeod, P. M., and Chang, E., *Skin punch biopsies and lymphocytes in the diagnosis of lipidoses.* Can J Neurol Sci, 1975. 2:67–73.

33. O'Brien, J. S., Bernett, J., Veath, M. L., and Paa, D., *Lysosomal storage disorders. Diagnosis by ultrastructural examination of skin biopsy specimens.* Arch Neurol, 1975. 32:592–599.

34. Holleran, W. M., Ginns, E. I., Menon, G. K., Grundmann, J. U., Fartasch, M., McKinney, C. E., Elias, P. M., and Sidransky, E., *Consequences of beta-glucocerebrosidase deficiency in epidermis. Ultrastructural and permeability barrier alterations in Gaucher disease.* J Clin Invest, 1994. 93:1756–1764.

35. Rafi, M. A., de Gala, G., Zhang, X. L., and Wenger,

D. A., *Mutational analysis in a patient with a variant form of Gaucher's disease caused by SAP-2 deficiency.* Somat Cell Mol Genet, 1993. 19:1–7.

36. Venencie, P. Y., Pauwels, C., Malherbe, V., Perie, G., and Landrieu, P., *Angiokeratoma and fucosidosis. Immunohistochemical and ultrastructural study.* Ann Dermatol Venereol, 1995. 122:432–435.

37. Prindiville, D. E., and Stern, D., *Oral lesions in fucosidosis.* J Oral Surg, 1976. 34:603–608.

38. Fleming, C., Rennie, A., Fallowfield, M., and McHenry, P. M., *Cutaneous manifestations of fucosidosis.* Br J Dermatol, 1997. 136:594–597.

39. Provenzale, J. M., Barboriak, D. P., and Sims, K., *Neuroradiologic findings in fucosidosis, a rare lysosomal storage disease.* AJNR Am J Neuroradiol, 1995. 16(Suppl 4):809–813.

40. Breier, F., Hobisch, G., Fang-Kircher, S., Braun, F., Paschke, E., and Jurecka, W., *Histology and electron microscopy of fucosidosis of the skin. Subtle clues to diagnosis by electron microscopy.* Am J Dermatopathol, 1995. 17:379–383.

41. Porfiri, B., Ricci, R., Seminara, D., and Segni, G., *Ultrastructural studies of type II fucosidosis.* Arch Dermatol Res, 19081. 270:57–66.

42. Johnson, K., and Dawson, G., *Molecular defect in processing alpha-fucosidase in fucosidosis.* Biochem Biophys Res Commun, 1985. 27:90–97.

43. Kornfield, M., Snyder, R. D., and Wenger, D. A., *Fucosidosis with angiokeratoma. Electron microscopic changes in the skin.* Arch Pathol Lab Med, 1977. 101:478–485.

44. Burck, U., Moser, H. W., Goebel, H. H., Gruttner, R., and Held, K. R., *A case of lipogranulomatosis Farber: Some clinical and ultrastructural aspects.* Eur J Pediatr, 1985. 143:203–208.

45. Chanoki, M., Ishii, M., Fukai, K., Kobayashi, H., Hamada, T., Murakami, K., and Tanaka, A., *Farber's lipogranulomatosis in siblings: Light and electron microscopic studies.* Br J Dermatol, 1989. 121:779–785.

46. Qualman, S. J., Moser, H. W., Valle, D., Moser, A. E., Antonarakis, S. E., Boitnott, J. K., and Zinkham, W. H., *Farber disease: Pathologic diagnosis in sibs with phenotypic variability.* Am J Med Genet Suppl, 1987. 3:233–241.

47. Koga, M., Ishihara, T., Uchino, F., and Fujikwaki, T., *An autopsy case of Farber's lipogranulomatosis in a Japanese boy with gastrointestinal involvement.* Acta Pathol Jpn, 1992. 42:42–48.

48. Abenoza, P., and Sibley, R. K., *Farber's disease: A fine structural study.* Ultrastruct Pathol, 1987. 11:397–403.

49. Hamanaka, S., Hara, A., and Otsuka, F., *A case of Farber's disease—histochemical, electron microscopic and biochemical studies.* Nippon Hifuka Gakkai Zasshi, 1991. 101:629–634.

50. Kim, Y. J., Park, S. J., Park, C. K., Kim, S. H., and Lee, C. W., *A case of Farber lipogranulomatosis.* J Korean Med Sci, 1998. 13:95–98.

51. Kattner, E., Schafer, A., and Harzer, K., *Hydrops fetalis: Manifestation in lysosomal storage diseases including Farber's disease.* Eur J Pediatr, 1997. 156:292–295.

52. Schmoeckel, C., and Hohlfed, M., *A specific ultrastructural marker for disseminated lipogranulomatosis (Farber).* Arch Dermatol Res, 1979. 266:187–196.

53. Zappatini-Tommasi, L., Dumontel, C., Guibaud, P., and Girod, C., *Farber's disease: An ultrastructural study. Report of a case and review of the literature.* Virchows Arch A Pathol Anat Histopathol, 1992. 420:281–290.

54. van Echten-Deckert, G., Klein, A., Linke, T., Heinemann, T., Weisgerber, J., and Sandhoff, K., *Turnover of endogenous ceramide in cultured normal and Farber fibroblasts.* J Lipid Res, 1997. 38:2569–2579.

Hyperlipidemias and the Skin

Xanthomas

Epidemiology. Xanthomas occur most frequently in patients with hyperlipidemia. Some types of xanthomas are associated relatively specifically with certain types of lipid abnormalities, whereas others have less specific associations and may even appear in patients who are normolipemic. Table 15–1 lists the types of primary hyperlipidemias. Some authors have proposed four types of xanthomas, including tendinous, tuberous, eruptive, and planar (including xanthelasma and xanthoma striatum palmaris) [1], each with characteristic clinical presentations [2].

Cutaneous Features. Tendinous xanthomas develop within the fascia and tendons, especially the Achilles tendon. They appear as firm nodules that are skin colored to yellow.

Tuberous xanthomas appear as large, yellowish nodules, often on the skin overlying the knees, elbows, interphalangeal joints, and buttocks. Some authors have described similar lesions on the palms, soles, and trunk [3].

Eruptive xanthomas appear as rapidly developing crops of yellow-red papules surrounded by erythematous halos. They are most common on the arms, legs, and buttocks [4]. Linear distributions related to Koebner's phenomenon have been reported [5]. Eruptive xanthomas tend to resolve when lipid levels return to normal [6]. Eruptive xanthomas are discussed further in Chapter 3.

Xanthelasma palpebrarum is the most common form of xanthoma. It is associated with hyperlipidemia in approximately 50% of cases [7]. Xanthelasma appear as 1–2 mm yellow papules, most prevalent on the upper eyelids and in the periorbital region.

Planar xanthomas have been reported in patients with multiple myeloma and leukemias [8, 9]. These are discussed briefly in Chapter 10. Xanthoma disseminatum, while not usually associated with hyperlipidemia, has been reported in a patient with type IIb hyperlipidemia [10].

Associated Disorders. Tendinous xanthomas are associated with type II hyperlipoproteinemia and elevated levels of low-density lipoprotein (LDL) cholesterol in many cases [11]. Rare cases are also associated with type III hyperlipoproteinemia [4].

Tuberous xanthomas are seen almost exclusively in patients with increased LDL cholesterol levels [12]. Type III hyperlipidemia is frequently seen in these patients [13]. Xanthomatous lesions on palmar creases tend to occur most commonly in patients with type III disease [1, 11]. Tuberous xanthomas have also been associated with types II and IV hyperlipoproteinemia [3, 14]. Tendinous xanthomas are associated with markedly increased levels of LDL cholesterol in nearly all cases [12].

Eruptive xanthomas are associated with type IV hyperlipoproteinemia and with markedly elevated levels of triglycerides [13]. This type of lipid disorder is seen frequently in patients with abnormal glucose metabolism, as well as in patients after exogenous estrogen therapy or ingestion of alcohol [1, 4, 15]. Eruptive xanthomas may also occur in association with types III and V hy-

Table 15–1. Hyperlipidemias

Type of Hyperproteinemia	Type of Xanthoma	Predominant Lipoprotein
Lipoprotein lipase deficiency	Eruptive xanthoma	Chylomicron
Apolipoprotein C-II deficiency	None	Chylomciron ± VLDL
Familial combined hyperlipidemia	Usually none	VLDL ± LDL
Familial hypertriglyceridemia	Usually none	VLDL
Familial hyperlipoproteinemia, type V	Eruptive xanthomas	VLDL and chylomicrons
Familial dysbetalipoproteinemia, type III	Tuberous, eruptive xanthomas, xanthelasma	VLDL and chylomicron remnants
Heterozygous familial hypercholesterolemia	Tendinous, tuberous xanthomas, xanthelasma	LDL
Homozygous familial hypercholesterolemia	Tendinous, tuberous xanthomas, xanthelasma	LDL

LDL = Low-density lipoprotein; VLDL = very-low-density lipoprotein.

From reference 4.

perlipoproteinemia [1, 11] (see also Chapter 3). Xanthelasma palpebrarum may occur in patients with hyperlipidemia, but at least 50% of patients with these lesions do not have any discernible lipid abnormalities [12, 16].

Histologic Features. Tuberous xanthomas are characterized by the presence of cells with extensive lipidization throughout the dermis [3]. Touton giant cells are less common than in other lipid-containing processes.

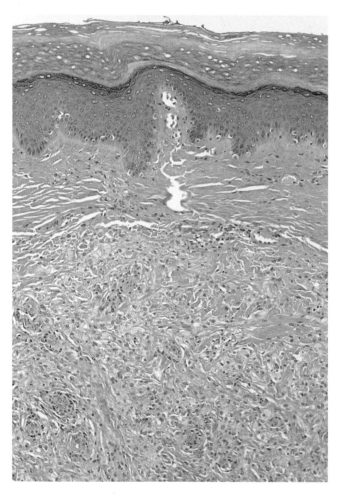

Fig. 15–1. Tuberous xanthoma demonstrates a dermal infiltrate of histiocytes that contain relatively slight amounts of lipid. There are few Touton giant cells and no epidermal changes.

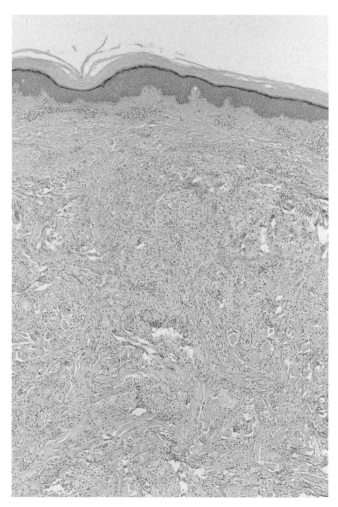

Fig. 15–2. Low magnification view of an eruptive xanthoma demonstrates an infiltrate of histiocytes in the upper reticular dermis.

There is usually no overlying epidermal change. Early lesions may have relatively little lipid within spindle-shaped and epithelioid histiocytes (Fig. 15–1). Tendinous xanthomas have identical histologic changes and are distinguished histologically from tuberous xanthomas based on the location of the xanthoma cells. Tuberous xanthomas demonstrate a reticular dermal infiltrate, and tendinous xanthomas have identical cells located in underlying fascia and tendons.

Eruptive xanthomas are characterized by a proliferation of cells within the upper reticular dermis (Fig. 15–2). A dense perivascular inflammatory infiltrate is usually present, and interstitial lymphocytes may be admixed with abundant histiocytes (Fig. 15–3). Early xanthomas may also have neutrophils in the dermis. Eruptive xanthomas have foamy histiocytes in the dermis, and occasional Touton giant cells may be present [5] (Fig. 15–4). There is a predilection for a perivascular distribution of foamy cells in early lesions. Acid mucopolysaccharides may be present within the superficial reticular dermis [17]. Extracellular lipid is present when serum lipid levels are very high and in acute cases. As lesions age, cells with abundant foamy cytoplasm become less prevalent as the lipid is resorbed. Fibrosis is more prominent in these older lesions.

Xanthelasmas are characterized by aggregates of foamy histiocytes present throughout the dermis (Fig. 15–5 and 15–6). Inflammatory cells are not generally present.

Special Studies. An oil red O stain performed on fresh tissue will demonstrate the presence of intracellular lipid in eruptive and tuberous xanthomas [5].

Pathogenesis. Xanthomas are thought to develop from the accumulation of free and esterified cholesterol

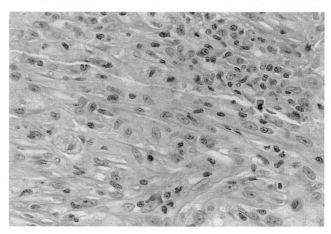

Fig. 15–4. High magnification reveals abundant histiocytes containing lipid, admixed with scattered inflammatory cells.

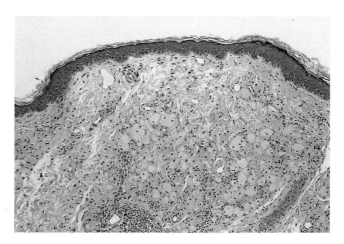

Fig. 15–5. Xanthelasma demonstrates a superficial infiltrate of lipid-laden histiocytes.

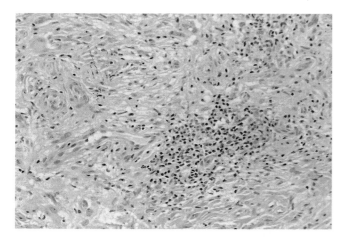

Fig. 15–3. Eruptive xanthomas are characterized by dense perivascular infiltrates of lymphocytes in addition to lipid-laden histiocytes.

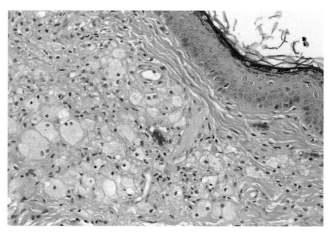

Fig. 15–6. Higher magnification of a xanthoma demonstrates cytoplasmic lipid characteristic of xanthelasmas, as well as other xanthomas.

within dermal histiocytes after the diffusion of high levels of lipoproteins through capillary walls [18].

Xanthoma Disseminatum

Epidemiology. Xanthoma disseminatum (XD) is a very rare disorder that is best classified as one of the non-X histiocytoses [19]. Most of the patients are nomolipemic. Approximately 100 cases are reported in the literature.

Cutaneous Features. Patients present with extensive discrete, scattered, symmetric yellow or red-brown papules and nodules. The neck and proximal extremities are sites of predilection, as are flexural surfaces. Eyelid involvement has been reported [20]. Mucous membranes are involved in up to 40% of patients [21, 22].

Associated Disorders. Xanthoma disseminatum is associated with diabetes insipidus in 40%–50% of cases [23], but in most cases this is mild and reversible [20]. Mucosal involvement of the larynx can result in obstruction necessitating surgery [22]. Other organs, including bones, liver, and conjunctiva, are only rarely involved [22, 24].

Histologic Features. The epidermis in XD is unremarkable or slightly flattened. A dense dermal infiltrate of histiocytes is present within the papillary and reticular dermis. The cells have centrally located nuclei and vesicular cytoplasm. Multinucleated cells may be present. Touton giant cells are only rarely present, and lipidization is not prominent in most cases. The following entities must be considered in the histologic differential diagnosis of XD:

- Benign cephalic histiocytosis
- Eruptive xanthoma
- Langerhans' cell histiocytoses
- Reticulohistiocytoma
- Reticulohistiocytosis
- Xanthogranuloma

Special Studies. In most cases, CD1a immunostaining is helpful in distinguishing XD, in which the proliferating cells are negative, from Langerhans' cell histiocytoses (see Chapter 10), in which case the cells strongly and diffusely express the CD1a antigen. Antibodies directed against S100 protein demonstrate a similar staining pattern and are useful in making this distinction. XD cells often express CD68 and factor XIIIa [19]. Electron microscopy is helpful in distinguishing XD from the Langerhans' cell histiocytoses. Langerhans' cells with Birbeck's granules are not seen in XD [25], but are the primary cells in Langerhans' cell histiocytoses.

Pathogenesis. The pathogenesis for XD, which is a proliferation of monocytes and macrophages, remains unknown [19].

References

1. Vermeer, B. J., van Gent, C.M., Goslings, B., and Polano, M. K., *Xanthomatosis and other clinical findings in patients with elevated levels of very low density lipoproteins.* Br J Dermatol, 1979. 100:657–666.
2. Love, J. R., and Dubin, H. V., *Xanthomas and lipoproteins.* Cutis, 1978. 21:801–805.
3. Cho, H. R., Lee, M. H., and Haw, C. R., *Generalized tuberous xanthoma with type IV hyperlipoproteinemia.* Cutis, 1997. 59:315–318.
4. Cruz, P. D., East, C., and Bergstresser, P. R., *Dermal, subcutaneous and tendon xanthomas: Diagnostic markers for specific lipoprotein disorders.* J Am Acad Dermatol, 1988. 19:95–111.
5. Miwa, N., and Kanzaki, T., *The Koebner phenomenon in eruptive xanthoma.* J Dermatol, 1992. 19:48–50.
6. Crowe, M. J., and Gross, D. J., *Eruptive xanthoma.* Cutis, 1992. 50:31–32.
7. Bergman, R., *The pathogenesis and clinical significance of xanthelasma palpebrarum.* J Am Acad Dermatol, 1994. 30:236–242.
8. Marcoval, J., Moreno, A., Bordas, X., Gallardo, F., and Peyri, J., *Diffuse plane xanthoma: Clinicopathologic study of 8 cases.* J Am Acad Dermatol, 1998. 39: 439–442.
9. Derrick, E. K., and Price, M. L., *Plane xanthomatosis with chronic lymphatic leukaemia.* Clin Exp Dermatol, 1993. 18:259–260.
10. Woollons, A., and Darley, C. R., *Xanthoma disseminatum: A case with hepatic involvement, diabetes insipidus and type IIb hyperlipidaemia.* Clin Exp Dermatol, 1998. 23:277–280.
11. Hessel, L. W., Vermeer, B. J., Polano, M. K., De Jonge, H., De Pagter, H. A., and van Gent, C. M., *Primary hyperlipoproteinemia in xanthomatosis.* Clin Chim Acta, 1976. 69:405–416.
12. Hata, Y., Shigematsu, H., Tsushima, M., Oikawa, T., Yamamoto, M., Yamauchi, Y., and Hirose, N., *Serum lipid and lipoprotein profiles in patients with xanthomas: A correlative study on xanthoma and atherosclerosis (I).* Jpn Circ J, 1981. 45:1236–1242.
13. Kusic, M., Stankovic, K., and Gavrilovic, M., *Xanthomatosis in patients with hyperlipoproteinemia.* Zb Vojnomed Akad, 1982. 24:14–18.
14. Bulkley, B. H., Buja, L.M., Ferrans, V. J., Bulkley, G. B., and Roberts, W. C., *Tuberous xanthoma in homozygous type II hyperlipoproteinemia. A histologic, histochemical, and electron microscopic study.* Arch Pathol, 1975. 99:293–300.
15. Kock, S., *Eruptive xanthoma as an early manifestation of type I diabetes mellitus.* Dtsch Med Wochenschr, 1996. 121:323.

16. Vermeer, B. J., and Gevers Leuven, J., *New aspects of xanthomatosis and hyperlipoproteinemia*. In *Metabolic Disorders and Nutrition Correlated with Skin*. B. J. Vermeer et al., Eds. 1991, Karger, Basal, pp. 63–72.
17. Cooper, P. H., *Eruptive xanthoma: A microscopic simulant of granuloma annulare*. J Cutan Pathol, 1986. 13:207–215.
18. Parker, F., *Xanthomas and hyperlipidemias*. J Am Acad Dermatol, 1985. 13:1–30.
19. Zelger, B. W. H., Sidoroff, A., Orchard, G., and Cerio, R., *Non-Langerhans cell histiocytoses*. Am J Dermatopathol, 1996. 18:490–504.
20. Zelger, B., Cerio, R., Orchard, G., Fritsch, P., and Wilson-Jones, E., *Histologic and immunohistochemical study comparing xanthoma disseminatum and histiocytosis X*. Arch Dermatol, 1992. 128:1207–1212.
21. Mishkel, M. A., Cockshott, W. P., Nazir, D. J., Rosenthal, D., Spaulding, W. P., and Wynn-Williams, A., *Xanthoma disseminatum—clinical, metabolic, pathologic, and radiologic aspects*. Arch Dermatol, 1977. 113:1094–1100.
22. Maloney, J. R., *Xanthoma disseminatum: Its otolaryngological manifestations*. J Laryngol Otol, 1979. 93:201–210.
23. Altman, J., and Winkelmann, R. K., *Xanthoma disseminatum*. Arch Dermatol, 1962. 86:582–596.
24. Battaglini, J., and Olson, T., *Disseminated xanthosiderohistiocyosis, a variant of xanthoma disseminatum, in a patient with plasma cell dyscrasia*. J Am Acad Dermatol, 1984. 11:750–755.
25. Kumarkiri, M., Sudoh, M., and Miura, Y., *Xanthoma disseminatum—report of a case, with histological and ultrastructural studies of skin lesions*. J Am Acad Dermatol, 1981. 4:291–299.

Nutritional Imbalances and the Skin

Phrynoderma

Epidemiology. Because vitamin A is lipid soluble and is stored in fat, vitamin A deficiency is usually found only in patients with malnutrition or other causes of severe nutritional deficiencies, including diabetes mellitus [1]. It has also been described in children after severe measles infection [2]. Phrynoderma has been reported after bowel-bypass surgery for morbid obesity [3, 4]. It is very rare.

Cutaneous Features. Patients demonstrate hyperkeratotic follicular papules. Slight erythema may be present surrounding the follicular orifices.

Associated Disorders. Patients with phrynoderma experience night-blindness [3]. Phrynoderma has been associated with a perforating folliculitis in a diabetic patient with vitamin A deficiency [1]. Phrynoderma has been associated with other nutritional deficiencies, including riboflavin, α-tocopherol [5], and essential fatty acids [6]. Acute vitamin A deficiency has also been reported in patients with severe measles [2].

Histologic Features. Histologic changes of phrynoderma consist of keratin plugging of hair follicles. Epidermal hyperkeratosis is present [3]. In severe cases, eccrine gland atrophy and squamous metaplasia may be present [7] (Fig. 16–1). The following entities must be considered in the histologic differential diagnosis of phrynoderma:

- Keratosis pilaris
- Lichen sclerosis et atrophicus
- Lichen spinulosus
- Lupus erythematosus
- Scurvy

Special Studies. Special studies performed on skin biopsy specimens are not helpful, but serum vitamin A levels help establish the diagnosis.

Pathogenesis. In the vast majority of cases, phrynoderma arises from decreased levels of vitamin A, usually due to malabsorption or other severe nutritional deficiency [3]. Vitamin A plays a central role in keratinocyte differentiation. It has been shown to increase rates of keratinocyte proliferation [8] and transit through the epidermis [9] and to play a vital role in terminal differentiation [10]. Decreased levels of vitamin A lead to premature production of 67 kD keratins and terminal differentiation [11]. Some investigators have speculated that the pathologic changes are more related to decreased essential fatty acids than to low levels of vitamin A [6]. Others have implicated a deficiency of vitamin E in the pathogenesis of the disease [12].

Hypervitaminosis A

Epidemiology. Hypervitaminosis A is an unusual condition that occurs most commonly due to excessive intake of carrots, liver, or vitamin supplements [13]. Occasional patients with oral retinoid therapy may develop a similar condition [14].

Cutaneous Features. The clinical appearance of hypervitaminosis A has been compared with that of con-

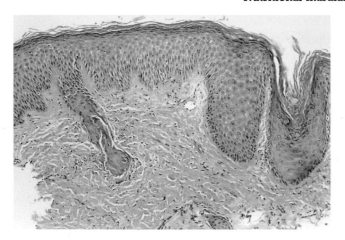

Fig. 16–1. Phrynoderma is characterized by follicular plugging and, in some cases, squamous metaplasia of the eccrine coils.

tact dermatitis and pellagra [15]. Cheilitis, dryness of mucous membranes, desquamation, hair loss, and xerosis are also reported [13, 14].

Associated Disorders. Hypervitaminosis A has been associated with increased serum lipid levels [14]. Vomiting and diarrhea may also occur.

Histologic Features. The histologic changes seen in hypervitaminosis A are nonspecific.

Special Studies. Special studies are not helpful in making a histologic diagnosis of hypervitaminosis A. Serologic tests usually confirm the diagnosis.

Pathogenesis. The relationship between cutaneous changes and increased circulating levels of vitamin A are still largely speculative.

Scurvy

Epidemiology. Scurvy is a rarely encountered disorder that is now seen predominantly in people with unusual dietary restrictions and habits [16, 17].

Cutaneous Features. Patients with scurvy present with a purpuric eruption. There is frequently follicular hyperkeratosis with surrounding small folliculocentric hemorrhage [18]. Corkscrew hairs are present, and gingival hemorrhage may also be observed [16].

Associated Disorders. Associated anomalies consist of myalgias and malaise [18]. Seventy-five percent of patients with scurvy also have a normochromic, normocytic anemia [16].

Scurvy occurs in patients with malabsorption, in alcoholics, and in patients with mental illness [16]. Pa-

tients receiving chronic dialysis also are at increased risk for developing scurvy [16].

Histologic Features. Hair follicle orifices are plugged with increased amounts of orthokeratotic keratin. Vessels surrounding hair follicles are ectatic and congested, and extravasated erythrocytes are present throughout the superficial portions of the dermis.

Special Studies. Serum levels of ascorbic acid are helpful in establishing the diagnosis of scurvy.

Pathogenesis. Scurvy is caused by decreased levels of ascorbic acid. Decreased levels of ascorbic acid lead to instability in the production of tropocollagen. This results in disintegration of connective tissue surrounding blood vessels [16]. The cause of the follicular plugging is not currently understood.

Pellagra

Epidemiology. Pellagra is an uncommon disease caused by a deficiency of niacin or its precursor amino acid, tryptophan. It classically presents with the triad of dermatitis, diarrhea, and dementia.

Cutaneous Features. Pellagra is characterized by scaly and hyperkeratotic erythematous macules that are distributed primarily in sun-exposed areas. Areas of repeated pressure or trauma are also preferentially involved. Affected skin is red-brown and has a sharply demarcated border. It is usually symmetric, involving the face, neck, hands, and forearms. The characteristic neck involvement has been termed "Casal's necklace." Legs can also be affected [19]. A burning sensation may be the initial cutaneous manifestation. Late lesions are characterized by extensive fissuring and hyperpigmentation.

Associated Disorders. In addition to the cutaneous manifestations, patients with pellagra classically present with diarrhea and dementia. Rectal inflammation and ulceration may accompany the gastrointestinal symptoms [20].

Pellagra is observed in patients with nutritional disorders. Pellagra is most frequently encountered in association with alcoholism and may be seen without the usual skin findings in these patients [21]. Pellagra has also been associated with isoniazid treatment in poorly nourished patients with tuberculosis [22] and after 5-fluorouracil treatment for cancer [23]. Treatment with carbamazepine has also resulted in pellagra [24]. Patients with anorexia nervosa have developed pellagra [25], and it has been seen rarely as a complication of long-standing hemodialysis [26].

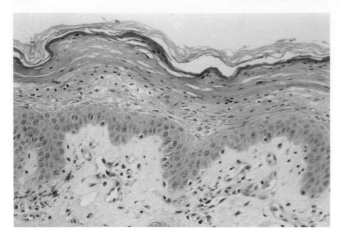

Fig. 16–2. Confluent parakeratosis and abrupt pallor of the upper half of a slightly acanthotic epidermis are present in pellagra.

Histologic Features. The histologic changes in pellagra are nonspecific and resemble those seen in other nutritional deficiency disorders. Confluent parakeratosis is present overlying psoriasiform epidermal hyperplasia. The upper portions of the epidermis demonstrate an abrupt pallor identical to that seen in necrolytic migratory erythema and acrodermatitis enteropathica. Slight spongiosis may be present. A mild lymphohistiocytic inflammatory infiltrate is present around the superficial vascular plexus (Fig. 16–2). The following entities must be considered in the differential diagnosis of pellagra:

- Acrodermatitis enteropathica
- Cystic fibrosis–associated dermatosis
- Hartnup's disease
- Necrolytic migratory erythema

Special Studies. Serum levels of nicotinamide and vitamin B$_6$ are helpful in establishing the diagnosis.

Pathogenesis. Pellagra is believed to be caused by an increase in the viscosity of extracellular matrix. Sun exposure releases various mediators that cannot diffuse due to the increased viscosity. Nicotinic acid, which is lacking in this condition, is essential for the degradation of glycosaminoglycans. Their accumulation leads to the increased viscosity [27].

Hartnup's Disease

Epidemiology. Hartnup's disease is a rare inherited metabolic disease. It consists of an abnormality in renal and/or intestinal transport of neutral amino acids. In some cases, autosomal dominant inheritance has been reported [28]. Although usually inherited, cases with adult onset have been reported [29].

Cutaneous Features. The cutaneous eruption of Hartnup's disease is indistinguishable from that seen in pellagra.

Associated Disorders. Patients with Hartnup's disease may be of small stature and have subnormal intelligence. Cerebellar ataxia and psychiatric disturbances have also been described [30]. Dystonia occurs in patients with Hartnup's disease. These anomalies are not, however, always present in patients with Hartnup's disease [28].

Histologic Features. The histologic features of the cutaneous eruption associated with Hartnup's disease are identical to those seen in patients with pellagra.

Special Studies. Special studies to evaluate amino acids in the urine are helpful in confirming the diagnosis [29].

Pathogenesis. The disease is caused by defective intestinal tryptophan absorption and/or impaired renal tubular resorption of neutral amino acids [31].

Richner-Hanhart Syndrome (Type II Oculotyrosinosis)

Epidemiology. Oculocutaneous tyrosinosis type II, or Richner-Hanhart syndrome, is a rare genodermatosis with an autosomal recessive inheritance pattern [32]. The genetic defect has been mapped to the long arm of chromosome 16 [33, 34].

Cutaneous Features. Patient with oculocutaneous tyrosinosis type II present with palmoplantar keratosis, usually during the first year of life. Punctate keratoses are most characteristic [35]. The keratoderma may begin as bullae and erosions, which gradually develop into white-yellow hyperkeratotic papules or plaques. Fingertips and thenar eminences are commonly involved, as are weight-bearing regions of the soles. The hyperkeratoses are frequently painful [36]. Late-onset hyperkeratosis of the palms and soles has been reported [32]. Leukokeratosis of the tongue has also been reported [37].

Associated Disorders. Patients with Richner-Hanhart syndrome often suffer from bilateral keratitis [32]. Photophobia, pain, excess tearing, and redness are also present [36]. Mental retardation is frequently seen, but is not invariable [32]. Impaired tyrosine degradation leads to axonal degeneration and other central nervous system changes [38]. An association with hepatolenticular degeneration (Wilson's disease has also been reported [39].

Histologic Features. The histologic changes in tyrosinosis type II include marked thickening of the stratum corneum with hyperkeratosis. Focal parakeratosis overlying the acrosyringia has been described [36]. Acanthosis is present, and individually keratinizing keratinocytes are frequently detected. Multinucleated keratinocytes may also be present.

Special Studies. Serum and urinary levels of tyrosine are helpful in establishing the diagnosis [32]. Electron microscopic examination reveals intracytoplasmic vacuoles within all keratinocytes and electron dense particles in the cytoplasm of superficial keratinocytes. Tyrosine crystals are present. Mitochondrial alterations and lysosomal defects are present in these cells [35]. Clumping of keratin filaments is frequently found [36].

Pathogenesis. The cause of Richner-Hanhart syndrome is a defect in soluble tyrosine aminotransferase in liver cells [35]. It is believed that intracellular tyrosine crystals damage lysosomal membranes and cause the release of lysosomal proteins that induce the cellular changes [37]. Tyrosine induces cross-linking of keratin, leading to abnormal tonofilament aggregation [36].

Kwashiorkor

Epidemiology. Kwashiorkor is a common problem worldwide, but is relatively uncommon in the United States. It is most common in children and tends to occur in less well-developed countries [40].

Cutaneous Features. The cutaneous features have been described as a "flaky paint dermatitis" or as an enamel paint sign [40, 41]. The eruption is often generalized and has an eczematous appearance with extensive desquamation [40]. The earliest changes are often present in areas subject to friction such as behind the knees, on the buttocks, and on the elbows [42]. Hypochromotrichia, alopecia, and glossitis are also described [43]. Atrophic scars may be present in later lesions [42].

Associated Disorders. Patients with kwashiorkor are severely malnourished. They often present with marked peripheral edema [40]. Weight loss, liver disease, neurologic disorders, and diarrhea are also present. Serologic studies demonstrate marked hypoalbuminemia [43].

Histologic Features. The are no specific histopathologic changes described in biopsy tissue taken from patients with kwashiorkor.

Special Studies. Serum albumin levels are helpful for making the diagnosis, but special skin biopsy studies are not necessary.

Pathogenesis. Kwashiorkor is caused by protein deficiency coupled with carbohydrate excess [43].

NOTE: Cystic fibrosis, which also causes a nutritional deficiency–induced cutaneous eruption, is discussed in Chapter 6.

References

1. Neill, S. M., Pembroke, A. C., du Vivier, A. W., and Salisbury, J. R., *Phyrnoderma and perforating folliculitis due to vitamin A deficiency in a diabetic.* J R Soc Med, 1988. 81:171–172.
2. Goskowicz, M., and Eichenfield, L. F., *Cutaneous findings of nutritional deficiences in children.* Curr Opin Pediatr, 1993. 5:441–445.
3. Weschler, H. L., *Vitamin A deficiency following small-bowel bypass surgery for obesity.* Arch Dermatol, 1979. 115:73–75.
4. Barr, D. J., Riley, R. J., and Greco, D. J., *Bypass phyrnoderma. Vitamin A deficiency associated with bowel-by-pass surgery.* Arch Dermatol, 1984. 120:919–921.
5. Christiansen, E. N., Piyasena, C., Bjorneboe, G. E., Bibow, K., Nilsson, A., and Wandel, M., *Vitamin E deficiency in phyrnoderma cases from Sri Lanka.* Am J Clin Nutr, 1988. 47:253–255.
6. Ghafoorunissa, Vidyasagar, R., and Krishnaswamy, K., *Phyrnoderma: Is it an EFA deficiency disease.* Eur J Clin Nutr, 1988. 42:29–39.
7. Logan, W. S., *Vitamin A and keratinization.* Arch Dermatol, 1972. 105:748–753.
8. Wilkinson, D. I., *Effect of vitamin A acid on the growth of keratinocytes in culture.* Arch Dermatol Res, 1978. 263:75–81.
9. Plewig, G., and Braun-Falco, O., *Kinetics of epidermis and adnexa following vitamin A acid in the human.* Acta Derm Venereol (Stockh), 1975. 74:87–98.
10. Fuchs, E., and Green, H., *Regulation of terminal differentiation of cultured human keratinocytes by vitamin A.* Cell, 1981. 25:617–625.
11. Kim, K. H., Schwartz, F., and Euchs, E., *Differences in keratin synthesis between normal epithelial cells and squamous cell carcinomas are mediated by vitamin A.* Proc Natl Acad Sci USA, 1984. 81:4280–4284.
12. Nadiger, H. A., *Role of vitamin E in the aetiology of phyrnoderma (follicular hyperkeratosis) and its interrelationship with B-complex vitamins.* Br J Nutr, 1980. 44:211–214.
13. Nagai, K., Hosoaka, H., Kubo, S., Nakabayahi, T., Amagasaki, Y., and Nakamura, N., *Vitamin A toxicity secondary to excessive intake of yellow-green vegetables, liver and laver.* J Hepatol, 1999. 31:142–148.
14. Shalita, A. R., *Mucocutaneous and systemic toxicity of*

retinoids: Monitoring and management. Dermatologica, 1987. 175(Suppl 1):151–157.

15. Hamann, K., and Avnstorp, C., *Chronic hypervitaminosis A with skin changes.* Hautarzt, 1982. 33:559–561.

16. Ghorbani, A. J., and Eichler, C., *Scurvy.* J Am Acad Dermatol, 1994. 30:881–883.

17. Ellis, C. N., Vanderveen, E. E., and Rasmussen, J. E., *Scurvy. A case caused by peculiar dietary habits.* Arch Dermatol, 1984. 120:1212–1214.

18. Adelman, H. M., Wallach, P. M., Gutierrez, F., Kreitzer, S. M., Seleznick, M. J., Espinoza, C. G., and Espinoza, L. R., *Scurvy resembling cutaneous vasculitis.* Cutis, 1994. 54:111–114.

19. Isaac, S., *The "gauntlet" of pellagra.* Int J Dermatol, 1998. 37:599.

20. Segal, I., Ou Tim, L., Demetriou, A., Paterson, A., Hale, M., and Lerious, M., *Rectal manifestations of pellagra.* Int J Colorectal Dis, 1986. 1:238–243.

21. Ishii, N., and Nishihara, Y., *Pellagra among chronic alcoholics: Clinical and pathological study of 20 necropsy cases.* J Neurol Neurosurg Psychiatry, 1981. 44:209–215.

22. Ishii, N., and Nishihara, Y., *Pellagra encephalopathy among tuberculous patients: Its relation to isoniazid therapy.* J Neurol Neurosurg Psychiatry, 1985. 48:628–634.

23. Stevens, H. P., Ostlere, L. S., Begent, R. H., Dooley, J. S., and Rustin, M. H., *Pellagra secondary to 5–fluorouracil.* Br J Dermatol, 1993. 128:578–580.

24. Heyer, G., Simon, M., and Schell, H., *Dose-dependent pellagroid skin reaction caused by carbamazepine.* Hautarzt, 1998. 49:123–125.

25. Rapaport, M. J., *Pellagra in a patient with anorexia nervosa.* Arch Dermatol, 1985. 121:255–257.

26. Waterlot, Y., Sabot, J. P., Marchal, M., and Vanherweghem, J. L., *Pellagra: Unusual cause of paranoid delirium in dialysis.* Nephrol Dial Transplant, 1986. 1:204–205.

27. Stone, O. J., *Pellagra—increased viscosity of extracellular matrix.* Med Hypotheses, 1993. 40:355–359.

28. Scriver, C. R., Mahon, B., Levy, H. L., Clow, C. L., Reade, T. M., Kronick, J., Lemieux, B., and Laberge, C., *The Hartnup phenotype: Mendelian transport disorder, multifactorial disease.* Am J Hum Genet, 1987. 40:401–412.

29. Oakley, A., and Wallace, J., *Hartnup disease presenting in an adult.* Clin Exp Dermatol, 1994. 19:407–408.

30. Mori, E., Yamadori, A., Tsutsumi, A., and Kyotani, Y., *Adult-onset Hartnup disease presenting with neuropsychiatric symptoms but without skin lesions.* Rinsho Shinkeigaku, 1989. 29:687–692.

31. Wong, P. W. K., and Pillai, P. M., *Clinical and biochemical observations in two cases of Hartnup disease.* Arch Dis Child, 1966. 41:383–388.

32. Podglajen-Wecxsteen, O., Delaporte, E., Piette, F., le Flohic, X., and Bergoend, H., *Oculocutanous type II tyrosinosis.* Ann Dermatol Venereol, 1993. 120:139–142.

33. Natt, E., Kao, F. T., Rettenmeier, R., and Scherer, G., *Assignment of the human tyrosine aminotransferase gene to chromosome 16.* Hum Genet, 1986. 72:225–228.

34. Barton, D. E., Yang-Feng, T. L., and Francke, U., *The human tyrosine aminotransferase gene mapped to the long arm chromosome 16 (region 16q22–q24) by somatic cell hybrid analysis and in situ hybridization.* Hum Genet, 1986. 72:221–224.

35. Larregue, M., De Giacomoni, P., Odievre, P., and Prigent, F., *Changes in the keratinocytes in oculo-cutaneous tyrosinosis: Richner-Hanhart syndrome.* Ann Dermatol Venereol, 1980. 107:1023–1030.

36. Tallab, T. M., *Richner-Hanhart syndrome: Importance of early diagnosis and early intervention.* J Am Acad Dermatol, 1996. 35:857–859.

37. Larregue, M., de Giacomoni, P., Bressiex, J. M., and Odievre, M., *Richner-Hanhart's syndrome or oculo-cutaneous tyrosinosis.* Ann Dermatol Venereol, 1979. 106:53–62.

38. Kobayashi, M., Nakamura, T., and Akai, K., *A neuropathological investigation of a case of tyrosinosis.* Acta Pathol Jpn, 1980. 30:285–292.

39. Thiel, H. J., and Weidle, E., *Tyrosinosis with hepatolenticular degeneration.* Klin Monatsbl Augenheilkd, 1983. 182:232–234.

40. Eastlack, J. P., Grande, K. K., Levy, M. L., and Nigro, J. F., *Dermatosis in a child with kwashiorkor secondary to food aversion.* Pediatr Dermatol, 1999. 16:95–102.

41. Buno, I. J., Morelli, J. G., and Weston, W. L., *The enamel paint sign in the dermatologic diagnosis of early-onset kwashiorkor.* Arch Dermatol, 1998. 134:107–108.

42. Latham, M. C., *The dermatosis of kwashiorkor in young children.* Semin Dermatol, 1991. 10:270–272.

43. Albers, S. E., Brozena, S. J., and Fenske, N. A., *A case of kwashiorkor.* Cutis, 1993. 51:445–446.

PART IV

Infectious Diseases and the Skin

CHAPTER
17

Bacterial Diseases

DIRECT BACTERIAL INFECTIONS

Meningococcemia

Epidemiology. Acute meningococcemia develops as an abrupt, often life-threatening condition that is most common in children, but does occur in patients of all ages. It gives rise to the clinical syndrome known as *purpura fulminans.*

A rare, chronic form of meningococcal infection occurs. This form of the disease is more common in adults than in children [1].

Cutaneous Features. Skin findings are present in more than 80% of patients with acute meningococcemia. Acute meningococcemia may present as a vasculitis, with hemorrhagic papules and pustules with necrotic centers. They are usually widespread and may show some predilection for distal extremities.

Purpura fulminans is characterized by the rapid onset of hemorrhagic macules, which progress to infarction within hours. Distal extremities are most dramatically involved.

Chronic meningococcemia is characterized by widespread erythematous and purpuric, crusted papules and pustules. Older lesions have a necrotic center [1].

Associated Disorders. The most frequent, and one of the most important, manifestations of meningococcemia is inflammation of the meninges that can lead to serious neurologic complications and death.

Arthralgias are frequently present in patients with both acute and chronic meningococcemia. These tend to be most pronounced during periods of fevers [2, 3].

Occasional patients with meningococcemia experience heart problems, including endocarditis and complete heart block [4, 5].

Histologic Features. Acute and chronic meningococcemia are both characterized by a leukocytoclastic vasculitis that is indistinguishable from leukocytoclastic vasculitis secondary to other causes [1]. It has been suggested that the inflammatory infiltrate is not as pronounced in leukocytoclastic vasculitis caused by meningococcal infection as it is in hypersensitivity-related vasculitides. In some cases, abundant organisms can be identified within vessel walls [6]. The histologic features of purpura fulminans include thrombosis of dermal blood vessels, with secondary hemorrhagic necrosis within the dermis and epidermis [7].

Special Studies. Direct immunofluorescence can be used to identify organisms directly in lesional skin [2].

Pathogenesis. Vascular damage and the subsequent inflammation present in meningococcemia are due, at least in part, to the direct invasion of vessel walls by bacteria [8]. *Neisseria meningitidis* produces an endotoxin causing release of cytokines, including interleukin-12, interferon-γ, tumor necrosis factor-α, and interleukin-1. These cytokines result in the consumption of proteins C and S and antithrombin III, which creates a significant bleeding diathesis [7].

Septic Vasculitis/Emboli

Epidemiology. Septic emboli occur in patients with sepsis and are occasinally associated with endocarditis, occur after trauma to blood vessels, and are present in immunocompromised patients [9].

Cutaneous Features. Cutaneous manifestations of septic emboli include hemorrhagic necrotic papules and nodules often located acrally and in sites of pressure. The tips of the fingers and toes, nose, and ears are common sites of involvement. The earliest changes may be faintly erythematous macules and papules. Pustules may also be present in some cases. Presentation with palpable purpura, in a pattern resembling leukocytoclastic vasculitis, is also described [9, 10].

Associated Disorders. Septic emboli are usually associated with underlying systemic infection. Subacute bacterial endocarditis may also be associated with these types of emboli [11]. Infection of nasal sinuses has also resulted in septic emboli [12]. Local trauma such as surgery to vessels can give rise to septic emboli by introducing exogenous bacteria and disrupting the endothelial lining, predisposing to clot formation [10, 13, 14]. *Pseudomonas, Streptococcus, Staphylococcus,* and *Gonococcus* are associated with septic vasculitis and embolization in most cases. Septic emboli also are more frequent in immunocompromised patients [9]. Angioinvasive fungi may also give rise to septic emboli (see Chapter 19).

Histologic Features. Early lesions of septic emboli demonstrate occlusion of dermal blood vessels with fibrin thrombi and clusters of organisms (Figure 17–1). Endothelial swelling may be quite marked. Inflammation is not marked, but scattered neutrophils may be present. Extravasation of erythrocytes into the surrounding dermis is commonly seen (Fig. 17–2). In later lesions, a neutrophilic infiltrate may become more

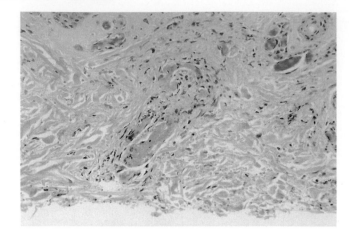

Fig. 17–2. Higher magnification demonstrates a minimally inflammatory vaso-occlusive process as is seen in early cases of septic vasculitis.

prominent. Necrosis of the surrounding dermis and overlying epidermis develops in the areas of vascular occlusion. In patients receiving cytoreductive therapy, the degree of inflammation is often less and may be essentially absent. The following entities must be considered in the histologic differential diagnosis of septic emboli:

- Cryoglobulinemia
- Disseminated intravascular coagulation
- Lupus anticoagulant
- Protein C/S deficiency
- Sneddon's syndrome
- Trombocytopenic thrombotic purpura

Special Studies. Tissue Gram stains may be helpful in determining the nature of the organisms found within vessel lumens. In most cases, however, they can be detected with routine histologic stains.

Pathogenesis. Clusters of organisms dislodge from larger colonies and spread hematogenously. In small vessels, the clusters are too large to easily pass through the channels, lodging within the vessel walls, causing occlusion of the vessels, secondary infarction, and the precipitation of a marked inflammatory response.

Syphilis

Epidemiology. Following a long period of slow decline, the incidence of syphilis rapidly increased from 1985 to 1990. In 1993, more than 26,000 cases of syphilis were reported in the United States [15]. The incidence in the United States was estimated at 20 per 100,000 in 1990 [16]. The incidence appears again to have decreased from 1993 to 1998 [17]. By 1998, the

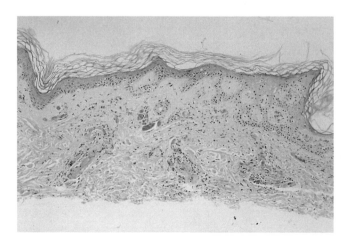

Fig. 17–1. Fibrin thrombi are present in vessels throughout the dermis, with relatively little surrounding inflammation in early lesions of septic vasculitis.

incidence had decreased to 3.2 cases per 100,00 people [18]. The increased incidence is most prominent among young, heterosexual adults. Syphilis is approximately 44 times more common in African Americans than in white Americans [18]. There has also been a dramatic increase in the incidence of congenital syphilis since about 1985 [15].

Cutaneous Features. A primary chancre, or ulceration, appears at the site of treponemal penetration within 3–5 weeks of exposure in the vast majority of patients. It begins as a dusky, erythematous macule that progresses to a sharply demarcated papule with a rolled border and an eroded surface [19]. Chancres are usually nontender. In men, the glans penis is the most common location for a primary chancre. In women, the primary chancre may be seen on the labia majora, labia minora, cervix, fourchette, urethra, or perineum. Chancres appear more edematous and are more frequently ulcerated in women. Oral chancres are occasionally found. This initial lesion resolves spontaneously and without scarring within 2 months.

Secondary syphilis has many different clinical appearances. Cutaneous eruptions are present in more than 90% of patients with secondary syphilis. The eruption may be localized or widespread. Most patients present with erythematous macules or macules and papules. In some cases, an annular configuration of the papules may be present. Lichenoid papules are present in some patients and may have a folliculocentric appearance [20]. Nodules are reported in some patients [21]. Pruritus is present in a few cases. Condyloma lata, which are broad, flat growths located mainly on folds of moist skin, are present in 10% of patients with secondary syphilis. Mucous patches, which are 4–5 mm soft, gray erosions located on the tonsils, tongue, and gums, occur in 10% of these patients and alopecia in approximately 1% of patients with secondary syphilis [22]. The alopecia may have the characteristic "moth-eaten" appearance. Telogen effluvium has also been described in patients with secondary syphilis [15]. Rarely, papules may appear along the hair line in a pattern known as *corona veneris* [23].

Bullae and vesicles are uncommon, but may rarely occur in secondary syphilis [24]. Lues maligna is an explosive, severe form of secondary syphilis that is characterized by an eruption of papules and pustules that rapidly become necrotic ulcers. These lesions usually involve the face and the scalp. This form of the disease is most common in immunocompromised or debilitated patients [15].

Tertiary syphilis develops in about one-third of untreated patients. These patients develop gummata and cardiovascular or neurologic symptoms. The cutaneous lesions may appear as erythematous to violaceous annular, scaling plaques, may be ulcerated, or may appear psoriasiform [25].

Congenital syphilis often presents with desquamation over the palms and soles [26]. The commonly described anomalies seen in children with congenital syphilis include mulberry molars, notched incisors, frontal bossing, "saddle nose" deformity, and interstitial keratitis. Eighth nerve deafness may be seen, as can periostitis. Annular lesions have also been described in this population [27]. Thickening of the skin over the palms and soles is present. Similar thickenings may be present at the corners of the mouth and often develop thick fissures known as *rhagades*. These lesions heal with radiating scars.

Associated Disorders. Lymphadenopathy may be present at the time that a chancre develops. The inguinal region is the most frequent site for the typical unilateral lymphadenopathy.

Secondary syphilis can involve virtually any organ. Consititutional symptoms including headaches and fevers are present in many patients. Among the most commonly encountered signs are iritis, periostitis, arthritis, acute glomerulonephritis, and hepatitis [28–33]. Cardiovascular involvement is occasionally manifested by the presence of an aortic aneurysm [34]. Thrombocytosis has also been reported in these patients [35].

Involvement of the central nervous system occurs in almost half of patients with primary or secondary syphilis and is manifested by elevated cerebrospinal fluid protein levels or white blood cell counts. Approximately one-fourth of these patients have a reactive VDRL in this fluid, and the organism can be cultured from up to one-third of them [15, 36].

Bone changes including metaphyseal dystrophy are present in approximately 85% of babies with congenital syphilis [26]. These neonates also suffer from hepatosplenomegaly, respiratory distress, and jaundice.

One potentially severe consequence of syphilis infection is the Jarisch-Herxheimer reaction. This occurs after the initial dose of antibiotic treatment and is most commonly seen in patients with secondary syphilis. The reaction includes shaking, chills, fever, malaise, arthralgias, myalgias, and headaches and occurs within 6–8 hours after treatment. Hospitalization is often required for patients who develop this reaction.

Histologic Features. Histologic changes in syphilis vary widely with the type of lesion biopsied. A primary chancre demonstrates epidermal (or epithelial) hyperplasia adjacent to an ulcer. There is a dense, mixed inflammatory infiltrate that usually has abundant plasma cells. There is exocytosis of lymphocytes into the surface epithelium. Organisms are often abundant and easily found with special stains (see later).

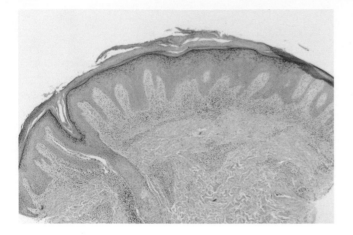

Fig. 17–3. Secondary syphilis often demonstrates a psoriasiform and lichenoid inflammatory reaction pattern.

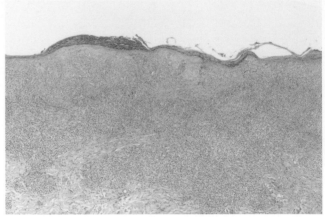

Fig. 17–5. Secondary syphilis may be characterized by a dense, superficial, and deep mixed inflammatory infiltrate.

In biopsy material taken from macules in secondary syphilis, the most frequent finding is that of an infiltrate of lymphocytes and histiocytes surrounding vessels of the superficial vascular plexus. The overlying epidermis is frequently uninvolved. Plasma cells are relatively uncommon [37].

In biopsy material taken from lesions with clinical scaling, parakeratosis and acanthosis are more frequently encountered. In these cases, extensive exocytosis of lymphocytes is usually present, along with a band-like inflammatory infiltrate along the dermal–epidermal junction (Fig. 17–3). Plasma cells are often present, but are rarely the predominant cell type within the inflammatory infiltrate. There may be damage to the basal layer of the epidermis and pigment incontinence. Biopsy specimens appear both psoriasiform and lichenoid [37] (Fig. 17–4).

Other cases of secondary syphilis demonstrate a deeper inflammatory infiltrate, usually surrounding eccrine ducts. In these cases, clusters of plasma cells may be present, in addition to lymphocytes and histiocytes (Figs. 17–5 and 17–6). Epidermal changes similar to those described earlier may be seen in conjunction with the deeper changes. Granulomas are present in a minority of cases and may be surrounded by plasma cells [37]. In other cases, the granulomatous appearance may resemble sarcoidosis, with a paucity of inflammatory cells surrounding the granulomas (Fig. 17–7). The following entities must be considered in the histologic differential diagnosis of syphilis:

- Lichen planus
- Lichen striatus
- Mycosis fungoides
- Pityriasis rosea
- Psoriasis

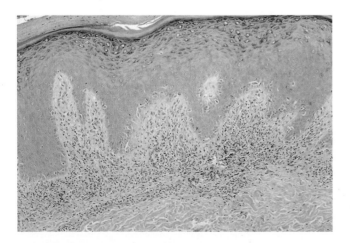

Fig. 17–4. A dense band-like inflammatory infiltrate with destruction of basal keratinocytes and pigment incontinence is present in many cases of secondary syphilis.

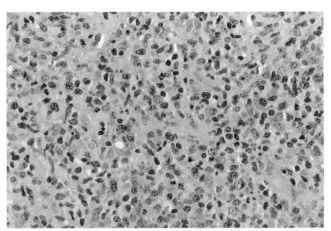

Fig. 17–6. Plasma cells are often admixed with lymphocytes and histiocytes in secondary syphilis.

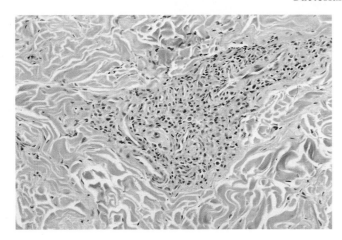

Fig. 17–7. Some cases of secondary syphilis demonstrate granulomas in the deeper reticular dermis.

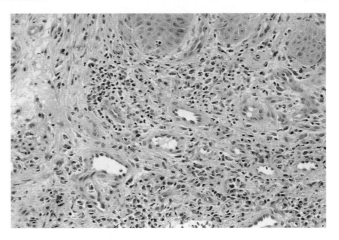

Fig. 17–9. A mixed inflammatory infiltrate containing abundant plasma cells is usually present in condyloma latum.

Condyloma lata demonstrate epidermal hyperplasia with exocytosis of neutrophils. Spongiosis is usually present, and ulceration is a common finding (Fig. 17–8). Endothelial swelling and proliferation are pres-ent, but these are nonspecific findings. Plasma cells are often present surrounding the vessels of the superficial vascular plexus [37] (Fig. 17–9).

Histologic changes seen in alopecia due to secondary syphilis include plugging within the infundibular portions of the hair follicles; a sparse, perivascular, and perifollicular infiltrate of lymphocytes; and occasional plasma cells and a shift toward increased numbers of telogen hairs. Clumping of melanin pigment within the follicles and in the surrounding dermis may lead to confusion with traction alopecia [38].

Special Studies. Warthin-Starry, Steiner, Dieterle, and other silver stains are helpful in detecting organisms.

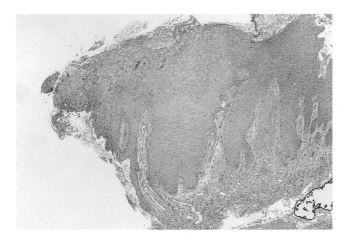

Fig. 17–8. Condyloma latum demonstrates epidermal hyperplasia, ulceration, and a prominent inflammatory infiltrate.

Organisms can be identified in virtually all primary chancres [39]. Only one-third to two-thirds of all cases of secondary syphilis will, however, demonstrate organisms [40]. Furthermore, as melanin granules and elastic tissue fibers also stain black with these stains, extreme care must be taken when interpreting the results. In both situations, most organisms are found along the dermal–epidermal junction [39]. Serologic tests are more sensitive and more specific for making the diagnosis of secondary syphilis. In primary chancres, serologic tests are less reliable, and dark-field examination of the tissue or of scrapings may be helpful in detecting organisms. It has also been demonstrated that serologic studies for syphilis are less reliable in human immunodeficiency virus (HIV)–positive patients.

Pathogenesis. Syphilis is caused by infection with *Treponema pallidum*. This spirochete measures 0.10–0.18 by 6–20 μm and has a characteristic corkscrew appearance (Fig. 17–10). It is usually transmitted by sexual intercourse, where it is estimated that there is a 35% risk of infection in people exposed to sexual contact with others with early syphilis [41].

Lyme Disease

Epidemiology. Lyme disease is caused by infection with *Borrelia burgdorferi*. The deer-tick *Ixodes* transmits the disease to humans. It is difficult to determine an exact incidence for the disease, given the lack of uniformity in disease reporting, as well as the marked variation in reproducibility of serologic tests. There is marked regional variation within the United States concerning the incidence of the disease. Most cases in the United States occur in the Northeast and Midwest. The incidence in Westchester County, New York, has been estimated to be approximately 1.2 cases per 100

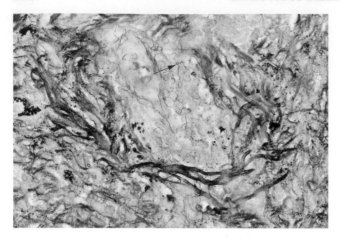

Fig. 17–10. Abundant corkscrew-shaped organisms are demonstrated (arrow) within the papillary dermis on this Warthin-Starry stain performed on tissue from a patient with secondary syphilis.

person-years [42]. Similar regional variations occur in Europe, where seropositivity rates are high in Sweden, the Netherlands, Croatia, and Switzerland and lower in Greece, Estonia, and Poland [43].

Cutaneous Features. There are several cutaneous manifestations of Lyme disease, perhaps dependent, in part, on the subtype of organism responsible for the disease. In the United States, the most common clinical manifestation is that of erythema migrans. This manifestation is also referred to as *erythema chronicum migrans* in some sources. Erythema migrans presents as an annular, erythematous patch with central clearing, most commonly located on the trunk. For reporting purposes, the Centers for Disease Control and Prevention requires that this patch be at least 5 cm in diameter [44]. There is often a thin rim of peripheral scale. The patch continues to enlarge for days to weeks and then stabilizes before resolving without cutaneous sequelae. Vesicles are rarely encountered [45]. A clinically identical eruption has been described in patients who have no serologic evidence of *Borrelia burgdurferi* infection [46].

In the European countries, the most common manifestation of *Borrelia* infection is acrodermatitis chronica atrophicans (ACA). Early lesions appear as erythematous macules and later progress to violaceous infiltrative plaques and nodules. Late lesions resolve with atrophy characteristic of the entity [47]. Less commonly, *Borrelia* infection has been associated with localized morphea/scleroderma [48]. Organisms have not been demonstrated within biopsied lesional skin in most patients with morphea residing in the United States. Although most series suggest that Lyme disease and ACA are separate and not interdependent, clear transition from one form of cutaneous disease to the other has been documented [49].

Lymphocytoma cutis, also known as *lymphadenitis benigna cutis* in the European literature, has been described as a cutaneous manifestation of *Borrelia burgdorferi* infection [50]. Lymphocytoma cutis occurs most frequently on the head and neck, but can be located anywhere. It presents as one or several erythematous, often tender, nodules with no overlying surface changes. Lymphocytoma cutis associated with *Borrelia burgdorferi* infection is clinically indistinguishable from lymphocytoma associated with arthropod bite reactions and as a reaction pattern to some drugs (see Chapter 26).

In a single case, infection with *Borrelia burgdorferi* has been shown to trigger dermatomyositis [51]. Erythema multiforme and "persistent erythema" have also been reported as initial manifestations of Lyme disease [52]. These associations are still unproved, however, as they exist only in single case reports.

Associated Disorders. Periarticular fibrous nodules have been described in patients with late-stage disease. These are seen especially in association with ACA [53, 54].

The central nervous system and musculoskeletal system are the most frequent extracutaneous sites of involvement in Lyme disease. Neural complications may include cranial polyneuritis, acute transverse myelitis, and facial nerve palsies [55, 56].

Myocarditis may occur more frequently in patients with long-standing Lyme disease than is currently believed [57]. Rheumatic complications are rarely associated with Lyme disease; however, if cases remain untreated for prolonged periods, deformities of fingers and toes may result [58]. Involvement of joints appears to be more common in the United States than in Europe. Symmetric oligoarthritis and monoarthritis are the most common patterns seen [59].

Parotitis has been described in one patient with Lyme disease [60]. Borrelial fasciitis in association with peripheral eosinophilia has been described in a few patients with Lyme disease. This appears to be relatively uncommon presentation [61].

Histologic Features. Erythema migrans is characterized by a lymphohistiocytic inflammatory response located in the superficial dermis when biopsy specimens are taken from the erythematous border of the lesion and deeper within the dermis when the central portion of a lesion is biopsied [62] (Figs. 17–11 and 17–12). Plasma cells are seen in some, but not all, cases, and eosinophils may be present in small numbers. The histologic findings are often nonspecific, and, although they may be supportive of a diagnosis of Lyme disease, they are rarely diagnostic.

The histologic findings in ACA include an infiltrate of lymphocytes, histiocytes, and plasma cells surrounding vessels of the superficial vascular plexus [47].

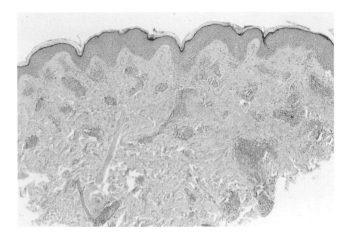

Fig. 17–11. Lyme disease is characterized by a superficial and deep perivascular inflammatory infiltrate.

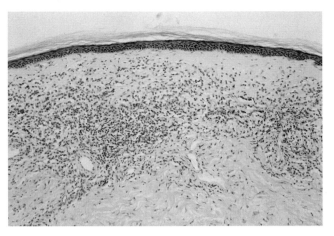

Fig. 17–13. Acrodermatitis chronica atrophicans is characterized by a dense superficial infiltrate of lymphocytes and plasma cells underlying an atrophic epidermis.

Later lesions demonstrate the characteristic epidermal atrophy with effacement of the rete ridges and degeneration of elastic and collagen fibers (Fig. 17–13) [63].

Lymphocytoma cutis, irrespective of the underlying etiology, is characterized by a dense infiltrate of lymphocytes and histiocytes filling the dermis. The epidermis is unremarkable and is often separated from the inflammatory infiltrate by a grenz zone. Follicular centers may be present within the inflammatory infiltrate. Plasma cells and occasional eosinophils are present in most cases. Tingible body macrophages are usually found within the lymphoid nodules and are very helpful in establishing a reactive, as opposed to a neoplastic, etiology for the cellular infiltrate. The inflammatory infiltrate frequently extends into the subcutaneous fat (see Chapter 26).

Special Studies. Organisms can be detected within the dermis in the region of the superficial vascular plexus by a Warthin-Starry or Steiner silver stain. They may be located within endothelial cells [64].

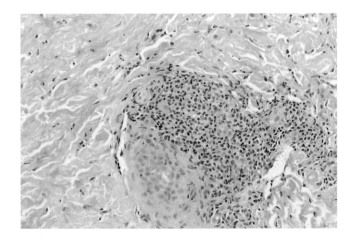

Fig. 17–12. Lymphocytes, histiocytes, and occasional plasma cells may be seen in the infiltrate in Lyme disease.

Culture is a more sensitive technique. Organisms can be isolated from approximately 40% of cases of erythema migrans, regardless of which portion of the lesion is submitted for culture [65].

Polymerase chain reaction has also been shown to be a useful technique for demonstrating the presence of organisms; however, cross-reaction with nonpathogenic organisms may occur [66]. Specific immune complexes have been detected in patients with acute Lyme disease using an enzyme-linked immunoassay. The reported specificities and sensitivities are quite high, but the test is not yet widely available [67].

Pathogenesis. *Borrelia burgdorferi*, *Borrelia garini*, and *Borrelia afzelii* have all been reported to cause Lyme disease. All three species are carried by ticks and transmitted to humans through bites [68]. *Borrelia burgdorferi sensu lato* is most commonly implicated in cases of erythema migrans in the United States. *Borrelia afzelii* is associated with ACA, primarily in Europe [58]. It has been suggested that the pathologic changes found in ACA may be related to a tissue injury mediated by T cells leading to sclerosis [69].

NOTE: Bacillary angiomatosis is discussed in Chapter 18.

Mycobacterial Infections—Tuberculosis

Epidemiology. Tuberculosis can involve the skin in many ways, including direct exogenous infection, contiguous spread from adjacent infected tissue, or hematogenous spread. Following a long, steady decline in incidence, there has been a recent resurgence in the incidence of pulmonary and extrapulmonary tuberculosis, in part attributed to the acquired immunodeficiency syndrome (AIDS) epidemic [70, 71]. Direct exogenous infection has been related to tattooing, external injury, and prosectors [72, 73].

Cutaneous Features. Cutaneous tuberculosis is quite rare, accounting for approximately 2.4% of all cases of tuberculosis in one study [70]. It can involve the skin with several presentations, known as lupus vulgaris, miliary tuberculosis, tuberculosis orificialis, tuberculosis verrucosa cutis, and scrofuloderma. Multiple forms of the disease can occur simultaneously [74].

Lupus vulgaris is the most common form of cutaneous tuberculosis [75]. It is caused by reinfection of the skin in patients with high immunity to the organism, and usually presents as a slowly growing verrucous plaque that begins as a flesh-colored to red papule. On diascopic examination, the lesion may have an "apple jelly" color. More than 80% of lesions are on the head and neck. It follows hematogenous or lymphatic spread from visceral tuberculosis [76]. Up to 30% of patients with lupus vulgaris have a history of scrofuloderma [77]. Lupus vulgaris is seen most commonly in young adults.

Scrofuloderma represents direct extension of disease to the skin from an underlying focus of infection, most commonly a lymph node. It has also been detected overlying tuberculous bones and joints. The cervical lymph nodes are most commonly affected. Scrofuloderma begins as a firm, mobile nodule that attaches to the skin, suppurates, and ulcerates.

Tuberculosis verrucosa appears as a slowly growing plaque on the back of the hands or fingers in people who have high immunity. It is most frequently seen in autopsy workers. Draining sinus tracts may be present [78].

Orificial tuberculosis is a rare manifestation of tuberculosis that is seen in immunocompromised patients who generally have widely disseminated disease. The cutaneous features are nonspecific, often resembling periorificial dermatitis, and are frequently missed [79]. Miliary, or disseminated, tuberculosis presents with generalized papules over the entire skin surface.

Associated Disorders. Infection with *Mycobacterium tuberculosis* can affect virtually any organ system. Abscesses within the central nervous system and tuberculous meningitis can be especially devastating [80, 81]. Abdominal tuberculosis and tubercular infection of the pancreas can also have ominous prognoses [82, 83]. Lupus vulgaris has been detected at the site of bacille Calmette-Guérin vaccine [84]. Rare cases of lupus vulgaris have been associated with squamous cell carcinoma arising at the same site [85].

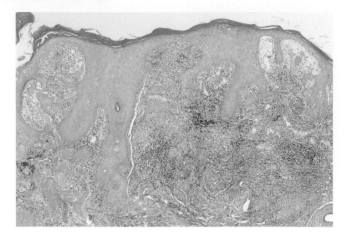

Fig. 17–14. Lupus vulgaris is characterized by epidermal hyperplasia and a dense underlying granulomatous inflammatory reaction.

Histologic Features. Lupus vulgaris is characterized by epidermal hyperplasia and a granulomatous infiltrate within the dermis (Fig. 17–14). Granulomas are well formed and may have central foci of caseation (Fig. 17–15). In many cases, however, caseation may not be present. Multinucleated giant cells are usually present, but are not abundant.

Scrofuloderma appears as an ulcerated epidermis with a marked abscess within the superficial dermis. Abundant necrosis and neutrophilic infiltrate are present. At the periphery of the lesion, well-formed granulomas with central areas of caseation are present (Fig. 17–16).

Tuberculosis verrucosa cutis has marked epidermal hyperplasia and overlying hyperkeratosis (Fig. 17–17). Caseating granulomas are present throughout the midreticular dermis (Fig. 17–18). Miliary tuberculosis is characterized by poorly formed granulomata with

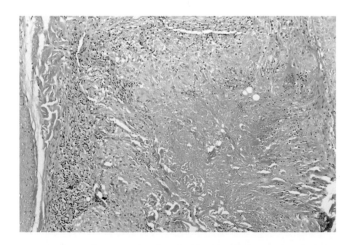

Fig. 17–15. Caseating granulomas are frequently present in lupus vulgaris.

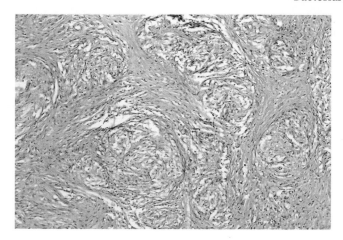

Fig. 17–16. Abundant granulomas are present throughout the dermis at the periphery of a lesion of scrofuloderma.

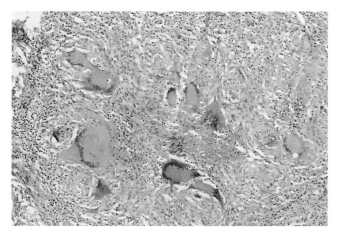

Fig. 17–18. Abundant multinucleated giant cells, caseation, and granulomatous inflammation are present in the dermis in tuberculosis verrucosa cutis.

abundant caseation extending diffusely throughout the dermis [86].

Special Studies. Acid-fast stains such as Ziehl-Nielsen and Fite-Faraco are used to identify *Mycobacterium tuberculosis*. The ease with which they can be identified depends on the type of tuberculosis examined. Organisms are scant in lupus vulgaris. In scrofuloderma, organisms are often found in smears from the lesion, but may not be easily detectable on tissue sections due to the necrosis. Organisms are usually found in tuberculosis verrucosa cutis but are not as numerous. Multi-

ple organisms are easily detectable in miliary tuberculosis [86]. Dieterle stains have also been useful in detecting these organisms [87]. Culture is the preferred method for making an unequivocal diagnosis. Polymerase chain reaction technology has also proved to be a valuable diagnostic aid in detecting mycobacterial proteins; however, cross-reactivity with other organisms has been reported and lessens the value of this technique [88].

Pathogenesis. Tuberculosis is caused by infection by *Mycobacterium tuberculosis*, an acid-fast bacillus. Infection can be through person-to-person contact or traumatic implantation.

Mycobacterium Other than *tuberculosis*

Many other mycobacteria cause cutaneous infections. They are subclassified based on culture characteristics, including production of color in different light settings (Table 17–1). *Mycobacterium marinum* gives rise to "fish tank granuloma" [89]. The disease is seen in both children and adults [90]. Most patients present with an ulcer, located on an extremity, often after trauma in an aquatic setting. Approximately 90% of cases involve an upper extremity [91]. Sporotrichoid, or linearly arrayed lesions, may be present along the affected extremity in more than 80% of cases [91]. In some cases, bursitis may be associated with this infection.

   Mycobacterium ulcerans is associated with the development of "buruli ulcers." These ulcers are most common in children [92]. Early lesions appear as small ulcerations, located almost exclusively on extremities. Advanced lesions demonstrate a characteristic undermined margin [92].

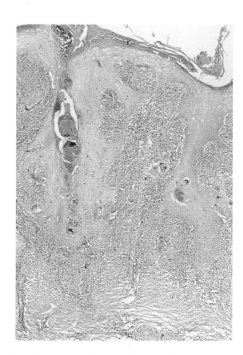

Fig. 17–17. Florid epidermal hyperplasia and a dense inflammatory response are seen in tuberculosis verrucosa cutis.

Table 17–1. Runyon Classification of *Mycobacterium* Species Other than Tuberculosis

Photochromagens
   M. kansasii
   M. marinum
   M. simiae
   M. szulgai
Scotochromagens
   M. flavescens
   M. gordonae
   M. scrofulaceum
   M. xenopi
Nonphotochromagens
   M. avium-intracellulare complex
   M. gastri
   M. heamophilum
   M. malmoense
   M. nonchromogenicum-triviale
   M. terrae
Rapid growers
   M. chelonei
   M. fortuitum

From reference 151.

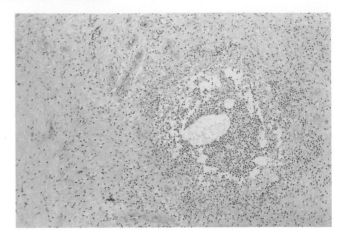

Fig. 17–19. An early lesion of *mycobacterium avium-intracellulare* demonstrates areas of necrosis with a neutrophil-rich inflammatory infiltrate.

Mycobacterium avium-intracellulare complex infection is seen in both immunosuppressed and immunocompetent patients [93], although it occurs with greatly increased frequency in patients with AIDS. There is no specific skin lesion associated with this mycobacterial infection, although the organisms may be seen in skin samples as incidental findings.

Mycobacterium haemophilum has been reported to cause lytic bone lesions in patients with AIDS [94]. Other organisms that may rarely cause cutaneous disease include *M. kansasii*, *M. fortuitum/chelonae* complex , and *M. scrofulaceum* [71].

The histologic changes associated with atypical mycobacteria are similar to those in *Mycobacterium tuberculosis* infections. Granulomatous inflammation is present within the dermis. Early lesions may display an abundance of neutrophils (Fig. 17–19). The epidermis may be hyperplastic or ulcerated, depending on the clinical situation. In fish tank granulomas, caseating necrosis is unusual, and organisms are present in approximately 63% of cases [91]. Buruli ulcers have an unusual coagulative necrosis within the dermis, and minimal inflammation, despite the presence of multiple organisms in most cases. A septal panniculitis occurs in most cases [95].

Each of the organisms that gives rise to cutaneous infection can be identified with acid-fast stains such as Ziehl-Nielsen and Fite-Faraco (Fig. 17–20), or with polymerase chain reaction.

Leprosy

Epidemiology. Leprosy is a common, worldwide infectious disease with an estimated prevalence of 11–12 million cases [96]. Most cases currently occur in Africa and Asia. The prevalence is very low in North America, but relatively high in South America [97]. Leprosy is transmitted by close and prolonged person-to-person contact. Rare cases are transmitted through other channels such as infected syringes or needles [98]. Transmission to human beings from armadillos has also been reported [99].

Cutaneous Features. The cutaneous manifestations of leprosy are largely determined by intrinsic host immunity to the organism. There are many classifications for leprosy that attempt to adequately separate these clinical differences [97]. One such classification scheme is as follows:

• Indeterminate
• Tuberculoid tuberculoid

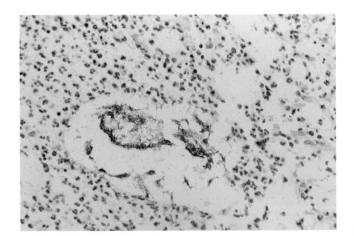

Fig. 17–20. An acid-fast stain demonstrates clusters of organisms in this case of *mycobacterium avium-intracellulare.*

- Borderline tuberculoid
- Borderline borderline
- Borderline lepromatous
- Lepromatous lepromatous leprosy

In general, all of the classification schemes organize the disease in terms of patient immunologic responses to the infection, ranging from the brisk host response in tuberculoid tuberculoid to the minimal response seen in lepromatous leprosy.

Indeterminate leprosy is a manifestation of early disease that has not yet fully evolved into a classifiable subtype. It appears as a single, poorly defined hypopigmented macule that may not be associated with abnormal sensation.

Tuberculoid tuberculoid leprosy presents as a few hypopigmented or erythematous macules or indurated plaques with sharp margins. There is loss of temperature, touch, and pain, and the cutaneous changes may be associated with enlarged nerves.

Borderline tuberculoid leprosy presents as hypopigmented and erythematous macules and indurated plaques that are similar to those in the tuberculoid tuberculoid form of the disease, but more numerous.

Borderline borderline leprosy presents with cutaneous lesions that have features of both borderline tuberculoid and borderline lepromatous diseases. The hypopigmented plaques and macules are bilateral and asymmetrical. Nerves are thickened and tender.

Borderline lepromatous leprosy presents with numerous, bilateral erythematous and hypopigmented macules and patches that tend to be symmetric. They are poorly marginated and blend imperceptibly into the surrounding skin. As the disease progresses, the cutaneous patches become progressively more indurated and progress to plaques. Nerves are quite enlarged and may be tender. In advanced cases, patients develop leonine facies. Mucous membranes are frequently involved [97].

Less common forms of the disease include histioid leprosy, which has multiple skin-colored subcutaneous nodules most commonly on the lower back, and polyneuritic leprosy that presents with neurologic signs without skin lesions [97].

The type 1 lepra reaction is a delayed-type hypersensitivity reaction to the organism. It is characterized by erythema and edema, ulceration, and very tender nerves. It usually occurs in patients who have begun treatment, but can also appear in patients who are not treated.

The type 2 erythema nodosum leprosum reaction is a type III hypersensitivity reaction to the same organism and occurs in up to 70% of patients with lepromatous leprosy. This reaction is characterized by the sudden appearance of cutaneous or subcutaneous nodules on the extensor surfaces of the body that ulcerate. Peripheral nerves are thickened and/or tender [97]. Lucio's phenomenon is a variation of this type of reaction and is characterized by painful ulcerations on the skin. Initial hemorrhage progresses to blister and ulceration. It occurs mainly in Mexicans with lepromatous leprosy.

Associated Disorders. Fever, chills, malaise, and loss of appetite frequently accompany a type 1 lepra reaction [97]. Conjunctivitis, keratitis, hepatosplenomegaly, orchitis, and lymphadenopathy may be seen in patients with a type 2 erythema nodosum leprosum reaction [97].

Histologic Features. Indeterminate leprosy is characterized by a nonspecific lymphohistiocytic infiltrate around vessels of the superficial vascular plexus and cutaneous appendages (Fig. 17–21).

Skin from tuberculoid tuberculoid leprosy demonstrates well-formed granulomas within the dermis. The granulomas are composed of histiocytes and multinucleated giant cells. A brisk lymphocytic response is present around the granulomas and within nerves, leading to their destruction. Plasma cells are often present. Granulomas may be present along the nerves in an oblong configuration (Fig. 17–22).

Borderline tuberculoid leprosy is characterized by changes similar to those seen in tuberculoid tuberculoid leprosy. Dermal nerves are markedly edematous and appear inflamed (Fig. 17–23).

Borderline borderline leprosy demonstrates less well-formed granulomas and only a scant surrounding lymphocytic inflammatory response. A *grenz* zone is often present within the papillary dermis. Granulomatous inflammation is present around and within the cutaneous nerves, resulting in their destruction.

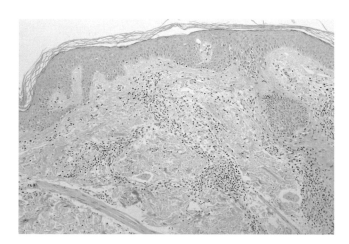

Fig. 17–21. Indeterminate leprosy demonstrates a slight superficial lymphohistiocytic inflammatory infiltrate around vessels of the superficial vascular plexus.

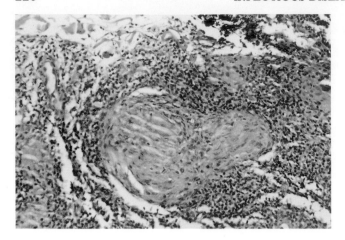

Fig. 17-22. Well-formed granulomas are surrounded by a dense infiltrate of lymphocytes and plasma cells in tuberculoid tuberculoid leprosy.

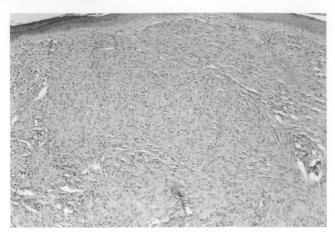

Fig. 17-25. Lepromatous lepromatous leprosy is characterized by sheets of histiocytes throughout the dermis, with a prominent Grenz zone and little accompanying inflammation.

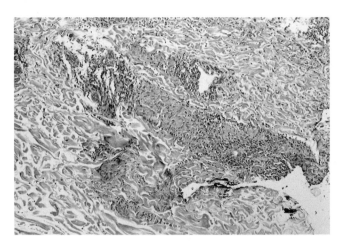

Fig. 17-23. Oblong granulomas surrounding dermal nerves are prevalent in borderline tuberculoid leprosy.

Borderline lepromatous leprosy has diffuse granulomata within the reticular dermis, sparing the papillary dermis. The granulomas are poorly formed and resemble sheets of histiocytes with admixed lymphocytes (Fig. 17-24). Nerves are markedly edematous and infiltrated by inflammatory cells.

Lepromatous lepromatous leprosy is characterized by sheets of histiocytes with granular cytoplasm diffusely spread throughout the dermis. There is a prominent *grenz* zone (Fig. 17-25). There are very few lymphocytes and plasma cells in the inflammatory response (Fig. 17-26). Nerves appear as "onion peels" and are edematous, inflamed, and destroyed [97].

Special Studies. *Mycobacterium leprae* can be detected with modified acid-fast stains. A Fite-Faraco stain is the

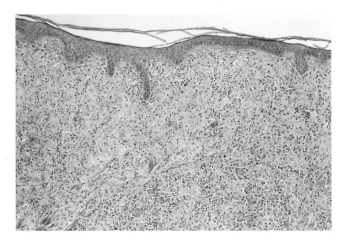

Fig. 17-24. Borderline lepromatous leprosy demonstrates a diffuse proliferation of dermal histiocytes, with a grenz zone and little tendency to form granulomas.

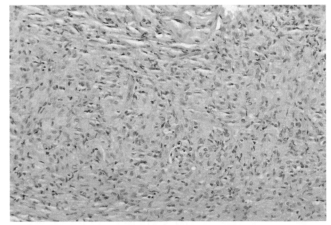

Fig. 17-26. A monomorphous sheet of histiocytes with abundant cytoplasm is present in lepromatous lepromatous leprosy.

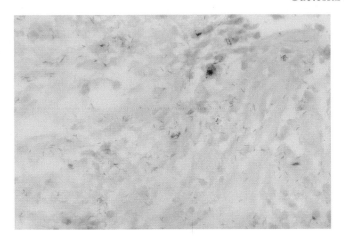

Fig. 17–27. Abundant acid-fast bacilli are demonstrated with a Fite-Faraco stain in lepromatous lepromatous leprosy.

most sensitive stain for detecting this organism in skin biopsy material (Fig. 17–27). Organisms are almost never seen in tuberculoid tuberculoid leprosy and are generally abundant and easy to find in lepromatous lepromatous leprosy. Rare organisms are present in indeterminate leprosy and borderline tuberculoid leprosy. In borderline borderline leprosy and borderline lepromatous leprosy, organisms are easily recognizable, as is the case in histioid leprosy. Histiocytes distended with easily visible organisms have been called "globi."

Pathogenesis. Leprosy is caused by *Mycobacterium leprae*, which is an obligate intracellular bacillus. It enters the body through abraded skin or mucosa. Rarely, the respiratory or gastrointestinal systems may provide a portal of entry for the organism [100].

It has been suggested that a defect in cell-mediated immunity, possibly due to a problem with macrophage-activating factor, may play a central role in the defective immunologic response found in patients with lepromatous lepromatous leprosy [96, 101–103].

SEQUELAE

Erythema Induratum

Epidemiology. Erythema induratum is a disease that is much more prevalent in women. It is most common in young to middle-aged women, although it can occur in teenagers and in older patients as well. Almost all patients with the disease demonstrate a moderate to strong degree of hypersensitivity to *Mycobacterium tuberculosis* [104]. Some authors believe erythema induratum to be a variant of nodular vasculitis [105].

Cutaneous Features. Erythema induratum presents as erythematous to violaceous, tender, indurated dermal or subcutaneous nodules that are predominantly on the lower extremities of women [106]. The arms may be involved infrequently. Ulceration is commonly present.

Associated Disorders. Many patients with erythema induratum will demonstrate a positive tuberculin hypersensitivity test. Many of these patients will fail to demonstrate active tuberculosis. Erythema induratum has been reported in patients with concomitant papulonecrotic tuberculid and lichen scrofulosorum [107, 108].

Histologic Features. Erythema induratum is characterized by a lobular panniculitis. Granulomas, necrosis, and vasculitis are variably present. Diffuse panniculitis, involving lobules with extension into the septa, is the most common pattern (Fig. 17–28). The granulomas are present in most but not all cases, can occur in any location, and are characterized by central, caseating necrosis in more than half of cases. Neutrophilic abscesses may be present in these areas. Multinucleated giant cells are common, and scattered plasma cells and eosinophils are present in most cases (Fig. 17–29). Muscular arteries and smaller vessels may demonstrate transmural inflammation with neutrophils [106] (Fig. 17–30). In rare cases, inflammation may be confined to the region of the inflamed blood vessel, giving rise to the pattern known as *nodular vasculitis*, but this pattern is seen in only a minority of cases [104]. The vascular inflammation is most often neutrophilic, but can be granulomatous in some cases.

Extension into the overlying dermis is seen in many cases. Usually, this inflammation is restricted to a lymphohistiocytic response, with no granulomas, plasma cells, or eosinophils [104].

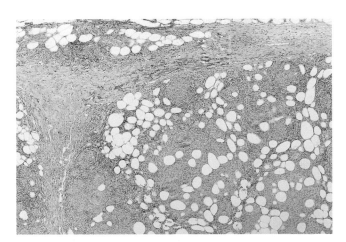

Fig. 17–28. Erythema induratum is characterized by a diffuse lobular panniculitis.

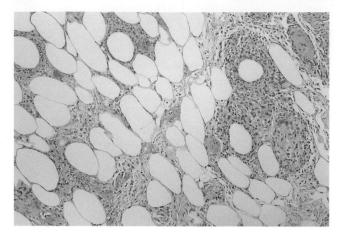

Fig. 17–29. Granulomas are frequently present in addition to a dense, mixed inflammatory infiltrate.

Special Studies. Polymerase chain reaction technology is very useful in detecting mycobacterial DNA in at least some cases of erythema induratum. Stains for acid-fast bacilli are generally negative [106].

Pathogenesis. The exact etiology of erythema induratum remains uncertain. It has recently been demonstrated that DNA from mycobacteria is present within lesional skin in up to one-fourth of cases [106, 109]. Further work with T lymphocytes from patients with erythema induratum demonstrates a hyperresponsiveness to mycobacterial proteins [105]. Thus, erythema induratum should probably best be considered a form of hypersensitivity to *Mycobacteria tuberculosis*, much like papulonecrotic tuberculid and lichen scrofulosorum [110]. It should be noted, however, that this is still quite controversial, and that not all practicing dermatologists are convinced of the intimate association between mycobacteria and erythema induratum. It has

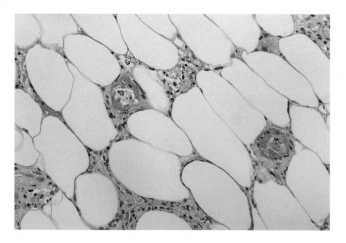

Fig. 17–30. Arteritis is present in some cases of erythema induratum.

been suggested that primary vasculitis is the initial event in erythema induratum [104, 111].

Papulonecrotic Tuberculid

Epidemiology. A tuberculid reaction is defined as an inflammatory response to an occult focus of tuberculosis that occurs in patients with high immunity and that resolves completely with effective antituberculous treatment. Papulonecrotic tuberculoid is an extremely rare disease affecting young adults [112] and is associated with pulmonary tuberculosis in most cases. It is even less common in children [112].

Cutaneous Features. Papulonecrotic tuberculid presents as dusky red papules distributed symmetrically on the extensor surfaces of the extremities. The papules, which are relatively sparse, become necrotic and resolve with atrophic scars over a period of weeks [112]. Involvement of the ears is common. Less commonly, pustules, lichenoid papules, umbilicated papules, punctate keratoses, and vesicles have been reported [113, 114].

Associated Disorders. Associated disorders are related to the systemic tuberculosis seen in most patients and include respiratory disease, hepatosplenomegaly, fever, conjunctivitis, and lymphadenopathy. Anemia is sometimes present, as is an elevated white cell count [112].

Histologic Features. The histologic features of early papulonecrotic tuberculid demonstrate a leukocytoclastic vasculitis that is indistinguishable from leukocytoclastic vasculitis related to other conditions. Subsequent wedge-shaped infarction is commonly seen [115, 116]. Later lesions demonstrate lymphocytes surrounding and invading dermal vessels in conjunction with a poorly formed granulamatous infiltrate [117]. Eosinophils may be present, but plasma cells are unusual.

Special Studies. Routine acid-fast stains fail to reveal organisms in papulonecrotic tuberculid. Polymerase chain reaction has been reported to be negative in many cases [112], but DNA from mycobacteria are found in at least 50% of cases [109].

Pathogenesis. It has been suggested that an Arthus-type hypersensitivity reaction is responsible for papulonecrotic tuberculid [112]; however, some investigators have failed to find immune complexes in skin lesions [118].

Lichen Scrofulosorum

Epidemiology. Lichen scrofulosorum is a very rare hypersensitivity reaction to *Mycobacterium tuberculosis* that is seen in patients with active disease. Lichen scrofulosorum appears to be seen almost exclusively in patients from developing nations.

Cutaneous Features. Patients with lichen scrofulosorum present with widespread lichenoid papules in the setting of known tuberculosis. These 0.5–3 mm papules are more prevalent on the trunk and extremities and may be folliculocentric. In rare cases, an annular configuration has been described.

Associated Disorders. In rare cases, more than one type of hypersensitivity reaction can be present simultaneously. Coexisting lichen scrofulosorum and erythema induratum have been described [107].

Although usually associated with pulmonary tuberculosis, lichen scrofulosorum may occur secondary to osseous tuberculosis or tuberculosis affecting cervical lymph nodes [119, 120]. Lichen scrofulosorum has been reported in several patients after bacille Calmette-Guérin vaccination [121]. It has also been described in AIDS patients with active pulmonary tuberculosis and cervical scrofuloderma [122].

Histologic Features. Lichen scrofulosorum is characterized by noncaseating granulomas distributed around hair follicles and eccrine ducts within the dermis. The epidermis may or may not be acanthotic [123, 124]. Small foci of caseating necrosis have been reported in rare cases [120]. In many cases, it is not possible to distinguish sarcoidosis from lichen scrofulosorum on histologic grounds.

Special Studies. Although acid-fast stains are usually indicated to search for organisms, organisms are not present in lesions of lichen scrofulosorum.

Pathogenesis. Lichen scrofulosorum is thought to be a delayed-type hypersensitivity reaction to *Mycobacterium tuberculosis* [123]. Organisms are not present at the site of the hypersensitivity reaction.

Toxic Shock Syndrome

Epidemiology. The first series of patients with toxic shock syndrome (TSS) demonstrated a strong relationship between tampon use and recent menstruation. Thus, most cases occurred in women of childbearing age [125]. As the causes of the disease have become better understood, this strong association has attenuated, and the frequency of the disease has decreased. Toxic shock syndrome occurs in persons of all ages, races, and sex [126].

Cutaneous Features. Most patients with TSS present with a scarlatiniform or diffuse macular erythroderma,

which rapidly desquamates. The diffuse erythema is most prevalent on the trunk. Palmar edema and erythema are also prominent. Peeling of the palms and soles is seen later in the course of the disease, and a telogen effluvium has been reported during the convalescent phase of the disease [127]. In advanced cases, the clinical appearance is that of disseminated intravascular coagulation, with multiple thromboses and infarction.

Associated Disorders. Constitutional symptoms associated with TSS include fevers, headaches, hypotension, myalgias, vomiting, diarrhea, and pharyngitis [128]. In florid, rapidly progressive disease, patients develop acute renal failure, liver involvement, disseminated intravascular coagulation, and shock [129]. Involvement of the central nervous system has also been reported [130].

Toxic shock syndrome has been described in the postoperative setting, after a urinary tract diversion procedure, and in infected burn wounds [131–133]. *Staphylococcus* infections in abscesses and bursitis and occurring postpartum have also been implicated in TSS [126]. Toxic shock syndrome has also been reported in association with HIV, intravenous drug use, and infected allergic contact dermatitis [130].

Histologic Features. The epidermis may be spongiotic and slightly acanthotic in early lesions of TSS. Ballooning degeneration may be present. Keratinocyte necrosis is present at all levels of the epidermis. Neutrophils and eosinophils are present in the region surrounding the dying keratinocytes. The papillary dermis is characterized by diffuse, prominent edema. Capillaries in the superficial dermis are invaded by inflammatory cells, including predominantly lymphocytes with admixed histiocytes and plasma cells, and fibrin thrombi are present in many of the vessels [127, 134]. Neutrophils and nuclear dust may be present, but are less prominent than the lymphocytes.

Special Studies. Direct immunofluorescence examination reveals granular deposits of IgM and C3 in and around the vessels of the superficial vascular plexus, suggesting true immune complex–mediated vascular damage [127].

Pathogenesis. Toxic shock syndrome is caused by a toxin produced by *Staphylococcus aureus* [125]. Phage group I organisms are preferentially implicated and cause the symptoms by producing an epidermal toxin, toxine 1 (TSS-T1), or enterotoxins B or C [125, 135]. These toxins act as superantigens that bind to major histocompatibility antigens and stimulate cytokine production (tumor necrosis factor and interleukin-1) by macrophages [132, 136]. It is thought that the skin eruption is due to a hypersensitivity reaction caused by the TSS-T1 [137].

A similar TSS-like eruption has been described after infection with group A *Streptococcus*. The disease is caused by exotoxins A, B, and C [138]. In these cases, there is a 80% incidence of soft tissue involvement [139].

Staphylococcal Scalded Skin Syndrome

Epidemiology. Staphylococcal scalded skin syndrome (SSSS) is predominantly a disease of children and also occurs in adults with renal failure. Most patients are less than 5 years of age [132, 140]. It is also seen in adults and is associated with a very high mortality rate in this setting [141]. Most affected adults suffer from immunosuppression or renal failure [141, 142]. A case of SSSS acquired congenitally has been reported [143]. A rare, chronic form of the disease, lasting for over 2 years, has also been reported [144].

Cutaneous Features. Diffuse erythema followed by flaccid bullae and wrinkling or widespread erosions are characteristic skin changes in patients with SSSS. Scarlatiniform erythema, accentuated in flexural areas, is seen in many cases [130]. Nikolsky's sign is usually present. There is no mucosal involvement, as there is ordinarily no granular layer, the target region for exotoxin binding, in mucosal epithelium.

Associated Disorders. Constitutional symptoms associated with SSSS include fever, irritability, and skin tenderness. Staphylococcal scalded skin syndrome is associated with impaired renal clearance of exotoxins, occurring most commonly in infants and in patients with impaired renal function.

Other immunosuppressive conditions, including organ transplantation, chronic alcoholism, malignancy, and AIDS, have predisposed some individuals toward developing SSSS [130, 140, 141, 145, 146]. Rare cases of SSSS have been reported in immunocompetent adults [147]. In one patient, an oral corticosteroid was implicated [148].

Histologic Features. Histologic features of SSSS include a noninflammatory subcorneal blister (Fig. 17–31). Focal acantholysis within the granular layer is seen. Within the dermis, there is a minimal lymphocytic infiltrate surrounding the vessels of the superficial vascular plexus. In some cases, the only change may be the loss of the granular layer, making the diagnosis very difficult.

Special Studies. Organisms are not present in skin biopsy specimens, so special stains are of no help in making a diagnosis of SSSS. Polymerase chain reaction

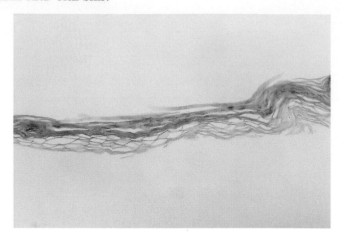

Fig. 17–31. Staphylococcal scalded skin syndrome demonstrates a superficial blister with separation of the granular layer and stratum corneum, as is seen in this section made from exfoliated epidermis.

has proved useful in detecting exotoxins [149]. Immunologic methods for identifying the toxins have also been described [142].

Pathogenesis. Staphylococcal scalded skin syndrome is caused by exfoliatin, or epidermolytic toxins A and B, produced by *Staphylococcus aureus*, phage group II, types 71 and 55 [132]. The toxins have been shown to stimulate T-cell proliferation [150]. Lack of immunity to the toxins and poor renal clearance of the toxins are thought to contribute to the development of the disease [132].

NOTE: Erythema nodosum is discussed in Chapter 19. Acute post-streptococcal glomerulonephritis and impetigo are addressed in Chapter 8.

References

1. Ploysangam, T., and Sheth, A. P., *Chronic meningococcemia in childhood: Case report and review of the literature.* Pediatr Dermatol, 1996. 13:483–487.
2. Olcen, P., Eeg-Olofsson, O., Fryden, A., Kernell, A., and Ansehn, S., *Benign meningococcemia in childhood. A report of five cases with clinical and diagnostic remarks.* Scand J Infect Dis, 1978. 10:107–111.
3. Pinals, R. S., *Meningococcemia presenting as acute polyarthritis.* J Rheumatol, 1977. 4:420–424.
4. Detsky, A. S., and Salit, I. E., *Complete heart block in meningococcemia.* Ann Emerg Med, 1983. 12:391–393.
5. Dennis, J., Edwards, L. D., Fisher, T. N., and Makeever, L., *Endocarditis on a Björk-Shiley mitral prosthesis due to Neisseria meningitidis.* Scand J Thorac Cardiovasc Surg, 1977. 11:205–209.
6. Sotto, M. N., Langer, B., Hoshino-Shimizu, S., and de

Brito, T., *Pathogenesis of cutaneous lesions in acute meningococcemia in humans: Light, immunofluorescent, and electron microscopic studies of skin biopsy specimens.* J Infect Dis, 1976. 133:506–514.

7. Darmstadt, G. L., *Acute infectious purpua fulminans: Pathogenesis and medical management.* Pediatr Dermatol, 1998. 15:169–183.

8. Kingston, M. E., and Mackey, D., *Skin clues in the diagnosis of life-threatening infections.* Rev Infect Dis, 1986. 8:1–11.

9. Shelley, W. B., and Zolin, W. D., *Disseminate intradermal bacterial colonization presenting as palpable purpura in lymphoblastic leukemia.* J Am Acad Dermatol, 1983. 8:714–717.

10. Goette, D. K., *Unilateral palpable purpura. A manifestation of septic emboli from an infected aortofemoral bypass graft eroding the jejunum.* Arch Dermatol, 1981. 117:430–431.

11. Vinson, R. P., Chung, A., Elston, D. M., and Keller, R. A., *Septic microemboli in a Janeway lesion of bacterial endocarditis.* J Am Acad Dermatol, 1996. 35:984–985.

12. Sanchez, T. G., Cahali, M. B., Murakami, M. S., Butugan, O., and Miniti, A., *Septic thrombosis of orbital vessels due to cutaneous nasal infection.* Am J Rhinol, 1997. 11:429–433.

13. McCready, R. A., Siderys, H., Pittman, J. N., Herod, G. T., Halbrook, H. G., Fehrenbacher, J. W., Beckman, D. J., et al., *Septic complications after cardiac catheterization and percutaneous transluminal coronary angioplasty.* J Vasc Surg, 1991. 14:170–174.

14. Martin, A., and Copeman, P. W., *Aorto-jejunal fistula from rupture of Teflon graft, with septic emboli in the skin.* BMJ 1967. 2:155–156.

15. Sanchez, M. R., *Infectious syphilis.* Semin Dermatol, 1994. 13:234–242.

16. *Primary and secondary syphilis—United States, 1981–1990.* MMWR, 1991. 40:314–323.

17. *Primary and secondary syphilis—United States, 1997.* MMWR, 1998. 47:493–497.

18. Brown, T. J., Yen-Moore, A., and Tyring, S. K., *An overview of sexually transmitted diseases. Part 1.* J Am Acad Dermatol, 1999. 41:511–529.

19. Crissey, J. T., and Denenholz, D. A., *Clinical picture of infectious syphilis.* Clin Dermatol, 1984. 2:39–61.

20. Carbia, S. G., Lagodin, C., Abbruzzese, M., Sevinsky, L., Casco, R., Casas, J., and Woscoff, A., *Lichenoid secondary syphilis.* Int J Dermatol, 1999. 38:53–55.

21. Papini, M., Bettachhi, A., and Guiducci, A., *Nodular secondary syphilis.* Br J Dermatol, 1998. 138:704–705.

22. Lukehart, S. A., *Immunology and pathogenesis of syphilis.* in *Sexually Transmitted Diseases*, T. C. Quin, Ed. 1992, Raven, New York, pp. 141–163.

23. Morton, R. S., *The treponematoses.* in *Textbook of Dermatology*, R. H. Champion, J. L. Burton, and F. J. G. Ebling, Eds. 1992, Blackwell Scientific Publications, Oxford. pp. 1085–1126.

24. Lawrence, P., and Saxe, N., *Bullous secondary syphilis.* Clin Exp Dermatol, 1992. 17:44–46.

25. Varela, P., Alves, R., Velho, G., Santos, C., Massa, A., and Sanches, M., *Two recent cases of tertiary syphilis.* Eur J Dermatol, 1999. 9:300–302.

26. Liu, C. C., So, W. C., Lin, C. H., and Yeh, T. F., *Congenital syphilis: Clinical manifestations in premature infants.* Scand J Infect Dis, 1993. 25:741–745.

27. Agarwal, U. S., Malpini, S., and Mathur, N. K., *Annular lesions in congenital syphilis.* Genitourin Med, 1992. 68:195–196.

28. Deschenes, J., Seamone, C. D., and Baines, M. G., *Acquired ocular syphilis: Diagnosis and treatment.* Ann Ophthalmol, 1992. 24:134–138.

29. Hansen, K., and Hvid-Jacobsen, K., *Bone lesions in early syphilis detected by bone scintigraphy.* Br J Vener Dis, 1984. 60:265–268.

30. Darmstadt, G. L., and Harris, J. P., *Luetic hearing loss: Clinical presentation, diagnosis and treatment (review).* Am J Otolaryngol, 2989. 10:410–421.

31. Winters, H. A., Notar-Francesco, V., Blomberg, K., Rawstrom, S. A., Vetrano, J., Prego, V., Kuan, J., and Raufman, J. P., *Gastric syphilis: Five recent cases and a review of the literature.* Ann Intern Med, 1992. 15:314–319.

32. Balikocioglu, A., Quaidoo, E., Vuletin, J. C., and Trotman, B. W., *Hepatitis and glomerulonephritis in secondary syphilis.* J Assoc Acad Minor Phys, 1991. 2:72–75.

33. Bukharovich, A. M., Sokol, A. N., Knigovskii, A. M., and Khil'ko, I. N., *Liver involvement in early secondary syphilis.* Vestn Dermatol Venereol, 1989. 9:58–61.

34. Fulton, J. O., Zilla, P., Ed Groot, K. M., and Oppell, U. O., *Syphilitic aortic aneurysm eroding through the sternum.* Eur J Cardiothorac Surg, 1996. 10:922–924.

35. Horn, T. D., *Thrombocytosis in a patient with secondary syphilis.* Arch Dermatol, 1985. 121:1241–1242.

36. Strom, T., and Schneck, S. A., *Syphilitiic meningomyelitis.* Neurology, 1991. 41:325–326.

37. Pandhi, R. K., Singh, N., and Ramam, M., *Secondary syphilis: A clinicopathologic study.* Int J Dermatol, 1995. 34:240–243.

38. Jordaan, H. F., and Louw, M., *The moth-eaten alopecia of secondary syphilis. A histopathologic study of 12 patients.* Am J Dermatopathol, 1995. 17:158–162.

39. Engelkens, H. J., ten Kate, F. J., Judanarso, J., Vuzevski, V. D., van Lier, J. B., Godshalk, J. C., van der Sluis, J. J., et al., *The localisation of treponemes and characterisation of the inflammatory infiltrate in skin biopsies from patients with primary or secondary syphilis, or early infectious yaws.* Genitourin Med, 1993. 69:102–107.

40. Engelkens, H. J., ten Kate, F. J., Vuzevski, V. D., van der Sluis, J. J., and Stolz, E., *Primary and secondary syphilis: A histopathological study.* Int J STD AIDS, 1991. 2:280–284.

41. Hook, E. W., and Marra, C. M., *Acquired syphilis in adults.* N Engl J Med, 1992. 326:1060–1069.

42. Campbell, G. L., Fritz, C. L., Fish, D., Nowakowski, J., Nadelman, R. B., and Wormser, G. P., *Estimation of the incidence of Lyme disease.* Am J Epidemiol, 1998. 148:1018–1026.

43. Santino, I., Dastoli, F., Sessa, R., and Del Piano, M., *Ge-*

ographical incidence of infection with Borrelia burgdorferi in Europe. Panminerva Med, 1997. 39:208–214.

44. Lyme disease—United States, 1996. MMWR 1997. 46:531–535.

45. Goldberg, N. S., Forseter, G., Nadelman, R. B., Schwartz, I., Jorde, U., McKenna, D., Holmgren, D., et al., Vesicular erythema migrans. Arch Dermatol, 1992. 128:1495–1498.

46. Felz, M. W., Chandler, F. W. Jr., Oliver, J. H. Jr., Rahn, D. W., and Schriefer, M. E., Solitary erythema migrans in Georgia and South Carolina. Arch Dermatol, 1999. 135:1317–1326.

47. Buechner, S. A., Rufli, T., and Erb, P., Acrodermatitis chronic atrophicans: A chronic T-cell-mediated immune reaction against Borrelia burgdorferi? Clinical, histologic, and immunohistochemical study of five cases. J Am Acad Dermatol, 1993. 28:399–405.

48. Buechner, S. A., Winkelmann, R. K., Lautenschlager, S., Gilli, L., and Rufli, T., Localized scleroderma associated with Borrelia burgdorferi infection. Clinical, histologic, and immunohistochemical observations. J Am Acad Dermatol, 1993. 29:190–196.

49. Patmas, M. A., Lyme disease: The evolution of erythema chronicum migrans into acrodermatitis chronica migrans. Cutis, 1993. 52:169–170.

50. Albrecht, S., Hofstadter, S., Artsob, H., Chaban, O., and From, L., Lymphadenosis benigna cutis resulting from Borrelia infection (Borrelia lymphocytoma). J Am Acad Dermatol, 1991. 24:621–625.

51. Horowitz, H. W., Sanghera, K., Goldberg, N., Pechman, D., Kamer, R., Duray, P., and Weinstein, A., Dermatomyositis associated with Lyme disease: Case report and review of Lyme myositis. Clin Infect Dis, 1994. 18:166–171.

52. Schuttelaar, M. L., Laeijendecker, R., Heinhuis, R. J., and Van Joost, T., Erythema multiforme and persistent erythema as early cutaneous manfiestations of Lyme disease. J Am Acad Dermatol, 1997. 37:873–875.

53. Espana, A., Torrelo, A., Guerrero, A., Suarez, J., Rocamora, A., and Ledo, A., Periarticular fibrous nodules in Lyme borreliosis. Br J Dermatol, 1991. 125:68–70.

54. Marsch, W. C., Mayet, A., and Wolter, M., Cutaneous fibroses induced by Borrelia burgdorferi. Br J Dermatol, 1993. 128:674–678.

55. Huisman, T. A., Wohlrab, G., Nadal, D., Bolthauser, E., and Martin, E., Unusual presentations of neuroborreliosis (Lyme disease) in childhood. J Comput Assist Tomogr, 1999. 23:39–42.

56. Vanzieleghem, B., Lemmerling, M., Carton, D., Achten, E., Vanlangenhove, P., Matthys, E., and Kunnen, M., Lyme disease in a child presenting with bilateral facial nerve palsy: MRI findings and review of the literature. Neuroradiology, 1998. 40:739–742.

57. Klein, J., Stanek, G., Bittner, R., Horvat, R., Holzinger, C., and Glogar, D., Lyme borreliosis as a cause of myocarditis and heart muscle disease. Eur Heart J, 1991. 12(Supppl D):73–75.

58. Gerster, J. C., and Peter, O., Rheumatic manifestations related to acrodermatitis chronica atrophicans. A review of four cases. Rev Rhum Engl Ed, 1998. 65:567–570.

59. Chary-Valckenaere, I., Jaulhac, B., Monteil, H., and Pourel, J., Diagnosis of Lyme disease. Current difficulties and prospects. Rev Rhum Engl Ed, 1995. 62:271–280.

60. Kawagishi, N., Takahashi, H., Hashimoto, Y., Miyamoto, K., and Iizuka, H., A case of Lyme disease with parotitis. Dermatology, 1998. 197:386–387.

61. Granter, S. R., Barnhill, R. L., and Duray, P. H., Borrelial fasciitis: Diffuse fasciitis and peripheral eosinophilia associated wtih Borrelia infection. Am J Dermatopathol, 1996. 18:465–473.

62. Van Mierlo, P., Jacob, W., and Dockx, P., Erythema chronica migrans: An electron-microscopic study. Dermatology, 1993. 186:306–310.

63. de Koning, J., Tazelaar, D. J., Hoogkamp-Korstanje, J. A., and Elema, J. D., Acrodermatitis chronica atrophicans: A light and electron microscopic study. J Cutan Pathol, 1995. 22:23–32.

64. Chary-Valckenaere, I., Jaulhac, B., Champigneulle, J., Piemont, Y., Mainard, D., and Pourel, J., Ultrastructural demonstration of intracellular localization of Borrelia burgdorferi in Lyme arthritis. Br J Rheumatol, 1998. 37:468–470.

65. Jurca, T., Ruzic-Sabljic, E., Lotric-Furlan, S., Maraspin, V., Cimperman, J., Picken, R. N., and Strle, F., Comparison of peripheral and central biopsy sites for the isolation of Borrelia burgdorferi sensu lato from erythema migrans skin lesions. Clin Infect Dis, 1998. 27:636–638.

66. Mouritsen, C. L., Wittwer, C. T., Litwin, C. M., Yang, L., Weis, J. J., Martins, T. B., Jaskowski, T. D., et al., Polymerase chain reaction detection of Lyme disease: Correlation with clinical manifestations and serologic responses. Am J Clin Pathol, 1996. 105:647–654.

67. Schutzer, S. E., Coyle, P. K., Reid, P., and Holland, B., Borrelia burgdorferi–specific immune complexes in acute Lyme disease. JAMA, 1999. 282:1942–1946.

68. Scarpa, C., Trevisan, G., and Sinco, G., Lyme borreliosis. Dermatol Clin, 1994. 12:669–685.

69. Aberer, E., The dermatologic spectrum of Lyme borreliosis. Wien Med Wochenschr, 1995. 145(7–8): 121–128.

70. del Carmen Farina, M., Gezundez, I., Pique, E., Esteban, J., Martin, L., Requena, L., Barat, A., et al., Cutaneous tuberculosis: A clinical, histopathologic, and bacteriologic study. J Am Acad Dermatol, 1995. 33: 433–440.

71. Wolinsky, E., Mycobacterial diseases other than tuberculosis. Clin Infect Dis, 1992. 15:1–10.

72. Goette, D. K., Jacobson, K. W., and Dory, R. D., Primary inoculation tuberculosis of the skin. Prosector's paronychia. Arch Dermatol, 1978. 114:567–569.

73. Sahn, S. A., and Pierson, D. J., Primary cutaneous inoculation drug-resistant tuberculosis. Am J Med, 1974. 57:676–678.

74. Kakakhel, K., Simultaneous occurrence of tuberculous gumma, tuberculosis verrucosa cutis, and lichen scrofulosorum. Int J Dermatol, 1998. 37:867–869.

75. Savin, J. L., Mycobacterial infections, In Textbook of Dermatology, R. H. Champion, J. L. Burton, and F. J. G. Ebling, Eds. 1992, Blackwell Scientific Publications, Oxford. pp. 1033–1063.

76. Brown, F. S., Anderson, R. H., and Burnett, J. W., *Cutaneous tuberculosis.* J Am Acad Dermatol, 1982. 6:101–106.

77. Tappeiner, G., and Wolf, K., *Tuberculosis and other mycobacterial infections.* In *Dermatology in General Medicine*, T. B. Fitzpatrick et al., Eds. 1993, McGraw-Hill, New York, pp. 2370–2391.

78. Hernandez-Martin, A., Fernandez-Lopez, E., Roman, C., de Unamuno, P., and Armijo, M., *Verrucous plaque on the back of a hand.* Cutis, 1997. 60:235–236.

79. Nachbar, F., Classen, V., Nachbar, T., Meurer, M., Schirren, C. G., and Degitz, K., *Orificial tuberculosis: Detection by polymerase chain reaction.* Br J Dermatol, 1996. 135:106–109.

80. Oshinowo, A. G., Blount, B. W., and Golusinski, L. L., *Tuberculous cerebellar abscess.* J Am Board Fam Pract, 1998. 11:459–464.

81. Yaramis, A., Gurkan, F., Elevli, M., Soker, M., Haspolat, K., Kirbas, G., and Tas, M. A., *Central nervous system tuberculosis in children: A review of 214 cases.* Pediatrics, 1998. 102:E49.

82. Aston, N. O., *Abdominal tuberculosis.* Word J Surg, 1997. 21:492–499.

83. Ladas, S. D., Vaidakis, E., Lariou, C., Anastasiou, K., Chalevelakis, G., Kintzonidis, D., and Raptis, S. A., *Pancreatic tuberculosis in non-immunocompromised patients: Reports of two cases, and a literature review.* Eur J Gastroenterol Hepatol, 1998. 10:973–976.

84. Izumi, A. K., and Matsunaga, J., *BCG vaccine induced lupus vulgaris.* Arch Dermatol, 1982. 118:171–172.

85. Hagiwara, K., Uezato, H., Miyazato, H., and Nonaka, S., *Squamous cell carcinoma arising from lupus vulgaris on an old burn scar: Diagnosis by polymerase chain reaction.* J Dermatol, 1996. 23:883–889.

86. Daikos, G. L., Uttamchandani, R. B., Tuda, C., Fischl, M. A., Miller, N., Cleary, T., and Saldana, M. J., *Disseminated miliary tuberculosis of the skin in patients with AIDS: Report of four cases.* Clin Infect Dis, 1998. 27:205–208.

87. Brady, J. G., Schutze, G. E., Seibert, R., Horn, H. V., Marks, B., and Parham, D. M., *Detection of mycobacterial infections using the Dieterle stain.* Pediatr Dev Pathol, 1998. 1:309–313.

88. Tan, S. H., Tan, B. H., Goh, C. L., Tan, K. C., Tan, M. F., Ng, W. C., and Tan, W. C., *Detection of mycobacterium tuberculosis DNA using polymerase chain reaction in cutaneous tuberculosis and tuberculids.* Int J Dermatol, 1999. 38:122–127.

89. Saadatmand, B., Poulton, J. K., and Kauffman, C. L., *Mycobacterium marinum with associated bursitis.* J Cutan Med Surg, 1999. 3:218–220.

90. Speight, E. L., and Williams, H. C., *Fish tank granuloma in a 14-month old girl.* Pediatr Dermatol, 1997. 14:209–212.

91. Edelstein, H., *Mycobacterium marinum skin infections. Report of 31 cases and review of the literature.* Arch Intern Med, 1994. 154:1359–1364.

92. Burchard, G. D., and Bierther, M., *Buruli ulcer: Clinical pathological study of 23 patients in Lambarene, Gabon.* Trop Med Parasitol, 1986. 37:1–8.

93. Ichiki, Y., Hirose, M., Akiyama, T., Esaki, C., and Kitajima, Y., *Skin infection caused by Mycobacterium avium.* Br J Dermatol, 1997. 136:260–263.

94. Lefkowitz, R. A., and Singson, R. D., *Considering Mycobacterium haemophilum in the differential diagnosis for lytic bone lesions in AIDS patients who present with ulcerating skin lesions.* Skeletal Radiol, 1998. 27:334–336.

95. Hayman, J., and McQueen, A., *The pathology of Mycobacterium ulcerans infection.* Pathology, 1985. 17:594–600.

96. Van Voorhis, W. C., Kaplan, G., Nunes Sarno, E., Horowitz, M. A., Steinman, R. M., Levis, W. R., Nogueira, N., Hair, L. S., et al., *The cutaneous infiltrates of leprosy. Cellular characteristics and the predominant T-cell phenotypes.* N Engl J Med, 1982. 307:1593–1597.

97. Sehgal, V. N., *Leprosy.* Dermatol Clin, 1994. 12:629–644.

98. Sehgal, V. N., *Inoculation leprosy: Current status.* Int J Dermatol, 1988. 27:6–9.

99. Job, C. K., Harris, E. B., Allen, J. L., and Hastings, R. C., *Thorns in armadillo ears and noses and their role in the transmission of leprosy.* Arch Pathol Lab Med, 1986. 110:1025–1028.

100. Sehgal, V. N., *Clinical Leprosy.* 3rd ed., 1993, New Delhi, Jaypee Brothers.

101. Nathan, C. F., Kaplan, G., Levis, W. R., Nusrat, A., Witmer, M. D., Sherwin, S. A., Job, C. K., et al., *Local and systemic effects of intradermal recombinant interferon-γ in patients with lepromatous leprosy.* N Engl J Med, 1986. 315:6–15.

102. Modlin, R. L., *Cytokine responses in leprosy lesions.* Nippon Rai Gakkai Zasshi, 1995. 64:85–88.

103. Sieling, P. A., and Modlin, R. L., *Cytokine patterns at the site of mycobacterial infection.* Immunobiology, 1994. 191:378–387.

104. Schneider, J. W., and Jordaan, H. F., *The histopathologic spectrum of erythema induratum of Bazin.* Am J Dermatopathol, 1997. 19:323–333.

105. Ollert, M. W., Thomas, P., Korting, H. C., Schraut, W., and Braun-Falco, O., *Erythema induratum of Bazin. Evidence of T-lymphocyte hyperresponsiveness to purified protein derivative of tuberculin: Report of two cases and treatment.* Arch Dermatol, 1993. 129:469–473.

106. Schneider, J. W., Jordaan, H. F., Geiger, D. H., Victor, T., Van Helden, P. D., and Rossouw, D. J., *Erythema induratum of Bazin. A clinicopathological study of 20 cases and detection of Mycobacterium tuberculosis DNA in skin lesions by polymerase chain reaction.* Am J Dermatopathol, 1995. 17:350–356.

107. Park, Y. M., Hong, J. K., Cho, S. H., and Cho, B. K., *Concomitant lichen scrofulosorum and erythema induratum.* J Am Acad Dermatol, 1998. 38:841–843.

108. Milligan, A., Chen, K., and Graham-Brown, R. A. C., *Two tuberculids in one patient: A case report of papulonecrotic tuberculid and erythema induratum occurring together.* Clin Exp Dermatol, 1990. 15:21–23.

109. Victor, T., Jordaan, H. F., Van Niekerk, D. J. T., Louw,

M., Jordaan, A., and Van Helden, P. D., *Papulonecrotic tuberculid: Identification of M. tuberculosis DNA by polymerase chain reaction.* Am J Dermatopathol, 1993. 14:491–495.

110. White, W. L., *On Japanese baseball and erythema induratum of Bazin.* Am J Dermatopathol, 1997. 19:318–322.

111. Black, M. M., *Panniculitis.* J Cutan Pathol, 1985. 12:366–380.

112. Jordaan, H. F., Schneider, J. W., Schaaf, H. S., Victor, T. S., Geiger, D. H., Van Helden, P. D., and Rossouw, D. J., *Papulonecrotic tuberculid in children. A report of eight patients.* Am J Dermatopathol, 1996. 18:172–185.

113. Pasricha, J. S., Gupta, R., and Khare, A. K., *Umbilicated papules as a manifestation of tuberculid.* Indian J Dermatol Venereol Leprol, 1984. 50:267–268.

114. Premlatha, S., Augustine, S. M., Yesudian, U., and Thambia, A. S., *Punctate palmoplantar keratosis acuminata: An unusual form of tuberculid.* Int J Dermatol, 1982. 21:470–471.

115. Morrison, J. G. L., and Fourie, E. D., *The papulonecrotic tuberculide: From Arthus reaction to lupus vulgaris.* Br J Dermatol, 1974. 91:263–270.

116. Wilson-Jones, E., and Winkelmann, R. K., *Papulonecrotic tuberulid: A neglected disease in Western countries.* J Am Acad Dermatol, 1986. 14:815–826.

117. Jordaan, H. F., Van Niekerk, D. J. T., and Louw, M., *Papulonecrotic tuberculid: A clinical, histopathological and immunohistochemical study of 15 patients.* Am J Dermatopathol, 1994. 16:474–485.

118. Iden, D. L., Rogers, R. S., and Schroeter, A. L., *Papulonecrotic tuberculid secondary to Mycobacterium bovis.* Arch Dermatol, 1978. 114:564–566.

119. Breathnach, S. M., and Black, M. M., *Atypical tuberculide (acne scrofulosorum) secondary to tuberculous lymphadenitis.* Clin Exp Dermatol, 1981. 6:339–344.

120. Hudson, P. M., *Tuberculide (lichen scrofulosorum) secondary to osseous tuberculosis.* Clin Exp Dermatol, 1976. 1:391–394.

121. Warner, J., *Lichen scrofulosorum following B. C. G.* Br J Dermatol, 1966. 78:549.

122. Arianayagam, A. V., Ash, S., and Jones, R. R., *Lichen scrofulosorum in a patient with AIDS.* Clin Exp Dermatol, 1994. 19:74–76.

123. Smith, N. P., Ryan, T. J., Sanderson, K. V., and Sarkany, I., *Lichen scrofulosorum. A report of four cases.* Br J Dermatol, 1976. 94:319–325.

124. Graham-Brown, R. A., and Sarkany, I., *Lichen scrofulosorum with tuberculous dactylitis.* Br J Dermatol, 1980. 103:561–564.

125. Davis, J. P., Chesney, P. J., Wand, P. J., LaVenture, M., and Team, I. A. L., *Toxic-shock syndrome. Epidemiologic features, recurrence, risk factors, and prevention.* N Engl J Med, 1980. 303:1429–1435.

126. Reingold, A. L., Hargett, N. T., Dan, B. B., Shands, K. N., Strickland, B. Y., and Broome, C. V., *Nonmenstrual toxic shock syndrome: A review of 130 cases.* Ann Intern Med, 1982. 96:871–874.

127. Vuzevski, V. D., van Joost, T., Wagenvoort, J. H. T., and Michiels Dey, J. J., *Cutaneous patholgoy in toxic shock syndrome.* Int J Dermatol, 1989. 28:94–97.

128. Todd, J., and Fishaut, M., *Toxic-shock syndrome associated with phage-group I staphylococci.* Lancet, 1978. 2:1116–1118.

129. Shands, K. M., Schmid, G. P., and Dan, B. B., *Toxic-shock syndrome, a newly recognized disease entity.* Mayo Clin Proc, 1980. 66:663–665.

130. Manders, S. M., *Toxin-mediated streptococcal and staphylococcal disease.* J Am Acad Dermatol, 1998. 39:383–398.

131. Graham, D. R., O'Brien, M., Hayes, J. M., and Raab, M. G., *Postoperative toxic shock syndrome.* Clin Infect Dis, 1995. 20:895–899.

132. Resnick, S. D., *Staphylococcal toxin-mediated syndromes in childhood.* Semin Dermatol, 1992. 11:11–18.

133. McCahill, P. D., Whittle, D. I., and Jacbos, S. C., *Toxic shock syndrome: A complication of continent urinary diversion.* J Urol, 1992. 147:681–682.

134. Hurwitz, R. M., and Ackerman, A. B., *Cutaneous pathology of the toxic-shock syndrome.* J Am Acad Dermatol, 1985. 7:563–578.

135. Findla, R. F., and Odom, R. B., *Toxic-shock syndrome.* Int J Dermatol, 1982. 21:117–121.

136. Leung, D. Y., Travers, J. B., and Norris, D. A., *The role of superantigens in skin disease.* J Invest Dermatol, 12995. 105(Suppl 1):37S–42S.

137. Schlievert, P. M., *Alteration of immune function by staphylococcal pyrogenic exotoxin type C: Possible role in toxic-shock syndrome.* J Infect Dis, 1983. 147:391–398.

138. Wood, T. F., Potter, M. A., and Jonasson, O., *Streptococcal toxic shock-like syndrome. The importance of surgical intervention.* 1993. 217:109–114.

139. Wolf, J. E., and Rabinowitz, L. G., *Streptococcal toxic shock-like syndrome.* Arch Dermatol, 1995. 131:73–77.

140. Gemmell, C. G., *Staphylococcal scalded skin syndrome.* J Med Microbiol, 1995. 43:318–327.

141. Roeb, E., Schonfelder, T., Matern, S., Sieberth, H. G., Lenz, W., Lutticken, R., and Reinert, R. R., *Staphylococcal scalded skin syndrome in an immunocompromised adult.* Eur J Clin Microbiol Infect Dis, 1996. 15:499–503.

142. Cribier, B., Piemont, Y., and Grosshans, E., *Staphylococcal scalded skin syndrome in adults. A clinical review illustrated with a new case.* J Am Acad Dermatol, 1994. 30:319–324.

143. Loughead, J. L., *Congenital staphylococcal scalded skin syndrome: Report of a case.* Pediatr Infect Dis J, 1992. 11:413–414.

144. Shelley, E. D., Shelley, W. B., and Talanin, N. Y., *Chronic staphylococcal scalded skin syndrome.* Br J Dermatol, 1998. 139:319–324.

145. Strauss, G., Mogensen, A. M., Rasmussen, A., and Kirkegaard, P., *Staphylococcal scalded skin syndrome in a liver transplant patient.* Liver Transplant Surg, 1997. 3:435–436.

146. Farrell, A. M., Ross, J. S., Umasankar, S., and Bunker, C. B., *Staphylococcal scalded skin syndrome in an HIV-1 seropositive man.* Br J Dermatol, 1996. 134:962–965.

147. Hardwick, N., Parry, C. M., and Sharpe, G. R., *Staphylococcal scalded skin syndrome in an adult. Influence of immune and renal factors.* Br J Dermatol, 1995. 132:468–471.

148. Shirin, S., Gottlieb, A. B., and Stahl, E. B., *Staphylococcal scalded skin syndrome in an immunocompetent adult: Possible implication of low-dosage prednisone.* Cutis, 1998. 62:223–224.

149. Oono, T., Kanzaki, H., Yoshioka, T., and Arata, J., *Staphylococcal scalded skin syndrome in an adult. Identification of exfoliative toxin A and B genes by polymerase chain reaction.* Dermatology, 1997. 195:268–270.

150. Monday, S. R., Vath, G. M., Ferens, W. A., Deobald, C., Rago, J. V., Gahr, P. J., Monie, D. D., Iandolo, J. J., et al., *Unique superantigen activity of staphylococcal exfoliative toxins.* J Immunol, 1999. 162:4550–4559.

151. Koneman, E. W., Allen, S. D., Dowell, Jr., V., R., and Sommer, H. M., *Color Atlas and Textbook of Diagnostic Microbiology.* 1983, Philadelphia, J. B. Lipppincott Company.

CHAPTER
18

Viral Diseases

DIRECT INFECTION

Human Papillomavirus

Epidemiology. Human papillomavirus (HPV) infection is ubiquitous. Up to 77 subtypes of HPVs have been described and give rise to many types of cutaneous lesions [1]. The major subtypes affecting the skin are summarized in Table 18–1. Children and young adults have the highest rates of infection in the general population. From 2% to 20% of children may be infected with HPV [2]. Meat, fish, and poultry handlers are also at high risk for infection with HPV [2], and the warts that subsequently develope have similar clinical appearances to verrucae vulgares and verrucae planae. These workers also develop myrmecia-type warts within increased frequency.

Verruca vulgaris, myrmecia (or deep palmoplantar warts), and verruca plana (or flat warts) are extremely common and are seen in patients of all ages and at all body sites. Epidermodysplasia verruciformis is a rare disease. Afflicted patients develop thousands of HPV-induced warts resembling verruca plana that predispose them to subsequent carcinomas, generally in sun-exposed sites. Many types of HPV have been identified within these pateints.

Condyloma acuminatum, or genital wart, is a sexually transmitted disease with a prevalence of 106.5/10,000 population in some studies [3]. The peak incidence is between ages 19 and 24 years. Bowenoid papulosis is also caused by HPV infection and is transmitted sexually. It has a similar age distribution.

Patients who have received organ transplants and are thus immunosuppressed have a markedly increased incidence of HPV-induced lesions. Warts occur in 92% of patients more than 5 years post-transplantation. DNA studies demonstrate that the distribution of HPV subtypes is similar to those in the general population [4]. Similarly, patients with human immunodeficiency virus (HIV) infection are also predisposed to developing HPV-induced warts.

Cutaneous Features. Verruca vulgaris is the most common type of HPV-induced tumor. Verrucae vulgares present as small, exophytic papillomatous growths with variable hyperkeratosis. In some cases, there is an erythematous base. Occasionally, small, punctate black specks can be seen within the lesion, representing ectatic and thrombosed papillary dermal blood vessels. Although they can occur at any body site, the feet, hands, and fingers are common locations.

Myrmecia, or deep palmoplantar warts, are common, especially in children. These lesions are both exophytic and endophytic and may be painful as they compress the underlying dermis due to surface pressure. Rare cases have been reported in which the epidermal proliferation has extended into the underlying bone [5].

Patients with epidermodysplasia verruciformis present with hundreds to thousands of verruca plana [6]. Flat warts are minimally elevated pink to flesh-colored papules, closely set and with minimal surface change.

In men, condyloma acuminatum arises along the inner lining of the prepuce, the corona, urinary meatus,

Table 18–1. Cutaneous Lesions Associated with Human Papillomavirus (HPV)*

Cutaneous Lesion	HPV Subtypes
Myrmecia	1
Verruca vulgaris	2, 4, (7*)
Verruca plana	3, (10, 28)
Epidermodysplasia verruciformis†	3, 5, 8,
Condyloma acuminatum	6, 11, 16, 18
Butcher's warts	7
Cervical/penile/vulvar carcinoma	16, 18
Bowenoid papulosis	16, 18
Verrucous carcinoma	16, 18
Epidermal cysts	60

*Less common associations are in parentheses.

†More than 60 subtypes of HPV have been identified in patients with epidermodysplasia verruciformis.

and glans of the penis. In women, they are most common along the posterior part of the vaginal introitus and on the adjacent vulva or perineum [7]. Anal involvement is also frequent. In both sexes, condyloma acuminatum may occur in any perineal location as well as along the inguinal crease. Condyloma most often have a gently lobulated, exophytic and endophytic appearance. Condyloma are extremely variable in terms of number and size.

Bowenoid papulosis presents as multiple skin-colored to erythematous and hyperpigmented papules and plaques on the genitalia and surrounding skin, resembling condyloma clinically. Rarely, HPV-induced epidermal cysts have been reported on the soles of the feet [8].

Verrucous carcinoma, also known as oral florid papillomatosis, carcinoma cuniculatum, or Buschke-Lowenstein giant condyloma, depending on site, presents as a markedly papillomatous, exophytic growth in the oral cavity or anogenital region [9]. These tumors tend to be large at the time of presentation.

Associated Disorders. Epidermodysplasia verruciformis is associated with altered cell-mediated immunity leading to a lack of cell-mediated response to HPV infection [6]. Patients are at greatly increased risk for developing cutaneous squamous cell carcinomas. Laryngeal papillomas are also caused by HPV infeciton.

Human papillomavirus infection is associated with cervical carcinoma. In up to 90% of cases, HPV types 16 and 18 are found [1, 10]. Similarly, HPV16 and HPV18 infections have been associated with as many as 50% of squamous cell carcinomas of the anal mucosa [1, 11]. Occasional cases of squamous cell carcinoma at other sites, especially the hands and feet, have been associated with HPV16 infection [12]. Human papillomavirus types 31, 33, 35, 39, 45, and 52 have also

been correlated with malignant transformation [13]. Human papillomavirus subtypes 5 and 8 have been associated with cutaneous squamous cell carcinomas in patients with epidermodysplasia verruciformis [14].

Histologic Features. Verruca vulgaris appears as an exophytic papillomatous epidermal proliferation. Tiers of parakeratosis are present overlying the papillomatous processes, with orthokeratotic keratin between these tips. Occasionally, blood may be present within the keratin layer at the tips of the processes. The keratinocytes within the stratum granulosum demonstrate abnormal clumping of the keratohyaline granules (Fig. 18–1). They appear large and somewhat rounded or angulated. The granular layer is increased in thickness. The epidermis is acanthotic. In many cases, there is a symmetric architecture in which the rete ridges turn in toward the center of the lesion. Keratinocytes within the stratum malpighii often have clear to light-pink and ample cytoplasm. Mitotic figures are common, although atypical mitoses are not seen. Papillary dermal blood vessels are widely ectatic, tortuous, and often easily seen immediately beneath the dermal–epidermal junction. There is a wide variation in the degree of immune response underlying these lesions, with some patients demonstrating a florid lymphocytic infiltrate and others having essentially no dermal inflammatory response.

Myrmecia are characterized by large, eosinophilic cytoplasmic inclusions located in the cytoplasm of keratinocytes (Figs. 18–2 and 18–3). They are present in suprabasilar cells and are most prominent in the cells within the granular layer. Myrmecia have an endophytic growth pattern, extending into the papillary dermis.

Verruca plana are characterized by a flat epidermal surface. There is overlying hyperkeratosis, but para-

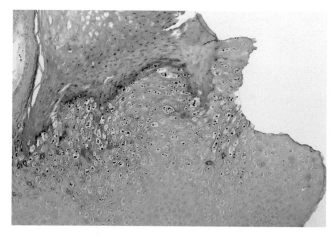

Fig. 18–1. Verruca vulgaris is characterized by papillomatous epidermal hyperplasia with marked clumping of keratohyaline granules.

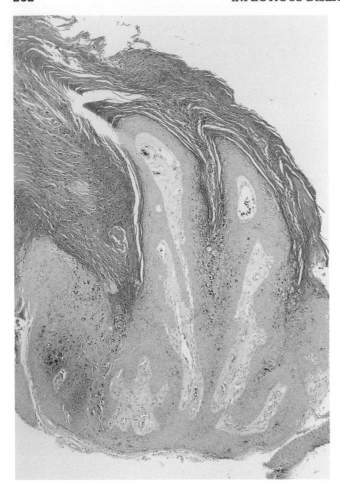

Fig. 18–2. There is marked epidermal hyperplasia in myrmecia.

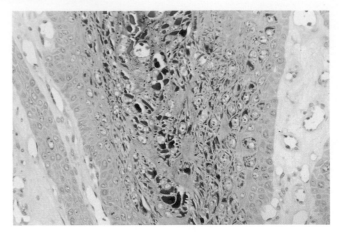

Fig. 18–3. Eosinophilic inclusions are large and angulated in myrmecia.

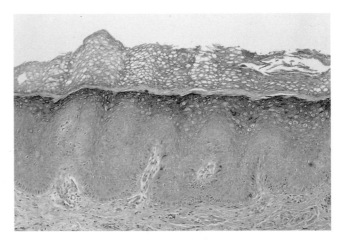

Fig. 18–4. Verruca plana is characterized by hyperkeratosis without parakeratosis and vacuolization of keratinocytes within the granular layer.

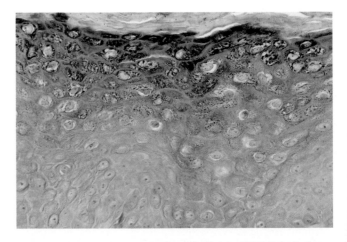

Fig. 18–5. Marked perinuclear halos are present in keratinocytes within the granular layer in verruca plana.

keratosis is usually absent (Fig. 18–4). The cells within the uppermost layers of the epidermis are characterized by pyknotic, hyperconvoluted nuclei and perinuclear haloes [15] (Fig. 18–5). When verruca plana occur in patients with epidermodysplasia verruciformis, they cause characteristic changes within the keratinocyte nuclei. The nuclei are markedly enlarged and have a unique blue-gray color.

Condyloma acuminatum is characterized by an endophytic and exophytic lobulated architecture. The epidermis is acanthotic and may display psoriasiform epidermal hyperplasia (Fig. 18–6). The granular layer is increased, with focal clumping of keratohyaline granules. Koilocytes, which are large keratinocytes with pyknotic, convoluted nuclei and perinuclear haloes, are present in the upper layers of the epidermis and are characteristic of this type of viral infection (Fig. 18–7).

Verrucous carcinoma is a difficult diagnosis to make on biopsy. The surface is papillomatous, with overlying parakeratosis and orthokeratosis. The epidermis is markedly acanthotic, with rounded rete ridges extend-

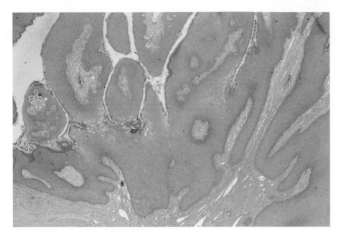

Fig. 18–6. Condyloma acuminata have a lobulated, papillomatous epidermis that is markedly acanthotic.

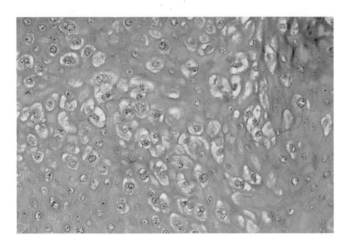

Fig. 18–7. Koilocytes are present within the granular layer in condyloma acuminatum.

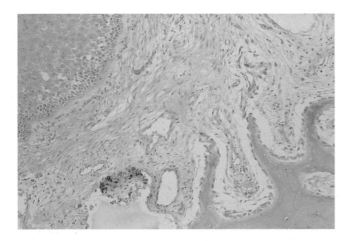

Fig. 18–8. Verrucous carcinoma is characterized by an acanthotic epidermis with pushing borders within the dermis

ing deeply into the underlying dermis with a blunt pushing, but not infiltrative border (Fig. 18–8). Superficial ulceration is common. Mitotic activity is present throughout the epidermis, but atypical mitoses are not common. Cytologic atypia is minimal [9]. Koilocytosis and other changes in the keratohyaline granules are found in many cases of verrucous carcinoma.

Special Studies. Human papillomavirus DNA is detectable on formalin-fixed, paraffin-embedded tissue sections with polymerase chain reaction technology. This technique is useful for determining precisely the subtype of HPV infection. Such information can be helpful in determining the potential for malignant transformation [16]. In situ hybridization can also distinguish among certain HPV subtypes and provides anatomic localization of the virus in the skin.

Pathogenesis. Human papillomaviruses are double-stranded DNA viruses that replicate within the nucleus of infected cells. Their E6/E7 oncoproteins are implicated in malignant transformation by incorporating into the host genome, activating cyclins E and A, and interfering with the functions of cellular proteins RB and p53, leading to mutagenesis [1, 17]. In patients with epidermodysplasia verruciformis, it is believed that ultraviolet irradiation serves as a "second hit" in patients with a defective immune system to prevent affected patients from responding appropriately to infection with the specific HPV-induced tumors. This results in formation of carcinomas [18]. The E4 protein from the HPV1 genome is responsible for creating the cytoplasmic inclusions in myrmecia [19].

Herpes Viruses

Epidemiology. Herpes simplex virus (HSV) is a very common virus that affects people of all ages. Type I HSV frequently appears as a "cold sore" and is not commonly associated with sexual transmission. Type II HSV is frequently transmitted sexually. Type I herpes can, however, involve the genitalia and type II the oral mucosa.

Varicella-zoster virus (VZV) most commonly affects children and gives rise to chickenpox. It is very highly contagious and demonstrates a seasonal variation in incidence, with most cases occurring in the winter and spring. It may also affect adults, especially those who suffer from immune dysfunctions [20].

The same virus also gives rise to herpes zoster, which occurs most commonly in adults. Many patients have some type of immune dysfunction [20]. Herpes zoster virus is uncommon in children [20, 21], and rare cases have been acquired congenitally [22]. There is no gender predilection. It is estimated that 300,000 cases of herpes zoster occur annually in the United States [23]. Up to 20% of adults experience herpes zoster at some time in their lives, with the incidence increasing with age [24]. The disease may be triggered by surgery, trauma, irradiation, immunosuppression, development of cancer, or infectious processes such as tuberculosis and syphilis [20].

Cutaneous features. Herpes simplex virus occurs most commonly in the vicinity of mucocutaneous junctions. Small, grouped vesicles on erythematous bases appear in crops and are accompanied by burning, itching, and pain. Individual vesicles persist for several days and heal with crust formation but without scarring. Local recurrences are quite common. Both skin and mucosal surfaces can be affected. The larynx and esophagus can also be involved in severe cases. In patients with atopic dermatitis, seborrheic dermatitis, and other chronic inflammatory dermatoses, herpes infection can lead to widespread cutaneous dissemination, a condition known as eczema herpeticum or Kaposi's varicelliform eruption. Ulcerated verrucous plaques may develop in patients with HIV infection and chronic herpes infections [25].

Primary inoculation can occur on fingers, giving rise to herpetic Whitlow. These ulcerations occur frequently in exposed health-care workers.

Varicella is characterized by a generalized exanthem that lasts for 4–8 days. The eruption characteristically begins on the face and scalp and extends to involve the trunk. Extremities are usually relatively spared. Crops of small, fluid-filled vesicles are present on an erythematous base. Lesions typically heal with scarring. The disease may be more florid and persist for a longer period of time in immunosuppressed patients. In HIV-infected patients, chronic infection may result in verrucous plaques [26].

Most patients with zoster (shingles) present with a unilateral vesiculobullous eruption along a dermatomal distribution. Macules and papules may be present before discrete vesicles appear, and pain precedes or accompanies the skin changes. New lesions continue to appear for 4–7 days. Although any part of the body may be affected, there is some predilection for dermatomes T3 through L3 [27]. The cutaneous eruption is accompanied by pain in 90% of patients and flu-like symptoms in approximately 10% of patients. One-third of patients have a prodromal syndrome of fever and malaise [28]. Recurrent attacks are common.

In some cases, more than one separate dermatome may be simultaneously affected [29]. Disseminated zoster is defined as the presence of more than 50 lesions outside of a single dermatome and is more common in the immunocompromised and the elderly.

Associated Disorders. Herpes simplex virus infection is rarely complicated by systemic involvement. Primary infection is rarely associated with a neuritis. In rare cases, childhood infection with herpes simplex may become disseminated, resulting in hepatitis, encephalitis, gastroenteritis, and pneumonitis. Recurrent HSV has been associated with erythema multiforme [30].

Intrauterine herpes is contracted in utero from mothers infected with primary herpes simplex during pregnancy. Multiple congenital anomalies may develop, including encephalitis, chorioretinitis, and intracerebral califications. Cutaneous vesicles may also be present in the neonate at the time of birth.

Neonatal herpes is acquired by the infant during passage through an infected birth canal. The ensuing disease ranges from limited skin infection to systemic disease, including hepatitis, pneumonia, and severe coagulation disorders. Approximately 3%–5% of babies born to mothers with active recurrent herpes infection will develop neonatal herpes. The risk is almost 50% in babies born to mothers with active primary genital herpes [31].

Varicella is rarely associated with systemic illness, but in florid cases can involve the lungs and central nervous system. The central nervous system is most commonly involved and manifests as Reye's syndrome, cerebral ataxia, encephalitis, meningoencephalitis, and Guillain-Barré syndrome [32]. Pneumonia occurs in 1/400 adult patients with primary VZV infection [33]. Other complications, including myocarditis, glomerulonephritis, pancreatitis, hepatitis, and arthritis, are much less common [34]. When infection occurs during pregnancy, intrauterine death may occur [35].

Herpes zoster occurs commonly in association with immunosuppression. It has been reported after varicella immunization [36].

Herpes zoster is associated with frequent neurologic involvement. These complications include postherpetic neuralgia, myelitis [37], and Guillain-Barré syndrome [38]. The incidence of acute meningoencephalitis is very low [39]. Neurologic involvement has also been implicated in postherpetic urinary retention [40]. Ophthalmologic complications are common and may include proptosis, conjunctival hemorrhages, keratitis of the cornea, uveitis, and optic neuropathy [20]. Rare cases of herpes zoster causing pancreatitis [41] and gastritis [42] have been reported.

As is the case with herpes simplex infection, varicella zoster infection has been associated with erythema multiforme [43]. A sarcoidal-like reaction has been reported within post-herpes zoster scars [44]. Acquired reactive perforating collagenosis has also appeared in this setting [45]. An acneiform eruption has also been described in the site of previous herpes zoster infection [46]. Herpes zoster may be a presenting manifestation of HIV infection.

Histologic Features. Herpes simplex infection is histologically indistinguishable from HZV infection and VZV infection. The epidermis is characterized by marked spongiosis, resulting in microvesiculation. There is reticular degeneration of the epidermis (Fig. 18–9). Infected cells demonstrate nuclear inclusions. These cells are characterized by nuclei with margination of the chromatin and a steel-gray appearance in their centers (Fig. 18–10). Multinucleation of keratinocytes is present, and there is molding of adjacent nuclei. Infected cells demonstrate ballooning degeneration. Hair follicles are frequently infected with the virus particles [47]. Within the dermis, there is moderate to brisk host response. Herpes infections of the skin may be associated with a leukocytoclastic vasculitis. It has been suggested that primary infections are associated with the most intense inflammatory response.

Cases of HZV infection associated with hematologic malignancies may demonstrate a specific infiltrate of neoplastic cells into the site of the infection. Both lymphomatous and leukemic infiltrates have been described [48–50].

Granulomatous inflammatory reactions are seen occasionally in patients after HZV and HSV infections [29, 51]. Other patients develop a pseudolymphomatous inflammatory response [52]. In rare cases, the granulomatous response may be associated with vasculitis and histologically resemble polyarteritis nodosa [53, 54]. Keloids, granuloma annulare, lichen planus, and sinus histiocytosis with massive lymphadenopathy have also been described as occurring within the sites of HZV scars [55].

Special Studies. In situ hybridization is a very sensitive and specific tool for detecting herpes family viruses in formalin-fixed, paraffin-embedded tissue sections [56]. Polymerase chain reaction has proved to be quite reliable in distinguishing HSV from VZV, even using

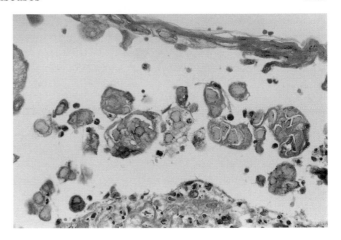

Fig. 18–10. Multinucleated cells and steel-gray nuclear inclusions are abundant in herpes simplex and varicella-zoster infections.

formalin-fixed, paraffin-embedded tissue. It is not, however, necessary to perform this examination in most clinical settings [57, 58].

Although immunostaining for herpes antigens has some utility in establishing a diagnosis of herpes infection, extensive cross-reactivity limits the ability of this technique to distinguish between HSV and VZV. It is a useful technique for distinguishing between other viruses of the herpes family.

Pathogenesis. Herpes simplex virus is caused by one of several subtypes of herpesvirus. Herpesvirus type 1 is most often associated with perioral infections. Herpesvirus type 2 is most often acquired through sexual transmission and gives rise to genital infections. Neither organism is site specific, however, and infections with either virus can be present in any mucocutaneous location.

Varicella is caused by VZV, a member of the herpes family of viruses. Herpes zoster is caused by the reactivation of the VZV that persists in the dorsal root or trigeminal ganglia [47]. It has been suggested that in herpes zoster, the damage to keratinocytes may be due to the cell-mediated host response to the virus in addition to the viral cytopathic changes [59].

Cytomegalovirus

Epidemiology. Cytomegalovirus (CMV) rarely causes significant cutaneous disease. Clinically apparent skin disease is essentially limited to immunocompromised patients who have systemic illness caused by CMV. Even in these situations, skin disease is exceptional [60].

Cutaneous Features. As documented cases of CMV-induced skin disease are rare, precise characterization of the cutaneous findings is not possible. One patient

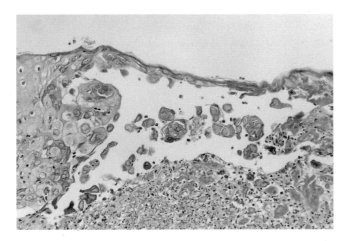

Fig. 18–9. The epidermis is disintegrating in multiple levels in herpes simplex or varicella zoster infection.

had a macular and papular eruption [61]. Another developed necrotic lesions [62]. A morbilliform eruption was described in one patient with CMV disease, and another had a vesiculobullous eruption [63, 64]. Perineal ulcers have also been associated with CMV infection. In these cases, while invariably present, it was thought that concurrent infection with HSV was the cause of the ulceration [65].

Associated Disorders. Cytomegalovirus infection of the skin has been reported in patients with organ transplants, Hodgkin's disease, and acquired immunodeficiency virus (AIDS) [64, 66, 67]. Additional cases have been described in patients after severe burns [66]. Clinically apparent disease caused by CMV is most frequent in the liver, kidneys, and lungs.

Histologic Features. The histologic features of cutaneous CMV infection are characterized by intranuclear and intracytoplasmic inclusions within endothelial cells, monocytes, and occasional pericytes. In nuclei, a progressively enlarging basophilic body grows to squeeze actual nuclear material to a thin, eccentrically placed crescent. There is a surrounding halo often imparting an "owl's eye" appearance. Subsequent production of numerous small virions occurs. These accumulate in the cytoplasm as small basophilic stipples and are released into the connective tissue upon cell rupture (Fig. 18–11). These inclusions are occasionally accompanied by a leukocytoclastic vasculitis involving vessels of the superficial vascular plexus. Although it is debatable whether CMV infects epidermal keratinocytes, the virus has been rarely, but confidently noted in eccrine glandular epithelium.

Special Studies. Electron microscopy, culture, direct immunofluorescence, immunoperoxidase, and in situ

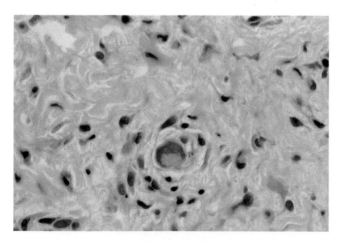

Fig. 18–11. Cytomegalovirus inclusions are present within endothelial cells and pericytes.

hybridization have all been used to confirm the diagnosis of cutaneous CMV infection [64, 68].

Pathogenesis. The presence of CMV within the skin is not necessarily associated with clinical disease. Its occult presence has been demonstrated with newer, more sensitive probes [68]. It is not yet understood when or if the presence of organisms will induce cutaneous changes and what other factors are necessary to cause these changes.

Molluscum Contagiosum

Epidemiology. Molluscum contagiosum and variola virus are the only two poxviruses that specifically infect human beings. Infection with molluscum contagiosum occurs most commonly in children, although in recent years it has become much more prevalent in immunosuppressed patients [69]. It is also seen in genital regions as a sexually transmitted disease in immunocompetent patients. Papules caused by molluscum contagiosum are among the most common cutaneous manifestations in HIV-infected individuals [70]. Up to 9% of HIV-infected patients demonstrate molluscum contagiosum infection in some studies [69].

Cutaneous Features. Molluscum contagiosum presents as one or several papules that are usually several millimeters in diameter and have a central area of umbilication. The papules have a waxy appearance and are skin colored. Molluscum can be found in any location on children and is frequently seen in the anogenital region of adults. In immunocompromised individuals, hundreds of papules can be present, and much larger nodules may also develop [71]. These nodules may coalesce into plaques and ulcerate. Facial involvement is more characteristic in HIV-infected patients [69]. Rarely, molluscum contagiosum can affect the oral cavity in these patients [72].

Associated Disorders. Molluscum contagiosum is a frequent cutaneous manifestation in immunocompromised patients. Infection with the virus has been reported to coexist within the same cutaneous lesion as *Cryptococcus neoformans* in an AIDS patient [73].

Molluscum contagiosum has been reported to induce erythema annulare centrifugum [74] (see Chapter 19). Molluscum contagiosum does not disseminate and give rise to systemic illness.

Histologic Features. The molluscum contagiosum virus infects keratinocytes. Often, the epidermis forms invaginations at the sites of molluscum infection. These central depressions can resemble a hair follicle or even a keratoacanthoma. Viral particles aggregate into large, eosinophilic cytoplasmic inclusions that compress the

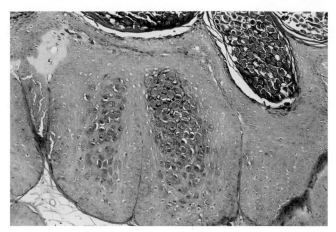

Fig. 18–12. Bright eosinophilic inclusions are present above the basal layer in molluscum contagiosum.

keratinocyte nuclei [75]. These viral particles are easily seen on routine histologic sections. They spare the basal layer of keratinocytes and are present in increasing numbers at higher levels of the epidermis. At the surface of the epidermis and within the stratum corneum, the viral inclusions become more basophilic and are frequently extracellular (Fig. 18–12).

A brisk host response is frequently seen in response to molluscum contagiosum. This is especially true when the epidermis is disrupted and viral particles come into contact with the dermis. In rare cases, the inflammatory response is vigorous enough and contains enough lymphocyte atypia to have been described as a pseudolymphoma [76]. In a single case, metaplastic ossification of the dermis was seen adjacent to multiple sites of molluscum contagiosum infection [77].

Special Studies. Scanning electron microscopy reveals the molluscum virus to have multiple forms, including spherical, ellipsoidal, and brick shapes. Each of the forms has long, linked cord-like structures connected to the core of the virus [78]. It has also been demonstrated that the molluscum viral particles are contained within a viral sac within infected keratinocytes [79].

Pathogenesis. Molluscum contagiosum is a double-stranded DNA poxvirus that replicates within keratinocytes.

Human Immunodeficiency Virus

Epidemiology. Human immunodeficiency virus infection is associated with a vast spectrum of cutaneous diseases, as shown in Table 18–2. In this section, we discuss the exanthem associated with initial seroconversion and several other cutaneous manifestations that are associated intimately with HIV infection. Other

Table 18–2. Cutaneous Disorders Associated with Human Immunodeficiency Virus Infection

Disease	Absolute CD4/µl Count
Tumors	
Basal cell carcinoma	
Bowenoid papulosis	
Kaposi's sarcoma	
Lymphoma	
Oral/anal squamous cell carcinoma	
Infections	
Atypical mycobacteria	<300
Bacillary angiomatosis	
Candida	<100
Condyloma acuminatum	>300
Cryptococcocus	
Cryptosporidiosis	
Cytomegalovirus	
Demodex folliculorum	
Dermatophytosis	
Herpes simplex	<100
Histoplasmosis	
Impetigo	
Leishmaniasis	
Molluscum contagiosum	>300
Mycobacterium tuberculosis	
Onychomycosis	
Oral hairy leukoplakia	<300
Pityrosporum obiculare	<300
Pneumocystis carinii	
Scabies	<100
Sporotrichosis	
Syphilis	
Toxoplasmosis	
Varicella-zoster	<100
Verruca vulgaris	
Miscellaneous	
Asteatotic eczema	<400
Atopic dermatitis	
Drug eruptions	
Eosinophilic folliculitis	<250
Erythema elevatum diutinum	
Exanthem of seroconversion	
Ichthyosis	
Lichen planus	
Papular eruption of AIDS	
Pityriasis rubra pilaris	>300
Pruritus	
Psoriasis	<200
Reiter s syndrome	
Seborrheic dermatitis	<100
Thrombocytopenic purpura	
Tricomegaly of eyelids	<100
Vasculitis	
Xerosis	>300
Yellow nail syndrome	

From references 114, 137, 165–167.

diseases that can occur in patients with HIV infection are presented elsewhere in this volume.

Infection with HIV is associated with a febrile illness and an acute exanthem of seroconversion in 28%–67% of people [80–82]. Oral hairy leukoplakia is observed in 15%–25% of patients with HIV infection [83, 84]. It is much more prevalent in HIV-infected men than in HIV-infected women [84]. It is often associated with significant immunosuppression.

Kaposi's sarcoma occurs in a classic form typically on the lower extremities of elderly men of Mediterranean descent. This form of the disease is not ordinarily associated with systemic disease. There is also an endemic form of the disease that was reported in Africa and an iatrogenic form associated with immunomodulatory therapies [85]. These forms of the disease are not discussed further in this chapter. A commonly seen form of the disease in the United States is AIDS-related Kaposi's sarcoma. It has been estimated that 10%–50% of patients with AIDS develop Kaposi's sarcoma. The advent of new antiretroviral medications has greatly reduced the incidence of AIDS-associated Kaposi's sarcoma. This is more common in homosexual and bisexual men with AIDS than in women or intravenous drug abusers with AIDS [85–87]. Kaposi's sarcoma is best defined as a multifocal angioproliferative neoplasm [86].

Eosinophilic folliculitis is another cutaneous manifestation of HIV infection. It tends to occur in relatively advanced stages of the disease when circulating CD4-positive cells are less than 250/mm^3 [88] and may not represent a discrete clinical entity. This disease is thought to be distinct from Ofuji's diease (eosinophilic pustular folliculitis) based on different epidemiologic characteristics. Ofuji's disease is most prevalent in Japan, affects mainly people who are otherwise healthy, and is characterized by sterile papules and pustules grouped in a seborrheic distribution. Although eosinophilic folliculitis was originally believed to be unique for HIV-infected people, it has subsequently been described in other immunocompromised patients [89]. It likely represents part of the prurigo folliculitis syndrome associated with late-stage HIV infection.

Bacillary angiomatosis (BA) was originally described as occurring exclusively in patients with HIV infection [90, 91]. A similar process has now, however, been described in patients with immunosuppression due to many causes. Rare cases have been reported in immunocompetent patients [92, 93].

Lymphomas develop in approximately 10% of HIV-positive patients. They are most commonly intermediate- to high-grade B-cell lymphomas [94]. The B-cell lymphomas tend to present in extranodal sites such as body cavities and the central nervous system, but they can also involve the skin. A range of cutaneous T-cell lymphomas has also been described in these patients [95, 96]. Human T-cell lymphotrophic virus type 1 (HTLV-1)–associated adult T-cell leukemia-lymphoma was reported in a patient with co-infections with HTLV-1 and HIV [97]. Hodgkin's disease has also been reported in HIV-positive patients [95]. Lymphomas are described more fully in Chapter 10.

Cutaneous Features

Exanthem of seroconversion. The exanthem associated with HIV seroconversion may be macular or papulovesicular and is most prominent on the upper trunk. Lesions have been described as oval shaped, and a necrotic center is occasionally present. Involvement of the palms and soles occurs. The eruption is often accompanied by fever and malaise [98].

Oral hairy leukoplakia. Oral hairy leukoplakia is characterized by bilateral, thickened, white plaques on the lateral sides and dorsum of the tongue [99]. The surface of the tongue appears corrugated. The buccal mucosa is also involved in a minority of cases [100].

Kaposi's sarcoma. Kaposi's sarcoma presents as erythematous to violaceous patches. In most cases, only a few patches are present initially, and more develop as the disease progresses. In some cases, a distribution along lines of cleavage has been described [101]. The patches are often oval. Although lesions may generalize and may develop on any body surface, the midface is frequently affected. As the disease progresses, patches become progressively thicker and evolve into plaques and even tumors. Ulceration may be present in tumor-stage lesions.

Eosinophilic folliculitis. Eosinophilic folliculitis presents as widespread erythematous, folliculocentric papules that are intensely pruritic. Pustules are common. Occasional urticarial papules are present. Later lesions evolve into coalsecent plaques and prurigo papules. The trunk, head, and neck and proximal extremities are most heavily involved [88, 102].

Bacillary angiomatosis. Cutaneous lesions of BA may be single or widespread [103]. They most commonly appear as dome-shaped, red papules that may enlarge with time and may have a rubbery consistency. Central ulceration is common. There is a striking resemblance to pyogenic granuloma or angioma for any single lesion. Mucosal surfaces are commonly involved. Lesions resolve without scarring and leave only minimal hyperpigmentation. Less commonly, BA may present with subcutaneous nodules that have no overlying surface changes. Rare black patients may present with hyperpigmented, indurated plaques [104].

Associated Disorders.
Oral hairy leukoplakia has been described in other patients who are immunocompromised, including patients with chronic lymphocytic leukemia [105], multiple myeloma [106], systemic lupus erythematosus [107], and ulcerative colitis [108] and in those taking corticosteroids long term [109].

Kaposi's sarcoma is associated with immunocompromised states other than HIV infection. It develops in some patients after organ transplantation [110]. In addition, involvement of lymph nodes and viscera, especially the lungs and colon, is well documented [111, 112].

Eosinophilic folliculitis has been reported in a patient undergoing immunosuppressive treatment for Waldenström's macroglobulinemia [89]. A similar-appearing, but nonrelated entity known as eosinophilic pustular folliculitis (Ofuji's disease) occurs primarily in infants, is most prevalent in Japan, and is presumed to be unrelated to the eosinophilic folliculitis seen in patients with AIDS [113]. Most patients with eosinophilic folliculitis have a concomitant peripheral eosinophilia [114].

Bacillary angiomatosis may be found in lymph nodes and in the liver, giving rise to peliosis hepatis [115]. Osseous defects have been reported underlying the vascular proliferations [116]. Angiomatous proliferations have been detected in the respiratory tract and gastrointestinal tract, as well [117].

Histologic Features. Histologic features of the exanthem of seroconversion are not specific. Biopsy specimens demonstrate a normal epidermis and a mild superficial perivascular lymphocytic infiltrate [80]. Other authors have noted focal mild spongiosis, vacuolar changes in the basal layer of the epidermis, and, rarely, foci of epidermal necrosis [118]. In one series, the lymphocytic infiltrate was also found in an interstitial pattern, and a perifollicular inflammatory infiltrate was present in some cases [119].

Oral hairy leukoplakia. Cytopathic changes are usually present in biopsied lesions of oral hairy leukoplakia. Inclusions or homogenization within nuclei of infected keratinocytes and extensive cytoplasmic ballooning with a ground-glass appearance are frequently present [120]. Perinuclear clearing is often pronounced, and the nuclei may appear pyknotic [121]. The affected mucosa is markedly acanthotic and demonstrates overlying hyperkeratosis and parakeratosis. The surface of the mucosa is papillomatous. There is virtually no inflammatory response. Although the histologic changes are characteristic, they are not entirely specific (Figs. 18–13 and 18–14). The following entities must be considered in the histologic differential diagnosis of oral hairy leukoplakia:

- Candidiasis
- Normal mucosa
- Oral leukoedema
- Verruca vulgaris
- White sponge nevus

Kaposi's sarcoma. Kaposi's sarcoma is characterized by an increased number of individually arrayed spindle-shaped endothelial cells, initially in the upper reticular dermis. Poorly formed, jagged, and irregularly

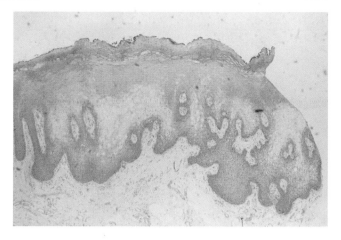

Fig. 18–13. The mucosal epithelium is acanthotic and pale staining in oral hairy leukoplakia.

dilated blood vessels are prominent (in most cases, although in some cases they may be relatively inconspicuous) throughout the dermis [122] (Figs. 18–15 and 18–16). These newly formed blood vessels may protrude into a preexisting vessel, giving rise to the "promontory sign" [123]. Dermal blood vessels are surrounded by a lymphocytic infiltrate. Plasma cells, if present, may be a helpful diagnostic clue [123]. Endothelial cells do not display significant cytologic atypia or mitotic activity in early lesions. The following entities must be considered in the histologic differential diagnosis of early patch-stage lesions of Kaposi's sarcoma:

- Acquired tufted angioma
- Angiosarcoma
- Capillary hemangioma
- Dermatofibroma
- Granuloma annulare, nonpalisaded
- Lymphangioma
- Targetoid hemosiderotic hemangioma

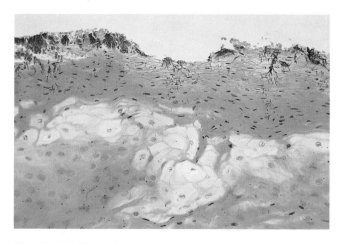

Fig. 18–14. Extensive cytoplasmic vacuolization and thick parakeratosis are often present in oral hairy leukoplakia.

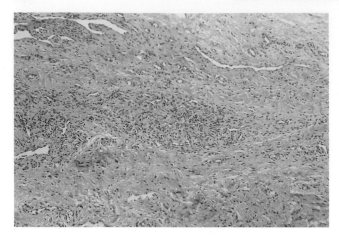

Fig. 18–15. Patch-stage Kaposi's sarcoma demonstrates clusters of poorly formed vascular spaces in the midreticular dermis.

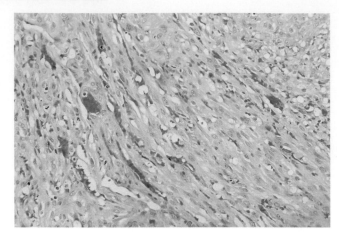

Fig. 18–17. Later lesions of Kaposi's sarcoma demonstrate large tumor nodules of spindle-shaped cells surrounding slit-like vascular spaces.

Plaques demonstrate vascular proliferations that completely fill the reticular dermis with poorly formed slit-like vascular spaces. There is increased cellularity compared with patch-stage lesions, and areas of spindle cells may be present in the reticular dermis, between the irregularly shaped vessels. These small collections of spindle-shaped cells are relatively monomorphous and display little cytologic atypia. Apoptotic endothelial cells are present in plaques and tumor nodules [124]. Extravasation of erythrocytes is present in most cases. Degenerating red cells may appear as hyaline globules [125].

Tumor nodules of Kaposi's sarcoma demonstrate sheets of spindle cells filling the dermis and extending into the subcutaneous fat. Although there is marked hypercellularity in these lesions, cytologic atypia of the spindle cells is still relatively mild. Mitotic activity varies from moderate to brisk (Figs. 18–17 and 18–18). The following entities must be considered in the histologic differential diagnosis of tumor stage lesions of Kaposi's sarcoma:

- Angiosarcoma
- Atypical fibroxanthoma
- Bacillary angiomatosis
- Hemangiopericytoma
- Leiomyosarcoma
- Malignant fibrous histiocytoma
- Pyogenic granuloma
- Spindle cell hemangioendothelioma

A lymphangiomatous variant of Kaposi's sarcoma has been described in which interanastamosing vascular channels percolate diffusely throughout the dermis

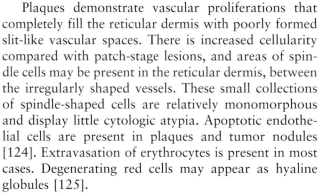

Fig. 18–16. Higher magnification demonstrates marked increase in cellularity around slit-like vascular spaces in early lesions of Kaposi's sarcoma.

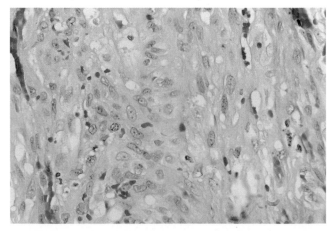

Fig. 18–18. Tumor cells show only slight atypia in tumor-stage Kaposi's sarcoma.

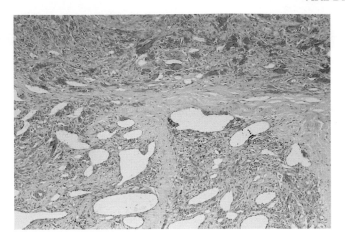

Fig. 18–19. Large ectatic, interanastamosing spaces are present in the lymphangiomatous variant of Kaposi's sarcoma.

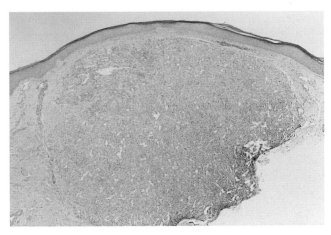

Fig. 18–21. A dermal nodular proliferation of small, well-formed blood vessels underlying a flattened epidermis is seen in bacillary angiomatosis, showing a striking resemblance to pyogenic granuloma.

and into the subcutaneous fat. These channels are lined by bland-appearing endothelial cells [123] (Fig. 18–19).

Eosinophilic folliculitis. Eosinophilic folliculitis is characterized by a perivascular and follicular inflammatory infiltrate consisting of predominantly eosinophils. Extension of the eosinophils into the follicular epithelium is essential to make a specific diagnosis of eosinophilic folliculitis. Plasma cells are also over-represented. Lymphocytes represent a minority population. There is spongiosis of the follicular epithelium and the adjacent sebaceous glands [88]. The inflammatory infiltrate is concentrated at the level of the follicular isthmus [126] (Fig. 18–20).

Bacillary angiomatosis. The histologic features of BA greatly resemble those of pyogenic granuloma. A well-circumscribed proliferation of well-formed, thin-walled vessels is present within the superficial and deep dermis (Fig. 18–21). The overlying epidermis is usually

flattened and forms a collarette around the vascular proliferation. Ulceration may occur. The stroma is initially quite edematous, and it becomes fibrotic in older lesions [103]. Endothelial cells may demonstrate prominent swelling and protrude into the vascular spaces. They may appear cytologically atypical, and mitoses are commonly seen. The presence of neutrophils and nuclear dust is seen in most cases and may be a very helpful clue in arriving at the correct diagnosis (Fig. 18–22). Neutrophils often cluster in areas of amphophilic granular material that represents masses of the organisms.

Special Studies. Polymerase chain reaction is helpful in detecting Epstein-Barr virus in cases of oral hairy leukoplakia [105]. The technique has been performed with re-

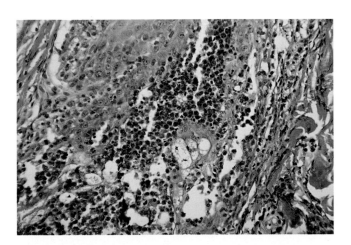

Fig. 18–20. Abundant eosinophils are present within the follicular infundibulum in eosinophilic folliculitis.

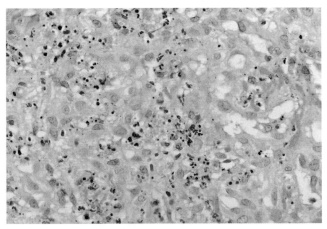

Fig. 18–22. Neutrophils, karyorrhectic debris, and amorphous material are present between endothelial cells in bacillary angiomatosis.

liability on scrapings of oral epithelial cells, but a positive finding is neither 100% sensitive nor 100% specific for the disease [127]. In situ hybridization studies enable direct localization of the viral particles in the infected epithelial cells and has been used with great success, as has routine immunohistochemistry [121, 128]. Detection of viral particles with electron microscopy has also been reported to be very sensitive [129].

Polymerase chain reaction technology is also helpful in identifying herpesvirus-8 in AIDS-related Kaposi's sarcoma. Although this is helpful in understanding the pathogenesis of the disease, it is not necessary for establishing a diagnosis of Kaposi's sarcoma. Occasionally, immunoperoxidase using antibodies against type IV collagen or other basement membrane zone antigens is helpful in demonstrating neovascularization. In subtle cases, this is helpful in distinguishing Kaposi's sarcoma from early and mild cases of granuloma annulare.

Silver stains such as Warthin-Starry and Steiner are helpful in highlighting organisms in BA. As they are often abundant in this disease, it is usually possible to identify them as clusters of coccobacilli (Fig. 18–23). The organisms can also be identified with electron microscopy. Serologic tests for antibodies directed against *Bartonella henselae* can also be used.

Pathogenesis. Oral hairy leukoplakia is believed to be caused by Epstein-Barr virus. A permissive environment, thought to be caused by co-infection with human papilloma virus, allows Epstein-Barr virus to replicate within epithelial cells and leads to the clinical findings [130]. Continued shedding of the virus appears to be necessary for development of clinical findings [131]. Others are less convinced that there is a role for HPV in this process [132].

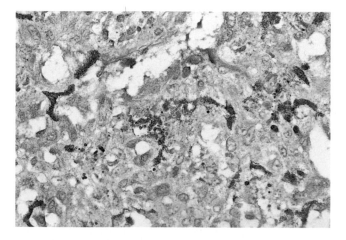

Fig. 18–23. Clusters of organisms are usually easy to detect in bacillary angiomatosis.

Kaposi's sarcoma has been intimately associated with herpesvirus-8 infection [133–135]. This virus has several known genes that enable it to alter the host environment and that may be important in the etiology of Kaposi's sarcoma [135]. The proliferating cell type is believed to be an endothelial cell that expresses CD34 and, less commonly, stains with factor VIII–related antigen.

Eosinophilic folliculitis has been thought to be related to immune dysregulation [136]. Although many organisms, including bacteria, *Pityrosporum*, and *Demodex* [137], have been implicated in the pathogenesis, none is present in all cases and shown to be causative. In one study, less than 25% of cases demonstrated organisms [126].

Bacillary angiomatosis is caused by infection with *Bartonella henselae* or, less commonly, *Bartonella quintana*. *Bartonella henselae* has the ability to colonize vascular tissue and to stimulate vasoproliferation, which may be the mechanism responsible for the observed findings in this disease [138].

SECONDARY MANIFESTATIONS OF VIRAL INFECTION

Papular Acrodermatitis of Childhood (Gianotti-Crosti Syndrome)

Epidemiology. Papular acrodermatitis of childhood, or Gianotti-Crosti syndrome, is an acrally distributed papulovesicular eruption that occurs after viral illness. It is most common in children with a mean age of about 2 years [139], although rare cases have been reported in adults [140]. The disorder is not rare, although its exact incidence is not known. It is a self-limited hypersensitivity reaction to a wide range of viruses [141].

Cutaneous Features. Papular acrodermatitis of childhood is characterized by the abrupt appearance of flat-topped 2–4 mm papules or vesicles distributed symmetrically on the face, buttocks, and extremities often over the extensor surfaces of the joints. The eruption is usually asymptomatic or only mildly pruritic and lasts from several weeks to months.

Associated Disorders. Lymphadenopathy is commonly seen in patients with Gianotti-Crosti syndrome, and hepatomegaly is rarely also present [139]. Gianotti-Crosti syndrome has been associated with many viral infections. Hepatitis B virus was the first virus to be associated [142], but this association is seen in only a minority of cases [139]. Other associated viral illnesses include respiratory syncytial virus [143], parain-

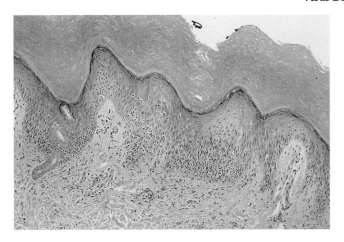

Fig. 18–24. Gianotti-Crosti syndrome is characterized by a nonspecific spongiotic dermatitis with a superficial lymphocytic infiltrate.

fluenza virus [144], herpesvirus-6 [145], poxvirus and parvovirus B19 [146], coxsackie viruses [147], Epstein-Barr virus [148], CMV [149], hepatitis C [150], and HIV [151]. It has also been reported after influenza virus vaccination [140]. Infection with group A β-hemolytic *Streptococcus* has also been implicated in triggering papular acrodermatitis of childhood [143].

Histologic Features. The histologic changes in papular acrodermatitis of childhood are not specific. In most cases, there is a superficial perivascular lymphocytic inflammatory infiltrate, accompanied by mild spongiosis and exocytosis of lymphocytes into the overlying epidermis (Fig. 18–24). Less commonly, a lichenoid inflammatory pattern with basal keratinocyte vacuolization may be present, and in rare cases lymphocytic vasculitis has been described [152]. The following entities must be considered in the differential diagnosis of Gianotti-Crosti syndrome:

- Arthropod bite reaction
- Atopic dermatitis
- Contact dermatitis
- Dermatophytosis
- Nummular dermatitis
- Seborrheic dermatitis
- Viral exanthem

Special Studies. Special studies are not helpful in arriving at a diagnosis of papular acrodermatitis of childhood.

Pathogenesis. The pathogenesis remains unknown. Gianotti-Crosti syndrome is believed to represent a nonspecific hypersensitivity reaction to a large number of antigens [151].

Hepatitis C

Epidemiology. The incidence of hepatitis C infection varies widely with geographic location. A high percentage of patients infected with the hepatitis C virus demonstrate cutaneous manifestations. Of these, lichen planus is one of the most frequent associations. In one European study, 16% of patients with lichen planus demonstrated antibodies to hepatitis C virus [153]. In another study, 78% of patients with oral or cutaneous lichen planus demonstrated antibodies to hepatitis C virus.

Cutaneous Features. The cutaneous manifestations that have most frequently been associated with hepatitis C infection include leukocytoclastic vasculitis and lichen planus [154]. These entities are discussed more fully in Chapter 4. Less common entities associated with hepatitis C infection include porphyria cutanea tarda (see Chapter 5) [155], erythema nodosum, erythema multiforme (see Chapter 23), and polyarteritis nodosa (see Chapter 4) [156]. Although urticaria has been described as occurring in patients with hepatitis C infection [157], controlled studies suggest that there is no statistical association [158].

Lichen planus associated with hepatitis C has the same morphologic characteristics as idiopathic lichen planus. The cutaneous eruption is characterized by the appearance of flat- lopped, polygonal papules that have a violaceous hue. They can appear in any location on the body, but have a predilection for flexural surfaces, especially on the wrists.

Oral involvement is frequently seen in patients with lichen planus related to hepatitis C infection [159]. The incidence of hepatitis C infection in patients with oral lichen planus has been determined to be at least 25% in some studies [159, 160]. Hypertrophic [161] and generalized [162] lichen planus have also been associated with hepatitis C virus infection.

Associated Disorders. Hepatitis C is associated with chronic hepatitis, and many of the sequelae including cirrhosis and liver failure arise from this frequently destructive process involving the liver. Mixed cryoglobulinemai is also associated with hepatitis C infection [154].

Histologic Features. The histologic features of lichen planus associated with hepatitis C are indistinguishable from those of idiopathic lichen planus. There is orthokeratotic hyperkeratosis, acanthosis, and wedge-shaped hypergranulosis. The rete ridges demonstrate a sawtoothed appearance at their bases (Fig. 18–25). There is extensive basal vacuolization, and the dermal–epidermal junction is obscured by a dense band-like in-

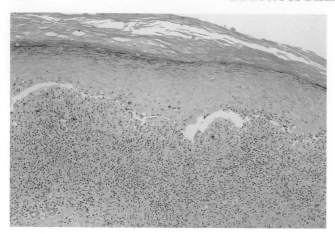

Fig. 18–25. Hyperkeratosis, wedge-shaped hypergranulosis, and acanthosis are present in hepatitis C–related lichen planus.

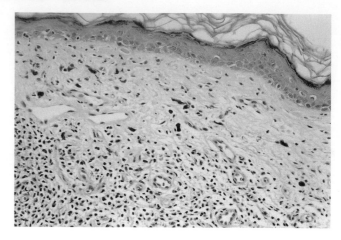

Fig. 18–27. Old lesions of lichen planus often demonstrate an atrophic epidermis with abundant pigment incontinence seen within histiocytes in the papillary dermis.

flammatory infiltrate. Dying keratinocytes, known by many names including Civatte bodies, cytoid bodies, dyskeratotic cells, and colloid bodies, are present, mostly along the dermal–epidermal junction, although additional dying cells can be seen at higher levels of the epidermis and in the dermis. The inflammatory infiltrate consists of lymphocytes and histiocytes (Fig. 18–26). It is usually confined to the papillary dermis, and the deeper portions of the dermis are not involved. Eosinophils and plasma cells are not commonly seen, and their presence favors another lichenoid process such as a drug eruption. The following entities must be considered in the histologic differential diagnosis of lichen planus:

- Lichenoid drug eruption
- Lichenoid keratosis

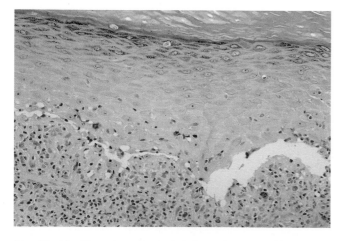

Fig. 18–26. Abundant dying keratinocytes, subepidermal splits, and a dense infiltrate of lymphocytes and histiocytes is seen in lichen planus related to hepatitis C infection.

- Lichen sclerosis et atrophicus (early)
- Lichen striatus
- Lupus erythematosus
- Mycosis fungoides
- Pityriasis lichenoides chronica
- Pityriasis lichenoides et varioliformis acuta
- Syphilis

An atrophic, as opposed to an acanthotic, epidermis is seen in some cases of lichen planus and is frequently seen in older, resolving lesions. In darker skinned persons, abundant melanin may be seen within papillary dermal melanophages in well-developed lesions (Fig. 18–27).

Special Studies. Special studies are not required to make a diagnosis of lichen planus.

Pathogenesis. Hepatitis C virus has not been detected in cutaneous lesions of lichen planus using immunolabeling methods. It is thus hypothesized that the cutaneous eruption is a nonspecific hypersensitivity reaction to the infection rather than a direct effect of the virus [163]. The association between hepatitis C virus and lichen planus is not related to a subtype of hepatitis C [164].

NOTE: Kawasaki disease is discussed in Chapter 4.

References

1. zur Hausen, H., *Papillomavirus infections—a major cause of human cancers.* Biochim Biophys Acta, 1996. 1288:F55–78.

2. Kilkenny, M., and Marks, R., *The descriptive epidemiology of warts in the community*. Austral J Dermatol, 1996. 37:80–86.

3. Chuang, T., Perry, H. U., Kurland, L. T., and Ilstrup, D. M., *Condyloma acuminata in Rochester, Minn, 1950–1978: Epidemiology and clinical features*. Arch Dermatol, 1984. 120:469–475.

4. Dyall-Smith, D., Trowell, H., and Dyall-Smith, M. L., *Benign human papillomavirus infection in renal transplant recipients*. Int J Dermatol, 1991. 30:785–789.

5. McLoughlin, S. J., Shaw, S. J., Turner, S., and Sylvester, B. S., *Deep palmo-plantar wart causing extensive bone erosion: Brief report*. J Hand Surg (Br), 1990. 15:129–130.

6. Weber, B. P., Fierlbeck, G., and Kempf, H. G., *Multiple metachronous skin squamous cell carcinomas and epidermodysplasia verruciformis in the head region: A human papilloma virus-associated disease*. Eur Arch Otorhinolaryngol, 1994. 251:342–346.

7. Sehgal, V. N., Koranne, R. V., and Srivastava, S. B., *Genital warts. Current status*. Int J Dermatol, 1989. 28:75–85.

8. Kashima, M., Adachi, M., Honda, M., Niimura, M., and Nakabayashi, Y., *A case of peculiar plantar warts. Human papillomavirus type 60 infection*. Arch Dermatol, 1994. 130:1418–1420.

9. Martin, F., Dalac, S., and Lambert, D., *Verrucous carcinoma. Nosologic aspects, apropos of 4 cases*. Ann Dermatol Venereol, 1995. 122:399–403.

10. McCance, D. J., Campion, M. J., Clarkson, P. K., Chesters, P. M., Jenkins, D., and Singer, A., *Prevalence of human papilloma virus type 16 DNA sequences in cervical intraepithelial neoplasia and invasive carcinoma of the cervix*. Br J Obstet Gynaecol, 1985. 92:1101–1105.

11. Gal, A. A., Saul, S. H., and Stoler, M. H., *In situ hybridization analysis of human papillomavirus in anal squamous cell carcinoma*. Mod Pathol, 1989. 2:439–443.

12. McGrae, J. D. Jr., Greer, C. E., and Manos, M. M., *Multiple Bowen's disease of the fingers associated with human papilloma virus type 16*. Int J Dermatol, 1993. 32:104–107.

13. Weaver, M. G., Abdul-Karin, F. W., Dale, G., Sorensen, K., and Huang, Y. T., *Detection and localization of human papillomavirus in penile condylomas and squamous cell carcinomas using in situ hybridization with biotinylated DNA viral probes*. Mod Pathol, 1989. 2:94–100.

14. Pfister, H., *Human papillomaviruses and skin cancer*. Semin Cancer Biol, 1992. 3:263–271.

15. Gross, G., Pfister, H., Hagedorn, M., and Gissman, L., *Correlation between human papillomavirus (HPV) type and histology of warts*. J Invest Dermatol, 1982. 78:160–164.

16. Blauvelt, A., Duarte, A. M., Prusksachatkunakorn, C., Leonardi, C. L., and Schachner, L. A., *Human papillomavirus type 6 infection involving cutaneous nongenital sites*. J Am Acad Dermatol, 1992. 27:876–879.

17. Pfister, H., *The role of human papillomavirus in anogenital cancer*. Obstet Gynecol Clin North Am, 1996. 23:579–595.

18. Majewski, S., and Jablonska, S., *Epidermodysplasia verruciformis as a model of human papillomavirus-induced genetic cancer of the skin*. Arch Dermatol, 1995. 131:1312–1318.

19. Rogel-Gaillard, C., Pehau-Arnaudet, G., Breitburd, F., and Orth, G., *Cytopathic effect in human papillomavirus type 1–induced inclusion warts: In vitro analysis of the contribution of two forms of the viral E4 protein*. J Invest Dermatol, 1993. 101:843–851.

20. Liesegang, T. J., *The varicella-zoster virus: Systemic and ocular features*. J Am Acad Dermatol, 1984. 11:165–191.

21. Elmer, K. B., and George, R. M., *Herpes zoster in a 7-month old infant: A case report and review*. Cutis, 1999. 63:217–218.

22. Mogami, S., Muto, M., Mogami, K., and Asagami, C., *Congenitally acquired herpes zoster infection in a newborn*. Dermatology, 1997. 194:276–277.

23. Ragozzino, M. W., Melton, L. J. I., Kurland, L. T., Chu, C. P., and Perry, H. O., *Risk of cancer after herpes zoster: A population-based study*. N Engl J Med, 1982. 307:393–397.

24. Juel-Jensen, B. E., and MacCallum, F. O., *Herpes Simplex Varicella and Zoster: Clinical Manifestations and Treatment*. 1972, Philadelphia, J. B. Lippincott.

25. Smith, K. J., Skelton, III, H. G., James, W. D., and Angritt, P., *Warty lesions secondary to DNA viruses in HIV infected patients (abstract)*. J Cutan Pathol, 1990. 17:317.

26. LeBoit, P. E., Limova, M., Benedict Yen, T. S., Palefsky, J. M., White, Jr., C. R., and Berger, T. G., *Chronic verrucous varicella-zoster virus infection in patients with the acquired immunodeficiency syndrome (AIDS)*. Am J Dermatopathol, 1992. 14:1–7.

27. Hope-Simpson, R. E., *The nature of herpes zoster: A long-term study and a new hypothesis*. Proc R Soc Med, 1965. 58:9–20.

28. Goh, C. L., and Khoo, L., *A retrospective study of the clinical presentation and outcome of herpes zoster in a tertiary dermatology outpatient referral clinic*. Int J Dermatol, 1997. 36:667–672.

29. Vu, A. Q., Radonich, M. A., and Heald, P. W., *Herpes zoster in seven disparate dermatomes (zoster multiplex): Report of a case and review of the literature*. J Am Acad Dermatol, 1999. 40:868–869.

30. Brice, S. L., Leahy, M. A., Ong, L., Krecji, S., Stockert, S. S., Huff, J. C., and Weston, W. L., *Examination of non-involved skin, previously involved skin, and peripheral blood for herpes simplex virus DNA in patients with recurrent herpes- associated erythema multiforme*. J Cutan Pathol, 1994. 21:408–412.

31. Arnold, H. L. Jr., Odom, R. B., and James, W. D., *Viral diseases*. In *Diseases of the Skin. Clinical Dermatology*. 1990, W. B. Saunders Company, Philadelphia, pp. 439.

32. McKendall, R. R., and Klawans, H. L., *Nervous system complications of varicella-zoster virus*. In *Handbook of Clinical Neurology*, P. J. Vinken and G. W. Bruyn, Eds. 1978, Elsevier, Amsterdam. p. 161.

33. Krugman, S., Goodrich, C. H., and Ward, R., *Primary varicella pneumonia.* N Engl J Med, 1957. 257:843–848.

34. McCrary, M. L., Severson, J., and Tyring, S. K., *Varicella zoster virus.* J Am Acad Dermatol, 1999. 41:1–14.

35. Sauerbrei, A., *Varicella-zoster virus infections in pregnancy.* Intervirology, 1998. 41:191–196.

36. Liang, M. G., Heidelberg, K. A., Jacobson, R. M., and McEvoy, M. T., *Herpes zoster after varicella immunization.* J Am Acad Dermatol, 1998. 38:761–763.

37. Baik, J. S., Kim, W. C., Heo, J. H., and Zheng, H. Y., *Recurrent herpes zoster myelitis.* J Korean Med Sci, 1997. 12:360–363.

38. Shishov, A. S., Virych, I. E., Bagrov, F. I., and Latysheva, I. T., *The Guillain-Barré syndrome in herpes zoster patients.* Zh Nevropatol Psikhiatr Im S S Korsakova, 1996. 96:26–29.

39. Appelbaum, E., Kreps, S. I., and Sunshine, A., *Herpes zoster encephalitis.* Am J Med, 1962. 32:25–31.

40. Yamanishi, T., Yasuda, K., Sakakibara, R., Hattori, T., Uchiyama, T., Minamide, M., and Ito, H., *Urinary retention due to herpes virus infections.* Neurourol Urodyn, 1998. 17:613–619.

41. Pulik, M., Teillet, F., Teillet-Thiebaud, F., Lionnet, F., Genet, P., and Petitdidier, C., *Varicella-zoster virus pancreatitis in hematologic diseases.* Ann Med Interne (Paris), 1995. 146:292–294.

42. McCluggage, W. G., Fox, J. D., Baillie, K. E., Coyle, P. V., Jones, F. G., and O'Hara, M. D., *Varicella zoster gastritis in a bone marrow transplant recipient.* J Clin Pathol, 1994. 47:1054–1056.

43. Weisman, K., Petersen, C. S., Blichmann, C. W., Nielsen, N. H., and Hultberg, B. M., *Bullous erythema multiforme following herpes zoster and varicella-zoster virus infection.* J Eur Acad Dermatol Venereol, 1998. 11:147–150.

44. Corazza, M., Bacilieri, S., and Strumia, R., *Post-herpes zoster scar sarcoidosis.* Acta Derm Venereol, 1999. 79:95.

45. Bang, S. W., Kim, Y. K., and Whang, K. U., *Acquired reactive perforating collagenosis: Unilateral umbilicated papules along the lesions of herpes zoster.* J Am Acad Dermatol, 1997. 36:778–779.

46. Stubbings, J. M., and Goodfield, M. J., *An unusual distribution of an acneiform rash due to herpes zoster infection.* Clin Exp Dermatol, 1993. 18:92–93.

47. Muraki, R., Iwasaki, T., Sata, T., Sato, Y., and Kurata, T., *Hair follicle involvement in herpes zoster: Pathway of viral spread from ganglia to skin.* Virchows Arch, 1996. 428:275–280.

48. Turner, R. J., Sviland, L., and Lawrence, C. M., *Acute infiltration by non-Hodgkin's B-cell lymphoma of lesions of disseminated herpes zoster.* Br J Dermatol, 1998. 139:295–298.

49. Bahadoran, P., Lacour, J. P., Del Giudice, P., Perrin, C., Dubois, D., Samak, R., and Ortonne, J. P., *Cutaneous localizations of chronic lymphoid leukemia in a zona area.* Ann Dermatol Venereol, 1996. 123:471–473.

50. Cerroni, L., Zenahlik, P., and Kerl, H., *Specific cutaneous infiltrates of B-cell chronic lymphocytic leukemia arising at the site of herpes zoster and herpes simplex scars.* Cancer, 1995. 76:26–31.

51. Serfling, U., Penneys, N. S., Zhu, W. Y., Sisto, M., and Leonardi, C., *Varicella-zoster virus DNA in granulomatous skin lesions following herpes zoster. A study by the polymerase chain reaction.* J Cutan Pathol, 1993. 20:28–33.

52. Roo, E., Villegas, C., Lopez-Bran, E., Jiminez, E., Valle, P., and Sancez-Yus, E., *Postzoster cutaneous pseudolymphoma.* Arch Dermatol, 1994. 130:661–663.

53. Rodriguez-Pereira, C., Suarez-Penaranda, J. M., del Rio, E., and Forteza-Vila, J., *Cutaneous granulomatous vasculitis after herpes zoster infection showing polyarteritis nodosa-like features.* Clin Exp Dermatol, 1997. 22:274–276.

54. Snow, J. L., El-Azhary, R. A., Gibson, L. E., Estes, S. A., Espy, M. J., and Smith, T. F., *Granulomatous vasculitis associated with herpes virus: A persistent, painful, postherpetic papular eruption.* Mayo Clin Proc, 1997. 72:851–853.

55. Requena, L., Kutzner, H., Escalonilla, P., Ortiz, S., Schaller, J., and Rohwedder, A., *Cutaneous reactions at sites of herpes zoster scars: An expanded spectrum,* Br J Dermatol, 1998. 138:161–168.

56. Annunziato, P., Lungu, O., Gershon, A., Silvers, D. N., LaRussa, P., and Silverstein, S. J., *In situ hybridization detection of varicella zoster virus in paraffin-embedded skin biopsy samples.* Clin Diagn Virol, 1996. 7:69–76.

57. Rubben, A., Baron, J. M., and Grussendorf-Conen, E. I., *Routine detection of herpes simplex virus and varicella zoster virus by polymerase chain reaction reveals that initial herpes zoster is frequently misdiagnosed as herpes simplex.* Br J Dermatol, 1997. 137:259–261.

58. Nahass, G. T., Mandel, M. J., Cook, S., Fan, W., and Leonardi, C. L., *Detection of herpes simplex and varicella-zoster infection from cutaneous lesions in different clinical stages with the polymerase chain reaction.* J Am Acad Dermatol, 1995. 32:730–733.

59. Tanaka, K., Tsuda, S., and Sasai, Y., *Scanning and transmission electron microscopic studies of lesional epidermis in herpes zoster.* J Dermatol, 1994. 21:560–570.

60. Swanson, S., and Feldman, P. S., *Cytomegalovirus infection initially diagnosed by skin biopsy.* Am J Clin Pathol, 1987. 87:113–116.

61. Walker, J. D., and McChesney, T., *Cytomegalovirus infection of the skin.* Am J Dermatopathol, 1982. 4:263–265.

62. Curtis, J. L., and Egbert, B. M., *Cutaneous cytomegalovirus vasculitis: An unusual clinical presentation of a common opportunistic pathogen.* Hum Pathol, 1982. 13:1138–1141.

63. Lin, C. S., Penha, P., Krishnan, M. N., and Zak, F. G., *Cytomegalic inclusion disease of the skin.* Arch Dermatol, 1981. 117:282–284.

64. Bhawan, J., Gellis, S., Ucci, A., and Chang, T. W., *Vesicular bullous lesions caused by cytomegalovirus infection in an immunocompromised adult.* J Am Acad Dermatol, 1984. 11:743–747.

65. Horn, T. D., and Hood, A. F., *Cytomegalovirus is pre-

dictably present in perineal ulcers from immunosuppressed patients. Arch Dermatol, 1990. 126:642–644.

66. Feldman, P. S., Walker, A. N., and Baker, R., *Cutaneous lesions heralding disseminated cytomegalovirus infection.* J Am Acad Dermatol, 1982. 7:545–548.

67. Minars, N., Silverman, J. F., Escobar, M. R., and Martinez, A. J., *Associated skin manifestations in a renal transplant patient.* Arch Dermatol, 1977. 113:1569–1571.

68. Myerson, D., Hackman, R. C., Nelson, J. A., Ward, D. C., and McDougall, J. K., *Widespread presence of histologically occur cytomegalovirus.* Hum Pathol, 1984. 15:430–439.

69. Husak, R., Garbe, C., and Orfanos, C. E., *Mollusca contagiosa in HIV infection. Clinical manifestation, relation to immune status and prognostic value in 39 patients.* Hautarzt, 1997. 48:103–109.

70. Reynaud-Mendel, B., Janier, M., Gerbaka, J., Hakin, C., Rabian, C., Chastang, C., and Morel, P., *Dermatologic findings in HIV-1–infected patients: A prospective study with emphasis on CD4+ cell count.* Dermatology, 1996. 192:325–328.

71. Vozmediano, J. M., Manrique, A., Petraglia, S., Romero, M. A., and Nieto, I., *Giant molluscum contagiosum in AIDS.* Int J Dermatol, 1996. 35:45–47.

72. Itin, P. H., and Lautenschlager, S., *Viral lesions of the mouth in HIV-infected patients.* Dermatology, 1997. 194:1–7.

73. Sulica, R. L., Kelly, J., Berberian, B. J., and Glaun, R., *Cutaneous cryptococcosis with molluscum contagiosum coinfection in a patient with acquired immunodeficiency syndrome.* Cutis, 1994. 53:88–90.

74. Furue, M., Akasu, R., Ohtake, N., and Tamaki, K., *Erythema annulare centrifugum induced by molluscum contagiosum.* Br J Dermatol, 1993. 129:646–647.

75. Lombardo, P. C., *Molluscum contagiosum and acquired immunodeficiency syndrome.* Arch Dermatol, 1985. 121:834–835.

76. de Diego, J., Berridi, D., Saracibar, N., and Requena, L., *Cutaneous pseudolymphoma in association with molluscum contagiosum.* Am J Dermatopathol, 1998. 20:518–521.

77. Naert, F., and Lachapelle, J. M., *Multiple lesions of molluscum contagiosum with metaplastic ossification.* Am J Dermatopathol, 1989. 11:238–241.

78. Mihara, M., *Three-dimensional ultrastructural study of molluscum contagiosum in the skin using scanning-electron microscopy.* Br J Dermatol, 1991. 125:557–560.

79. Shelley, W. B., and Burmeister, V., *Demonstration of a unique viral structure: The molluscum viral colony sac.* Br J Dermatol, 1986. 115:557–562.

80. Balsev, E., Thomsen, H. K., and Weisman, K., *Histopathology of acute human immunodeficiency virus exanthem.* J Clin Pathol, 1990. 43:201–202.

81. Kinloch de Loes, S., de Sassure, P., Saurat, J. H., Stalder, H., Hirschel, B., and Perrin, L. H., *Symptomatic primary infection due to human immunodeficiency virus type 1: Review of 31 cases.* Clin Infect Dis, 1993. 17:59–65.

82. Tindall, B., Barker, S., Donovan, B., Barnes, T., Roberts, J., Kronenberg, C., Gold, J., et al., *Characterization of the acute clinical illness associated with human immunodeficiency virus infection.* Arch Intern Med, 1988. 148:945–949.

83. Reichart, P. A., Langford, A., Gelderblom, H. R., Pohle, H. D., Becker, J., and Wolf, H., *Oral hairy leukoplakia: Observations in 95 cases and review of the literature.* J Oral Pathol Med, 1989. 18:410–415.

84. Husak, R., Garbe, C., and Orfanos, C. E., *Oral hairy leukoplakia in 71 HIV-seropositive patients: Clinical symptoms, relation to immunologic status, and prognostic significance.* J Am Acad Dermatol, 1996. 35:928–934.

85. Tappero, J. W., Conant, M. A., Wolfe, S. F., and Berger, T. G., *Kaposi's sarcoma. Epidemiology, pathogenesis, histology, clinical spectrum, staging criteria and therapy.* J Am Acad Dermatol, 1993. 28:371–395.

86. Jin, Y.-T., Tsai, S.-T., Yan, J.-J., Hsiao, J.-H., Lee, Y.-Y., and Su, I.-J., *Detection of Kaposi's sarcoma–associated herpesvirus-like DNA sequence in vascular lesions.* Am J Clin Pathol, 1996. 105:360–363.

87. Katz, M. H., Hessol, N. A., Buchbinder, S. P., Hirozawa, A., O'Malley, P., and Holmberg, S. D., *Temporal trends of opportunistic infections and malignancies in homosexual men with AIDS.* J Infect Dis, 1994. 170:198–202.

88. Rosenthal, D., LeBoit, P. E., Klumpp, L., and Berger, T. G., *Human immunodeficiency virus–associated eosinophilic follicultiis.* Arch Dermatol, 1991. 127:206–209.

89. Bull, R. H., Harland, C. A., Fallowfield, M. E., and Mortimer, P. S., *Eosinophilic folliculitis: A self-limited illness in patients being treated for haematological malignancy.* Br J Dermatol, 1993. 129:178–182.

90. Stoler, M. H., Bonfiglio, T. A., Steigbigel, R. T., and Pereira, M., *An atypical subcutaneous infection associated with acquired immune deficiency syndrome.* Am J Clin Pathol, 1983. 80:714–718.

91. Cockerell, C. J., Whitlow, M. A., Webster, G. F., and Friedman-Kien, A. E., *Epithelioid angiomatosis: Distinct vascular disorder in patients with the acquired immunodeficiency syndrome or AIDS-related complex.* Lancet, 1987. ii:654–656.

92. Cockerell, C. J., Bergstresser, P. R., Myrie-Williams, C., and Tierno, P. M., *Bacillary epithelioid angiomatosis occurring in an immunocompetent individual.* Arch Dermatol, 1990. 126:787–790.

93. Tappero, J. W., Koehler, J. E., Berger, T. G., Cockerell, C. J., Lee, T. H., Busch, M. P., Stites, D. P., et al., *Bacillary angiomatosis and bacillary splenitis in immunocompetent adults.* Ann Intern Med, 1993. 118:363–365.

94. Crane, G. A., Variakojis, D., Rosen, S. T., Sands, A. M., and Roenigk, J., Roenigk, Jr., H. H., *Cutaneous T-cell lymphoma in patients with human immunodeficiency virus infection.* Arch Dermatol, 1991. 127:989–994.

95. Nahass, G. T., Kraffert, C. A., and Penneys, N. S., *Cutaneous T-cell lymphoma associated with the acquired immunodeficiency syndrome.* Arch Dermatol, 1991. 127:1020–1022.

96. Myskowski, P. L., *Cutaneous T-cell lymphoma and human immunodeficiency virus.* Arch Dermatol, 1991. 127:1045–1047.

97. Shibata, D., Brynes, R. K., Rabinowitz, A., et al., *Human T-cell lymphotropic virus type I (HTLV-1)–associated adult T-cell leukemia-lymphoma in a patient infected with human immunodeficiency virus type 1 (HIV-1).* Ann Intern Med, 1989. 111:871–875.

98. Hulsebosch, H. J., Claessen, F. A. P., van Ginkel, C. J., Kuiters, G. R., Goudsmit, J., and Lange, J. M., *Human immunodeficiency virus exanthem.* J Am Acad Dermatol, 1990. 23:483–486.

99. Triantos, D., Porter, S. R., Scully, C., and Teo, C. G., *Oral hairy leukoplakia: Clinicopathologic features, pathogenesis, diagnosis, and clinical significance.* Clin Infect Dis, 1997. 25:1392–1396.

100. Ficarra, G., Romagnoli, P., Piluso, S., Milo, D., and Adler-Storthz, K., *Hairy leukoplakia with involvement of the buccal mucosa.* J Am Acad Dermatol, 1992. 27:855–858.

101. Gottlieb, G. J., and Ackerman, A. B., *Kaposi's sarcoma: An extensively disseminated form in young homosexual men.* Hum Pathol, 1982. 13:882–892.

102. Premlatha, S., Augustine, S. M., Yesudian, U., and Thambia, A. S., *Punctate palmoplantar keratosis acuminata: An unusual form of tuberculid.* Int J Dermatol, 1982. 21:470–471.

103. Cockerell, C. J., and LeBoit, P. E., *Bacillary angiomatosis: A newly characterized, pseudoneoplastic, infectious, cutaneous vascular disorder.* J Am Acad Dermatol, 1990. 22:501–512.

104. Webster, G. F., Cockerell, C. J., and Friedman-Kien, A. E., *The clinical spectrum of bacillary angiomatosis.* Br J Dermatol, 1992. 126:535–541.

105. Nicolatou, O., Nikolatos, G., Fisfis, M., Belegrati, M., Papdaki, T., Oikonomaki, E., and Kalmantis, T., *Oral hairy leukoplakia in a patient with acute lymphocytic leukemia.* Oral Dis, 1999. 5:76–79.

106. Blomgren, J., and Back, H., *Oral hairy leukoplakia in a patient with multiple myeloma.* Oral Surg Oral Med Oral Pathol Oral Radiol Endod, 1996. 82:408–410.

107. Miranda, C., and Lozada-Nur, F., *Oral hairy leukoplakia in an HIV-negative patient with systemic lupus erythematosus.* Compend Contin Educ Dent, 1996. 17:412.

108. Fluckiger, R., Laifer, G., Itin, P., and Meyer, B. L., Meyer, B., *Oral hairy leukoplakia in a patient with ulcerative colitis.* Gastroenterology, 1994. 106:506–508.

109. Zakrzewska, J. M., Aly, Z., and Speight, P. M., *Oral hairy leukoplakia in an HIV-negative asthmatic patient on systemic steroids.* J Oral Pathol Med, 1995. 24:282–284.

110. Stribling, J., Weitzner, S., and Smith, G. V., *Kaposi's sarcoma in renal allograft recipients.* Cancer, 1978. 42:442–446.

111. Ioachim, H. L., Adsay, V., Giancotti, F. R., Dorsett, B., and Melamed, J., *Kaposi's sarcoma of internal organs.* Cancer, 1995. 75:1376–1385.

112. Moskowitz, L. B., Hensley, G. T., Gould, E. W., and Weiss, S. D., *Frequency and anatomic distribution of lymphadenopathic Kaposi's sarcoma in the acquired immunodeficiency syndrome: An autopsy series.* Hum Pathol, 1985. 16:447–456.

113. Teraki, Y., Konohana, I., Shihara, T., Nagashima, M., and Nishikawa, T., *Eosinophilic pustular folliculitis (Ofuji's disease). Immunohistochemical analysis.* Arch Dermatol, 1993. 129:1015–1019.

114. Zalla, M. J., Su, W. P. D., and Fransway, A. F., *Dermatologic manifestations of human immunodeficiency virus infection.* Mayo Clin Proc, 1992. 67:1089–1108.

115. Perkocha, L. A., Geaghan, S. M., Yen, T. S. B., Nishimura, S. L., Chan, S. P., Garcia-Kennedy, R., Hda, G., et al., *Clinical and pathological features of bacillary peliosis hepatitis in association with human immunodeficiency infection.* N Engl J Med, 1990. 323:1581–1586.

116. Koehler, J. E., LeBoit, P. E., Egbert, P. M., and Berger, T. G., *Cutaneous vascular lesions and disseminated cat-scratch disease in patients with the acquired immunodeficiency syndrome (AIDS) and AIDS-related complex.* Ann Intern Med, 1988. 109:449–455.

117. LeBoit, P. E., *Bacillary angiomatosis.* Mod Pathol, 1995. 8:218–222.

118. Goldman, G. D., Milstone, L. M., and Shapiro, P. E., *Histologic findings in acute HIV exanthem.* J Cutan Pathol, 1995. 22:371–373.

119. Barnadas, M. A., Alegre, M., Baselga, E., Randazzo, L., Margall, N., Rabella, N., Curell, R., et al., *Histopathological changes of primary HIV infection. Description of three cases and review of the literature.* J Cutan Pathol, 1997. 24:507–510.

120. Fernandez, J. F., Benito, M. A., Lizaldez, E. B., and Montanes, M. A., *Oral hairy leukoplakia: A histopathologic study of 32 cases.* Am J Dermatopathol, 1990. 12:571–578.

121. Greenspan, J. S., De Souza, Y. G., Regezi, J. A., Daniels, T. E., Greenspan, D., MacPhail, L. A., and Hilton, J. F., *Comparison of cytopathic changes in oral hairy leukoplakia with in situ hybridization for EBV DNA.* Oral Dis, 1998. 4:95–99.

122. Niedt, G. W., Myskowski, P. L., Urmacher, C., Niedzwiecki, D., Chapman, D., and Safai, B., *Histology of early lesions of AIDS-associated Kaposi's sarcoma.* Mod Pathol, 1990. 3:64–70.

123. Chor, P. J., and Santa Cruz, D. J., *Kaposi's sarcoma. A clinicopathologic review and differential diagnosis.* J Cutan Pathol, 1992. 19:6–20.

124. McNutt, N. S., Fletcher, V., and Conant, M. A., *Early lesions of Kaposi's sarcoma in homosexual men: An ultrastructural comparison with other vascular proliferations in skin.* Am J Pathol, 1983. 3:62–77.

125. Fukunaga, M., and Silverberg, S. G., *Hyaline globules in Kaposi's sarcoma: A light microscopic and immunohistochemical study.* Mod Pathol, 1991. 4:187–190.

126. McCalmont, T. H., Altemus, D., Maurer, T., and Berger, T. G., *Eosinophilic folliculitis. The histologic spectrum.* Am J Dermatopathol, 1995. 17:439–446.

127. Scully, C., Porter, S. R., Di Alberti, L., Jalal, M., and Maitland, N., *Detection of Epstein-Barr virus in oral scrapes in HIV infection, in hairy leukoplakia, and in*

healthy non-HIV–infected people. J Oral Med Pathol, 1998. 27:480–482.

128. Mabruk, M. J., Flint, S. R., Coleman, D. C., Shiels, O., Toner, M., and Atkins, G. J., *A rapid microwave–in situ hybridization method for the definitive diagnosis of oral hairy leukoplakia: Comparison with immunohistochemistry.* J Oral Pathol Med, 1996. 25:170–176.

129. Epstein, J. B., Fatahzadeh, M., Matisic, J., and Gnderson, G., *Exfoliatve cytology and electron microscopy in the diagnosis of hairy leukoplakia.* Oral Surg Oral Med Oral Pathol Oral Radiol Endod, 1995. 79:564–569.

130. Webster-Cyriaque, J., and Raab-Traub, N., *Transcription of Epstein-Barr virus latent cycle genes in oral hairy leukoplakia.* Virology, 1998. 248:53–65.

131. Itin, P. H., *Oral hairy leukoplaia—10 years on.* Dermatology, 1993. 187:159–163.

132. Brandwein, M., Nuovo, G., Ramer, M., Orlowskin, W., and Miller, L., *Epstein-Barr virus reactivation in hairy leukoplakia.* Mod Pathol, 1996. 9:298–303.

133. Moore, P. S., and Chang, Y., *Detection of herpesvirus-like DNA sequences in Kaposi's sarcoma in patients with and those without HIV infection.* N Engl J Med, 1995. 332:1181–1185.

134. Chang, Y., Cesarman, E., Pessin, M. S., Lee, F., Culpepper, J., Knowles, D. M., and Moore, P. S., *Identification of herpesvirus-like DNA sequences in AIDS-associated Kaposi's sarcoma.* Science, 1994. 266:1865–1869.

135. Chang, Y., and Moore, P. S., *Kaposi's sarcoma (KS)–associated herpesvirus and its role in KS.* Infect Agents Dis, 1996. 5:215–222.

136. Magro, C. M. J., and Croswon, A. N., *Eosinophilic pustular follicular reaction: A paradigm of immune dysregulation.* Int J Dermatol, 1994. 33:172–178.

137. Fisher, B. K., and Warner, L. C., *Cutaneous manifestations of the acquired immunodeficiency syndrome. Update 1987.* Int J Dermatol, 1987. 26:615–630.

138. Dehio, C., *Interactions of Bartonella henselae with vascular endothelial cells.* Curr Opin Microbiol, 1999. 2:78–82.

139. Taieb, A., Plantin, P., Du Pasquier, P., Guillet, G., and Maleville, J., *Gianotti-Crosti syndrome: A study of 26 cases.* Br J Dermatol, 1986. 115:49–59.

140. Cambiaghi, S., Scarabelli, G., Pistritto, G., and Gelmetti, C., *Gianotti-Crosti syndrome in an adult after influenza virus vaccination.* Dermatology, 1995. 191: 340–341.

141. Caputo, R., Gelmetti, C., Ermacora, E., Gianni, E., and Silvestri, A., *Gianotti-Crosti syndrome: A retrospective analysis of 308 cases.* J Am Acad Dermatol, 1992. 26: 207–210.

142. Crosti, A., and Gianotti, F., *Ulteriore alla conoscenza dell'acrodermatite papulosa infantile.* G Ital Dermatol, 1964. 105:477–504.

143. Draelos, Z. K., Hansen, R. C., and James, W. D., *Gianotti-Crosti syndrome associated with infections other than hepatitis B.* JAMA, 1986. 256:2386–2388.

144. Hergueta Lendinez, R., Pozo Garcia, L., Alejo Garcia, A., Romero Cachza, J., and Gonzalez Hachero, J., *Gianotti-Crosti syndrome due to a mixed infection produced by the mumps virus and the parainfluenza virus type 2.* An Esp Pediatr, 1996. 44:65–66.

145. Yasumoto, S., Tsujita, J., Imayama, S., and Hori, Y., *Case report: Gianotti-Crosti syndrome associated with human herpesvirus-6 infection.* J Dermatol, 1996. 23: 499–501.

146. Carrascosa, J. M., Just, M., Ribera, M., and Ferrandiz, C., *Papular acrodermatitis of childhood related to poxvirus and parvovirus B19 infection.* Cutis, 1998. 61:265–267.

147. James, W. D., Odom, R. B., and Hatch, M. H., *Gianotti-Crosti–like eruption assocaited with coxsackie A-16 infection.* J Am Acad Deramtol, 1982. 6:862–866.

148. Drago, F., Crovato, F., and Rebora, A., *Gianotti- Crosti syndrome as a presenting sign of EBV-induced acute infectious mononucleosis.* Clin Exp Dermatol, 1997. 22:301–302.

149. Haki, M., Tsuchida, M., Kotsuji, M., Iijima, S., Tamura, K., Koike, K., Izumis, I., et al., *Gianotti-Crosti syndrome associated with cytomegalovirus antigenemia after bone marrow transplantation.* Bone Marrow Transplant, 1997. 20:691–693.

150. Gelmetti, C., *Present concepts of Gianotti-Crosti disease and syndrome.* In *Dermatology, Progress and Perspectives: The Proceedings of the 18th World Congress of Dermaotlogy*, Burgdorf, W. H. C. and S. I. Katz, Eds. 1992, Parthenon Publishing Group, New York, pp. 485–487.

151. Blauvelt, A., and Turner, M. L., *Gianotti-Crosti syndrome and human immunodeficiency virus infection.* Arch Dermatol, 1994. 130:481–483.

152. Spear, K. L., and Winkelmann, R. K., *Gianotti-Crosti syndrome: A review of 10 cases not associated with hepatitis B.* Arch Dermatol, 1984. 120:891–896.

153. Imhof, M., Popal, H., Lee, J. H., Zeuzem, S., and Milbradt, R., *Prevalence of hepatitis C virus antibodies and evaluation of hepatitis C virus genotypes in patients with lichen planus.* Dermatology, 1997. 195:1–5.

154. Daoud, M. S., Gibson, L. E., Daoud, S., and el-Azhary, R. A., *Chronic hepatitis C and skin diseases: A review.* Mayo Clin Proc, 1995. 70:559–564.

155. Pereyo, N. G., Lesher, Jr., J. L., and Davis, L. S., *Hepatitis C and its association with lichen planus and porphyria cutanea tarda.* J Am Acad Dermatol, 1995. 1995:32.

156. Pawlotsky, J. M., Dhumeaux, D., and Bagot, M., *Hepatitis C virus in dermatology. A review.* Arch Dermatol, 1995. 131:1185–1193.

157. Reichel, M., and Mauro, T. M., *Urticaria and hepatitis C (letter).* Lancet, 1990. 336:822–823.

158. Cribier, B. J., Santinelli, F., Schmitt, C., Stoll-Keller, F., and Grosshans, E., *Chronic urticaria is not significantly associated with hepatitis C or hepatitis G infection.* Arch Dermatol, 1999. 135:1335–1339.

159. Dupond, A. S., Lacour, J. P., Lafont, C., and Ortonne, J. P., *Prevalence of hepatitis C virus in oral erosive lichen.* Ann Dermatol Venereol, 1998. 125:676–678.

160. Mignogna, M. D., Lo Muzio, L., Favia, G., Mignogna, R. E., Carbone, R., and Bucci, E., *Oral lichen planus and HCV infection: A clinical evaluation of 263 cases.* Int J Dermatol, 1998. 37:575–578.

161. Schissel, D. J., and Elston, D. M., *Lichen planus associated with hepatitis C.* Cutis, 1998. 61:90–92.

162. Bellman, B., Reddy, R., and Falanga, V., *Generalized lichen planus associated with hepatitis C virus immunoreactivity.* J Am Acad Dermatol, 1996. 35:770–772.

163. Boyd, A. S., Nanney, L. B., and King, L. E. Jr., *Immunoperoxidase evaluation of lichen planus biopsies for hepatitis C virus.* Int J Dermatol, 1998. 37:260–262.

164. Lodi, G., Carrozzo, M., Hallett, R., D'Amico, E., Piatelli, A., Teo, C. G., Gandolfo, S., et al., *HCV genotypes in Italian patients with HCV-related oral lichen planus.* J Oral Pathol Med, 1997. 26:381–384.

165. Goodman, D. S., Tepllitz, E. D., Wishner, A., Klein, R. S., Burk, P. G., and Hershenbaum, E., *Prevalence of cutaneous disease in patients with acquired immunodeficiency syndrome (AIDS) or AIDS-related complex.* J Am Acad Dermatol, 1987. 17:210–220.

166. Kaplan, M. H., Sadick, N., McNutt, N. S., Meltzer, M., Sarngadharan, M. G., and Pahwa, S., *Dermatologic findings and manifestations of acquired immunodeficiency syndrome (AIDS).* J Am Acad Dermatol, 1987. 16:485–506.

167. Dover, J. S., and Johnson, R. A., *Cutaneous manifestations of human immunodeficiency virus infection. Part II.* Arch Dermatol, 1991. 127:1549–1558.

CHAPTER
19

Fungal and Algal Diseases

A vast number of fungi have been identified and cultured from the skin of infected patients. Those fungi that are most commonly encountered in the practice of dermatopathology in North America and Europe are the focus of this chapter. Fungi that rarely cause human disease are not addressed.

Aspergillosis

Epidemiology. There are several species of *Aspergillus* that cause infection. These organisms cause disease in a variety of ways, including pulmonary disease, disseminated disease, and localized cutaneous disease. Involvement of the skin is seen most commonly in the setting of an immunocompromised host. Premature infants also have an increased risk for developing invasive *Aspergillus* infection [1].

Cutaneous Features. In most cases, cutaneous aspergillosis is a sequela of hematogenous dissemination from primary pulmonary infection or from direct extension from underlying infection of the orbit or sinus tracts [2]. Involvement of the skin is uncommon, however, even in disseminated disease [3]. Direct cutaneous infection is seen after localized trauma and may occur in the setting of an indwelling intravenous line in an immunosuppressed patient [4].

Cutaneous infection may have several different clinical appearances. Multiple erythematous to violaceous, indurated papules and plaques may later progress to ulcerations and eschars [5].

Associated Disorders. Many cases of chronic granulomatous disease are associated with *Aspergillus* infection [1, 6]. Cutaneous aspergillosis has been reported as a complication in a patient with pyoderma gangrenosum [7]. The relationship is probably due to a loss of skin integrity or to the immunosuppression involved with treating the condition and rather than to any primary process related to the disease itself.

Histologic Features. Except for direct observation and identification of the organisms, the changes seen in *Aspergillus* infection of the skin are nonspecific. *Aspergillus* infection frequently involves arteries or veins, leading to subsequent infarction of the dependent skin (Fig. 19–1). The affected vessels are often thrombosed and may or may not have a surrounding inflammatory infiltrate consisting of neutrophils and lymphocytes (Fig. 19–2). The absence of significant inflammation is typical in patients undergoing cytoreductive therapies. Later lesions demonstrate necrosis of the dermis and epidermis and much more extensive inflammation. Organisms may also be present freely within the dermis and are associated with inflammation and occasionally granuloma formation.

Aspergillus organisms are seen as hyphae in tissue sections. They are 3–6 μm in width and are septate and branched. The branching is at acute angles, and branches are the same caliber as the parent hyphae [8] (Fig. 19–3). Transepidermal elimination of *Aspergillus* organisms has been reported [9].

Special Studies. The most reliable and sensitive method to make a definitive diagnosis of *Aspergillus*

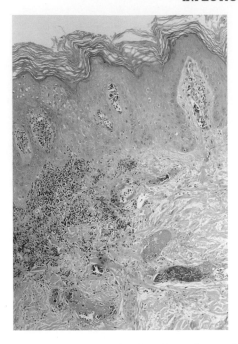

Fig. 19–1. *Aspergillus* is occluding dermal vessels, leading to congestion and dermal hemorrhage.

infection remains culture [3]. Although histologic sections display the characteristic branching, it is not always possible to reliably distinguish *aspergillus* from *Fusarium* and *Pseudoallescheria boydii*. All of these organisms stain strongly with periodic acid–Schiff and Gomori's methenamine silver stains.

Pathogenesis. *Aspergillus flavus* is the most common species to infect people, followed by *Apergillus fumigatus* and *Aspergillus niger*. They are ubiquitous organisms that may be inhaled or traumatically implanted. They are most likely to cause disease in patients with altered immunity.

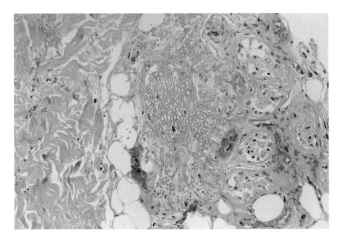

Fig. 19–2. *Aspergillus* is completely distending and occluding blood vessels in the reticular dermis.

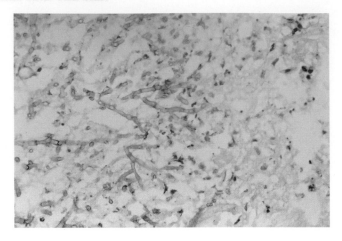

Fig. 19–3. PAS after diastase digestion stain reveals characteristic branching pattern and septation of *Aspergillus*.

Zygomycosis (Mucormycosis)

Epidemiology. Zygomycosis is an uncommon infection that is most prevalent in patients with underlying illnesses such as diabetes mellitus, metabolic acidosis, or immunodeficiencies [10]. It has also been reported in immunocompetent patients. Rhinocerebral, disseminated, and limited cutaneous forms of the infection have been described. Although the disseminated and rhinocerebral forms are the most common, limited cutaneous infection is becoming more prevalent. The reasons for this change in pattern are not fully understood [11]. Primary cutaneous zygomycosis is still relatively rare and usually follows local trauma or the presence of an occlusive dressing [10, 12]. Dissemination of the infection is uncommon in these patients, but does occur. The mortality rate for the rhinocerebral and disseminated forms ranges from 78% to 100%, whereas primary cutaneous zygomycosis is not associated with increased mortality [13]. Patients with zygomycosis and acquired immunodeficiency syndrome (AIDS) have an especially ominous prognosis [14].

Cutaneous Features. Primary cutaneous zygomycosis presents as a solitary ulcer, often at a site of previous trauma or injection site. Other cases have an ecthyma-like appearance with marked erythema and edema [15] or a pyoderma-like appearance [16]. Subcutaneous nodules have been described after subcutaneous injections [17]. An exceptional patient has been described in whom the cutaneous lesions had a zosteriform appearance [18].

The rhinocerebral form of the disease appears as erythematous, cellulitis-like streaks in the region of the nose and eyes. There is often extreme tenderness, and the patients may appear acutely ill.

Associated Disorders. Rhinocerebral infection is seen in patients with underlying disease. Diabetic ketoacidosis is a major risk factor. Other risk factors include neutropenia, malnutrition, and iron overload, as is seen patients undergoing hemodialysis [19]. Co-infection with other opportunistic fungi such as *Aspergillus* has been described in immunosuppressed patients [20].

Osteomyelitis has been described as a complication of primary cutaneous infection [21]. Cardiac zygomycosis is an uncommon complication of disseminated disease, and other organs, including the gastrointestinal tract, spleen, liver, and adrenal glands, can be similarly affected [22].

Histologic Features. The organisms that give rise to zygomycosis are angioinvasive fungi (Fig. 19–4). Vessels may be completely occluded by the organisms, and there is frequently a surrounding inflammatory infiltrate throughout the dermis, composed of neutrophils, lymphocytes, and eosinophils. Thrombi are usually present, and later lesions will demonstrate secondary changes related to infarction.

Zygomycoses are indistinguishable on tissue sections. They appear as 5–20 μm diameter hyphae that are pauciseptate and branch at right angles [23]. Their thin walls tend to stain on routine histologic sections, but there is no staining of the central portions of the organisms, giving them a ribbon-like appearance (Fig. 19–5).

Special Studies. Culture is the most sensitive and specific method for making a definitive diagnosis. Periodic acid–Schiff stains and Gomori's methenamine silver stains highlight the organisms.

Pathogenesis. Zygomycosis is a disease caused by infection with any of the members of the *Mucorales* or

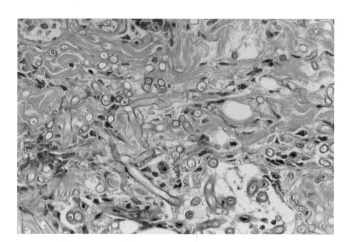

Fig. 19–4. Mucormycoses are present as large, ribbon-like organisms within the dermis.

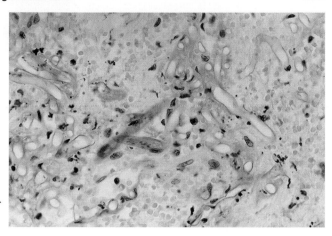

Fig. 19–5. PAS after diastase digestion stain reveals the characteristic central clearing displayed by mucormycoses.

Entomophthorales fungi. These are usually airborne infectious agents and infect the respiratory tract initially in most patients [19].

Cryptococcosis

Epidemiology. The opportunistic yeast *Cryptococcus neoformans* causes cryptococcosis. It is most commonly encountered in immunosuppressed patients, including those with organ transplants, malignant neoplasms, and AIDS. In some studies, up to 85% of infected patients are immunodeficient [24]. From 6% to 13% of patients with AIDS develop infections with *Cryptococcus*. This infection most commonly affects the central nervous system in this group [25]. Long-term corticosteroid therapy has also been implicated in increasing susceptibility to infection [26]. Virtually all immunosuppressed patients with skin involvement are infected systemically [25]. In immunocompetent patients, isolated skin involvement has been reported [27]. Cryptococcosis is not ordinarily transmitted between persons [24].

Cutaneous Features. Cutaneous manifestations are present in 10%–26% of patients with systemic infection [28, 29]. Many different clinical appearances have been described. The most common findings include umbilicated papules (resembling molluscum contagiosum) and nodules [25]. Pustules may also be present [29], as can cellulitis [30]. The head and neck are affected most commonly. Large ulcerations are sometimes encountered [26]. Less commonly, erythematous and hemorrhagic or violaceous plaques suggestive of bullous erysipelas have also been described [26]. A clinical resemblance to varicella has been reported in patients with AIDS and *Cryptococcus* infection [31]. In some patients with AIDS, cutaneous sites of *Cryptococcus* have been reported that resemble the "rodent ulcer" appearance of basal cell carcinoma [28].

Associated Disorders. Cryptococcosis is associated with immunosuppression from many causes, including underlying malignant neoplasms, organ transplants, systemic corticosteroid therapy, and AIDS. Because of this relationship, co-infection with *Cryptococcus* and other opportunistic organisms has been reported.

Histologic Features. The most common histologic features of cryptococcosis include a dense, diffuse dermal infiltrate (Fig. 19–6). The inflammatory infiltrate is characterized by granulomas that are sometimes caseating, surrounded by abundant neutrophils and lymphocytes and scattered lymphocytes. Abundant multinucleated giant cells are usually present. The organisms are present diffusely throughout the dermis, most commonly in an extracellular location (Fig. 19–7). They are usually 4–10 μm in diameter. The capsules surrounding the organisms are of variable size and may appear gelatinous. Gelatinous forms have been identified primarily in patients with more significant immunodeficiencies. In many cases of cutaneous cryptococcosis, innumerable organisms are present in the dermis in the absence of any significant inflammation. This pattern is most commonly seen in patients with coexisting human immunodeficiency virus (HIV) infection.

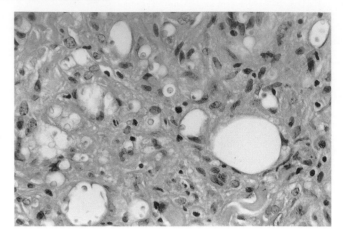

Fig. 19–7. Cryptococci are present within cells and extracellularly and are characterized by a large, unstained capsule.

Special Studies. *Cryptococcus neoformans* stains with periodic acid–Schiff and Gomori's methenamine silver stains (Fig. 19–8). The thick capsule also stains brightly with mucicarmine, a staining characteristic that is unique to this organism and often helpful in making the diagnosis. The capsule will also stain with Alcian blue and colloidal iron stains. Culture is the most sensitive and most accurate method for diagnosis, although in its gelatinous form cutaneous cryptococcosis is reliably diagnosed on histologic sections.

Pathogenesis. Almost all cases of infection occur secondary to inhalation of aerosolized organisms [24]. They are commonly found in pigeon excretions. Multiple strains of *Cryptococcus neoformans* have been isolated. Serotype D is responsible for human disease in most cases [32]. Direct traumatic implantation with the organisms rarely occurs.

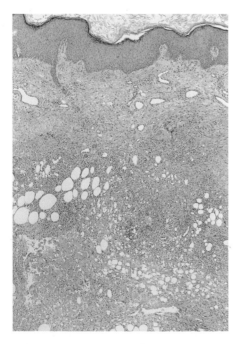

Fig. 19–6. A dense, diffuse dermal inflammatory infiltrate is seen in most cases of cryptococcosis.

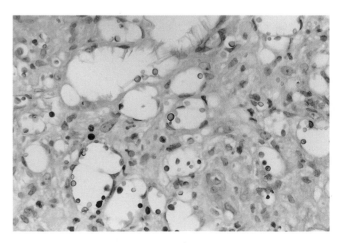

Fig. 19–8. PAS after diastase digestion stain highlights the capsule of cryptococci.

Histoplasmosis

Epidemiology. Histoplasmosis is endemic in many parts of the United States and does not produce clinically apparent disease in the 90%–95% of infected patients [33]. It is especially prevalent along the Mississippi and Ohio River valleys. The prevalence among normal, healthy adults in the middle southern states has been estimated to be 69% [34]. Of those with clinical disease, most suffer limited respiratory involvement, and only a small percentage develop disseminated disease or chronic pulmonary complications. Disseminated disease is uncommon. In one hospital-based series, the incidence of dissemination was 14% [35]. Disseminated disease is much more common in patients with altered immune systems such as those with AIDS, organ transplants, underlying neoplasia, or congenital immunodeficiencies [36–40]. Disseminated histoplasmosis is present in approximately 0.5%–5% of patients with AIDS living in endemic areas [40, 41].

Cutaneous Features. The skin is the most commonly affected extrapulmonary site in the rare patients with disseminated histoplasmosis and is involved in approximately 11% of these cases [42]. In rare cases, primary cutaneous histoplasmosis has been reported. It has been estimated to be present in approximately 1% of all infected patients who demonstrate clinical disease [35].

Histoplasmosis does not produce a specific cutaneous lesion. Disseminated cutaneous disease presents as a generalized papular eruption with ulcers and erythematous, scaly plaques [38]. Some papules may be follicular [43]. In some patients, hyperkeratosis may be prominent [41]. Verrucous plaques are present in some cases [44]. Occasional cases present with a cellulitic appearance [36]. An unusual presentation of disseminated histoplasmosis is that of a panniculitis in which organisms have been isolated directly from the lesions [45].

Primary cutaneous histoplasmosis is much less common. The reported cases have presented as isolated nodules, some with ulceration and with a cellulitis or erysipelas-like eruption [46].

Associated Disorders. Most patients with histoplasmosis are either asymptomatic or suffer from self-limited respiratory infections, with mild symptoms. In patients with disseminated disease, fever, chills, weight loss, hepatosplenomegaly, and lymphadenopathy may be present. Oropharyngeal and genital ulcerations may be seen [47]. Anemia has been reported in these patients [38]. The gastrointesintal tract is occasionally involved and is characterized by small-bowel obstruction, mucosal erythema, and friability or rectal masses [48]. Renal involvement is exceptional, but has been reported [49]. Endocarditis is also encountered in rare cases [50]. In immunocompromised patients, co-infection with *Cryptococcus* and other organisms has been reported [51].

Histologic Features. Disseminated histoplasmosis is characterized by a perivascular neutrophilic infiltrate with accompanying lymphocytes and histiocytes. Well-formed granulomas are uncommon. Leukocytoclasia may be seen. Organisms are present within the cytoplasm of histiocytes and occasionally free in the dermis [43] (Fig. 19–9). Rare cases demonstrating transepidermal elimination of the organisms have been reported [41]. Organisms are also present within the oral cavity, and these lesions may also be biopsied.

Primary cutaneous involvement is characterized by pseudoepitheliomatous hyperplasia in some cases. The dermal inflammatory infiltrate is granulomatous, with abundant multinucleated giant cells. Organisms are present within histiocytes and free within the superficial portions of the dermis.

The organisms are 2–4 μm spherical organisms and may demonstrate single buds. Hyphal forms are not usually present in tissue sections taken from the skin [33].

Special Studies. Histoplasma capsulatum is easily identified with periodic acid–Schiff and Gomori's methenamine silver stains (Fig. 19–10).

Pathogenesis. Histoplasmosis is caused by inhalation of the dimorphic fungus *Histoplasma capsulatum.* [52]. Chicken coops and bird roosts are sites that harbor high levels of this organism [40].

Blastomycosis (North American)

Epidemiology. North American blastomycosis is endemic to the south central and midwestern United States. It can affect people of all ages and both sexes,

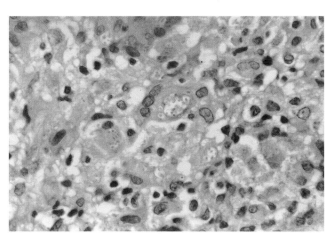

Fig. 19–9. Abundant intracellular organisms are present within histiocytes in histoplasmosis.

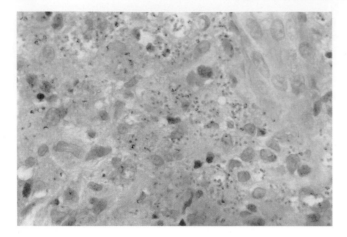

Fig. 19–10. PAS after diastase digestion stain highlights the intracellular organisms in histoplasmosis.

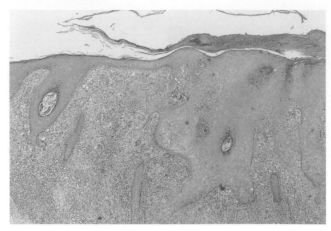

Fig. 19–11. Epidermal hyperplasia overlying a dense dermal inflammatory infiltrate is often seen in blastomycosis.

but is much more common in men and in young to middle-aged patients [53]. Many infected patients remain completely asymptomatic and unaware that they have been infected. Others develop a short-lasting, flu-like illness. Another group of patients develops a more acute, florid pneumonia. Still others develop a more chronic, low-grade respiratory illness, and a final group develops fulminant infection resulting in acute respiratory distress syndrome [54]. The clinical presentation of blastomycosis in immunosuppressed patients is similar to that in immunocompetent patients, unlike the situation with other dimorphic fungal infections [55].

Cutaneous Features. The skin is the most common site of extrapulmonary involvement. The most common presentation is that of a verrucous plaque with overlying crust and a stippled "salt and pepper" surface. Ulceration is also present in many cases [53]. Less commonly, cutaneous involvement may manifest as multiple papules or as pustules [56]. More than one skin lesion may be present. In many cases, skin involvement may be the only evidence of infection, although in these cases it is likely that the pulmonary infection is subclinical [57].

Associated Disorders. North American blastomycosis most frequently involves the lungs. Blastomycotic pneumonia is the most common manifestation. It can present with either acute symptoms or with more chronic, low-grade symptoms. The skin is the second most common site of involvement, followed by the skeletal system [58]. Prostatic [59] and central nervous system involvement are also involved in many cases [53]. Septic arthritis due to blastomycosis is also seen. In most cases this is monoarticular [60]. Less commonly, the heart, adrenal glands, and lymph nodes can be infected [56]. Choroidal blastomycosis can be seen in patients with disseminated blastomycosis [61].

Histologic Features. Histologic sections of cutaneous North American blastomycosis demonstrate pseudoepitheliomatous hyperplasia that may be quite florid (Fig. 19–11). A dense, dermal infiltrate is present and composed of abundant neutrophils, lymphocytes, and histiocytes. Later lesions demonstrate granulomatous foci, and multinucleated giant cells may be present, but these are not seen in all cases (Fig. 19–12). Caseation may be present within the granulomas.

These dimorphic fungi appear as 8–15 μm yeasts in tissue sections. They have single, broad-based buds and thick-walled, double-contoured cell walls that are refractile [56]. A single case of necrotizing arthritis has been reported in association with blastomycosis infection [62].

Special Studies. Periodic acid–Schiff and Gomori's methenamine silver stains highlight the fungi in tissue

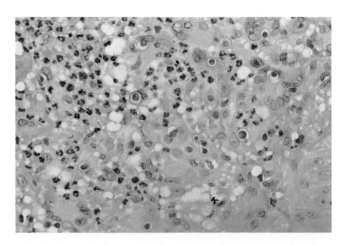

Fig. 19–12. Blastomycosis organisms can be identified within the dense granulomatous inflammatory infiltrate.

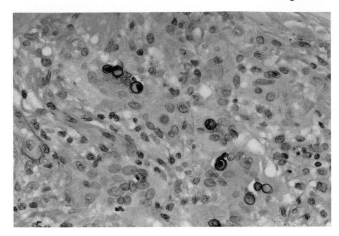

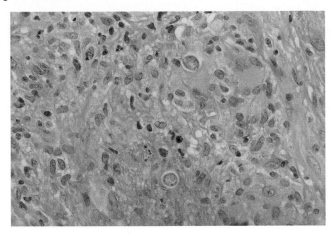

Fig. 19–13. PAS after diastase digestion stain demonstrates the broad-based budding characteristic of blastomycosis.

Fig. 19–14. Abundant, large coccidiodomycoses are visible on routine sections, admixed within a dense, granulomatous dermal infiltrate.

sections (Fig. 19–13). Mucin stains may be weakly positive [56]. Direct immunofluorescence tests are available that are specific for the organism.

Pathogenesis. North American blastomycosis is due to infection with the dimorphic fungus *Blastomyces dermatitidis* [56]. Infection is due to inhalation of airborne spores. Rare cases of direct inoculation have been reported [56].

Coccidioidomycosis

Epidemiology. Coccidioidomycosis is concentrated in the southwestern portions of the United States. The incidence of the disease has increased precipitously in the past decade [63]. In most cases, the disease remains limited to the respiratory system; however, in less than 1% of cases, disseminated disease occurs. Filipinos, Mexicans, American Indians, blacks, pregnant females, and infants and the elderly are at increased risk for developing systemic disease [64]. Immunocompromised patients are also at markedly increased risk for developing disseminated disease [65].

Cutaneous Features. It is presumed that all patients who present with cutaneous manifestations suffer from disseminated coccidioidomycosis infection [64]. Rare patients may develop cutaneous disease through traumatic implantation.

Cutaneous coccidioidomycosis may take the form of a verrucous plaque, a subcutaneous abscess, pustules, papules, or plaques [66, 67]. Erythema nodosum is reported in up to 20% of patients with pulmonary coccidioidomycosis [67].

Associated Disorders. Most patients with coccidioidomycosis develop an acute, self-limited respiratory infection. This progresses to a chronic pneumonia in

less than 1% of cases [64]. Miliary involvement of the lungs also develops in less than 1% of cases.

Hematogenous dissemination is a very rare complication seen in patients with coccidioidomycosis infection. In these patients, the meninges, bones, and joints are involved, in addition to the skin.

Histologic Features. Histologic sections reveal a dense, diffuse dermal inflammatory infiltrate. Granulomas are common and frequently display central caseation and a brisk neutrophilic infiltrate. Abundant histiocytes and multinucleated giant cells are present in most cases. Eosinophils are usually present and often abundant. Organisms may be present within histiocytes or located free within the dermis (Fig. 19–14). Although epidermal hyperplasia is usually present, this is not an invariable finding.

In tissue sections, coccidioidomycosis appears as large, 30–100 μm spherules, containing multiple 2–5 μm endospores. In most cases, the spherules are easily seen on routinely stained sections.

Special Studies. Periodic acid–Schiff and Gomori's methenamine silver stains may highlight the organisms.

Pathogenesis. The disease is contracted by inhalation of *Coccidioides immitis*, which is endemic in the desert soils of the southwestern United States.

Protothecosis

Epidemiology. Protothecosis is an uncommon infectious process caused by a unicellular alga. Patients can have localized cutaneous disease, prothecal olecranon bursitis, or systemic disease [68]. The saprophytic organisms are found in ponds and streams. Human disease is most common in immunocompromised patients after traumatic implantation [69]. The majority of cases in the United States have been reported in the southeastern states.

Cutaneous Features. Cutaneous protothecosis is the most common form of the disease in immunosuppressed patients [70] and accounts for 33%–62% of reported cases [71, 72]. It can appear as a papular or eczematous process or as a single ulcer [69]. Less common presentations include cellulitis, vesicles, and verrucous nodules [72]. One patient had a recurrent eruption that clinically resembled chromomycosis [69]. The scalp and extremities are the most common sites for cutaneous involvement [73]. The lesions will not heal spontaneously and may persist without progression for years. They heal with scarring. Pruritus has been described in association with the cutaneous eruption [73].

Associated Disorders. Protothecosis occurs most commonly in immunosuppressed patients. It has been associated with diabetes, renal transplantation, hepatitis, alcoholism, systemic lupus erythematosus, AIDS, and underlying carcinoma [69, 71, 72, 74]. It has also been described in patients receiving long-term systemic corticosteroids [74]. Nasopharyngeal involvement has been reported after prolonged endotracheal intubation [75].

Protothecal olecranon bursitis occurs after traumatic implantation and is usually seen in the context of an immunocompetent patient. Protothecosis can rarely cause disseminated disease [68]. Saprophytic contamination of the gastrointestinal tract has also been reported [72].

Histologic Features. Histologic sections demonstrate a marked granulomatous inflammatory response within the dermis. Abundant neutrophils may be present. Eosinophils are present in most cases. The overlying epidermis is acanthotic in some cases, but not in all.

The organisms may be present within the cytoplasm of histiocytes or lying free within the dermal collagen (Fig. 19–15). They appear as thick-walled, round organisms ranging in size from 4 to 15 μm in diameter that form morula bodies (endosporulation). It can be difficult to identify the organisms on routine sections because they appear as clear morula, failing to pick up the hematoxylin or eosin.

Special Studies. Protothecal organisms stain well with Gomori's methenamine silver and periodic acid–Schiff, but do not stain with mucicarmine (Fig. 19–16). Culture is the most sensitive and specific way to make a definitive diagnosis; however, the organisms have a very characteristic appearance on routine tissue sections.

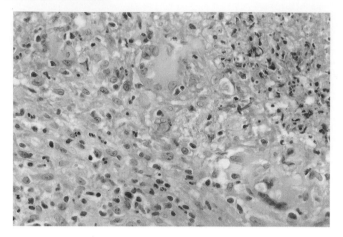

Fig. 19–15. Endosporulation of protothecosis is apparent on routine histologic sections.

Pathogenesis. Members of the genus *Prototheca*, which are achloric unicellular algae [68], cause protothecosis. There are several species, but only *Prototheca wickerhamii* and *Prototheca zopfi* have been associated with human disease.

Related Hypersensitivity Reactions

Erythema Annulare Centrifugum.
Erythema annulare centrifugum (EAC) is a related hypersensitivity reaction.

Epidemiology. The incidence of EAC has been estimated at 1/100,000. Although it has been associated with a large number of entities, as described later, in most cases it is not associated with underlying disease [76].

Cutaneous Features. One or several large, annular erythematous patches are present on the trunk and prox-

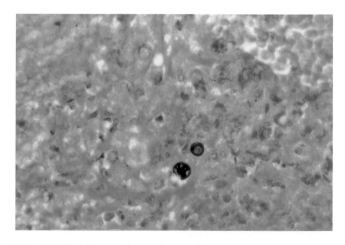

Fig. 19–16. Gomori's methenamine silver stain demonstrates the characteristic morula-like appearance of protothecosis.

imal extremities. The face, hands, and feet are involved infrequently. The patches grow centrifugally and demonstrate a thin rim of scale just inside the advancing edge (trailing scale). A deep variant of EAC has also been described that has a similar appearance but generally lacks the peripheral scale. The slowly advancing patches last for weeks to years and resolve without sequelae.

Associated Disorders. Erythema annulare centrifugum is associated with internal malignant neoplasm in a small minority of cases. It has been described in association with malignant carcinoids [77], non-small cell carcinomas of the lung [78], and hematologic malignancies including Langerhans' cell histiocytosis [79], hypereosinophilic syndrome [80], leukemia [81], and Hodgkin's disease [82, 83]. It has also been reported in association with metastatic prostate adenocarcinoma [84].

Erythema annulare centrifugum is more frequently associated with infectious processes, especially dermatophytosis. Infections with fungi [85], bacteria [86, 87], rickettsia [88], and viruses [89, 90] have all been related to the appearance of EAC.

Erythema annulare centrifugum has also been observed after ingestion of a wide range of medications, including cimetidine [91], hydroxychloroquine [92], piroxicam [93], hydrochlorothiazide [94], and gold [95]. As each of these observations represents a single case report, the incidence of drug-associated EAC is undoubtedly quite low.

Erythema annulare centrifugum has been observed in association with Hashimoto's thyroiditis [96], Graves' disease [97], liver disease [98], appendicitis [99], and pregnancy [100]. These associations are infrequent.

Histologic Features. There are two forms of EAC that have slightly different histologic appearances [101]. The superficial form is characterized by slight, focal epidermal spongiosis underlying small tufts of parakeratosis at the advancing edge of the lesion. The stratum corneum is otherwise unremarkable. A moderately intense infiltrate of predominantly lymphocytes and histiocytes tightly surrounds vessels of the superficial vascular plexus in a pattern that has been described as "tight cuffing" or "coat sleeve–like." There is relatively little interstitial inflammation (Figs. 19–17 and 19–18). Eosinophils are present only rarely. In the deep form of the disease, the epidermal changes are not present, and the inflammatory infiltrate extends down to involve the deeper dermal blood vessels in addition to the superficial ones.

Special Studies. Special studies are not helpful in making a diagnosis of EAC. Often, however, it is helpful

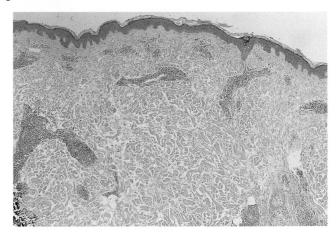

Fig. 19–17. Erythema annulare centrifugum demonstrates a superficial and deep perivascular inflammatory infiltrate, with a characteristic "tight cuffing" around the dermal blood vessels.

to review a periodic acid–Schiff stain to exclude dermatophyte infection.

Pathogenesis. The pathogenesis of EAC is unknown. A hypersensitivity reaction to various antigens has been proposed as the cause of this cutaneous eruption [94].

Id Reaction (Autosensitization Reaction)

Epidemiology. An id reaction is a cutaneous hypersensitivity reaction to a distant antigen. In many cases, this represents a chronic fungus infection, such as dermatophytosis with secondary bacterial infection. Organisms are not present within the lesions of the id reaction, and treatment of the underlying infectious process results in resolution of the hypersensitivity process.

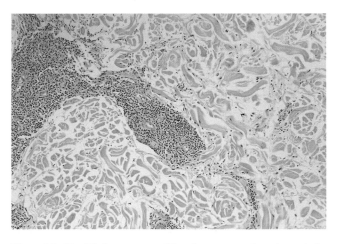

Fig. 19–18. Higher magnification reveals the tight perivascular aggregation of lymphocytes and histiocytes in erythema annulare centrifugum.

Cutaneous Features. Id reactions may display many clinical patterns. Most of them are described as appearing eczematous, with erythema, scaling, and microvesiculation. The palms and soles are most frequently involved in these generalized eruptions. In other cases, id reactions may be papular and urticarial [102] or psoriasiform [103]. Other authors describe Sweet's-like, erythema multiforme-like, and erythema nodosum-like lesions [104, 105].

Associated Disorders. Id reactions occur in association with many exogenous or endogenous antigens. The most common association is with dermatophyte infection, especially tinea pedis in conjunction with bacterial superinfection [105]. Other associated infections include mycobacteria, bacteria, and viruses.

Histologic Features. As might be expected from the varied clinical presentations, the histologic patterns of an id reaction may be manifold. The most common pattern is that of a spongiotic dermatitis. Parakeratosis is present overlying a spongiotic epidermis. Spongiotic microvesicles are often present. There is slight to marked acanthosis, and a lymphohistiocytic infiltrate is present within the epidermis (Fig. 19–19). In the dermis, lymphocytes, histiocytes, and scattered eosinophils may be present around vessels of the superficial vascular plexus. These findings are not specific and can be seen in many eczematous processes.

The histologic changes seen in Sweet's-like, erythema multiforme-like, or erythema nodosum-like id reactions are indistinguishable from the histologic changes seen in spontaneously occurring forms of these diseases. They are described elsewhere.

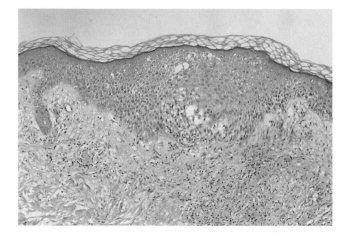

Fig. 19–19. An id reaction most often has the histologic appearance of a spongiotic dermatitis with no further specific histologic changes.

Special Studies. Special studies are not necessary for diagnosing an id reaction. In some cases, it is helpful to perform a periodic acid–Schiff stain in order to exclude a primary cutaneous fungal infection that can demonstrate similar histologic changes.

Pathogenesis. Id reactions are thought be hypersensitivity reactions to distant antigens. The exact process by which they develop is not understood.

Erythema Nodosum

Epidemiology. Erythema nodosum is a type of hypersensitivity reaction that may occur in association with multiple systemic processes or as an independent process with no detectable underlying conditions. Up to 83% of cases occur in women, with a peak incidence between the ages of 18 and 34 years [106, 107]. The thighs and anterior lower legs are the most commonly affected sites. Bilateral involvement is present in about half of the cases [106]. Although less common, erythema nodosum does occur in children [108].

Cutaneous Features. Erythema nodosum presents as one or more tender, nonulcerated, erythematous subcutaneous nodules. There are no overlying surface changes. The nodules persist from weeks to months and resolve spontaneously without sequelae. A more chronic form of the disease exists in which nodules are longer lasting and appear at varied sites.

Associated Disorders. Erythema nodosum is most commonly associated with infectious processes [106]. Streptococcal infections are especially common in this setting. Approximately 28% of cases of erythema nodosum were associated with streptococcal infection in one study [107, 108]. Other associated infections include mycobacteria, *Yersinia*, infectious mononucleosis, hepatitides B and C, and scabies [107, 109].

Erythema nodosum in the United States is associated frequently with oral contraceptive use. It is also associated with exogenous estrogen therapy and pregnancy [110, 111]. Many drugs have been associated with erythema nodosum.

Other associations include sarcoidosis, Crohn's disease, non-Hodgkin's lymphoma, carcinoma, Sjögren's syndrome, Sweet's syndrome, radiation, and discoid lupus erythematosus [106, 107, 112–115]. There is no identifiable association in up to half of cases of erythema nodosum [116].

Histologic Features. Erythema nodosum is a septal panniculitis. Interlobular septa are widened and either edematous or fibrotic. The septal inflammatory infiltrate is

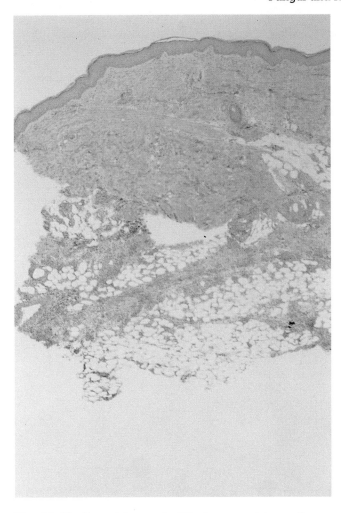

Fig. 19–20. A septal panniculitis is present in erythema nodosum.

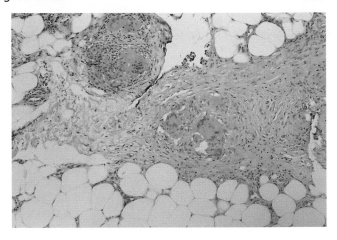

Fig. 19–22. Granulomas are present in more than half of cases of erythema nodosum.

predominantly lymphohistiocytic (Fig. 19–20). In most cases, the inflammatory infiltrate, while centered in the septa, extends into the periphery of the adjacent fatty lobules (Fig. 19–21). Eosinophils are present in up to half of cases [117] (Fig. 19–22). Histiocytes, which may cluster into small granulomatous foci, are present in approximately 75% of cases [117]. Foreign body–type giant cells may also be observed. Small vessel leukocytoclastic vasculitis may be present in up to 30% of biopsy specimens [106]. Other authors do not believe vasculitis to be a part of the process [117, 118]. Scattered neutrophils are present within the septa in early cases. These neutrophils are not necessarily distributed within or around blood vessels.

Inflammation is present in the dermis in most cases. It is composed of lymphocytes and histiocytes surrounding the superficial and deep vascular plexuses and is usually relatively sparse.

Special Studies. Special studies are not required to make a diagnosis of erythema nodosum.

Pathogenesis. The pathogenesis of erythema nodosum is not known. Most investigators believe it to be a hypersensitivity reaction that occurs in response to a wide range of antigens.

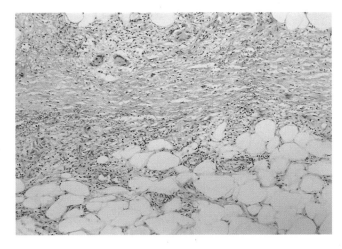

Fig. 19–21. Erythema nodosum is characterized by fibrosis of the interlobular septa with a mixed inflammatory infiltrate containing lymphocytes, eosinophils, occasional neutrophils, and histiocytes.

References

1. Groll, A. H., Jaeger, G., Allendorf, A., Herrmann, G., Schloesser, R., and von Loewenich, V., *Invasive pulmonary aspergillosis in a critically ill neonate: Case report and review of invasive aspergillosis during the first 3 months of life.* Clin Infect Dis, 1998. 27:437–452.

2. Galimberti, R., Kowalczuk, A., Hidalgo Parra, I., Gonzalez Ramos, M., and Flores, V., *Cutaneous aspergillosis: A report of six cases.* Br J Dermatol, 1998. 139: 522–526.

3. Meyer, R. D., *Cutaneous and mucosal manifestations of the deep mycotic infections.* Acta Derm Venereol (Stockh), 1986. 121:57–72.

4. Stiller, M. J., Teperman, L., Rosenthal, S. A., Riordan, A., Potter, J., Shupack, J. L., and Gordon, M. A., *Primary cutaneous infection by Aspergillus ustus in a 62-year-old liver transplant recipient.* J Am Acad Dermatol, 1994. 31:344–347.

5. Bohler, K., Metze, D., Poitschek, C., and Jurecka, W., *Cutaneous aspergillosis.* Clin Exp Dermatol, 1990. 15:446–450.

6. Dohil, M., Prendiville, J. S., Crawford, R. I., and Speert, D. P., *Cutaneous manifestations of chronic granulomatous disease. A report of four cases and review of the literature.* J Am Acad Dermatol, 1997. 36:899–907.

7. Harmon, C. B., Su, W. P. D., and Peters, M. S., *Cutaneous aspergillosis complicating pyoderma gangrenosum.* J Am Acad Dermatol, 1993. 29:656–658.

8. Chandler, F. W., and Watts, J. C., *Aspergillosis. In Pathologic diagnosis of fungal infections.* 1987, American Society of Clinical Pathologists Press, Chicago, pp. 55–74.

9. Hartman, P. D., and Kaplan, R. P., *Transepithelial elimination in cutaneous aspergillosis.* J Am Acad Dermatol, 1986. 15:1305–1307.

10. Linder, N., Keller, N., Huri, C., Kuint, J., Goldshmidt-Reuven, A., and Barzilai, A., *Primary cutaneous mucormycosis in a premature infant: Case report and review of the literature.* Am J Perinatol, 1998. 15:35–38.

11. Marchevsky, A. M., Bottone, E. J., Geller, S. A., and Giger, D. K., *The changing spectrum of disease, etiology, and diagnosis of mucormycosis.* Hum Pathol, 1980. 11:457–464.

12. Veliath, A. J., Rao, R., Prabhua, M. R., and Aurora, A. L., *Cutaneous phycomycosis (mucormycosis) with fatal pulmonary dissemination.* Arch Dermatol, 1976. 112:509–512.

13. Adam, R. D., Hunter, G., DiTomasso, J., and Comerci, G. Jr., *Mucormycosis: Emerging prominence of cutaneous infections.* Clin Infect Dis, 1994. 19:67–76.

14. Mostaza, J. M., Barbado, F. J., Fernandez-Martin, J., Pena-Yanez, J., and Vazquez-Rodrguez, J. J., *Cutaneoarticular mucormycosis due to Cunninghamella bertholletiae in a patient with AIDS.* Rev Infect Dis, 1989. 11:316–318.

15. Wirth, F., Perry, R., Eskenazi, A., Schwalbe, R., and Kao, G., *Cutaneous mucormycosis with subsequent visceral dissemination in a child with neutropenia: A case report and review of the pediatric literature.* J Am Acad Dermatol, 1997. 36:336–341.

16. Geller, J. D., Peters, M. S., and Su, W. P. D., *Cutaneous mucormycosis resembling superficial granulomatous pyoderma in an immunocompetent host.* J Am Acad Dermatol, 1993. 29:462–465.

17. Verma, K. K., and Pandhi, R. K., *Subcutaneous mucormycosis in a nonimmunocompromised patient treated with potassium iodide.* Acta Derm Venereol, 1994. 74:215–216.

18. Woods, S. G., and Elewski, B. E., *Zosteriform zygomycosis.* J Am Acad Dermatol, 1995. 32:357–361.

19. Sugar, A. M., *Mucormycosis.* Clin Infect Dis, 1992. 14(Suppl 1):S126–S129.

20. Johnson, A. S., Ranson, M., Scarffe, J. H., Morgenstern, G. R., Shaw, A. J., and Oppenheim, B. A., *Cutaneous infection with Rhizopus oryzae and Aspergillus niger following bone marrow transplantation.* J Hosp Infect, 1993. 25:293–296.

21. Maliwan, N., Reyes, C. V., and Rippon, J. W., *Osteomyelitis secondary to cutaneous mucormycosis. Report of a case and a review of the literature.* Am J Dermatopathol, 1984. 6:479–481.

22. Virmani, R., Connor, D. H., and McAllister, H. A., *Cardiac mucormycosis. A report of five patients and review of 14 previously reported cases.* Am J Clin Pathol, 1982. 78:42–47.

23. Chandler, F. W., and Watts, J. C., *Zygomycosis. In Pathologic diagnosis of fungal infections.* 1987, American Society of Clinical Pathologists Press, Chicago, pp. 85–96.

24. Chandler, F. W., and Watts, J. C., *Cryptococcosis. in Pathologic Diagnosis of Fungal Infections.* 1987, American Society of Clinical Pathology Press, Chicago, pp. 161–175.

25. Murakawa, G. J., Kerschmann, R., and Berger, T., *Cutaneous Cryptococcus infection and AIDS. Report of 12 cases and review of the literature.* Arch Dermatol, 1996. 132:545–548.

26. Vogelaers, D., Petrovic, M., Deroo, M., Verplancke, P., Claessens, Y., Naeyaert, J. M., and Afschrift, M., *A case of primary cutaneous cryptococcosis.* Eur J Clin Microbiol Infect Dis, 1997. 16:150–152.

27. Vandersmissen, G., Meuleman, L., Tits, G., Verhaeghe, A., and Peetermans, W. E., *Cutaneous crytpococcosis in corticosteroid-treated patients without AIDS.* Acta Clin Belg, 1996. 51:111–117.

28. Ingleton, R., Koestenblatt, E., Don, P., Levy, H., Szaniawski, W., and Weinberg, J. M., *Cutaneous cryptococcosis mimicking basal cell carcinoma in a patients with AIDS.* J Cutan Med Surg, 1998. 3:43–45.

29. Manfredi, R., Mazzoni, A., Nanetti, A., Mastroianni, A., Coronado, O., and Chiodo, F., *Morphologic features and clinical significance of skin involvement in patients with AIDS-related cryptococcosis.* Acta Derm Venereol, 1996. 76:72–74.

30. Anderson, D. J., Schmidt, C., Goodman, J., and Pomeroy, C., *Cryptococcal disease presenting as cellulitis.* Clin Infect Dis, 1992. 14:666–672.

31. Yantsos, V. A., Carney, J., and Greer, D. L., *Review of the morphological variations in cutaneous cryptococcosis with a new case resembling varicella.* Cutis, 1994. 54:343–347.

32. Tortorano, A. M., Viviani, M. A., Rigoni, A. L., Cogliati, M., Roverselli, A., and Pagano, A., *Prevalence of serotype D in Cryptococcus neoformans isolates from HIV positive and HIV negative patients in Italy.* Mycoses, 1997. 40:297–302.

33. Chandler, F. W., and Watts, J. C., *Histoplasmosis capsulati.* In *Pathologic Diagnosis of Fungal Infections.* 1987, American Society of Clinical Pathologists Press, Chicago, pp. 123–139.

34. Leggiadro, R. J., Leudtke, G. S., Convey, A., Gibson, L., and Barrett, F. F., *Prevalence of histoplasmosis in a midsouthern population.* South Mcd J, 1991. 84:1360–1361.

35. Butler, J. C., Heller, R., and Wright, P. F., *Histoplasmosis during childhood.* South Med J, 1994. 87:476–480.

36. Cooper, P. H., Walker, A. W., and Beacham, B. E., *Cellulitis caused by Histoplasma organisms in a renal transplant recipient.* Arch Dermatol, 1982. 118:3–4.

37. Yilmaz, G. G., Yilmaz, E., Coskun, M., Karpuzoglu, G., Gelen, T., and Yegin, O., *Cutaneous histoplasmosis in a child with hyper-IgM.* Pediatr Dermatol, 1995. 12:235–238.

38. Bellman, B., Berman, B., Sasken, H., and Kirsner, R. S., *Cutaneous disseminated histoplasmosis in AIDS patients in south Florida.* Int J Dermatol, 1997. 36:599–603.

39. Angius, A. G., Viviani, M. A., Muratori, S., Cusini, M., Brignolo, L., and Alessi, E., *Disseminated histoplasmosis presenting with cutaneous lesions in a patient with acquired immunodeficiency syndrome.* J Eur Acad Dermatol Venereol, 1998. 10:182–185.

40. Hajjeh, R. A., *Disseminated histoplasmosis in persons infected with human immunodeficiency virus.* Clin Infect Dis, 1995. 21(Suppl 1):S108–S110.

41. Welykyj, S., Von Heimburg, A., Massa, M. C., Schmidt, K., Reddy, V., Gattuso, P., and O'Keefe, P., *Cutaneous lesions of histoplasmosis with transepidermal elimination in a patient with acquired immunodeficiency syndrome.* Cutis, 1991. 47:397–400.

42. Cohen, P. R., Bank, D. E., Silvers, D. N., and Grossman, M. E., *Cutaneous lesions of disseminated histoplasmosis in human immunodeficiency virus–infected patients.* J Am Acad Dermatol, 1990. 23:422–428.

43. Eidbo, J., Sanchez, R. L., Tschen, J. A., and Ellner, K. M., *Cutaneous manifestations of histoplasmosis in the acquired immune deficiency syndrome.* Am J Surg Pathol, 1993. 17:110–116.

44. Cohen, P. R., Held, J. L., Grossman, M. E., Ross, M. J., and Silvers, D. N., *Disseminated histoplasmosis presenting as an ulcerated verrucous plaque in a human immundeficiency virus–infected man. Report of a case possibly involving human-to-human transmission of histoplasmosis.* Int J Dermatol, 1991. 30:104–108.

45. Abildgaard, W. H. Jr., Hargrove, R. H., and Kalivas, J., *Histoplasma panniculitis.* Arch Dermatol, 1985. 121:914–916.

46. Giessel, M., and Rau, J. M., *Primary cutaneous histoplasmosis: A new presentation.* Cutis, 1980. 25:152–154.

47. Smith, M. B., Schnadig, V. J., Zaharopoulos, P., and Van Hook, C., *Disseminated Histoplasma capsulatum infection presenting as genital ulcerations.* Obstet Gynecol, 1997. 89:842–844.

48. Cappell, M. S., Mandell, W., Grimes, M. M., and Neu, H. C., *Gastrointestinal histoplasmosis.* Dig Dis Sci, 1988. 33:353–360.

49. Kedar, S. S., Eldar, S., Abrahamson, J., and Boss, J., *Histoplasmosis of kidneys presenting as chronic recurrent renal disease.* Urology, 1988. 31:490–494.

50. Blair, T. P., Waugh, R. A., Pollack, M., Ashworth, H. E., Young, N. A., Anderson, S. E., and Bem, T. P., *Histoplasma capsulatum endocarditis.* Am Heart J, 1980. 99:783–788.

51. Myers, S. A., and Kamino, H., *Cutaneous cryptococcosis and histoplasmosis coinfection in a patient with AIDS.* J Am Acad Dermatol, 1996. 34:898–900.

52. Hay, R. J., *Histoplasmosis.* Semin Dermatol, 1993. 12:310–314.

53. Bradsher, R. W., *Clinical features of blastomycosis.* Semin Respir Infect, 1997. 12:229–234.

54. Davies, S. F., and Sarosi, G. A., *Epidemiological and clinical features of pulmonary blastomycosis.* Semin Respir Infect, 1997. 12:206–218.

55. Recht, L. D., Davies, S. F., Eckman, M. R., and Sarosi, G. A., *Blastomycosis in immunosuppressed patients.* Am Rev Respir Dis, 1982. 125:359–362.

56. Chandler, F. W., and Watts, J. C., *Blastomycosis.* In *Pathologic Diagnosis of Fungal Infections.* 1987, American Society of Clinical Pathologists Press, Chicago, pp. 149–160.

57. Mercurio, M. G., and Elewski, B. E., *Cutaneous blastomycosis.* Cutis, 1992. 50:422–424.

58. Saccente, M., Abernathy, R. S., Pappas, P. G., Shah, H. R., and Bradsher, R. W., *Vertebral blastomycosis with paravertebral abscess: Report of eight cases and review of the literature.* Clin Infect Dis, 1998. 26:413–418.

59. Inoshita, T., Youngberg, G. A., Boelen, L. J., and Langston, J., *Blastomycosis presenting with prostatic involvement: Report of 2 cases and review of the literature.* J Urol, 1983. 130:160–162.

60. Abril, A., Campbell, M. D., Cotten, V. R. Jr., Steckleberg, J. M., El-Azhary, R. A., and O'Duffy, J. D., *Polyarticular blastomycotic arthritis.* J Rheumatol, 1998. 25:1019–1021.

61. Gottlieb, J. L., McAllister, I. L., Guttman, F. A., and Vine, A. K., *Choroidal blastomycosis. A report of two cases.* Retina, 1995. 15:248–252.

62. Houston, M. C., Marion, J. M., and Curry, W. A., *Necrotizing arteritis associated with blastomycosis.* South Med J, 1986. 79:519–520.

63. Vaz, A., Pineda-Roman, M., Thomas, A. R., and Carlson, R. W., *Coccidioidomycosis: An update.* Hosp Pract (Off Ed), 1998. 15:119–120.

64. Chandler, F. W., and Watts, J. C., *Coccidioidomycosis.* In *Pathologic Diagnosis of Fungal Infections.* 1987, American Society of Clinical Pathologists Press, Chicago, pp. 13–25.

65. Deresinski, S. C., and Stevens, D. A., *Coccidioidomycosis in compromised hosts.* Medicine (Baltimore), 1975. 54:377–395.

66. Schwartz, R. A., and Lamberts, R. J., *Isolated nodular cutaneous coccidioidomycosis. The initial manifestation of disseminated disease.* J Am Acad Dermatol, 1981. 4:38–46.

67. Bayer, A. S., Yoshikawa, T. T., Galpin, J. E., and Guze, L. B., *Unusual syndromes of coccidiodomycosis: Diagnostic and therapeutic considerations. A report of 10 cases and review of the English literature.* Medicine (Baltimore), 1976. 55:131–152.

68. Mayhall, C. G., Miller, C. W., Eisen, A. Z., Kobayahi, G. S., and Medoff, G., *Cutaneous protothecosis. Successful treatment with amphotericin B.* Arch Dermatol, 1976. 112:1749–1752.

69. McAnally, T., and Parry, E. L., *Cutaneous protothecosis presenting as recurrent chromomycosis.* 1985. 121:1066–1069.

70. Nelson, A. M., Neafie, R. C., and Connor, D. H., *Cutaneous protothecosis and chlorellosis, extraordinary "aquatic-borne" algal infections.* Clin Dermatol, 1987. 5:76–87.

71. Woolrich, A., Koestenblatt, E., Don, P., and Szaniawski, W., *Cutaneous protothecosis and AIDS.* J Am Acad Dermatol, 1994. 31:920–924.

72. Tyring, S. K., Lee, P. C., Walsh, P., Garner, F., and Little, W. P., *Papular protothecosis of the chest. Immunologic evaluation and treatment with a combination of oral tetracycline and topical amphotericin B.* Arch Dermatol, 1989. 125:1249–1252.

73. Kuo, D.-T., Hsueh, S., Wu, J.-L., and Wang, A.-M., *Cutaneous protothecosis. A clinicopathologic study.* Arch Pathol Lab Med, 1987. 111:737–740.

74. Polk, P., and Sanders, D. Y., *Cutaneous protothecosis in association with the acquired immunodeficiency syndrome.* South Med J, 1997. 90:831–832.

75. Iacoviello, V. R., DeGirolami, P. C., Lucarini, J., Sutker, K., Williams, M. E., and Wanke, C. A., *Protothecosis complicating prolonged endotracheal intubation: Case report and literature review.* Clin Infect Dis, 1992. 15:959–967.

76. Mahood, J. M., *Erythema annulare centrifugum: A review of 24 cases with special reference to its association with underlying disease.* Clin Exp Dermatol, 1983. 8:383–387.

77. Everall, J. D., Dowd, P. M., and Ardalan, B., *Unusual cutaneous associations of a malignant carcinoid tumour of the bronchus—erythema annulare centrifugum and white banding of the toe nails.* Br J Dermatol, 1975. 93:341–345.

78. Monsieur, I., Meysman, M., Noppen, M., De Greve, J., Delhove, O., Velckeniers, B., Jacobvitz, D., and Vincken, W., *Non-small cell lung cancer with multiple paraneoplastic syndromes.* Eur Respir J, 1995. 8:1231–1234.

79. Dodd, H. J., Kirby, J. D., Chambers, T. J., and Stansfeld, A. G., *Erythema annulare centrifugum and malignant histiocytosis—report of a case.* Clin Exp Dermatol, 1984. 9:608–613.

80. Shelley, W. B., and Shelley, E. D., *Erythema annulare centrifugum as the presenting sign of the hypereosinophilic syndrome: Observations on therapy.* Cutis, 1985. 35:53–55.

81. Zultak, M., Blanc, D., Merle, C., Maingon, P., and Rosenbaum, A., *Erythema annulare centrifugum and acute myeloblastic leukemia.* Ann Dermatol Venereol, 1989. 116:477–480.

82. Yaniv, R., Shpielberg, O., Shapiro, D., Feinstein, A., and Ben-Bassat, I., *Erythema annulare centrifugum as the presenting sign of Hodgkin's disease.* Int J Dermatol, 1993. 32:59–61.

83. Villette, B., and Tulliez, M., *Erythema annulare centrifugum and Hodgkin's disease.* Ann Dermatol Venereol, 1990. 117:889–890.

84. Dupre, A., Carrere, A., Bonafe, J. L., Viraben, R., Christol, B., and Lassere, J., *Erythema annulare centrifugum of the legs symptomatic of prostate adenocarcinoma: A specific paraneoplastic syndrome?* Ann Dermatol Venereol, 1979. 106:789–792.

85. Kikuchi, I., Ogata, K., and Inoue, S., *Pityrosporum infection in an infant with lesions resembling erythema annulare centrifugum.* Arch Dermatol, 1984. 120:380–382.

86. Borbujo, J., de Miguel, C., Lopez, A., de Lucas, R., and Casado, M., *Erythema annulare centrifugum and Escherichia coli urinary infection.* Lancet, 1996. 347:897–898.

87. Burkhart, C. G., *Erythema annulare centrifugum. A case due to tuberculosis.* Int J Dermatol, 1982. 21:538–539.

88. Betlloch, I., Amador, C., Chiner, E., Varona, C., Carbonell, C., and Vilar, A., *Erythema annulare centifugum in Q fever.* Int J Dermatol, 1991. 30:502.

89. Furue, M., Akasu, R., Ohtake, N., and Tamaki, K., *Erythema annulare centrifugum induced by molluscum contagiosum.* Br J Dermatol, 1993. 129:646–647.

90. Hammar, H., *Erythema annulare centrifugum coincident with Epstein-Barr virus infection in an adult.* Acta Pediatr Scand, 1974. 63:788–792.

91. Merrett, A. C., Marks, R., and Dudley, F. J., *Cimetidine-induced erythema annulare centrifugum: No cross-sensitivity with ranitidine.* BMJ (Clin Res Ed), 1981. 283 (6293):698.

92. Hudson, L. D., *Erythema annulare centrifugum: An unusual case due to hydroxychloroquine sulfate.* Cutis, 1985. 36:129–130.

93. Hogan, D. J., and Blocka, K. L., *Erythema annulare centrifugum associated with piroxicam.* J Am Acad Dermatol, 1985. 13:840–841.

94. Goette, D. K., and Beatrice, E., *Erythema annulare centrifugum caused by hydrochlorothiazide-induced interstitial nephritis.* Int J Dermatol, 1988. 27:129–130.

95. Tsuji, T., Nishimura, M., and Kimura, S., *Erythema annulare centrifugum associated with gold sodium thiomalate therapy.* J Am Acad Dermatol, 1992. 27:284–287.

96. Thess, F., Rigon, J. L., Cuny, J. F., Schmutz, J. L., Weber, M., and Beurey, J., *Erythema annulare centrifugum and Hashimoto's thyroiditis.* Ann Dermatol Venereol, 1986. 113:1087–1088.

97. Braunstein, B. L., *Erythema annulare centrifugum and Graves' disease.* Arch Dermatol, 1982. 118:623.

98. Tsuji, T., and Kadoya, A., *Erythema annulare centrifugum associated with liver disease.* Arch Dermatol, 1986. 122:1239–1240.

99. Sack, D. M., Carle, G., and Shama, S. K., *Recurrent acute appendicitis with erythema annulare centrifugum.* Arch Intern Med, 1984. 144:2090–2092.

100. Choonhakarn, C., and Seramethakun, P., *Erythema an-*

nulare centrifugum associated with pregnancy. Acta Derm Venereol, 1998. 78:237–238.

101. Bressler, G. S., and Jones, R. E. Jr., *Erythema annulare centrifugum.* J Am Acad Dermatol, 1981. 4:597–602.

102. Jordaan, H. F., and Schneider, J. W., *Papular urticaria: A histopathologic study of 30 patients.* Am J Dermatopathol, 1997. 19:119–126.

103. Gianni, C., Betti, R., and Crosti, C., *Psoriasiform id reaction in tinea corporis.* Mycoses, 1996. 39:307–308.

104. Magro, C. M., and Crowson, A. N., *A distinctive cutaneous reaction pattern indicative of infection by reactive arthropathy-associated microbial pathogens: The superantigen ID reaction.* J Cutan Pathol, 1998. 25:538–544.

105. Svejgaard, E., *Immunologic investigations of dermatophytoses and dermatophytosis.* Semin Dermatol, 1985. 4:201–221.

106. Bohn, S., Buchner, S., and Itin, P., *Erythema nodosum: 112 cases. Epidemiology, clinical aspects and histo-pathology.* Schweiz Med Wochenschr, 1997. 127:1168–1176.

107. Cribier, B., Caille, A., Heid, E., and Grosshans, E., *Erythema nodosum and associated diseases. A study of 129 cases.* Int J Dermatol, 1998. 37:667–672.

108. Labbe, L., Perel, Y., Maleville, J., and Taieb, A., *Erythema nodosum in children: A study of 27 patients.* Pediatr Dermatol, 1996. 13:447–450.

109. Picco, P., Gattorno, M., Vignola, S., Barabino, A., Marazzi, M. G., Bondi, E., Pistoia, V., and Buoncompagni, A., *Clinical and biological characteristics of immunopathological disease–related erytehma nodosum in children.* Scand J Rheumatol, 1999. 28:27–32.

110. Bartelsmeyer, J. A., and Petrie, R. H., *Erythema nodosum, estrogens, and pregnancy.* Clin Obstet Gynecol, 1990. 33:777–781.

111. Yang, S. G., Han, K. H., Cho, K. H., and Lee, A. Y., *Development of erythema nodosum in the course of oestrogen replacement therapy.* Br J Dermatol, 1997. 137:319–320.

112. Yamamoto, T., Yokoyama, A., Yamamoto, Y., and Mamada, A., *Erythema nodosum associated with Sjögren's syndrome.* Br J Rheumatol, 1997. 36:707–708.

113. Altomare, G. F., and Capella, G. L., *Paraneoplastic erythema nodosum in a patient with carcinoma of the uterine cervix.* Br J Dermatol, 1995. 132:667–668.

114. Takagawa, S., Nakamura, S., Yokozeki, H., and Nishika, K., *Radiation-induced erythema nodosum.* Br J Dermatol, 1999. 140:372.

115. Waltz, K. M., Long, D., Marks, J. G. Jr., and Billingsley, E. M., *Sweet's syndrome and erythema nodosum: The simultaneous occurrence of 2 reactive dermatoses.* Arch Dermatol, 1999. 135:62–66.

116. Alvarez-Lario, B., Piney, E., Rodriguez-Valverde, V., Pena Sagredo, J. L., and Peiro Callizo, E., *Eritema nodoso: Estudio de 103 casos.* Med Clin (Barc), 1987. 88:5–8.

117. Sanchez Yus, E., Sanz Vico, D., and de Diego, V., *Miescher's radial granuloma. A characteristic marker of erythema nodosum.* Am J Dermatopathol, 1989. 11: 434–442.

118. Ackerman, A. B., *Histologic Diagnosis of Inflammatory Skin Diseases.* 1978, Lea & Febiger, Philadelphia, pp. 196–197.

CHAPTER
20

Rickettsial Diseases

There are many species of *rickettsia* that give rise to human infections. Many of these are, however, quite rare in the United States. In addition, cutaneous manifestations are not a feature of all human rickettsial infections. A nonspecific macular and papular eruption is seen in many of them. This chapter addresses only the most common rickettsial infections with cutaneous involvement encountered in the United States. Table 20–1 lists many of the other rickettsial species that cause human disease.

Rocky Mountain Spotted Fever

Epidemiology. Rocky Mountain spotted fever (RMSF) is found in virtually all states within the United States. About half of all reported cases occur in North Carolina, Oklahoma, Tennessee, and South Carolina. The incidence is approximately 2 cases per 1 million population, and the disease is most common in children aged 5–9 years. Most cases occur during the spring and summer months. The mortality rate is difficult to assess, but a case-fatality ratio of 4.0% was found in one large study [1]. Older patients have a worse prognosis.

Cutaneous Features. Cutaneous manifestations are present in 80% of patients with RMSF [1]. These patients display a generalized purpuric skin eruption. Macules and papules are usually purpuric, but may blanch. Skin findings usually begin and are accentuated on the extremities [2]. Up to 10% of patients with RMSF have only minimal cutaneous findings, which may be transient and easily missed. The relative absence of cutaneous manifestations appears to be more frequent in men and in black patients [3]. Rare patients with a localized erythematous patch resembling the erythema chronicum migrans of Lyme disease have been described [4]. In some patients, complications of the cutaneous eruption progress to include massive skin necrosis [5] and even gangrene [6].

Associated Disorders. Patients with RMSF also demonstrate constitutional symptoms such as fever and bleeding diatheses [7]. Fever is present in 94% of patients, headache in 86%, and myalgias in 82% [1]. As RMSF is essentially a systemic vasculitis, clinical manifestations secondary to vascular involvement can be seen in virtually all organs, including the heart, brain, and kidneys [8]. Acute renal failure occurred in up to 20% of patients hospitalized with RMSF in some series [9].

Histologic Features. Rocky Mountain spotted fever is characterized by a lymphohistiocytic inflammatory infiltrate surrounding and invading the walls of dermal capillaries and postcapillary venules [2] (Fig. 20–1). Vascular thrombi and destruction of the vessel walls are present in most cases (Fig. 20–2). Focal leukocytoclastic vasculitis, with transmural neutrophils, fibrinoid necrosis, and nuclear dust is present in about 75% of cases. In the other cases, a solely lymphocytic inflammatory infiltrate is observed. In cases with a neutrophil-predominant inflammatory infiltrate, basal layer vacuolization and exocytosis of lymphocytes are also frequently present. Subepidermal blister formation and necrosis of the epidermis are seen in later lesions. Plasma cells are present within the dermal infiltrate in about 20% of cases and eosinophils in about 10% [2].

Table 20–1. Rickettsial Diseases in Humans

Disease	Organism	Geographic Distribution
Rocky Mountain spotted fever	R. ricketsii	Americas
Rickettsialpox	R. akari	North America, Korea
Ehrlichiosis	E. chaffeensis	Southeastern US, Europe, Africa
Boutonneuse fever	R. conorii	Meditteranean
South African tick-bite fever	R. conorii	Africa
Oriental spotted fever	R. japonica	Japan
Siberian tick typhus	R. sibirica	Russia
Queensland tick typhus	R. australis	Australia
Epidemic typhus	R. prowazekii	Africa, Central and South America
Brill-Zinsser disease	R. prowazekii	Worldwide
Murine typhus	R. typhi	Worldwide
Scrub typhus	R. tsutsugamushi	Southeast Asia
Q fever	Coxiella burnetii	Worldwide

Special Studies. Multiple immunologic methods of detecting *Rickettsia rickettsii* have been described. Although immunofluorescence methods are faster, immunoperoxidase detection systems have proved to be just as sensitive and specific in finding organisms on formalin-fixed, paraffin-embedded tissue [10, 11].

Organisms can also be identified using electron microscopy. They are found in both the cytoplasm and nuclei of endothelial cells and in the surrounding dermis [12].

Pathogenesis. It has been suggested that *Rickettsia rickettsii* causes damage to endothelial cells that then precipitates a lymphohistiocytic vasculitis. The vasculitis progresses to become leukocytoclastic in fully developed lesions [2].

Ehrlichiosis

Epidemiology. Ehrlichiosis is a tick-borne disease that is most prevalent in the south central and southeastern portions of the United States [13]. The disease is contracted most frequently in the spring and summer months and is strongly associated with exposures to ticks [14].

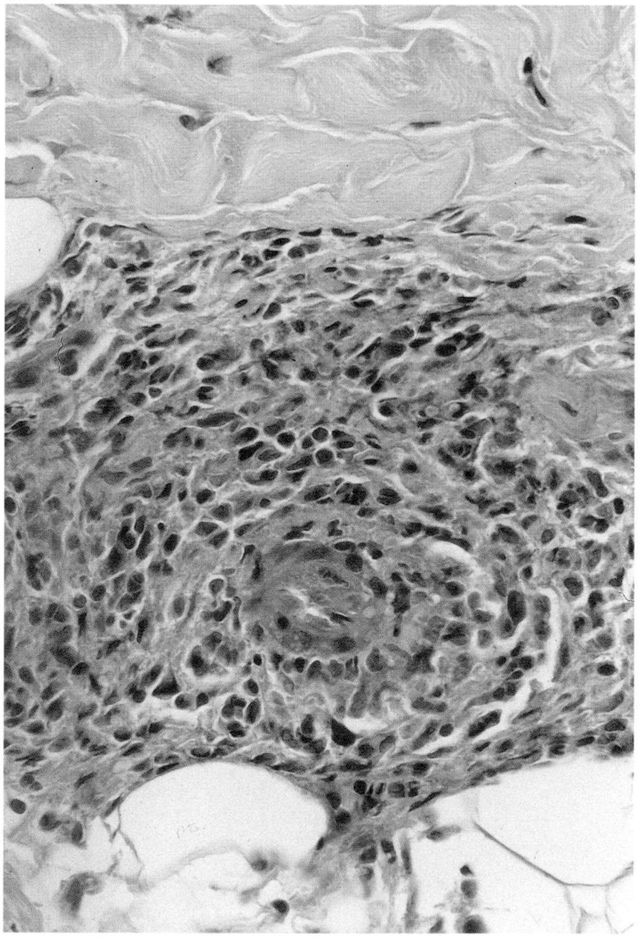

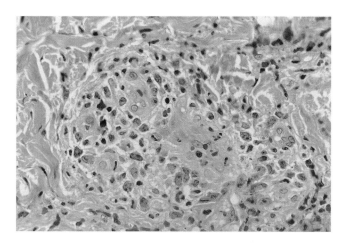

Fig. 20–1. A dense perivascular lymphocytic infiltrate characterizes the histologic changes seen in Rocky Mountain spotted fever.

Fig. 20–2. Vascular destruction, with fibrin thrombi and leukocytoclasis, is seen in many cases of Rocky Mountain spotted fever.

Cutaneous Features. Cutaneous eruptions occur in 10%–30% of patients infected with ehrlichiosis [15, 16]. When present, the cutaneous eruption appears from 5 to 21 days after the onset of illness. Many different clinical appearances have been described [17]. The exanthem is often macular and papular and occasionally petechial or vesicular [18]. The trunk and upper extremities are most frequently affected. A scarlatiniform eruption has been reported in children [19]. Palms and soles are affected in rare patients.

Associated Disorders. Patients with ehrlichiosis infection present with acute, unexplained fevers in 97% of cases, chills, and headaches in 81% of patients [15]. Laboratory examination reveals cytopenias and elevated serum enzyme values [17]. Severe thrombocytopenia has been reported [15]. Neurologic symptoms including severe headaches, meningismus, and altered mental status are seen in many infected patients. Less commonly, unilateral weakness and Bell's palsy have been described [20]. Myalgias and arthralgias are seen in about half of infected patients [15]. Co-infection with RMSF has been reported [13].

Histologic Features. The histologic findings of the cutaneous eruptions are not well described. A dense lymphohistiocytic perivascular infiltrate has been found in the dermis in the few biopsy specimens reported [15].

Special Studies. Polymerase chain reaction on blood samples is helpful in identifying the organism and establishing the correct diagnosis. In one study, 87% of patients with suspected disease were found to have *Ehrlichia* sequences in the blood [17]. Immunoperoxidase technology has been reported to detect these organisms, but only with great difficulty [15]. Immunofluorescent analysis is also helpful in making a diagnosis [21].

Pathogenesis. *Ehrlichia chaffeensis* is the organism responsible for ehrlichiosis [17]. It is a 1 μm length obligate intracellular coccobacillary bacterium [16]. Evidence is accruing that there may be more than one subtype of ehrlichial infection, with some patients experiencing monocytic involvement and others granulocytic [16, 22]. It remains unclear whether one or more closely related organisms are responsible for the different disease presentations. The monocytic disease is associated with prolonged exposure to the Lone Star tick *Amblyomma americanum* and to the granulocytic disease with the deer tick *Ixodes scapularis* [15].

Rickettsialpox

Epidemiology. Rickettsialpox is caused by *Rickettsia akari*, which is transmitted to humans from rodents by mites. It is an uncommonly encountered disease that

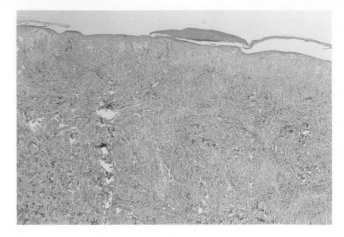

Fig. 20–3. A dense dermal inflammatory infiltrate is seen underlying a spongiotic epidermis in early lesions of rickettsialpox infection.

has been reported in urban areas throughout the United States and Russia. It is a self-limited disease.

Cutaneous Features. Rickettsialpox presents with an eschar that occurs at the initial site of the mite bite [23, 24]. After the eschar forms (clinically recognized as a "tache noir"), affected patients develop 5–40 macules, papules, and vesicles that can occur in any body location. The cutaneous presentation greatly resembles that of chickenpox [25]. The papules and vesicles resolve with occasional scarring.

Associated Disorders. Patients infected with rickettsialpox develop fevers, myalgias, headaches, and malaise 1 to 2 weeks after the initial bite. Lymphadenitis is frequently seen.

Histologic Features. The initial eschar seen in rickettsialpox demonstrates nonspecific histologic changes,

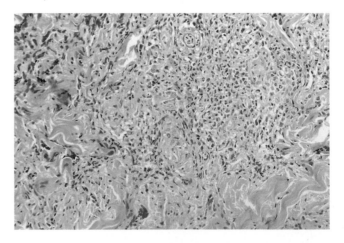

Fig. 20–4. A dense lymphocytic infiltrate is present around and within vessels in rickettsialpox, often leading to vascular thrombosis.

including extensive necrosis and a dense, mixed inflammatory infiltrate. The papules and vesicles that characterize rickettsialpox demonstrate intraepidermal spongiosis and marked papillary dermal edema that eventuates in subepidermal blisters in some cases [25]. A vacuolar interface dermatitis is present in most cases. A perivascular lymphocytic infiltrate is also present and may result in endothelial cell swelling, vascular wall destruction, and fibrin thrombi [23] (Figs. 20–3 and 20–4).

Special Studies. Direct immunofluorescence testing for the presence of *Rickettsia akari* on formalin-fixed, paraffin- embedded tissue sections has been described [25].

Pathogenesis. Rickettsialpox is caused by *Rickettsia akari*. It is transmitted from the rodent population to human beings via mites [25].

References

1. Dalton, M. J., Clarke, M. J., Holman, R. C., Krebs, J. W., Fishbein, D. B., Olson, J. G., and Childs, J. E., *National surveillance for Rocky Mountain spotted fever, 1981–1992: Epidemiologic summary and evaluation of risk factors for fatal outcome.* Am J Trop Med Hyg, 1995. 52:405–413.

2. Kao, G. F., Evancho, C. D., Ioffe, O., Lowitt, M. H., and Dumler, J. S., *Cutaneous histopathology of Rocky Mountain spotted fever.* J Cutan Pathol, 1997. 24:604–610.

3. Sexton, D. J., and Corey, G. R., *Rocky Mountain "spotless" and "almost spotless" fever: A wolf in sheep's clothing.* Clin Ifect Dis, 1992. 15:439–448.

4. Hughes, C., *Rocky Mountain "spotless" fever with an erythema migrans-like skin lesion.* Clin Infect Dis, 1995. 21:1328–1329.

5. Griffith, G. L., and Luce, E. A., *Massive skin necrosis in Rocky Mountain spotted fever.* South Med J, 1978. 71:1337–1340.

6. Kirkland, K. B., Marcom, P. K., Sexton, D. J., Dumler, J. S., and Walker, D. H., *Rocky Mountain spotted fever complicated by gangrene: Report of six cases and review.* Clin Infect Dis, 1993. 16:629–634.

7. Schimeca, P. G., Weinblatt, M. E., and Kochen, J. A., *Acquired coagulation inhibitor in association with Rocky Mountain spotted fever. With a review of other acquired coagulation inhibitors.* Clin Pediatr (Phila), 1987. 26: 459–463.

8. Bradford, W. D., Croker, B. P., and Tisher, C. C., *Kidney lesions in Rocky Mountain spotted fever: A light, immunofluorescence-, and electron-microscopic study.* Am J Pathol, 1979. 97:381–392.

9. Conlon, P. J., Procop, G. W., Fowler, V., Eloubeidi, M. A., Smith, S. R., and Sexton, D. J., *Predictors of prognosis and risk of acute renal failure in patients with Rocky Mountain spotted fever.* Am J Med, 1996. 101: 621–626.

10. Procop, G. W., Burchette, J. L. Jr., Howell, D. N., and Sexton, D. J., *Immunoperoxidase and immunofluorescent staining of Rickettsia rickettsii in skin biopsies. A comparative study.* Arch Pathol Lab Med, 1997. 121: 894–899.

11. White, W. L., Patrick, J. D., and Miller, L. R., *Evaluation of immunoperoxidase techniques to detect Rickettsia rickettsii in fixed tissue sections.* Am J Clin Pathol, 1994. 101:747–752.

12. Dimmitt, S. K., and Miller, D. K., *Rocky Mountain spotted fever. Ultrastructural findings.* Am J Clin Pathol, 1982. 78:131–134.

13. Sexton, D. J., Corey, G. R., Carpenter, C., Kong, L. Q., Gandhi, T., Breitschwerdt, E., Hegarty, B., Chen, S. M., et al., *Dual infection with Ehrlichia chaffeensis and a spotted fever group rickettsia: A case report.* Emerg Infect Dis, 1998. 4:311–316.

14. Goldman, D. P., Artenstein, A. W., and Bolan, C. D., *Human ehrliciosis: A newly recognized tick-borne disease.* Am Fam Physician, 1992. 46:199–208.

15. Marty, A. M., Dumler, J. S., Imes, G., Brusman, H. P., Smrkovski, L. L., and Frisma, D. M., *Ehrlichiosis mimicking thrombotic thrombocytopenic purpura. Case report and pathological correlation.* Hum Pathol, 1995. 26:920–925.

16. Mounzer, K. C., and Dinubile, M. J., *Ehrlichial infections.* Clin Dermatol, 1996. 14:289–293.

17. Everett, E. D., Evans, K. A., Henry, R. B., and McDonald, G., *Human ehrlichiosis in adults after tick exposure. Diagnosis using polymerase chain reaction.* Ann Intern Med, 1994. 120:730–735.

18. Rohrbach, B. W., Harkess, J. R., Ewing, S. A., Kudlac, J., McKee, G. L., and Istre, G. R., *Epidemiologic and clinical characteristics of persons with serologic evidence of E. canis infection.* Am J Public Health, 1990. 80:442–445.

19 Heymann, W. R., *Human ehrlichiosis: A rash in need of dermatologic evaluation.* Int J Dermatol, 1995. 34:618–619.

20. Grant, A. C., Hunter, S., and Partin, W. C., *A case of acute monocytic ehrlichiosis with prominent neurologic signs.* Neurology, 1997. 48:1619–1623.

21. Dawson, J. E., Fishbein, D. J., Eng, T. R., Redus, M. A., and Greene, N. R., *Diagnosis of human ehrlichiosis with the indirect fluorescent antibody test: Kinetics and specificity.* J Infect Dis, 1990. 162:91–95.

22. Walker, D. H., and Dmuler, J. S., *Human monocytic and granulocytic ehrlichiosis. Discovery and diagnosis of emerging tick-borne infections and the critical role of the pathologist.* Arch Pathol Lab Med, 1997. 121:785–791.

23. Brettman, L. R., Lewin, S., Holzman, R. S., Goldman, W. D., Marr, J. S., Kechijian, P., and Schinella, R., *Rickettsialpox: Report of an outbreak and a contemporary review.* Medicine, 1981. 60:363–372.

24. Wong, B., Singer, C., Armstrong, D., and Millian, S. J., *Rickettsialpox. Case report and epidemiologic review.* JAMA, 1979. 242:1998–1999.

25. Kass, E. M., Szaniawski, W. K., Levy, H., Leach, J., Srinivasan, K., and Rives, C., *Rickettsialpox in a New York City hospital, 1980 to 1989.* N Engl J Med, 1994. 331:1612–1617.

CHAPTER 21

Parasitic Infestations

Leishmaniasis

Epidemiology. Leishmaniasis is a protozoan that is transmitted to humans from rodents and dogs by the phlebotomus sandfly. There are three clinical forms of leishmaniasis: localized cutaneous leishmaniasis, visceral leishmaniasis, and mucocutaneous leishmaniasis [1]. These forms have different predilections for different geographic regions. Diffuse cutaneous leishmaniasis, leishmaniasis recidivans, and post–kala-azar dermal leishmaniasis are regarded as less common variants [2, 3].

Primary infection within the United States is extremely rare. Americans with a history of foreign travel are most at risk. About half of patients reported travel to Mexico or Central America [4].

Cutaneous Features. Localized cutaneous leishmaniasis in the western hemisphere is usually characterized by a single primary lesion, whereas multiple primary lesions are more commonly seen in the eastern hemisphere. One to 3 weeks after bite by an infected sandfly, a red papule or nodule appears at the affected site. It may progress to an ulcer that is surrounded by a violaceous border [2]. Lymphangitic spread is frequently seen. Satellite papules may appear around the primary papule. These primary lesions are relatively asymptomatic. The primary papule or nodule heals within 6–12 months, leaving a scar [5].

An id, or hypersensitivity, reaction may appear as generalized erythematous papules. Koebnerization has been reported.

Mucocutaneous changes of leishmaniasis present from years to decades after initial cutaneous manifestations. Mucocutaneous involvement is probably re-lated to hematogenous or lymphatic spread. The nasal septum is often involved and may perforate. Eye and genital involvement may occur [5].

Kala-azar, or visceral leishmaniasis, is caused by infection of the reticuloendothelial system by *Leishmania donovani*. At the time of active involvement, the skin may become markedly hyperpigmented due to increased melanocyte activity and xerosis. Brittle hair may lead to complete alopecia [2, 5]. Primary cutaneous lesions of leishmaniasis are rarely seen in patients with kala-azar, but have been described in human immunodeficiency virus (HIV)–infected patients. In these patients, symmetric papules on acral zones characterized the cutaneous manifestations [6].

Disseminated cutaneous leishmaniasis is characterized by the appearance of a single papule or nodule at the site of infection, followed rapidly by generalized papules and nodules. Leishmaniasis recidivans is characterized by the recurrence of plaques of leishmaniasis at the sites of scars from previous sites of infection. These lesions may appear psoriasiform. Dormant periods of up to 15 years have been reported [5].

Post–kala-azar leishmaniasis appears 1–3 years after recovery from visceral leishmaniasis. The cutaneous manifestations are those of hypopigmented macules that coalesce into patches. These patches are symmetric and are usually on the chest, neck, and back. These patches often progress into yellow-pink nodules. Nodules are seen most commonly on the face, earlobes, and trunk [5].

Associated Disorders. Kala-azar, or visceral leishmaniasis, is associated with fever, splenomegaly, emaciation, hyperglobulinemia, and pancytopenia [5].

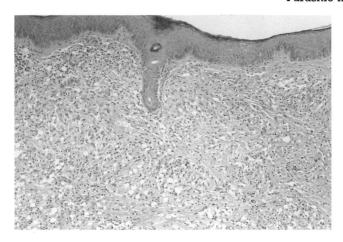

Fig. 21–1. Leishmaniasis is characterized by a diffuse, dense dermal inflammatory infiltrate with abundant histiocytes.

Histologic Features. Histologic features of localized cutaneous leishmaniasis include epidermal hyperplasia and ulceration. A dense dermal inflammatory infiltrate composed of neutrophils, lymphocytes, histiocytes, and plasma cells is present throughout the dermis (Fig. 21–1). Parasites are easy to see within the histiocytes and extracellularly early in the course of the disease in routine sections [1] (Fig. 21–2). The organisms are from 2 to 4 μm in diameter and are round to oval. A small rod-shaped kinetoplast can be seen in some cases. Later in the course of the disease, fibrosis is more apparent, neutrophils are less common, multinucleated giant cells more abundant, and organisms may be more difficult to find. Small granulomas may be present.

Diffuse cutaneous leishmaniasis has a distinctive histologic pattern characterized by an atrophic dermis overlying a dermis that is completely filled with foamy

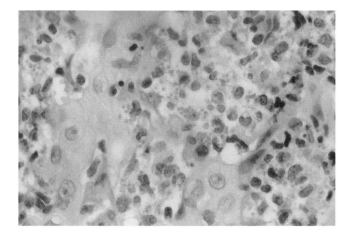

Fig. 21–2. Abundant intracellular organisms are present within the cytoplasm of histiocytes in early lesions of leishmaniasis.

histiocytes containing parasites [1]. The following entities must be considered in the histologic differential diagnosis of leishmaniasis:

- Granuloma inguinale
- Histoplasmosis
- Rhinoscleroma

Special Studies. Giemsa's stain is sometimes helpful in highlighting the organisms, which can be seen with routine hematoxylin and eosin–stained sections. Touch preparations performed on ulcerated plaques have also been reported to be helpful in identifying organisms and making the diagnosis [7]. Antibodies directed against *Leishmania* have been used with limited success. Although the sensitivity and specificity of these antibodies are slightly higher than those of routine stains, these antibodies are not yet ideal diagnostic tools [8].

Serologic tests for leishmaniasis range from 75% to 100% sensitive, depending upon the type of leishmaniasis; however, extensive cross-reactivity with other microorganisms limits the specificity and hence the utility of these tests [9].

Pathogenesis. Human beings are an accidental host for *leishmania*. The phlebotomus sandfly transmits the parasite from dogs or rodents to humans. Each of the different types of leishmaniasis is caused by a different organism. *Leishmania braziliensis braziliensis* and *Leishmania mexica* cause the mucocutaneous variant. *Leishmania donovani* is the most frequent cause of visceral leishmaniasis. *Leishmania tropica* and *Leishmania major* are frequently associated with cutaneous disease. It has been proposed that Langerhans' cells take up the parasites on the skin surface, transport them to draining lymph nodes, and initiate the specific host response to the organisms [10].

Acanthamebiasis

Epidemiology. *Acanthamoeba,* *Leptomyxida,* and *Naegleria* species are free-living amoebas normally found in water, soil, and dust [11, 12]. *Acanthamoeba* species only rarely invade the skin. It is almost always found in association with immunologically compromised hosts and is seen most commonly in HIV-infected patients.

Cutaneous Features. Primary cutaneous infection with *Acanthamoeba* has been reported in patients with acquired immunodeficiency syndrome (AIDS) [13]. Tender papules and subcutaneous nodules are present at the sites of infection [14]. Patients may have one to many erythematous nodules. Pustules and ulcers [11], as well as purpuric macules [15], have been reported.

Disseminated granulomatous infection of the skin has also been reported and may be fatal [16].

Associated Disorders. *Acanthamoeba* species are known to cause central nervous system disease, including granulomatous amebic encephalitis [17] and meningoencephalitis [18]. Involvement of the eyes with keratitis and conjunctivitis [12] and of the lungs are also reported [18]. Osteomyelitis secondary to acanthamebiasis has been reported in a child with AIDS [19].

Histologic Features. Acanthamebiasis of the skin leads to a dense, mixed inflammatory response. A necrotizing granulomatous process is often present [20]. Trophozoites are found near blood vessels within the areas of inflammation [21] (Fig. 21–3). Other cases may demonstrate pustules within the epidermis or leukocytoclastic vasculitis [11, 15]. The trophozoites are 20–30 μm in diameter. A clear halo and abundant spongy cytoplasm (Fig. 21–4) surround a central endosome. Cysts are smaller and have thick, double-contoured walls and dense, eosinophilic cytoplasm.

Special Studies. Periodic acid–Schiff stain and Gomori's methenamine silver stain will highlight the amebic cyst walls and aid in making the tissue diagnosis [22]. Precise identification of species requires molecular methods, including restriction endonuclease digestion of DNA and isoenzyme analyses [12]. Monoclonal antibodies against specific strains have been developed and show some diagnostic promise.

Pathogenesis. *Acanthamoeba castellanii* and *Acanthamoeba culbertsoni* are two of the more frequently implicated species in causing human disease. *Naegleria* species are also known to cause human disease. In most

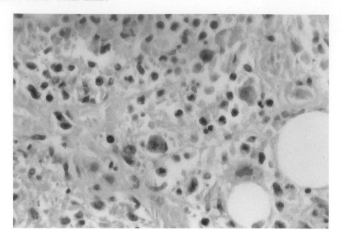

Fig. 21–4. Scattered acanthamoebaes are present in surrounding tissues, admixed with inflammatory cells.

cases, involvement of the skin is secondary to primary infection located in the lungs or sinuses [16].

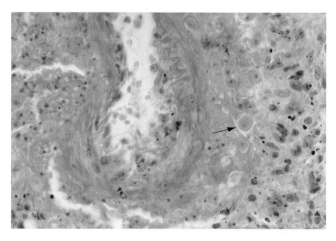

Fig. 21–3. Acanthamoebaes are present within and around the vessel walls, giving rise to a necrotizing vasculitis.

References

1. Sangueza, O. P., Sangueza, J. M., Stiller, M. J., and Sangueza, P., *Mucocutaneous leishmaniasis: A clinicopathologic classification.* J Am Acad Dermatol, 1993. 28:927–932.
2. Grevelink, S. A., and Lerner, E. A., *Leishmaniasis.* J Am Acad Dermatol, 1996. 34:257–272.
3. Watson, B. C., *Leishmaniasis. A worldwide problem.* Int J Dermatol, 1989. 28:305–307.
4. Herwaldt, B. L., Stokes, S. L., and Juranek, D. D., *American cutaneous leishmaniasis in U.S. travelers.* Ann Intern Med, 1993. 15:779–784.
5. Lerner, E. A., and Grevelink, S. A., *Leishmaniasis.* In *Cutaneous Medicine and Surgery,* K. A. Arndt et al., Eds. 1996, W. B. Saunders Company, Philadelphia, pp. 1163–1171.
6. Postigo, C., Llamas, R., Zarco, C., Rubio, R., Pulido, F., Costa, J. R., and Iglesias, L., *Cutaneous lesions in patients with visceral leishmaniasis and HIV infection.* J Infect, 1997. 35:265–268.
7. Berger, R. S., Perez-Figaredo, R. A., and Spielvogel, R. L., *Leishmaniasis: The touch preparation as a rapid means of diagnosis.* J Am Acad Dermatol, 1987. 16:1096–1105.
8. Kenner, J. R., Aronson, N. E., Bratthauer, G. L., Turnicky, R. P., Jackson, J. E., Tang, D. B., and Sau, P., *Immunohistochemistry to identify Leishmania parasites in fixed tissues.* J Cutan Pathol, 1999. 26:130–136.
9. Kar, K., *Serodiagnosis of leishmaniasis.* Crit Rev Microbiol, 1995. 21:123–152.
10. Moll, H., *Epidermal Langerhans cells are critical for immunoregulation of cutaneous leishmaniasis.* Immunol Today, 1993. 14:383–387.
11. Murakawa, G. J., McCalmont, T., Altman, J., Telang,

G. H., Hoffman, M. D., Kantor, G. R., and Berger, T. G., *Disseminated acanthamebiasis in patients with AIDS. A report of five cases and a review of the literature.* Arch Dermatol, 1995. 131:1291–1296.

12. Szenasi, Z., Endo, T., Yagita, K., and Nagy, E., *Isolation, identification and increasing importance of "free-living" amoebae causing human disease.* J Mcd Microbiol, 1998. 47:5–16.

13. Migueles, S., and Kumar, P., *Primary cutaneous acanthamoeba infection in a patient with AIDS.* Clin Infect Dis, 1998. 27:1547–1548.

14. Chandrasekar, P. H., Nandi, P. S., Fairfax, M. R., and Crane, L. R., *Cutaneous infections due to Acanthamoeba in patients with acquired immunodeficiency syndrome.* Arch Intern Med, 1997. 157:569–572.

15. Helton, J., Loveless, M., and White, C. R. Jr., *Cutaneous acanthamoeba infection associated wtih leukocytoclastic vasculitis in an AIDS patient.* Am J Dermatopathol, 1993. 15:146–149.

16. Gullett, J., Mills, J., Hadley, K., Podemskin, B., Pitts, L., and Gelber, R., *Disseminated granulomatous acanthamoeba infection presenting as an unusual skin lesion.* Am J Med, 1979. 67:891–896.

17. Martinez, A. J., *Infection of the central nervous system due to Acanthamoeba.* Rev Infect Dis, 1991. 13(Suppl 5):S399–402.

18. Martinez, A. J., Sotelo-Avila, C., Garcia-Tamayo, J., Moron, J. T., Willaert, E., and Stamm, W. P., *Meningoencephalitis due to Acanthamoeba SP. Pathogenesis and clinico-pathological study.* Acta Neuropathol (Berl), 1977. 37:183–191.

19. Selby, D. M., Chandra, R. S., Rakusan, T. A., Loechelt, B., Markle, B. M., and Visvesvara, G. S., *Amebic osteomyelitis in a child with acquired immunodeficiency syndrome: A case report.* Pediatr Pathol Lab Med, 1998. 18:89–95.

20. Hunt, S. J., Reed, S L., Mathews, W. C., and Torian, B., *Cutaneous Acanthamoeba infection in the acquired immunodeficiency syndrome: Response to multidrug therapy.* Cutis, 1995. 56:285–287.

21. Im, K., and Kim, D. S., *Acanthamoebiasis in Korea: Two new cases with clinical cases review.* Yonsei Med J, 1998. 39:478–484.

22. Tan, B., Weldon-Linne, C. M., Rhone, D. P., Penning, C. L., and Visvesvara, G. S., *Acanthamoeba infection presenting as skin lesions in patients with the acquired immunodeficiency syndrome.* Arch Pathol Lab Med, 1993. 117:1043–1046.

PART V

Drug-Induced Processes

CHAPTER
22

Drug-Induced Autoimmune Eruptions

Pemphigus

Epidemiology. Drug-induced pemphigus is a heterogeneous group of acantholytic blistering processes [1]. Pemphigus vulgaris and pemphigus foliaceus both have been induced by a variety of medications. It has been shown that half of patients with drug-induced pemphigus spontaneously recover after cessation of therapy [2]. In contrast, resolution occurs in only 15% of patients with a previous diagnosis of pemphigus in whom the administration of a drug triggers an exacerbation of disease [2].

Cutaneous Features. The clinical features of drug-induced pemphigus are indistinguishable from those of spontaneously occurring pemphigus. In pemphigus vulgaris-like disease, flaccid bullae develop surrounded by erythematous patches, usually within weeks of receiving the offending medication. These blisters spread easily and erode, with secondary infection and crust formation. A positive Nikolsky's sign is present [3]. The oral mucosa is frequently but not always involved.

Pemphigus foliaceus-like eruptions demonstrate more superficially located blisters, which appear more as erythematous scaling and mild erosion. Intact blisters are occasionally observed. This process is most prominent on the trunk and less commonly affects mucosal surfaces.

Associated Disorders. The following drugs are reported to cause a pemphigus-like drug eruption:

- Ampicillin
- Captopril
- Cephalosporin family
- Enalapril
- Penicillamine
- Penicillin
- Rifampin
- Thiopronine

Thiol-containing drugs are the largest category of therapeutic agents responsible for inducing pemphigus, accounting for more than 80% of reported cases [4]. This category includes drugs such as penicillamine, captopril, enalapril, and thiopronine [5]. Penicillamine is the drug most frequently implicated in precipitating pemphigus vulgaris. Captopril is also commonly implicated in inducing pemphigus [6]. Less commonly, cephalosporins and penicillin and its derivatives have been implicated [7]. Amide-containing drugs have also been implicated rarely in the induction of pemphigus [8].

Histologic Features. Histologic features of drug-induced pemphigus are indistinguishable from those seen in spontaneously occurring pemphigus [9]. Two separate categories of drug-induced pemphigus are seen. Some cases resemble pemphigus vulgaris histologically, and others appear identical to pemphigus foliaceus. In both groups, the primary histologic change is that of acantholysis.

In pemphigus foliaceus-like lesions, the site of acantholysis is within the granular layer of the stratum spin-

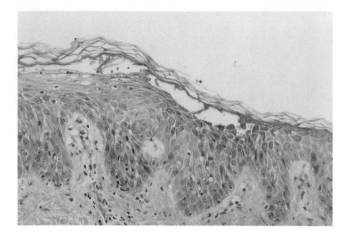

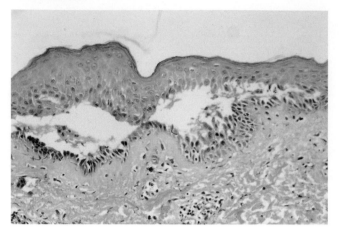

Fig. 22–1. Drug-induced pemphigus foliaceus demonstrates an acantholytic blister within the upper layers of the epidermis.

Fig. 22–2. Drug-induced pemphigus vulgaris shows a suprabasilar acantholytic blister.

osum. In these cases, the stratum corneum is frequently separated from the underlying epidermis, and individual acantholytic cells are present within the granular layer (Fig. 22–1). The remainder of the epidermis is often slightly spongiotic, and a mild infiltrate of eosinophils and lymphocytes may be present within the epidermis and in the underlying papillary dermis [3]. The following entities must be considered in the histologic differential diagnosis of a pemphigus foliaceus-like drug eruption:

- Friction blister
- Grover's disease
- Impetigo
- Pemphigus erythematosus
- Pemphigus foliaceus
- Staphylococcal scalded skin syndrome

In pemphigus vulgaris-like cases of drug-induced pemphigus, the acantholytic blister occurs in a suprabasilar distribution (Fig. 22–2). A row of basal keratinocytes remains attached to the underlying dermis, often separated from each other laterally, giving rise to a "tombstone" appearance (Fig. 22–3). Minimal acantholysis is present within the upper portions of the epidermis. A mildly spongiotic epidermis with an infiltrate of eosinophils and lymphocytes may be present, similar to pemphigus foliaceus-like cases. Acantholytic cells are sometimes present floating free within the blister cavity. The following entities must be considered in the histologic differential diagnosis of a pemphigus vulgaris-like drug eruption:

- Darier's disease
- Grover's disease
- Hailey-Hailey disease

- Herpes infection
- Pemphigus vulgaris
- Squamous cell carcinoma, acantholytic type
- Warty dyskeratoma

Special Studies. Immunofluorescence studies are helpful in some cases of drug-induced pemphigus. In some but not all cases of both pemphigus foliaceus and pemphigus vulgaris induced by drugs, circulating levels of autoantibodies are present in the sera of affected patients. These antibodies are directed against the same pemphigus foliaceus and pemphigus vulgaris antigen complexes, desmoglein 1 and desmoglein 3, respectively, as autoantibodies in the spontaneously occurring diseases [10]. Indirect immunofluorescence studies can detect the presence of these autoantibodies. Titers of circulating autoantibodies are often lower than those seen in spontaneously occurring pemphigus and do not

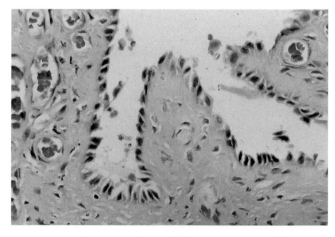

Fig. 22–3. "Tombstoning" of the basal keratinocytes is present in drug-induced pemphigus vulgaris.

correlate well with levels of disease activity. Direct immunofluorescence performed on perilesional skin will show an intercellular staining pattern with antihuman IgG [11].

Pathogenesis. It has been suggested that the sulfhydryl group present in penicillamine and several other groups of drugs in some way alters the intercellular substance between keratinocytes. This leads to the formation of an antigenic structure that elicits an autoimmune response [7]. It has been suggested that these thiol-containing drugs bind to the cellular membranes of keratinocytes, causing the formation of drug–cysteine instead of cysteine–cysteine bondings, initiating the process of acantholysis [12]. Others have suggested that plasminogen activator inhibitor levels stimulated by thiol-containing drugs lead to increased plasminogen activator in keratinocytes that results in the acantholysis seen in this entity [5]. Other authors have suggested that the drugs can induce a direct acantholytic effect on keratinocytes [13].

Pemphigoid

Epidemiology. Both bullous pemphigoid and cicatricial pemphigoid have been associated with drug ingestion. These drug-induced blistering processes are most frequently associated with neuroleptics (15.5% of patients) and diuretics (36.2% of cases) [14].

Cutaneous Features. Clinical features of drug-induced bullous pemphigoid are identical to those of the spontaneously occurring disease. Large, tense blisters arise on the trunk and extremities. There is often an erythematous base surrounding the blister. The blisters are not particularly fragile, and Nikolsky's sign is not present. In some cases, a more target-like appearance resembling erythema multiforme has been reported in patients with penicillin-induced bullous pemphigoid [15].

Cicatricial pemphigoid is also reported after administration of drugs and also is clinically indistinguishable from the sporadically occurring disease. Mucous membranes develop blisters that heal with scarring. Conjunctival involvement is prominent in many cases.

Associated Disorders. The following drugs have been implicated in causing bullous pemphigoid:

- Aldosterone antagonists
- Amiodarone
- Ampicillin
- Analgesics
- Benzodiazepines
- Benzothiadiazides
- Calcium channel blockers
- Cholesterol-lowering agents
- Enalapril
- Furosemide
- Neuroleptics
- Nonsteroidal antiinflammatory agents
- Penicillin
- Sulfhydryl-containing compounds
- Timolol

Furosemide is the drug that is most commonly implicated in inducing bullous pemphigoid [16, 17]. Photochemotherapy for treatment of psoriasis has also been reported to induce generalized bullous pemphigoid in a series of patients [18]. Penicillin [15] and its derivatives [19] are implicated in rare cases.

Use of clonidine has been associated with cicatricial pemphigoid [20], as has the use of topical glaucoma medication [21]. Timolol has also been associated with the development of ocular cicatricial pemphigoid [22].

Histologic Features. The histologic features of drug-induced bullous pemphigoid are identical to those of idiopathic bullous pemphigoid. A subepidermal blister is present in the absence of keratinocyte necrosis (Fig. 22–4). Mild to moderate amounts of epidermal spongiosis may be present, and a cellular inflammatory infiltrate, consisting of eosinophils and neutrophils, is present within the epidermis. The blister cavity is often filled with similar inflammatory cells (Fig. 22–5). Within the dermis, there is a superficial perivascular and diffuse inflammatory infiltrate consisting of lymphocytes and eosinophils. Eosinophils sometimes can be seen lined up adjacent to the dermal–epidermal junction (Fig. 22–6). The inflammatory infiltrate does not ordinarily extend into the deeper portions of the dermis. The following entities must be considered in the

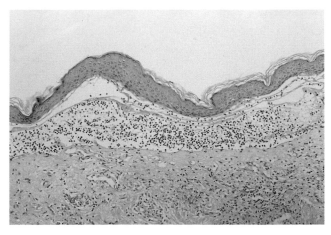

Fig. 22–4. An inflammatory subepidermal blister characterizes drug-induced bullous pemphigoid.

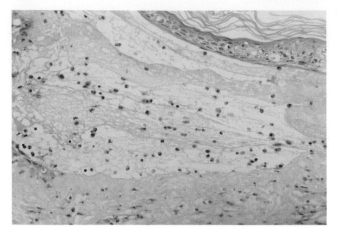

Fig. 22–5. Higher magnification demonstrates eosinophils within the blister cavity in drug-induced bullous pemphigoid.

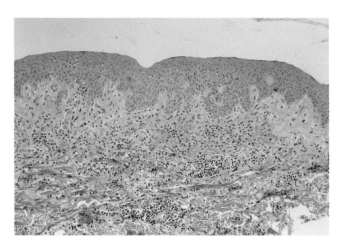

Fig. 22–6. Abundant eosinophils are often seen along the dermal–epidermal junction in areas away from the blister in drug-induced bullous pemphigoid.

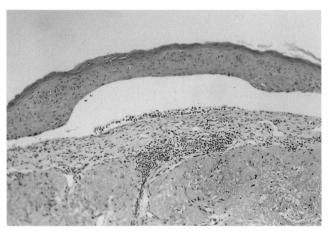

Fig. 22–7. Drug-induced cicatricial pemphigoid demonstrates an inflammatory subepidermal blister.

histologic differential diagnosis of drug-induced bullous pemphigoid and cicatricial pemphigoid:

- Bullous lupus erythematosus
- Bullous pemphigoid
- Cicatricial pemphigoid
- Epidermolysis bullosa acquisita
- Linear IgA bullous dermatosis
- Pemphigoides (herpes) gestationis
- Porphyria cutanea tarda
- Pseudoporphyria cutanea tarda

In patients with drug-induced cicatricial pemphigoid, the histologic changes again mimic the idiopathic form of the disease. A subepidermal blister is present, with a mixed inflammatory infiltrate present in the epidermis and dermis (Fig. 22–7). Often, neutrophils constitute the predominant cell type, although lymphocytes and eosinophils are present in varying amounts (Fig. 22–8). Increased dermal fibrosis secondary to scarring is present in older, well-developed lesions.

Special Studies. Direct immunofluorescence reveals linear deposition of IgG and C3 along the dermal–epidermal junction in cases of drug-induced pemphigoid. This is the same staining pattern that is seen in most cases of idiopathic bullous pemphigoid and cicatricial pemphigoid. Further investigation of one pa-

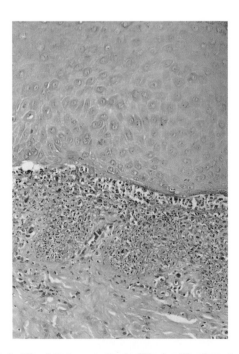

Fig. 22–8. The blister cavity is filled with abundant neutrophils admixed with other inflammatory cells in drug-induced cicatricial pemphigoid.

tient with drug-induced bullous pemphigoid showed that the antibodies are directed against a 230 kD protein located on the roof of the blister. This is identical to the pattern seen with spontaneously occurring bullous pemphigoid [23].

Linear IgA Bullous Dermatosis

Epidemiology. Linear IgA bullous dermatosis is a rare complication that can develop from the ingestion of a wide array of drugs and rarely with other systemic disorders.

Cutaneous Features. The cutaneous features of drug-induced linear IgA bullous dermatosis range from hemorrhagic blisters to asymptomatic red papules and plaques. In the classic case, a collarette of vesicles is present surrounding an erythematous patch. The blisters heal without scarring [24]. Mucosal involvement is not a feature of this condition. The cutaneous changes in linear IgA bullous dermatosis associated with drug ingestion are more varied in appearance than those seen in idiopathic linear IgA bullous dermatosis. Lesions of linear IgA may initially appear up to two weeks after the causative drug has been removed. In some cases, the cutaneous blisters can have a targetoid appearance and mimic erythema multiforme [25].

Associated Disorders. Many types of drugs have been associated with linear IgA bullous dermatosis, including the following:

- Captopril
- Cefamandole
- Diclofenac
- Interferon-γ
- Glibenclamide
- Interleukin-2
- Lithium carbonate
- Nonsteroidal antiinflammatory agents
- Piroxicam
- Sulfadimethoxynum
- Sodium hypochlorite
- Vancomycin

Antibiotics are most frequently associated, with vancomycin the most commonly reported drug in this category [24, 26]. Sulfa antibiotics have also been implicated [25]. Nonsteroidal antiinflammatory agents such as piroxicam also have been frequently associated [27], as has captopril [28]. Interleukin-2 therapy has also precipitated a case of linear IgA bullous dermatitis [29]. Irritant contact dermatitis after exposure to sodium hypochlorite has also been implicated in precipitating linear IgA bullous dermatosis [30].

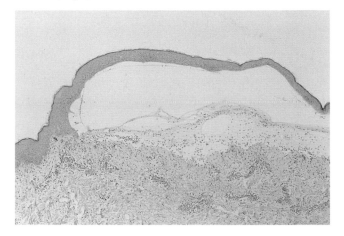

Fig. 22–9. Drug-induced linear IgA bullous dermatosis is characterized by an inflammatory subepidermal blister.

Linear IgA bullous dermatosis is also associated with a higher than expected rate of lymphoproliferative malignancies [31] and has also been reported as a complication of pregnancy [32] and in association with multiple sclerosis [33] and rheumatoid arthritis [34].

Histologic Features. Histologic changes in most cases include an inflammatory subepidermal blister, indistinguishable from the histologic appearance of spontaneously occurring linear IgA bullous dermatosis and bullous dermatosis of childhood. The blister cavity is filled with inflammatory cells, with neutrophils predominating in most cases and many eosinophils in some cases [24] (Figs. 22–9 and 22–10). Eosinophils are not ordinarily the predominant inflammatory cell type in the idiopathic form of the disease. Keratinocytes in the roof of early blisters are not necrotic. The inflammatory infiltrate is confined to the superficial portions of the dermis.

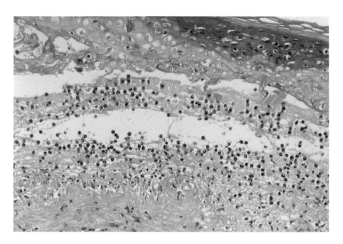

Fig. 22–10. The blister cavity is filled with abundant neutrophils in most cases of drug-induced linear IgA bullous dermatosis.

Special Studies. Direct immunofluorescence studies of skin from patients with drug-induced linear IgA bullous dermatosis demonstrated linear deposits of IgA at the basement membrane zone. C3 is less frequently found in this distribution. Indirect immunofluorescence is less commonly positive, and most patients lack circulating antibodies [35]. Immunoelectron microscopy has demonstrated immune complexes deposited within the lamina densa in patients with drug-induced linear IgA bullous dermatosis [24].

Pathogenesis. The method by which ingested drugs induce IgA-mediated subepidermal blisters has not been elucidated.

References

1. Mutasim, D. F., Pelc, N. J., and Anhalt, G. J., *Drug-induced pemphigus.* Dermatol Clin, 1993. 11:463–471.
2. Wolf, R., Tamir, A., and Brenner, S., *Drug-induced versus drug-triggered pemphigus.* Dermatologica, 1991. 182:207–210.
3. Fitzpatrick, J. E., *New histopathologic findings in drug eruptions.* Dermatol Clin, 1992. 10:19–36.
4. Ruocco, V., and Sacerdoti, G., *Pemphigus and bullous pemphigoid due to drugs.* Int J Dermatol, 1991. 30:307–312.
5. Lombardi, M. L., de Angelis, E., Rossano, F., and Ruocco, V., *Imbalance between plasminogen activator and its inhibitors in thiol-induced acantholysis.* Dermatology, 1993. 186:118–122.
6. Kaplan, R. P., Potter, T. S., and Fox, J. N., *Drug-induced pemphigus related to angiotensin-converting enzyme inhibitors.* J Am Acad Dermatol, 1992. 26:364–366.
7. Wilson, J. P., Koren, J. F., Daniel, R. C. 3rd, and Chapman, S. W., *Cefadroxil-induced ampicillin-exacerbated pemphigus vulargis: Case report and review of the literature.* Drug Intell Clin Pharm, 1986. 20:219–223.
8. Wolf, R., and Brenner, S., *An active amide group in the molecule of drugs that induce pemphigus: A casual or causal relationship?* Dermatology, 1994. 189:1–4.
9. Landau, M., and Brenner, S., *Histopathologic findings in drug-induced pemphigus.* Am J Dermatopathol, 1997. 19:411–414.
10. Brenner, S., Bialy-Golan, A., and Anhalt, G. J., *Recognition of pemphigus antigens in drug-induced pemphigus vulgaris and pemphigus foliaceus.* J Am Acad Dermatol, 1997. 36:919–923.
11. Korman, N. J., Eyre, R. W., Zone, J., and Stanley, J. R., *Drug-induced pemphigus: Autoantibodies directed against the pemphigus antigen complexes are present in penicillamine and captopril-induced pemphigus.* J Invest Dermatol, 1991. 96:273–276.
12. Wolf, R., and Ruocco, V., *Gaining more insight into the pathomechanisms of thiol-induced acantholysis.* Med Hypotheses, 1997. 48:107–110.
13. Yokel, B. K., Hood, A. F., and Anhalt, G. J., *Induction of acantholysis in organ explant culture by penicillamine and captopril.* Arch Dermatol, 1989. 125:1367–1370.
14. Bastuji-Garin, S., Joly, P., Picard-Dahan, C., Bernard, P., Vaillant, L., Pauwels, C., Salagnac, V., Lok, C., et al., *Drugs associated with bullous pemphigoid.* Arch Dermatol, 1996. 132:272–276.
15. Alcalay, J., David, M., Ingber, A., Hazaz, B., and Sandbank, M., *Bullous pemphigoid mimicking bullous erythema multiforme: An untoward side effect of penicillins.* J Am Acad Dermatol, 1988. 18:345–349.
16. Fellner, M. J., and Katz, J. M., *Occurrence of bullous pemphigoid after furosemide therapy.* Arch Dermatol, 1976. 112:75–77.
17. Koch, C. A., Mazzaferri, E. L., Larry, J. A., and Fanning, T. S., *Bullous pemphigoid after treatment with furosemide.* Cutis, 1996. 58:340–344.
18. Brun, P., and Baran, R., *Bullous pemphigoid induced by photochemotherapy of psoriasis. Apropos of 2 cases, with a review of the literature.* Ann Dermatol Venereol, 1982. 109:461–468.
19. Hodak, E., Ben-Shetrit, A., Ingber, A., and Sandbank, M., *Bullous pemphigoid—an adverse effect of ampicillin.* Clin Exp Dermatol, 1990. 15:50–52.
20. Van Joost, T., Faber, W. R., and Manhel, H. R., *Drug-induced anogenital cicatricial pemphigoid.* Br J Dermatol, 1980. 103:715–718.
21. Butt, Z., Kaufman, D., McNab, A., and McKelvie, P., *Drug-induced ocular cicatricial pemphigoid: A seris of clinico-pathological reports.* Eye, 1998. 12:285–290.
22. Fiore, P. M., Jacobs, I. H., and Goldberg, D. B., *Drug-induced pemphigoid. A spectrum of diseases.* Arch Ophthalmol, 1987. 105:1660–1663.
23. Smith, E. P., Taylor, T. B., Meyer, L. J., and Zone, J. J., *Antigen identification in drug-induced bullous pemphigoid.* J Am Acad Dermatol, 1993. 29:879–882.
24. Carpenter, S., Berg, D., Sidhu-Malik, N., Hall, R. P. III, and Rico, M. J., *Vancomycin-associated linear IgA dermatosis. A report of three cases.* J Am Acad Dermatol, 1992. 26:45–48.
25. Tonev, S., Vasileva, S., and Kadurina, M., *Depot sulfonamid associated with linear IgA bullous dermatosis with erythema multiforme-like clinical features.* J Eur Acad Deramtol Venereol, 1998. 11:165–168.
26. Whitworth, J. M., Thomas, I., Peltz, S. A., Sullivan, B. C., Wolf, A. H., and Cytryn, A. S., *Vancomycin-induced linear IgA bullous dermatosis (LABD).* J Am Acad Dermatol, 1996. 34:890–891.
27. Camilleri, M., and Pace, J. L., *Linear IgA bullous dermatosis induced by piroxicam.* J Eur Acad Deramtol Venereol, 1998. 10:70–72.
28. Klein, L. E., Shmunes, E., Carter, J. B., and Walsh, M. Y., *Linear IgA bullous dermatosis related to captopril treatment.* Cutis, 1989. 44:393–396.
29. Tranvan, A., Pezen, D. S., Medenica, M., Michelson, G. C., Vogelzang, N., and Soltani, K. M., *Interleukin-2 associated linear IgA bullous dermatosis.* J Am Acad Dermatol, 1996. 35:865–867.
30. Pellicano, R., Lomuto, M., Cozzani, E., Iannantuono, M., and De Simone, C., *Linear IgA bullous dermatosis*

after contact with sodium hypochlorite. Dermatology, 1997. 194:284–286.

31. Godfrey, K., Wojnarowska, F., and Leonard, J., *Linear IgA disease of adults: Association with lymphoproliferative malignancy and possible role of other triggering factors.* Br J Dermatol, 1990. 123:447–452.

32. Collier, P. M., Kelly, S. E., and Wojnarowska, F., *Linear IgA disease and pregnancy.* J Am Acad Dermatol, 1994. 30:407–411.

33. Abreu, A., Bowers, K., Mattson, D. H., and Gaspari, A. A., *Linear IgA bullous dermatosis in association with multiple sclerosis.* J Am Acad Dermatol, 1994. 31: 797–799.

34. Hayakawa, K., Shiohara, T., Yagita, A., and Nagashima, M., *Linear IgA bullous dermatosis associated with rheumatoid arthritis.* J Am Acad Dermatol, 1992. 26: 110–113.

35. Kucchlc, M. K., Stegemeir, E., Maynard, B., Gibson, L. E., Leiferman, K. M., and Peters, M. S., *Drug-induced linear IgA bullous dermatosis: Report of six cases and review of the literature.* J Am Acad Dermatol, 1994. 30: 187–192.

CHAPTER 23

Drug-Induced Interface Dermatoses

Erythema Multiforme

Epidemiology. Erythema multiforme is an acute, self-limited disease. It has an overall incidence of 0.03%–0.10% [1]. There are several variants of the disease that lead to confusion and controversy in classification [2]. The minor variant is reasonably well characterized and agreed on by most authors. Most patients afflicted with erythema multiforme minor are 20–40 years of age, but up to 20% of cases occur in children and adolescents [1]. There is a male predominance [3]. The disease characteristically lasts 3–4 weeks and resolves without sequelae. Disease recurrence is common, ranging from 22% to 37% [4].

Controversy revolves around the major variant(s) of the disease. Most authors believe that the Stevens-Johnson syndrome represents a similar disease process and is differentiated from the minor variant by the involvement of at least two mucosal surfaces [4]. The incidence of Stevens-Johnson syndrome is estimated to range from 1.1 cases [5] to 7.1 cases [6] per 1 million per year.

Debate exists whether toxic epidermal necrolysis also represents a major variant of erythema multiforme or is a separate entity [7]. Because the clinical distinctions between these entities are marked, toxic epidermal necrolysis is presented separately later in this chapter.

Cutaneous Features. Erythema multiforme minor is characterized by a polymorphous cutaneous eruption that is symmetrically distributed and typically appears first on the dorsal surfaces of hands and extensor surfaces of the extremities [4]. Involvement of the palms, soles, flexural surfaces, and face is less common. The classic lesion is that of an asymptomatic, round, erythematous macule or papule with three separate zones. A dusky, red central zone is surrounded by edema. Erythema is present at the periphery of the papules, and gentle pressure will cause blanching. This is the typical "iris" or "targetoid" lesion [2]. The papules may enlarge into edematous, erythematous plaques, and central, necrotic blisters occasionally develop. Other patients demonstrate atypical lesions that only have two zones. In some patients, macules with or without blisters are present. Zonation is not seen in these cases. These types of lesions may be more commonly associated with cases of erythema multiforme associated with drugs [2]. Rarely, mild mucosal involvement occurs in erythema multiforme minor [1]. In some cases of drug-induced erythema multiforme, a photodistribution has been described [8].

The Stevens-Johnson variant, or erythema multiforme of the major type, occurs most frequently in young men. It is a relatively uncommon disease, which affects from 1.1 to 7.1 people per 1 million per year [6]. Prodromal constitutional symptoms invariably precede onset of mucocutaneous manifestations. The lips are the most commonly involved site, with erosions and crusting in 95%–100% of cases. Bullae are less commonly observed. More extensive cases involve the pharynx, larynx, esophagus, and bronchial mucosa [9].

Ocular mucosa is involved in 70%–75% of cases and genital mucosa in slightly more than half of cases [10, 11]. Resolution of mucosal lesions takes 4–6 weeks and may be accompanied by scar formation.

Associated Disorders. Up to one-third of patients with erythema multiforme experience mild constitutional symptoms including malaise, fever, headache, rhinorrhea, and cough. These symptoms are more common in patients with erythema multiforme major than in those with the minor variant of the disease [11].

Erythema multiforme is also associated with many processes, including most commonly herpes simplex and *Mycoplasma pneumoniae* infections and drug exposures. Cases of erythema multiforme associated with herpes simplex tend to occur in young adults and children, whereas cases associated with drug exposures are more frequent in elderly patients [3]. It is difficult to establish an exact incidence, but about half of all cases are thought to be related to drug exposures [12]. The most commonly implicated drugs are sulfonamides and penicillins. Partial lists of associations are provided in Tables 23–1 to 23–3. Recurrent erythema multiforme is frequently associated with herpes simplex infection. Viral DNA has been found in involved skin of patients with erythema multiforme [13].

Histologic Features. Erythema multiforme is characterized by the presence of scattered dying keratinocytes at all levels of the epidermis. The overlying stratum

Table 23–1. Infectious Diseases Associated with Erythema Multiforme

Bacterial	Viral
Streptococcus	Vaccinia
Typhoid fever	Orf
Pseudomonas	Milker's nodule
Proteus	Mumps
Tularemia	Measles
Vibrio parahemolyticus	Influenza
Dental infections	Psittacosis
Vincent's angina	Varicella/herpes zoster
Pneumococcus	Lymphogranuloma
Yersinia infections	venereum
Legionnaire's disease	Enterovirus
Mycobacterial	Adenovirus
Tuberculosis	Hepatitis B and C
Bacille Calmette-Guérin	Epstein-Barr virus
Spirochetal	Parvovirus B19
Syphilis	Fungal
Mycoplasmal	Histoplasmosis
Mycoplasma pneumoniae	Coccidiodomycosis
Viral	Dermatophytes
Herpes simplex	Protozoal
Infectious mononucleosis	*Trichomonas*

From references 3 and 4.

Table 23–2. Drugs Associated with Erythema Multiforme

Antibiotics	Anticonvulsants
Ampicillin	Barbiturates
Cephalosporin	Carbamazepine
Chloramphenicol	Chlorpromazine
Chloroquine	Diphenylhydantoin
Clindamycin	Heptabarbital
Ciprofloxacin	Phenobarbital
Cotrimoxazole	Phenytoin
Ethambutol	Chemotherapeutics
Ethosuximide	Alkylating agents
Fluconazole	Busulfan
Griseofulvin	Cyclophosphamide
Isoniazid	Hydroxyurea
Ketotifen	Methotrexate
Lincomycin	Thiouracil
Nalidixic acid	Heavy metals
Nitrofurantoin	Arsenic
Novobiocin	Bismuth
Nystatin	Gold
Penicillins	Mercury
Pyrimethamine-sulfadoxine	Hormones
Quinidine	Danazol
Quinine	Estrogens
Rifampin	17-α-Hydroxyprogesterone
Streptomycin	Glucose-lowering agents
Sulfonamides	Chlorpropamide
Tetracycline	Tolbutamide
Thiabendazole	Miscellaneous
Antihypertensives	Acetlysalicylic acid
β-blockers	Allopurinol
Captopril	Atropine
Chlorthiazide	Cimetidine
Diltiazem	Clofibrate
Enalapril	Codeine
Furosemide	Dipyridamole
Indapamide	Iodine
Minodixil	Lithium
Propranolol	Methenamine
Verapamil	D-Penicillamine
Nonsteroidal antiinflammatory	Theophylline
Benoxaprofen	Thiopental
Diclofenac	Vitamin A
Diflunisal	
Ibuprofen	
Naproxen	
Phenylbutazone	
Piroxicam	
Sulindac	
Zomepirac	

From references 3 and 4.

corneum is unremarkable, and parakeratosis is not seen, except in older lesions. There is hydropic degeneration of basal keratinocytes and exocytosis of lymphocytes into the epidermis (Fig. 23–1). It has been demonstrated that the necrotic keratinocytes are concentrated around and within acrosyringia in cases of erythema multiforme attributed to drugs [14]. In older,

Table 23–3. Miscellaneous Conditions Associated with Erythema Multiforme

Immunizations	Lupus erythematosus
Diphtheria-pertussis	Sunlight
Polio	Foods
Typhoid	Sarcoidosis
Measles	Pregnancy
Poison ivy hyposensitization	Menstruation
Pollen hyposensitization	Inflammatory bowel disease
Neoplasms	
Leukemia	
Lymphoma	
Leiomyoma	
Carcinoma	

From references 3 and 4.

more well-developed lesions, a subepidermal blister is present and the epidermis may be largely necrotic. The dermis is characterized by a superficial perivascular inflammatory infiltrate consisting primarily of lymphocytes and histiocytes. Scattered eosinophils are present in the inflammatory infiltrate in most cases. They may be more abundant in drug-induced erythema multiforme [15]. Abundant neutrophils are not a feature of erythema multiforme [16]. It is not possible to differentiate between erythema multiforme minor and erythema multiforme major of the Stevens-Johnson type in tissue.

Special Studies. Rare patients have been reported to have granular deposits of IgM or C3 surrounding vessels of the superficial vascular plexus in the earliest of lesions [17]. In most cases of erythema multiforme, however, direct immunofluorescence examination is negative and is only useful for excluding autoimmune blistering processes in the differential diagnosis of erythema multiforme.

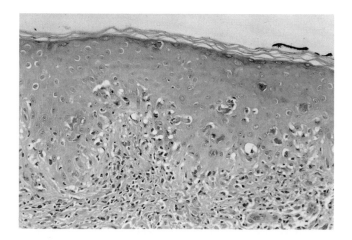

Fig. 23–1. Necrotic keratinocytes are present at all layers of the epidermis in erythema multiforme.

Pathogenesis. It has been postulated that erythema multiforme is caused by an immunologic reaction to a range of triggering antigens [18]. The finding of perforin, produced by cytotoxic T cells, in affected skin supports a cell-mediated process [19]. Perforin may mediate apoptosis leading to the epidermal changes seen in erythema multiforme [20].

Toxic Epidermal Necrolysis

Epidemiology. Toxic epidermal necrolysis (TEN) is also known as Lyell's syndrome. As discussed earlier, the relationship between this entity and erythema multiforme remains controversial. One clinically based classification suggested the designation of TEN for eruptions that involve detachment of the skin over 30% of the body surface with widespread purpuric macules or targets or detachment of large sheets of epidermis extending over more than 10% of the body surface [2]. Toxic epidermal necrolysis occurs in patients of all ages, but is most common in the elderly, who are more likely to be taking more medications [21]. There is a female predominance [22]. The overall incidence is approximately 1 case per 1 million people per year [21], and TEN accounts for 1% of cutaneous drug eruptions that require hospitalization [23]. A relationship between TEN and human leukocyte antigen (HLA) subtype B12 has been reported [24], as has an association with HLA-A29 [25]. The mortality rate among patients with TEN is approximately 30%, with sepsis being the main cause of death. Age and percentage of body surface area with necrolysis were the most important predictors of survival [26].

Cutaneous Features. Patients have an initial sensation of pain or burning on the face and upper extremities or other site of initial involvement that progresses to involve the entire body. Large, poorly defined macules with necrotic centers appear and rapidly coalesce to form large, flaccid bullae. In many cases, actual blisters may not form; rather, sheets of epidermis desquamate and are easily extended with gentle pressure (positive Nikolsky's sign). Hair-bearing scalp is never involved, nor is the skin of the areola. Mucous membranes, including the oropharynx, eyes, genitalia, and anus, are affected in 85%–95% of all patients with TEN and may precede the skin involvement by several days [27]. The skin will re-epithelialize, usually without scarring, within several weeks. Ocular sequelae may be severe and affect 40%–50% of survivors [28].

Associated Disorders. Patients with TEN often have constitutional symptoms such as fever, weakness, and malaise that precede onset of the cutaneous process by a few days. Multiple systems are involved in most patients with TEN. Extracutaneous involvement is sum-

Table 23–4. Extracutaneous Manifestations of Toxic Epidermal Necrolysis

Sites or Type of Manifestation	Incidence (%)
Gastrointestinal tract	
Esophagus	Unknown (common)
Liver	50
Pancreas	Rare
Pulmonary	10–20
Hematologic	
Anemia	100
Leukopenia	90
Neutropenia	30
Thrombocytopenia	15
Glomerulonephritis	Rare

marized in Table 23–4. The gastrointestinal tract is frequently affected by mucosal ulcerations. The esophagus is most frequently affected [29]. Hepatitis is seen in about 10% of cases and up to half of all patients with TEN have elevated transaminases. Less com-

Table 23–5. Drugs Associated with Toxic Epidermal Necrolysis

Antibiotics	Fenbufen
Ampicillin	Indomethacin
Chloramphenicol	Isoxicam
Erythromycin	Naprosyn
Ethambutol	Oxyphenbutazone
Gentamicin	Phenylbutazone
Griseofulvin	Sulindac
Isoniazid	Tolmetin
Mezlocillin	Zomepirac
Neomycin	Miscellaneous
Nitrofurantoin	Acetaminophen
Pyrimethamine	Allopurinol
Quinolones	Chlorpromazine
Rifampicin	Chlorpropamide
Streptomycin	Dapsone
Sulfadiazine	Diclofenac
Sulfadoxidine	Disulfiram
Sulfamethoxazole	Fluorouracil
Sulfasalazine	Gold salts
Sulfonylureas	Hydroxychloroquine
Tetracycline	Imipramine
Tobramycin	Levamisole
Vancomycin	Methotrexate
Anticonvulsants	Methlyprednisolone
Carbamazepine	Oxypurinol
Pentobarbitol	Penicillamine
Phenobarbitol	Pentamidine
Phenytoin	Pentazocine
Antihypertensives	Phenophthalein
Captopril	Quinine
Nonsteroidal anti-inflammatory	Thiabendazole
drugs	Vitamin B_6
Acetylsalicylic acid	
Benoxaprofen	

From references 25 and 31.

monly, pancreatitis is seen [30]. The respiratory mucosa may be similarly affected by the blistering process, resulting in required artificial ventilation for up to 10%–20% of patients [27]. Anemia is found in virtually all patients with TEN, and leukopenia is present in 90% [31].

Virtually all cases of TEN are caused by drugs or other exposures [27]. Some implicated drugs are listed in Table 23–5. The most common offending agents are sulfonamides, anticonvulsants, and allopurinol [31]. The presence of both TEN and systemic lupus erythematosus has been reported in several patients [31].

Histologic Features. Skin biopsy specimens demonstrate full-thickness epidermal necrosis and a subepidermal blister. A sparse lymphohistiocytic infiltrate is present, and scattered lymphocytes may be present within the necrotic epidermis (Fig. 23–2). Early lesions and areas adjacent to frank desquamation demonstrate hydropic degeneration of the basal layer with a mild lymphocytic exocytosis and occasional dying keratinocytes. Eccrine ducts are also affected, but hair follicles are less frequently involved. Biopsy tissues taken from these types of lesions are histologically indistinguishable from those from erythema multiforme and fixed drug eruption lesions.

Special Studies. Direct immunofluorescence tests are negative in the vast majority of cases and are not ordinarily recommended for making a diagnosis of TEN. Frozen section examination of sheets of desquamated epidermis is a useful method for differentiating TEN from staphylococcal scalded skin syndrome. In TEN, the entire epidermis is present in the desquamated sheets. In contrast, in staphylococcal scalded skin syndrome, the desquamated epidermis is limited to the stratum corneum and a small portion of the granular layer.

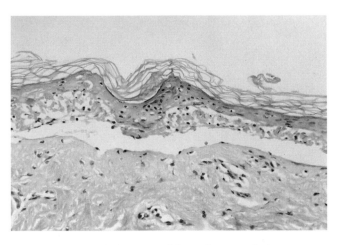

Fig. 23–2. Full-thickness epidermal necrosis is present, leading to subepidermal blister formation in toxic epidermal necrolysis.

Pathogenesis. Although the exact pathogenesis of TEN remains unknown, the disease is generally recognized to be a cellular immune reaction to drugs. It has been shown that there is a recruitment of antigen-primed and cytotoxic T cells in the skin and blister cavities of patients with TEN [32]. It is believed that cytokines play a major role in the observed epidermal necrolysis [31], in part supported by the presence of HLA-DR antigens expressed by affected keratinocytes [33]. Tumor necrosis factor-α has been implicated in causing the necrolysis [34]. Many cases of TEN, however, lack significant inflammation, and it has been suggested that the pathogenesis may be due to a direct toxic effect of drugs.

Fixed Drug Eruption

Epidemiology. Fixed drug eruptions (FDEs) account for up to 20% of all drug eruptions in one series of patients [35]. The male to female ratio of affected patients is 1:1.1 [36]. Patients with HLA-B22 have a higher incidence of experiencing an FDE [37]. Well over 100 drugs have been implicated in the induction of the FDE (see Table 23–6).

Cutaneous Features. Fixed drug eruptions initially present as a single or as several erythematous, pruritic macules with dusky centers that evolve into edematous plaques [38]. The macules are sharply bordered and very well demarcated from normal skin. Central vesicles and bullae may develop, and the initial eruption resolves with varying degrees of hyperpigmentation. With each recurrence of the process, macules reappear at the same sites, as well as additional ones in some cases. With each recurrence, the residual hyperpigmentation is more prominent. At the time of presentation, slightly more than half of all patients have more than one lesion [39]. The trunk and extremities are involved in about one-fourth of cases, followed in frequency by the lips and genitalia [39]. Palms and soles are also commonly affected [40]. Mucosal surfaces can be involved. In extreme cases, extensive blister formation can give rise to TEN-like appearance [41]. Less commonly, the FDE can mimic other dermatoses, including lichen planus, erythema multiforme, cheilitis, psoriasis, lupus erythematosus, erythema annulare centrifugum, pemphigus vulgaris, and chilblains [36]. It has been suggested that different inciting drugs give rise to involvement of different mucocutaneous sites, with cotrimoxazole and tetracycline responsible for lip and genital lesions, cotrimoxazole and phenytoin responsible for most cases of generalized disease, and analgin and pyrazolones most responsible for FDEs involving the trunk and extremities [39]. Other series have demonstrated similar, but not identical, drug and affected site relationships [42].

Table 23–6. Drugs Most Commonly Associated with Fixed Drug Eruptions	
Acetaminophen	Heroin
Ampicillin	Meprobamate
Anovulatory drugs	Minocycline
Aspirin	Morphine
Barbiturates	Nystatin
Carbamazepine	Oxyphenbutazone
Chlordiazepoxide	Penicillin
Ciprofloxacin	Phenacetin
Codeine	Phenolphthalein
Colchicine	Quinine derivatives
Dipyrone	Quiniodochlor
Erythromycin	Tetracycline
Griseofulvin	Trimethaprim-sulfamethoxazole

From references 38 and 44.

Associated Disorders. Systemic manifestations are quite uncommon. Malaise, fever, and weakness have been reported, as have nausea and diarrhea in exceptional cases [43]. Fixed drug eruptions have been associated with many types of drugs. A partial list is presented in Table 23–6. Similar eruptions have been associated with toothpastes, food coloring, and foods [44]. In several large series, cotrimoxazole was the drug most frequently implicated in causing an FDE, followed by analgin, tetracycline, and pyrazolones [36, 39].

Histologic Features. Fixed drug eruptions are characterized by hydropic degeneration of the basal keratinocytes and exocytosis of lymphocytes (Fig. 23–3). Spongiosis is focally prominent. Dyskeratotic cells are present in varying numbers and with confluence may give rise to subepidermal blisters. The blister cavity is filled with dying keratinocytes and a mixed inflamma-

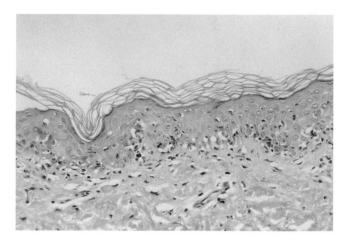

Fig. 23–3. Fixed drug eruptions are characterized by basal vacuolization, necrotic keratinocytes, and exocytosis of lymphocytes into the epidermis.

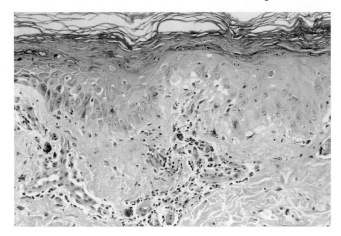

Fig. 23–4. Melanin is present within dermal macrophages in fixed drug eruptions.

tory infiltrate. Melanin is present in the papillary dermis, free, and within macrophages (Fig. 23–4). A mixed inflammatory infiltrate consisting of lymphocytes, histiocytes, neutrophils, and eosinophils is present [38].

Special Studies. There are no special studies that are helpful in making a diagnosis of FDE.

Pathogenesis. The exact pathogenesis of FDEs remains elusive, although the case for an immunologically mediated process is quite convincing. Antibodies, serum factors, tissue factors, and cell-mediated immunity have all been implicated [38]. Intercellular adhesion molecule-1 is known to be rapidly upregulated in lesional skin after exposure to inciting agents. This is thought to provide a localized initiating stimulus for activation of a subpopulation of T cells [45]. In addition, HLA-DR and γ-IP-10, two proteins upregulated by interferon-γ, are also markedly increased in affected skin, suggesting a central role for T cells in the pathogenesis of FDEs [46]. It has further been shown that an oligoclonal population of T cells is recruited to and is present within the epidermis in FDEs [47].

Drug-Induced Lupus Erythematosus

Epidemiology. Drug-induced lupus erythematosus occurs in rare patients who are exposed to various drugs. The signs and symptoms of the disease may be virtually indistinguishable from those of idiopathic systemic lupus erythematosus; however, in most cases, the disease resolves completely upon withdrawal of the offending drug.

Cutaneous Features. The cutaneous features of drug-induced lupus erythematosus are virtually indistinguishable from those of idiopathic lupus. An erythematous patch with follicular plugging on the cheeks and nose is the most

characteristic cutaneous finding. The cutaneous findings are discussed more fully in Chapter 1. In rare patients, the cutaneous eruption may resemble Sweet's syndrome, with erythematous, edematous plaques and papules [48].

Associated Disorders. A lupus erythematosus-like syndrome has been associated with a large number of drugs, some of which are listed in Table 23–7. The most commonly implicated drug, by far, is hydralazine.

Patients with drug-induced lupus erythematosus may suffer from the same systemic complications as those with idiopathic lupus erythematosus. These can include fevers, interstitial lung disease [49], joint pains, and hepatosplenomegaly. Increased thrombotic tendency may also appear in these patients [50], as can leukopenia [49]. A positive antinuclear antibody is found in most patients with the syndrome [51], and some patients have antihistone antibodies [48], anticardiolipin antibodies, and rheumatoid factor [49]. More specific details about systemic involvement in lupus erythematosus are discussed in Chapter 1.

Histologic Features. The histologic findings of drug-induced lupus erythematosus are identical to those seen in the idiopathic form of the disease. Lymphocytes are present along the dermal–epidermal junction, extending into the overlying epidermis and in some cases inducing dyskeratosis of basal keratinocytes (Fig. 23–5). Additionally, lymphocytes are aggregated around vessels of the superficial vascular plexus and cutaneous appendages and are present superficially and deeply within the reticular dermis (Fig. 23–6). Occasional plasma cells may be present. These findings are described in detail in Chapter 1. A neutrophil-rich subepidermal blistering process has been reported in patients with drug-induced lupus erythematosus [52]. These histologic changes can be seen in idiopathic bullous lupus erythematosus, as well as in Sweet's syndrome. In rare patients, leukocytoclastic vasculitis may be seen in histologic sections of affected skin [50].

Special Studies. Direct immunofluorescence examination reveals granular deposits of IgG, C3, and less com-

Table 23–7. Inciting Agents in Lupus Erythematosus-Like Drug Eruptions	
Chlorpromazine	Peroben
Hydralazine	Phenytoin
Isoniazid	Procainamide
Methimazole	Propylthiouracil
Nitrofurantoin	Sulfasalazine
Penicillamine	

From references 51 and 66.

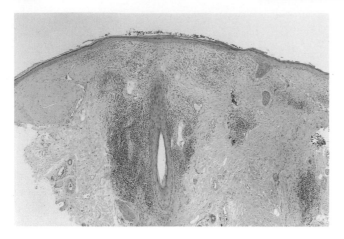

Fig. 23–5. Drug-induced lupus erythematosus is histologically identical to idiopathic lupus erythematosus, with an interface dermatitis and a superficial and deep perivascular and periappendageal lymphocytic infiltrate.

monly IgM and/or IgA along the dermal–epidermal junction in a pattern identical to that seen in idiopathic lupus erythematosus.

Pathogenesis. Drug-induced lupus erythematosus is seen in patients with slow acetyltransferase activity ("slow acetylators"), who accrue increased amounts of some drug breakdown products that precipitate the systemic immune complex–mediated disease [53].

Lichenoid Drug Eruptions

Epidemiology. Lichenoid drug eruptions are seen most commonly in patients taking gold therapy, antimalarials, and penicillamine. Also frequent, but less commonly, thiazide diuretics and β-adrenergic blocking

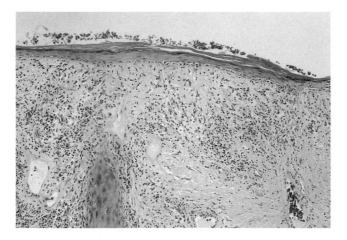

Fig. 23–6. Epidermal atrophy, interface dermatitis, and extensive basal vacuolization are present in this case of drug-induced lupus erythematosus.

agents are implicated [54]. The mean age of patients with a lichenoid drug eruption is 50–60 years [54]. The latent period between the onset of medication and the appearance of the cutaneous eruption is somewhat longer in lichenoid drug eruptions than in other types and is often as much as several months [55] to a year [56]. In most patients, the lichenoid eruption resolves with cessation of the offending drug, although this may take a period of months [57].

Cutaneous Features. Patients with a drug-induced lichenoid eruption may be clinically indistinguishable from those with idiopathic lichen planus. Multiple pruritic, violaceous flat-topped papules and plaques are present on the trunk and extremities. Flexural surfaces are favored. Some authors believe that drug-related eruptions display larger, more psoriasiform-appearing patches than occur in the idiopathic disease [57]. Wickham's striae are often not present in lichenoid drug eruptions [58]. In some patients, the lichenoid papules are most prevalent on sun-exposed skin [59]. In one case, the lichenoid eruption induced by nicergoline was reported to have a linear distribution that followed the lines of Blashko [60]. Oral and genital mucosas are involved in many cases, and ulceration may occur [61]. Alopecia and decreased sweating have been described in patients with lichenoid drug eruptions that involve hair follicles and eccrine structures [62].

Associated Disorders. Some of the drugs reported to induce lichenoid drug eruptions are listed in Table 23–8. A similar eruption has been reported after hepatitis B vaccination [63]. A lichenoid drug eruption has also been reported to occur secondary to contact with certain drugs and chemicals, most commonly in developers of color film and people who work with dental restorative materials [54]. Systemic involvement has not been reported in patients with drug-induced lichenoid eruptions.

Histologic Features. Histologic features of drug-induced lichenoid eruptions may be indistinguishable from those of idiopathic lichen planus. Both entities are associated with a dense band-like infiltrate of lymphocytes that abut and focally obscure the dermal–epidermal junction. Acanthosis, hypergranulosis, hyperkeratosis, and multiple dying keratinocytes are present (Fig. 23–7). The epidermis develops a "saw-toothed" rete ridge pattern. Hydropic degeneration of the basal layer may lead to blister formation. Exocytosis of lymphocytes into the epidermis is common, and satellite necrosis may be seen (Fig. 23–8). The presence of parakeratosis and/or dyskeratotic keratinocytes within the stratum corneum and granular layers of the epidermis is seen in more than half of the cases of drug-

Table 23–8. Drugs that Cause a Lichenoid Eruption

Antifungals	Hypoglycemics
Ketoconazole	Chlorpropamide
Antihypertensives	Tolazamide
Captopril	Miscellaneous
Diazoxide	Allopurinol
Enalapril	Amiphenazole
Methyl dopa	Carbamazepine
Propranolol	Crystal methamphetamine
Antimalarials	Cyanamide
Quinacrine	Cycloserine
Quinine	Dapsone
Pyrimethamine	Gold
Antituberculosis drugs	Iodides
Ethambutol	Lithium carbonate
Isoniazid	Nandrolone furylpropionate
Streptomycin	Nicergoline
Calcium channel blockers	Pravastatin
Nifedipine	Procainamide
Cinnarizine	Pyritinol
Flunarizine	Simvastatin
Chemotherapeutic agents	Tiopronin
Hydroxyurea	Phenothiazines
5-Fluorouracil	Chlorpromazine
Diuretics	Metopromazine
Chlorothiazine	
Furosemide	
Spironolactone	
Heavy metals	
Arsenicals	
Bismuth	
Mercury	

From references 54, 59–61, and 67–79.

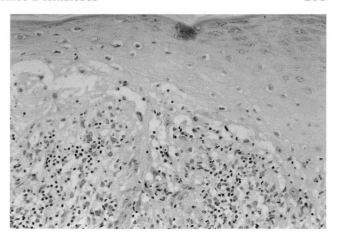

Fig. 23–8. Abundant dying keratinocytes are present along with a lichenoid lymphocytic infiltrate in drug-induced lichen planus.

a drug-induced eruption. Rare cases of lichenoid dermatitis with accompanying multinucleated giant cells have been related to drugs [65].

Special Studies. Special studies are not helpful in diagnosing a lichenoid drug eruption.

Pathogenesis. The pathogenesis of lichenoid drug eruptions is currently not known.

induced lichenoid eruptions. These changes are not ordinarily seen in idiopathic lichen planus [64]. The presence of eosinophils and/or plasma cells within the inflammatory infiltrate may also be evidence in favor of

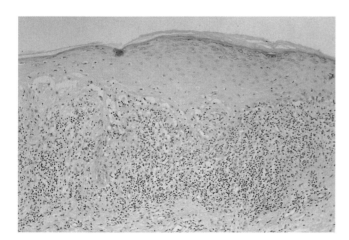

Fig. 23–7. Drug-induced lichen planus demonstrates hyperkeratosis, wedge-shaped hypergranulosis, and acanthosis with a dense, band-like dermal infiltrate of lymphocytes.

References

1. Hellgren, L., and Hersle, K., *Erythema multiforme. Statistical evaluation of clinical and laboratory data in 224 patients and matched healthy controls.* Acta Allergol, 1965. 21:45–51.
2. Bastuji-Garin, S., Rzany, B., Stern, R. S., Shear, N. H., Naldi, L., and Roujeau, J. C., *Clinical classification of cases of toxic epidermal necrolysis, Stevens-Johnson syndrome and erythema multiforme.* Arch Dermatol, 1993. 129:92–96.
3. Fabbri, P., and Panconesi, E., *Erythema multiforme ("minus" and "maius") and drug intake.* Clin Dermatol, 1993. 11:479–489.
4. Huff, J. C., Weston, W. L., and Tonnesen, M. G., *Erythema multiforme: A critical review of characteristics, diagnostic criteria, and causes.* J Am Acad Dermatol, 1983. 8:763–775.
5. Schopf, E., Stuhmer, A., Rzany, B., Victor, N., Zentgraf, R., and Kapp, J. F., *Toxic epidermal necrolysis and Stevens-Johnson syndrome. An epidemiologic study from West Germany.* Arch Dermatol, 1991. 127:839–842.
6. Strom, B. L., Carson, J. L., Halpern, A. C., Schinnar, R., Snyder, E. S., Shaw, M., Tilson, H. H., Joseph, M., et al., *A population-based study of Stevens-Johnson syndrome.* Arch Dermatol, 1991. 127:831–838.

7. Roujeau, J.-C., *The spectrum of Stevens-Johnson syndrome and toxic epidermal necrolysis: A clinical classification.* J Invest Dermatol, 1994. 102:28S-30S.

8. Shiohara, T., Chiba, M., Tanaka, Y., and Nagashima, M., *Drug-induced, photosensitive, erythema multiforme-like eruption: Possible role for cell adhesion molecules in a flare induced by Rhus dermatitis.* J Am Acad Dermatol, 1990. 22:647–650.

9. Bailey, J. H., *Lesion of the cornea and conjunctiva in erythema exudativum multiforme (Hebra).* Acta Ophthalmol, 1931. 6:362–79.

10. Tonneson, M., and Soter, N. A., *Erythema multiforme.* J Am Acad Dermatol, 1979. 1:357–364.

11. Ashby, D. W., and Lazar, T., *Erythema multiforme exudativum major (Stevens-Johnson syndrome).* Lancet, 1951. 1:1091–1095.

12. Fegan, D., and Glennan, J., *Cutaneous sensitivity to thiacetazone.* Lancet, 1991. 337:1036.

13. Brice, S. L., Leahy, M. A., Ong, L., Krecji, S., Stockert, S. S., Huff, J. C., and Weston, W. L., *Examination of non-involved skin, previously involved skin, and peripheral blood for herpes simplex virus DNA in patients with recurrent herpes-associated erythema multiforme.* J Cutan Pathol, 1994. 21:408–412.

14. Zohdi-Mofid, M., and Horn, T. D., *Acrosyringeal concentration of necrotic keratinocytes in erythema multiforme: A clue to drug etiology. Clinicopathologic review of 29 cases.* J Cutan Pathol, 1997. 24:235–240.

15. Patterson, J. W., Parsons, J. M., Blaylock, K., and Mills, A. S., *Eosinophils in skin lesions of erythema multiforme.* Arch Pathol Lab Med, 1989. 113:36–39.

16. Ackerman, A. B., Penneys, N. S., and Clark, W. H., *Erythema multiforme exudativum: A distinctive pathological process.* Br J Dermatol, 1971. 84:554–565.

17. Kazmierowski, J. A., and Wuepper, K. D., *Erythema multiforme: Immune complex vasculitis of the superficial cutaneous microvasculature.* J Invest Dermatol, 1978. 71:366–369.

18. Roujeau, J. C., *What is going on in erythema multiforme?* Dermatology, 1994. 188:249–250.

19. Sayama, K., Watanabe, Y., Tohyama, M., and Miki, Y., *Localization of perforin in viral vesicles and erythema muliforme.* Dermatology, 1994. 188:305–309.

20. Inachi, S., Mizutani, H., and Shimizu, M., *Epidermal apoptotic cell death in erythema multiforme and Stevens-Johnson syndrome.* Arch Dermatol, 1997. 133:845–849.

21. Schopf, E., *Skin reactions to co-trimazole.* Infection, 1987. 15(Suppl 5):254–258.

22. Lyell, A., *A review of toxic epidermal necrolysis in Britain.* Br J Dermatol, 1967. 79:662–671.

23. Alanko, K., Stubb, S., and Kauppinen, K., *Cutaneous drug reactions: Clinical types and causative agents.* Acta Derm Venereol (Stockh), 1989. 69:223–226.

24. Roujeau, J.-C., Huyn, N. T., Bracq, C., Guillaume, J. C., Revuz, J., and Touraine, R., *Genetic susceptibility to toxic epidermal necrolysis.* Arch Dermatol, 1987. 123:1171–1173.

25. Avakian, R., Flowers, F. P., Araujo, O. E., and Ramos-Caro, F. A., *Toxic epidermal necrolysis: A review.* J Am Acad Dermatol, 1991. 25:69–79.

26. Revuz, J., Penso, D., and Roujeau, J.-C., *Toxic epidermal necrolysis: Clinical findings and prognosis factors in 87 patients.* Arch Dermatol, 1987. 123:1160–1165.

27. Lyell, A., *Toxic epidermal necrolysis (the scalded skin syndrome): A reappraisal.* Br J Dermatol, 1979. 100:69–86.

28. Kauppinen, K., *Cutaneous reactions to drugs with special reference to severe bullous mucocutaneous eruptions and sulphonamides.* Acta Derm Venereol (Stockh), 1972. 52(Suppl):1–89.

29. Rasmussen, J. E., *Toxic epidermal necrolysis.* Med Clin North Am, 1980. 64:901–920.

30. Klein, S. M., and Dhan, M. A., *Hepatitis, toxic epidermal necrolysis and pancreatitis in association with sulindac therapy.* J Rheumatol, 1983. 10:512–513.

31. Roujeau, J.-C., Chosidow, O., Saiaig, P., and Guillaume, J.-C., *Toxic epidermal necrolysis (Lyell syndrome).* J Am Acad Dermatol, 1990. 23:1039–1058.

32. Correia, O., Delgado, L., Ramos, J. P., Resene, C., and Fleming Torrinha, J. A., *Cutaneous T-cell recruitment in toxic epidermal necrolysis. Further evidence of CD8+ lymphocyte involvement.* Arch Dermatol, 1993. 129:466–468.

33. Villada, G., Roujeau, J.-C., Clerici, T., Bourgault, I., and Revuz, J., *Immunopathology of toxic epidermal necrolysis. Keratinocytes, HLA-DR expression, Langerhans cell, and mononuclear cells: An immunopathologic study of five cases.* Arch Dermatol, 1992. 128:50–53.

34. Heng, M. C. Y., and Allen, S. G., *Efficacy of cyclophosphamide in toxic epidermal necrolysis. Clinical and pathophysiologic aspects.* J Am Acad Dermatol, 1991. 25:778–786.

35. Kauppinen, K., and Stubb, S., *Drug eruptions: Causative agents and clinical types.* Acta Derm Venereol, 1984. 64:320–324.

36. Mahboob, A., and Haroon, T. S., *Drugs causing fixed eruptions: A study of 450 cases.* Int J Dermatol, 1998. 37:833–838.

37. Pellicano, R., Ciavarella, G., Lommuto, M., and Di Giorgio, G., *Genetic susceptibility to fixed drug eruption: Evidence for a link with HLA-B22.* J Am Acad Dermatol, 1994. 30:52–54.

38. Korkij, W., and Soltani, K., *Fixed drug eruption. A brief overview.* Arch Dermatol, 1984. 120:520–524.

39. Sharma, V. K., Dhar, S., and Gill, A. N., *Drug related involvement of specific sites in fixed eruptions: A statistical evaluation.* J Dermatol, 1996. 23:530–534.

40. Talbot, M. D., *Fixed genital drug eruption.* Practitioner, 1980. 224:823–824.

41. Baird, B. J., and De Villez, R. L., *Widespread bullous fixed drug eruption mimicking toxic epidermal necrolysis.* Int J Dermatol, 1988. 27:170–174.

42. Thankappan, T. P., and Zachariah, J., *Drug-specific clinical pattern in fixed drug eruptions.* Int J Dermatol, 1991. 30:867–870.

43. Browne, S. G., *Fixed eruption in deeply pigmented subjects: Clinical observations on 350 patients.* BMJ, 1964. 2:1041–1044.

44. Abdul Gaffoor, P. M., and George, W. M., *Fixed drug eruptions occurring on the male genitals.* Cutis, 1990. 45:242–243.

45. Teraki, Y., Moriya, N., and Shiohara, T., *Drug-induced expression of intercellular adhesion molecule-1 on lesional keratinocytes in fixed drug eruption.* Am J Pathol, 1994. 145:550–560.

46. Smoller, B. R., Krueger, J., Gray, M. H., Luster, A., and Gottlieb, A., *Fixed drug eruptions: Evidence for a cytokine-mediated process.* J Cutan Pathol, 1991. 18.13–19.

47. Komatsu, T., Moriya, N., and Shiohara, T., *T cell receptor (TCR) repertoire and function of human epidermal T cells: Restricted TCR V alpha-V beta genes are utilized by T cells residing in the lesional epidermis in fixed drug eruption.* Clin Exp Dermatol, 1996. 104: 343–350.

48. Ramsey-Goldman, R., Franz, T., Solano, F. X., and Medsger, T. A. Jr., *Hydralazine induced lupus and Sweet's syndrome. Report and review of the literature.* J Rheumatol, 1990. 17:682–684.

49. Schattner, A., Sthoeger, Z., and Geltner, D., *Effect of acute cytomegalovirus infection on drug-induced SLE.* Postgrad Med J, 1994. 70:738–740.

50. Van neste, D., Pierard, G. E., and Hermanns, J. F., *Immune complex disease associated with Peroben intake.* Dermatologica, 1979. 158:417–426.

51. Searles, R. P., Plymate, S. R., and Troup, G. M., *Familial thioamide-induced lupus syndrome in thyrotoxicosis.* J Rheumatol, 1981. 8:498–500.

52. Fleming, M. G., Bergfeld, W. F., Tomecki, K. J., Tuthill, R. J., Norris, M., Benedetto, E. A., and Weber, L. A., *Bullous systemic lupus erythematosus.* Int J Dermatol, 1989. 28:321–326.

53. Shear, N. H., and Spielberg, S. P., *Pharmacogenetics and adverse drug reactions in the skin.* Pediatr Dermatol, 1983. 1:165–173.

54. Halvey, S., and Shai, A., *Lichenoid drug eruptions.* J Am Acad Dermatol, 1993. 29:249–255.

55. Powell, F. C., Rogers, R. S. I., and Dickson, E. R., *Primary biliary cirrhosis and lichen planus.* J Am Acad Dermatol, 1983. 9:540–545.

56. Hodl, S., *Side effects of beta receptor blockers on the skin: Review and personal observation.* Hautarzt, 1985. 36:549–557.

57. Halevy, S., Sandbank, M., Pick, A. I., and Feuerman, E. J., *Cowden's disease in three siblings: Electron-microscopic and immunologic studies.* Acta Derm Venereol, 1985. 65:126–131.

58. Bork, K., *Lichenoid eruptions.* in *Cutaneous Side Effects of Drugs.* 1988, W. B. Saunders, Philadelphia, pp. 170–171.

59. Lee, A. Y., and Jung, S. Y., *Two patients with isoniazid-induced photosensitive lichenoid eruptions confirmed by photopatch test.* Photodermatol Photoimmunol Photomed, 1998. 14:77–78.

60. Munoz, M. A., Perez-Bernal, A. M., and Camacho, F. M., *Lichenoid drug eruption following the Blaschko lines.* Dermatology, 1996. 193:66–67.

61. Massa, M. C., Jason, S. M., Gradini, R., and Welykyj, S., *Lichenoid drug eruption secondary to propranolol.* Cutis, 1991. 48:41–43.

62. Sulzberger, M. B., Herrmann, F., and Zak, F. G., *Studies of sweating. I. Preliminary report with particular emphasis on a sweat retention syndrome.* J Invest Dermatol, 1947. 9:221–242.

63. Saywell, C. A., Wittal, R. A., and Kossard, S., *Lichenoid reaction to hepatitis B vaccination.* Austral J Dermatol, 1997. 38:152–154.

64. Van den Haute, V., Antoine, J. L., and Lachapelle, J. M., *Histopathological discriminant criteria between lichenoid drug eruption and idiopathic lichen planus: Retrospective study on selected samples.* Dermatologica, 1989. 179:10–13.

65. Gonzalez, J. G., Marcus, M. D., and Santa Cruz, D. J., *Giant cell lichenoid dermatitis.* J Am Acad Dermatol, 1986. 15:87–92.

66. VanArsdel, P. P. Jr., *Allergy and adverse drug reactions.* J Am Acad Dermatol, 1982. 6:833–845.

67. Roten, S. V., Mainetti, C., Donath, R., and Saurat, J. H., *Enalpril-induced lichen planus-like eruption.* J Am Acad Dermatol, 1995. 32:293–295.

68. Reinhardt, L. A., Wilkin, J. K., and Kirkendall, W. M., *Lichenoid eruption produced by captopril.* Cutis, 1983. 31:98–99.

69. Aihara, M., Kitamura, K., and Ikezawa, Z., *Lichenoid drug eruptions due to nandrolone furylpropionate (Demelon).* J Dermatol, 1989. 16:330–334.

70. Franz, C. B., Massullo, R. E., and Welton, W. A., *Lichenoid drug eruption from chlorpropaminde and tolazamide.* J Am Acad Dermatol, 1990. 22:128–129.

71. Atkin, S. L., McKenzie, T. M., and Stevenson, C. J., *Carbamazepine-induced lichenoid eruption.* Clin Exp Dermatol, 1990. 15:382–283.

72. Schrallhammer-Benkler, K., Ring, J., Przybilla, B., Meurer, M., and Landthaler, M., *Acute mercury intoxication with lichenoid drug eruption followed by mercury contact allergy and development of antinuclear antibodies.* Acta Derm Venereol, 1992. 72:294–296.

73. Alzieu, P. H., Amoric, J. C., Bureau, B., Remond, L., Milpied, B., Stalder, J. F., and Litoux, P., *Lichenoid eruption induced by gold salts. An autonomous eruption.* Ann Dermatol Venereol, 1994. 121:798–801.

74. Roger, D., Rolle, F., Labrousse, F., Brosset, A., and Bonnetblanc, J. M., *Simvasatin-induced lichenoid drug eruption.* Clin Exp Dermatol, 1994. 19:88–89.

75. Deloach-Banta, L. J., *Lichenoid drug eruption: Crystal methamphetamine or adulterants?* Cutis, 1994. 53:97–98.

76. Shim, J. H., Kim, T. Y., Kim, H. O., and Kim, C. W., *Cycloserine-induced lichenoid drug eruption.* Dermatology, 1995. 191:142–144.

77. Kawana, S., *Drug eruption induced by cyanamide (carbimide): A clinical and histopathologic study of 7 patients.* Dermatology, 1997. 195:30–34.

78. Keough, G. C., Richardson, T. T., and Grabski, W. J., *Pravastatin-induced lichenoid drug eruption.* Cutis, 1998. 61:98–100.

79. Clark, C., and Douglas, W. S., *Lichenoid drug eruption induced by spironolactone.* Clin Exp Dermatol, 1998. 23:43–44.

CHAPTER 24

Photo-Related Drug Eruptions

There are two broad classes of cutaneous eruptions associated with medications that are induced by exposure to light. These are traditionally termed *phototoxic* and *photoallergic* drug eruptions. The clinical findings, histologic changes, and pathogenetic mechanisms of these types of reactions are quite different. Furthermore, the types of drugs that induce these very different reactions are quite dissimilar. Therefore, these reactions are described separately.

Phototoxic Drug Eruptions

Epidemiology. Phototoxic drug eruptions are far more common than are photoallergic drug eruptions. They can occur with the first exposure to a drug and are dose related [1]. The incidence of phototoxic drug eruptions varies widely, from as high as 25% from chlorpromazine [2] to less than 0.025% from fluoroquinolones [3]. These reactions are due to direct cellular damage to keratinocytes due to phototoxicity.

Cutaneous Features. Phototoxic drug eruptions clinically resemble sunburns. Although changes are not strictly limited to sun-exposed areas of the body, they are usually most evolved in these regions. The skin is erythematous and edematous. Overlying scale may be present in older lesions. Affected skin may be tender or pruritic. Some photosensitizing drugs can induce abundant postinflammatory pigmentary changes.

Associated disorders. The following drugs are associated with phototoxic drug eruptions [4–12]:

- Afloqualone
- Amiodarone
- Chlorpromazine
- Chlorpropamide
- Ciprofloxacin
- Coal tar derivatives
- Demeclocycline
- Diclofenac
- Doxycycline
- Ibuprofen
- Levaquin
- Lomefloxacin
- Phenothiazine
- Psoralens
- Trimethoprim

Histologic Features. Acute phototoxic drug eruptions are characterized by dyskeratotic keratinocytes. Vacuolization of keratinocytes within the basal layer may be present (Figs. 24–1 and 24–2). There is relatively little inflammatory infiltration within the papillary dermis. Papillary dermal edema is present in most cases. With more chronic eruptions, the epidermis becomes atrophic, with flattening of rete ridges. Keratinocyte disorder and reactive atypia may be present. Vascular ectasia within the superficial vascular plexus and the accumulation of acid mucopolysaccharides is occa-

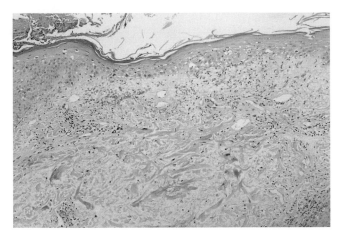

Fig. 24–1. Basal vacuolization, papillary dermal edema, and a mild lymphohistiocytic inflammatory infiltrate characterize phototoxic drug eruptions.

sionally seen, along with an increase in degenerating elastic tissue fibers [13]. The following entities must be considered in the histologic differential diagnosis of a phototoxic drug eruption:

- Dermatomyositis
- Erythema multiforme
- Graft-versus-host disease
- Lupus erythematosus
- Sunburn, idiopathic

Special Studies. Special studies are not required to make a diagnosis of a phototoxic drug eruption.

Pathogenesis. It is believed that the inducing drug is concentrated within the skin and absorbs ultraviolet energy [4]. It has been shown that some drugs such as

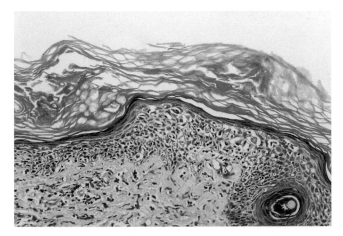

Fig. 24–2. Necrotic keratinocytes are present in phototoxic drug eruptions.

sulfonamides and vinblastin are transformed by exposure to ultraviolet B light, whereas others, such as tetracyclines, nalidixic acid, and phenothiazines, are transformed by ultraviolet A light [14]. These reactions can be oxygen dependent or oxygen independent [5]. Immunologic mechanisms are not believed to play a role in the pathogenesis of phototoxic drug eruptions [5].

Photoallergic Drug Eruptions

Epidemiology. Photoallergic drug eruptions are much less common than are phototoxic reactions [13]. They begin 5–21 days after onset of therapy and generally resolve rapidly with cessation of the inciting drug [4]. Subsequent exposures to the same drug will usually elicit a more rapid and florid cutaneous eruption. Photoallergic drug eruptions may follow ingestion or topical application of the offending agent.

Cutaneous Features. Two types of photoallergic reactions have been described. An immediate urticarial or papulovesicular reaction may occur, as can a more delayed, papular, eczematous eruption [15, 16]. In the acute phase, bullae may form. Lichenoid papules have also been described [1]. The erythematous, often scaly macules and papules are seen predominantly in sun-exposed regions, although in florid cases they will extend onto more sun-protected areas of the skin.

Associated Disorders. The following drugs are commonly associated with photoallergic drug eruptions [1, 4, 6, 17–20]:

- Afloqualone
- Benoxaprofen
- Chlorpromazine
- Griseofulvin
- Ketoprofen
- Nalidixic acid
- Piroxicam
- Psoralens
- Ranitidine
- Sulfonamides
- Tegafur
- Tetracycline
- Thiazides
- Vitamin B_6

Histologic Features. Urticaria-type photoallergic drug eruptions are histologically indistinguishable from other urticarial reactions. Vasodilation (which may be relatively minimal) and papillary dermal edema are the characteristic changes. A relatively sparse, mixed inflammatory infiltrate consisting of neutrophils, eosino-

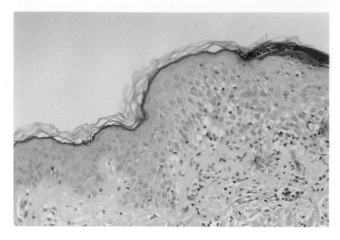

Fig. 24–3. Spongiosis and exocytosis of lymphocytes into the epidermis characterize photoallergic drug eruptions.

phils, and lymphocytes is detected around the vessels of the superficial vascular plexus.

The eczematous type of photoallergic drug eruption demonstrates histologic changes similar to those of other spongiotic dermatoses. Spongiosis within the epidermis, sometimes leading to microvesiculation, is present, and there is an exocytosis of lymphocytes into the overlying epidermis (Fig. 24–3). Eosinophils are characteristically present in increased numbers, enhancing the histologic similarities with allergic contact dermatitis (Fig. 24–4). Within the dermis, there is a superficial perivascular inflammatory infiltrate of lymphocytes and eosinophils centered on the vessels of the superficial vascular plexus. The following entities must be considered in the histologic differential diagnosis of photoallergic drug eruption:

- Arthropod bite reaction
- Contact dermatitis

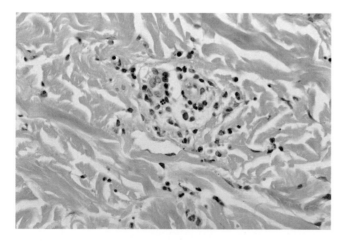

Fig. 24–4. A mixed inflammatory infiltrate with scattered eosinophils is characteristic of the dermal infiltrate in photoallergic drug eruptions.

- Dermatophyte infection
- Nummular dermatitis

Special Studies. Photopatch testing is helpful in proving that a specific drug is the cause of a photoallergic drug eruption, but is rarely employed.

Pathogenesis. Photoallergic drug eruptions are due to cell-mediated hypersensitivity reactions. It is believed that the inducing hapten is a photostable metabolite of the drug, which may combine with some protein within the skin to produce the target of the immunologic reaction [13]. Less light is required to induce a photoallergic reaction than a phototoxic one.

References

1. Wintroub, B. U., and Stern, R., *Cutaneous drug reactions: Pathogenesis and clinical classification.* J Am Acad Dermatol, 1985. 13:167–179.
2. Calnan, C. D., Frain Bell, W., and Cuthbert, J. W., *Occupational dermatitis from chlorpromazine.* Trans St. John's Hosp Derm Soc, 1962. 48:49–74.
3. Halkin, H., *Adverse effects of the fluoroquinolones.* Rev Infect Dis, 1988. 10(Suppl):S258–261.
4. Van Arsdel, P. P. Jr., *Allergy and adverse drug reactions.* J Am Acad Dermatol, 1982. 6:833–845.
5. Gonzalez, E., and Gonzalez, S., *Drug photosensitivity, idiopathic photodermatoses and sunscreens.* J Am Acad Dermatol, 1996. 35:871–885.
6. Tokura, Y., Ogai, M., Yagi, H., and Takigawa, M., *Afloqualone photosensitivity: Immunogenicity of afloqualone-photomodifed epidermal cells.* Photochem Photobiol, 1994. 60:262–267.
7. Layton, A. M., and Cunliffe, W. J., *Phototoxic eruptions due to doxycycline—a dose-related phenomenon.* Clin Exp Dermatol, 1993. 18:425–427.
8. Chandler, M. J., *Recurrence of phototoxic skin eruption due to trimethoprim.* J Infect Dis, 1986. 153:1001.
9. Arata, J., Horio, T., Soejima, R., and Ohara, K., *Photosensitivity reactions caused by lomefloxacin hydrochloride: A multicenter survery.* Antimicrob Agents Chemother, 1998. 42:3141–3145.
10. Encinas, S., Bosca, F., and Miranda, M. A., *Phototoxicity associated with diclofenac: A photophysical, photocehmical, and photobiological study on the drug and its photoproducts.* Chem Res Toxicol, 1998. 11:946–952.
11. Vargas, F., Matskevitch, V., and Sarabia, Z., *Photodegradation and in vitro phototoxicity of the antidiabetic drug chlorpropamide.* Arzneimmittelforschung, 1995. 45:1079–1081.
12. Bergner, T., and Przybilla, B., *Photosensitization caused by ibuprofen.* J Am Acad Dermatol, 1992. 26:114–116.
13. Epstein, J. H., *Phototoxicity and photoallergy in man.* J Am Acad Dermatol, 1983. 8:141–147.
14. Kaidbey, K. H., and Kligman, A. M., *Identification of*

systemic phototoxic drugs by human intradermal assay.
J Invest Dermatol, 1978. 70:272–274.

15. Stork, H., *Photoallergy and photosensitivity.* Arch Dermatol, 1965. 91:469–482.

16. Tanaka, M., Niizeki, H., Shimizu, S., and Miyakawa, S., *Photoallergic drug eruption due to pyridoxine hydrochloride.* J Dermatol, 1996. 23:708–709.

17. Epstein, J. H., *Photoallergy: A review.* Arch Dermatol, 1972. 106:741–748.

18. Bastien, M., Milpied-Homsi, B., Baudot, S., Dutarte, H.,

and Litoux, P., *Keoprofen–induced contact photosensitivity disorders: 5 cases.* Ann Dermatol Venereol, 1997. 124:523–526.

19. Usuki, A., Funasaka, Y., Oka, M., and Ichihashi, M., *Tegafur-induced photosensitivity—evaluation of provocation by UVB irradiation.* Int J Dermatol, 1997. 36:604–606.

20. Todd, P., Norris, P., Hawk, J. L., and Du Vivier, A. W., *Ranitidine-induced photosensitivity.* Clin Exp Dermatol, 1995. 20:146–148.

CHAPTER 25

Chemotherapy-Induced Drug Eruptions

Neutrophilic Eccrine Hidradenitis

Epidemiology. Neutrophilic eccrine hidradenitis is seen most commonly in patients undergoing chemotherapy. Although originally described in patients with acute leukemia receiving cytarabine therapy, the list of associated conditions has increased dramatically. An idiopathic form of the disease, unrelated to chemotherapy or to hematologic proliferative disorders, has been described and is called *idiopathic plantar hidradenitis* [1].

Cutaneous Features. The onset of cutaneous manifestations occurs within 1 to 2 weeks after the initiation of chemotherapy in most patients with neutrophilic eccrine hidradenitis. The eruption may recur after re-exposure to a similar drug [2].

Neutrophilic eccrine hidradenitis demonstrates a variety of morphologic patterns. Multiple erythematous papules and nodules, or fixed erythematous plaques confined to the extremities, are the most common presentations. These papules and plaques are typically quite tender. Other patients may demonstrate erythematous papules in a more widespread distribution, including the trunk and head and neck. Rare patients present with multiple erythema multiforme-like lesions in a generalized pattern involving extremities [2]. The eruption resolves without treatment in 1 to 4 weeks.

Associated Conditions. Neutrophilic eccrine hidradenitis has been associated with many chemotherapeutic agents, including cytarabine, bleomycin, mitox-

antrone, chlorambucil, and zidovudine. Despite the central and peripheral neutropenia associated with these treatments, neutrophils do accumulate around eccrine structures. Neutrophilic eccrine hidradenitis has also been reported in patients taking acetaminophen [3] and after infection [4]. Similar clinical and histologic changes have been described in patients receiving granulocyte colony-stimulating factor [5].

Histologic Features. Neutrophilic eccrine hidradenitis is characterized by a perieccrine infiltrate of neutrophils. In some cases, the inflammatory infiltrate may be quite sparse. Both glands and ducts demonstrate vacuolar degeneration and variable amounts of necrosis of the lining cells (Fig. 25–1). Mucin is often present around the damaged eccrine apparatus [6]. In some patients, apocrine glands may be similarly affected [7].

Another common histologic feature present in biopsy specimens that demonstrate neutrophilic eccrine hidradenitis is a chemotherapy-induced "dysmaturation" within the epidermis. Keratinocytes fail to undergo a normal maturation sequence after administration of some chemotherapeutic agents. This results in a pattern of mild to moderate cytologic atypia within the epidermis. The atypia is not as striking as that seen in most cutaneous keratinocytic neoplasms, but care should be taken not to interpret these changes as true malignant degeneration. These changes are not related to neutrophilic eccrine hidradenitis, per se, but are related to chemotherapy and can be seen in biopsy specimens from all patients who are undergoing such treatment.

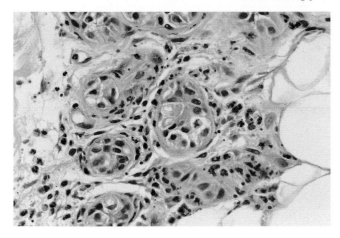

Fig. 25-1. Neutrophils and leukocytoclasis surrounding the eccrine apparatus characterize neutrophilic eccrine hidradenitis. Vacuolar degeneration of cells lining the glands and ducts is present.

Special Studies. Special studies are not required to make a diagnosis of neutrophilic eccrine hidradenitis; however, in some cases, multiple levels through the tissue block may be necessary to demonstrate the perieccrine nature of the neutrophilic infiltrate. As infectious processes may be part of the differential diagnosis, tissue Gram's and periodic acid–Schiff stains may be helpful in establishing the diagnosis.

Pathogenesis. The pathogenesis of neutrophilic eccrine hidradenitis is not known. Some workers have suggested that excretion and concentration of high levels of chemotherapeutic agents by the eccrine apparatus cause a direct toxic effect [7, 8].

Neutrophilic Dermatosis Associated with Granulocyte-Macrophage and Granulocyte Colony-Stimulating Factor

Epidemiology. Cutaneous reactions to granulocyte-macrophage colony-stimulating factor (GM-CSF) appear to be common. They can present as localized eruptions at the site of injection or as diffuse macular and papular eruptions [9]. Although not actually chemotherapeutic, GM-CSF and granulocyte colony-stimulating factor (GCSF) are used in conjunction with chemotherapeutic agents in order to hasten leukocyte recovery.

Cutaneous Features. A diffuse eruption of macules and papules occurs within 3–4 days of starting GM-CSF therapy [10]. This eruption may resolve with desquamation. The eruption resolves within 2 weeks of discontinuing therapy [9, 10]. In some patients, the papules are arranged in an annular configuration resembling granuloma annulare. There is occasionally an overlying scale [11]. Other patients receiving GM-CSF

experience a generalized erythroderma [12]. Both GCSF and GM-CSF have been associated with localized reactions at injection sites [9].

Associated Conditions. Treatments with GM-CSF is often associated with myalgia, fever, and bone pain. Less commonly, patients may develop autoimmune thyroiditis, bone marrow histiocytosis, and multiple myeloma [9].

Histologic Features. Histologic changes associated with GM-CSF are well documented [9]. The earliest changes include an infiltrate of lymphocytes and eosinophils into the papillary dermis, accompanied by mild edema (Fig. 25–2). Scattered, enlarged macrophages are also seen in biopsy specimens from early lesions. In some patients, neutrophils may be present in greater numbers than eosinophils. Nuclear dust is frequently present (Figs. 25–3 and 25–4). Basal layer vacuolization and mild spongiosis are seen in many cases. A slight lymphocytic exocytosis may also be present. Rare dying keratinocytes have been reported. Small amounts of dermal mucin may be seen in the papillary dermis and epidermis [10]. One week into treatment, the infiltration of dermal macrophages becomes much more striking, and pale staining intracytoplasmic elastin is present within these markedly enlarged cells (Fig. 25–5). The following entities must be considered in the histologic differential diagnosis of a GM-CSF–induced neutrophilic dermatosis:

- Leukemia cutis
- Leukocytoclastic vasculitis
- Palisaded and neutrophilic dermatosis of rheumatoid arthritis
- Pyoderma gangrenosum
- Sweet's syndrome

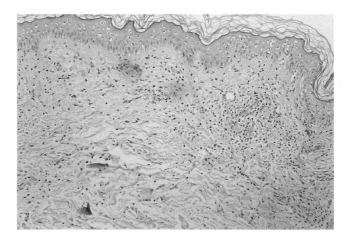

Fig. 25-2. Early lesions of GM-CSF–associated eruption demonstrate a mixed dermal infiltrate with mild papillary dermal edema.

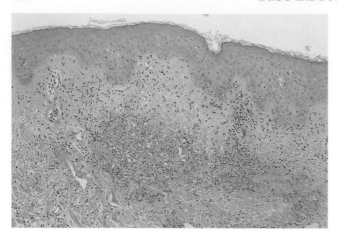

Fig. 25–3. A dense neutrophilic infiltrate is present in well-developed lesions of GM-CSF–associated eruption.

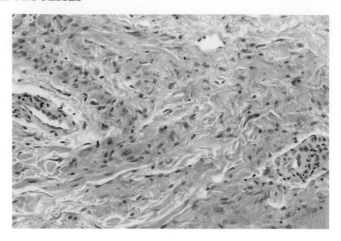

Fig. 25–5. Late lesions of GM-CSF–associated eruptions are characterized by collections of large histiocytes, giving a granulomatous appearance to the dermal infiltrate.

In a minority of patients with an eruption induced by GM-CSF, the inflammatory infiltrate is devoid of polymorphonuclear leukocytes and is composed entirely of lymphocytes and enlarged macrophages [11]. In some cases, the macrophages contain ingested elastin fibers [9].

Histologic changes seen with GCSF are slightly different. Biopsy material taken from affected skin demonstrates a spongiotic epidermis and an infiltrate of plump, enlarged macrophages within the papillary dermis [11]. Sparse lymphocytes are present around the superficial vascular plexus, and neutrophils are only variably present.

Special Studies. There are no special studies that help in making a diagnosis of GM-CSF–induced eruption.

Pathogenesis. High concentrations of GM-CSF in the skin may induce cytokine production, leading to activa-

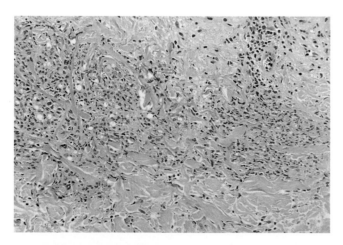

Fig. 25–4. Abundant karyorrhectic debris, neutrophils, and scattered histiocytes are present in well-developed lesions of GM-CSF–associated eruptions.

tion of macrophages and induction of chemotaxis. This hypothesis is supported by reports of upregulation of ELAM-1 (expression of a leukocyte-adhesion molecule 1), VCAM-1 (vascular cell adhesion marker), interleukin-1, and tumor necrosis factor-α in patients receiving GM-CSF [11]. Alternatively, GM-CSF and GCSF may be directly responsible for inducing neutrophil chemotaxis, independent of cytokine upregulation.

Acral Erythema

Epidemiology. Acral erythema is most frequently described in patients undergoing treatment with chemotherapy. It is most common in adults, but has been described in children [13]. The incidence of this condition is difficult to assess, but has been estimated as being between 6% and 42% of patients receiving chemotherapy [14–16]. The reaction occurs days to weeks after high-dose chemotherapy, but may not appear for many months after long-term, low-dose treatment [17].

Cutaneous Features. A prodrome of dysesthesia frequently precedes the onset of abrupt erythema and swelling. Both pain and a tingling sensation have been described. The finger pads of the distal phalanges are most severely affected. Areas of sparing may be present in some patients, and the erythema may extend onto the dorsal surfaces of the hands. Over the ensuing 1 to 2 weeks, the erythematous plaques resolve by desquamating [17]. Rarely, blisters occur over areas of pressure and trauma. A mild, morbilliform eruption on the trunk, head, and neck may accompany the acral changes [18].

Associated Conditions. Acral erythema occurs in patients receiving chemotherapy. It is most frequently associated with cytarabine, but also occurs in patients receiving methotrexate, hydroxyurea, mercaptopurine, cyclophosphamide, and mitotane [17]. The most frequent underlying condition is acute myelogenous leukemia [19].

Similar acral erythemas have been described after viral infections, with connective tissue diseases, and with human immunodeficiency virus [20]. It remains to be determined if the pathogenesis of the acral changes is the same in all of these conditions. It has been suggested that the increased incidence of acral erythema may be related to the popular use of GCSF, which enables the use of higher doses of chemotherapy [21].

Histologic Features. Histologic changes in acral erythema are nonspecific. Basal vacuolar degeneration of the epidermis is usually present, as is spongiosis. Scattered dying keratinocytes are present in most cases. There is a superficial perivascular lymphocytic inflammatory infiltrate accompanied by papillary dermal edema [19, 22]. The eccrine apparatus does not demonstrate histologic changes [17]. The following entities must be considered in the histologic differential diagnosis of acral erythema:

- Contact dermatitis
- Dyshidrotic dermatosis
- Erythema multiforme
- Gianotti-Crosti syndrome
- Graft-versus-host disease
- Lupus erythematosus
- Perniosis
- Polymorphous light eruption

Special Studies. Special studies are not required to make a diagnosis of acral erythema.

Pathogenesis. Direct toxic effects of chemotherapy on eccrine coils have been postulated as the cause of acral erythema [17].

Syringosquamous Metaplasia

Epidemiology. Eccrine squamous syringometaplasia has been reported in patients receiving any of a large number of chemotherapeutic agents for various types of cancer. The finding has not been associated with any particular drug regimen or type of tumor [23]. In one study, the cutaneous eruption began about 2 weeks after the onset of chemotherapy and resolved without scarring in 7–10 days [23].

Cutaneous Features. The usual presentation in patients with eccrine squamous syringometaplasia is that of asymptomatic, 1–3 mm erythematous papules and plaques, often limited to the extremities [23]. The papules may resemble miliaria. Less commonly, vesicles may be present, and the process may become generalized. Involvement of intertriginous areas by edematous, erythematous plaques has also been reported [23].

Associated Conditions. Eccrine squamous syringometaplasia occurs most frequently in the setting of patients undergoing chemotherapy for hematologic disorders, including Hodgkin's lymphoma, non-Hodgkin's lymphoma, acute myelogenous or lymphocytic leukemia, multiple myeloma, and myelodysplastic syndrome. Cytarabine is the most frequently implicated drug [6]. It has also been described in a patient with Ewing's sarcoma [23]. The condition has been described after bone marrow transplantation [24]. Eccrine squamous syringometaplasia has been reported to occur in association with acral erythema [25]. Eccrine squamous syringometaplasia may be an incidental finding.

Histologic Features. The invariable histologic finding in eccrine squamous metaplasia is squamous metaplasia of the eccrine ducts. The overlying epidermis frequently demonstrates basal vacuolization, interface dermatitis, and keratinocyte apoptosis. In a minority of cases, the epidermis is acanthotic. Cytologic atypia is often present within the metaplastic eccrine duct cells and may be extensive enough to resemble squamous cell carcinoma [6] (Figs. 25–6 and 25–7). There is cornification present within the ducts and into the acrosyringium. Surrounding the affected eccrine coils is a moderately intense lymphohistiocytic infiltrate that may be granulomatous when there is extensive keratinization. A loose fibroblastic stroma is present around the eccrine coils. The process does not involve eccrine

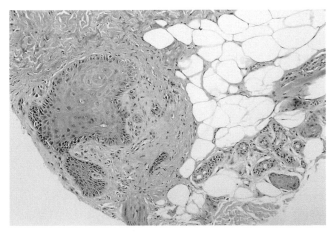

Fig. 25–6. Squamous metaplasia of the eccrine ducts is seen in syringosquamous metaplasia associated with chemotherapy.

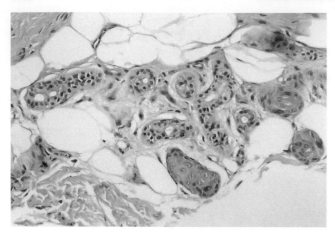

Fig. 25–7. Squamous metaplasia of an eccrine duct is seen in syringosquamous metaplasia related to chemotherapy.

glands. The following entities must be considered in the histologic differential diagnosis of eccrine squamous metaplasia:

- Neutrophilic eccrine hidradenitis
- Pressure necrosis
- Squamous cell carcinoma

Special Studies. There are no special studies that help make the diagnosis of eccrine squamous syringometaplasia.

Pathogenesis. It has been suggested that some chemotherapeutic agents concentrate in sweat glands and produce a locally toxic effect [26]. Others have documented eccrine excretion of alkylating agents [27].

References

1. Stahr, B. J., Cooper, P. H., and Caputo, R. V., *Idiopathic plantar hidradenitis: A neutrophilic eccrine hidradenitis occurring primarily in children.* J Cutan Pathol, 1994. 21:289–296.
2. Bernstein, E. F., Spielvogel, R. L., and Topolsky, D. L., *Recurrent neutrophilic eccrine hidradenitis.* Br J Dermatol, 1992. 127:529–533.
3. Kuttner, B. J., and Kurban, R. S., *Neutrophilic eccrine hidradenitis in the absence of underlying malignancy.* Cutis, 1988. 41:403–405.
4. Allegue, F., Rocamora, A., Martin-Gonzalez, M., Alonso, M. L., and Ledo, A., *Infectious eccrine hidradenitis.* J Am Acad Dermatol, 1985. 22:119–120.
5. Bachmeyer, C., Chaibi, P., and Aractingi, S., *Neutrophilic eccrine hidradenitis induced by granulocyte colony-stimulating factor.* Br J Dermatol, 1998. 139:354–355.
6. Fitzpatrick, J., *The cutaneous histopathology of chemotherapeutic reactions.* J Cutan Pathol, 1993. 20:1–14.
7. Brehler, R., Reimann, S., Bonsmann, G., and Metze, D., *Neutrophilic hidradenitis induced by chemotherapy involves eccrine and apocrine glands.* Am J Dermatopathol, 1997. 19:73–78.
8. Flynn, T. C., Harrist, T. J., Murphy, G. F., and Mihm, M. C. Jr., *Neutrophilic eccrine hidradenitis: A distinctive rash associated with cytarabine therapy and acute leukemia.* J Am Acad Dermatol, 1984. 11:584–590.
9. Scott, G. A., *Report of three cases of cutaneous reactions to granulocyte macrophage-colony-stimulating factor and a review of the literature.* Am J Dermatopathol, 1995. 17:107–114.
10. Horn, T. D., Burke, P. J., Karp, J. E., and Hood, A. F., *Intravenous administration of recombinant granulocyte-macrophage colony-stimulating factor causes a cutaneous eruption.* Arch Dermatol, 1991. 127:49–52.
11. Glass, L. F., Fotopoulos, T., and Messina, J. L., *A generalized cutaneous reaction induced by granulocyte colony-stimulating factor.* J Am Acad Dermatol, 1996. 34:455–459.
12. Mehregan, D. R., Fransway, A. F., and Edmonston, J. E., *Cutaneous reactions to granulocyte-monocyte colony-stimulating factor.* Arch Dermatol, 1992. 128:1055–1059.
13. Burke, M. C., Bernhard, J. D., and Michelson, A. D., *Chemotherapy-induced painful acral erythema in chilhood: Burgdorf's reaction.* Am J Pediatr Hematol Oncol, 1989. 11:44–55.
14. Lokich, J. J., and Moore, C., *Chemotherapy-associated palmar-plantar erythrodysesthesia syndrome.* Ann Intern Med, 1984. 101:798–800.
15. Peters, W. G., and Willemze, R., *Palmar-plantar skin changes and cytarabine.* Ann Intern Med, 1985. 103:805.
16. Vogelzang, N. J., and Ratain, M. J., *Cancer chemotherapy and skin changes.* Ann Intern Med, 1985. 103:303–304.
17. Baack, B. R., and Burgdorf, W. H. C., *Chemotherapy-induced acral erythema.* J Am Acad Dermatol, 1991. 24:457–461.
18. Kroll, S. S., Koller, C. A., Koled, S., and Dreizen, S., *Chemotherapy-induced acral erythema: Desquamating lesions involving the hands and feet.* Ann Plast Surg, 1989. 23:263–265.
19. Demicray, Z., Gurbuz, O., Alpdogan, T. B., Yucelten, D., Alpdogan, O., Kurtkaya, O., and Bayik, M., *Chemotherapy-induced acral erythema in leukemic patients: A report of 15 cases.* Int J Dermatol, 1997. 36:593–598.
20. Barzegar, C., Dubreuil, M. L., Revuz, J., and Cosnes, A., *Acral erythema and HIV infection.* Ann Dermatol Venereol, 1998. 125:595–597.
21. Komamura, H., Higashiyama, M., Hashimoto, K., Takeda, K., Kimura, H., Tani, Y., Ogawa, H., et al., *Three cases of chemotherapy-induced acral erythema.* J Dermatol, 1995. 22:116–121.
22. Levine, L. E., Medenica, M. M., Lorinez, A. L., Soltani, K., Raab, B., and Ma, A., *Distinctive acral erythema oc-*

curring during therapy for severe myelogenous leukemia. Arch Dermatol, 1985. 121:102–104.

23. Valks, R., Fraga, J., Porras-Luque, J., Figuera, A., Garcia-Diez, A., and Fernandez-Herrera, J., *Chemotherapy-induced eccrine squamous syringometaplasia. A distinctive eruption in patients receiving hematopoietic progenitor cells.* Arch Dermatol, 1997. 133:873–878.

24. Horn, T. D., *Antineoplastic chemotherapy, sweat and the skin.* Arch Dermatol, 1997. 133:905–906.

25. Rongioletti, F., Ballestrero, A., Bogliolo, F., and Rebora, A., *Necrotizing eccrine squamous syringometaplasia presenting as acral erythema.* J Cutan Pathol, 1991. 18:453–456.

26. Johnson, H. L., and Maibach, H. I., *Drug excretion in human eccrine sweat.* J Invest Dermatol, 1971. 56:182–188.

27. Horn, T. D., Beveridge, R. A., Egorin, M.J., Abeloff, M. J., and Hood, A. F., *Observations and proposed mechanisms in N, N′, N′-triethylene-phospamide (thiotepa)-induced hyperpigmentation.* Arch Dermatol, 1989. 125:524–527.

CHAPTER 26

Miscellaneous Drug Eruptions

Acute Generalized Exanthematous Pustulosis

Epidemiology. Acute generalized exanthematous pustulosis (AGEP) is a cutaneous eruption that is most commonly associated with antibiotic ingestion. β-Lactams are the most frequently implicated drugs in causing this type of eruption [1]. In one series, 80% of cases were associated with antibiotic usage [2]. The eruption is self-limited and resolves rapidly upon cessation of the drug. People of any age can be affected, and there is no gender predilection.

Cutaneous Features. Acute generalized exanthematous pustulosis is characterized by the rapid onset of less than 5 mm disseminated pustules within 24 hours after ingestion of the offending agent. The pustules arise on erythematous bases. Less commonly, purpuric, or erythema multiforme-like, lesions may be seen, and areas of edema are often present [1]. A positive Nikolsky's sign is often present [3]. The face and intertriginous areas are the most commonly affected sites. Most patients have more than 100 pustules [2]. Pustules resolve within 15 days.

Associated Disorders. Acute generalized exanthematous pustulosis is accompanied by acute onset of fever [1]. Leukocytosis is present in most patients and can be characterized by marked neutrophilia or eosinophilia. Hypocalcemia, related to hypoalbuminemia, is present in most patients with AGEP [2]. In one series, one-third of affected patients had renal failure [2].

Approximately 87% of cases of AGEP are associated with drug ingestion [2]. Some of the drugs implicated in causing AGEP are listed in Table 26–1. Several types of viral infection, including coxsackie virus B4 [4], enteroviruses [2], and cytomegalovirus [5], have been associated with AGEP.

Histologic Features. The major histologic finding of AGEP is the presence of subcorneal pustules. Surrounding spongiosis is present, with accompanying papillary dermal edema (Figs. 26–1 and 26–2). There is a superficial perivascular inflammatory infiltrate, characterized by lymphocytes, neutrophils, and eosinophils in about one-third of cases. Focal keratinocyte necrosis is seen in about 25% of cases [2]. The following entities must be considered in the histologic differential diagnosis of AGEP:

- Candidiasis
- Gonococcemia
- Impetigo
- Infantile acropustulosis
- Pustular psoriasis
- Subcorneal pustular dermatosis
- Transient neonatal pustular melanosis

Special Studies. Special studies are not required to make a diagnosis of AGEP. In some cases, patients with AGEP

Table 26–1. Drugs Implicated in Inducing Acute
Generalized Exanthematous Pustulosis

Acetazolamide	Itraconazole
Acetaminophen	Mercury
Acetylsalicylic acid	Metronidazole
Amoxacillin	Minocycline
Amoxapine	Nadoxolol
Ampicillin	Nifedipine
Bufexamac	Nifuroxazide
Carbamazepine	Nystatin
Carbutamide	Paracetamol
Cefaclor	Penicillin
Chromium picolinate	Progesterone
Clobazam	Quinidine
Clozapine	Roxithromycin
Diltiazem	Sulbutamide
Doxycycline	Sulfasalazine
Erythromycin	Terbinafine
Hydroxychloroquine	Vancomycin

From references 2 and 19–35.

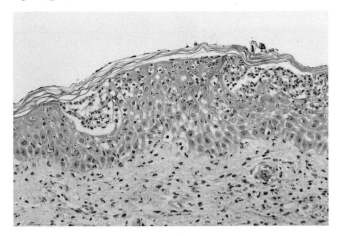

Fig. 26–2. Higher magnification demonstrates a subcorneal vacuole filled with neutrophils in acute generalized exanthematous pustulosis.

are febrile and may appear quite ill. Special stains for fungi and bacteria may be helpful in ruling out infectious causes.

Pathogenesis. It has been postulated that AGEP is an evolving process in which neutrophils localize around vessels in the superficial plexus in the initial stages. Papillary edema is the next stage, which then progresses to spongiosis and neutrophilic pustules within the epidermis [6]. It has been suggested that AGEP represents a delayed-type hypersensitivity reaction [7].

Drug-Induced Pseudolymphomas

Epidemiology. A disseminated drug eruption resembling mycosis fungoides or other types of cutaneous

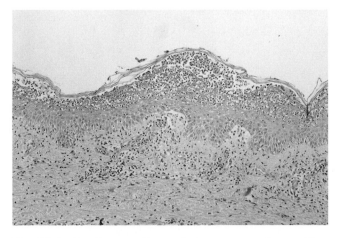

Fig. 26–1. A subcorneal pustule is present, along with a superficial perivascular infiltrate, in acute generalized exanthematous pustulosis.

lymphoma has been described, primarily in patients taking phenytoin or other anticonvulsants [8, 9]. This complication is extremely uncommon in this group of patients. It is seen equally in men and women and occurs in patients of all ages. In some series, this complication is more prevalent in black patients [10].

Cutaneous Features. In the pseudolymphoma associated with phenytoin, patients develop an exfoliative erythroderma [8]. Other patients develop isolated erythematous plaques or coalescent papules. The cutaneous eruption evolves months after therapy is begun. It should be noted that patients taking phenytoin or any of the other medications implicated in the "pseudolymphoma"-like presentation can also give rise to a drug-induced hypersensitivity syndrome. In these patients, there may be marked systemic symptoms, but a dense, "pseudolymphomatous" infiltrate is not noted in skin biopsy material.

The presence of isolated, erythematous nodules has also been described in patients taking anticonvulsant medications for months [9]. Less commonly, pustules, vesicles, and a morbilliform eruption may be present [10]. There is a predilection for acral sites of involvement in this group of patients.

Associated Disorders. Patients with phenytoin-induced pseudolymphoma may also develop lymphadenopathy and hepatosplenomegaly. Peripheral eosinophilia is also found in many of these patients [8]. Hepatitis may be present [11]. Some patients have accompanying fever, malaise, myalgias, arthralgias, and headaches [12]. Mild anemia and leukocytosis have also been reported [13]. Rare patients may also have nephritis or pneumonitis [14].

It has been suggested that patients with anticonvulsant-induced pseudolymphomas may be at higher

Table 26–2. Drugs Associated with Dense Lymphoid Infiltrates

Anticonvulsants	Antihistamines
Carbamazepine	Antidepressants
Diltiazem	Amitryptiline
Mesantoin	Clomipramine
Phenytoin	Fluoxetine
Phenobarbitol	Miscellaneous
Phenothiazines	Allpurinol
Primidone	Amiloride
Antihypertensives	Cyclosporine
β-Blockers	D-penicillamine
Calcium channel blockers	Gold
Angiotensin-converting	
enzyme inhibitors	

From references 8, 9, 13, 16, and 36–42.

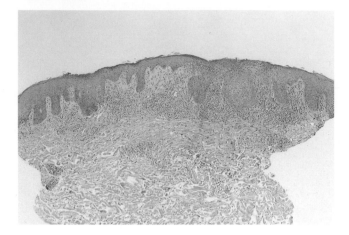

Fig. 26–3. Anticonvulsant-induced pseudolymphoma demonstrates a dense, band-like lymphocytic infiltrate with epidermotropism.

risk for subsequently developing lymphoma [10, 11]. Table 26–2 lists drugs that have been associated with cutaneous lymphoid reactions.

Histologic Features. Histologic features of the phenytoin-induced pseudolymphoma include the presence of Pautrier-like microabscesses within the epidermis. Spongiotic microvesicles are also present within the epidermis. The upper portion of the epidermis contains a dense infiltrate of lymphocytes that often demonstrate cytologic atypia (Fig. 26–3). The nuclei are enlarged and hyperconvoluted [8] (Fig. 26–4). The following entities must be considered in the histologic differential diagnosis of this pattern of atypical lymphoid infiltrate:

- Actinic reticuloid
- Gianotti-Crosti syndrome
- Lymphomatoid papulosis
- Mycosis fungoides
- Spongiotic dermatitis

Lymph nodes may demonstrate follicular hyperplasia, sinus histiocytosis, and the presence of similar-appearing atypical lymphocytes [15].

The nodular pattern of anticonvulsant-related pseudolymphoma is characterized by a dense dermal infiltrate of lymphocytes, with focal extension of the infiltrate into the overlying epidermis (Fig. 26–5). There is an admixture of small and large lymphocytes and histiocytes that extend deep in the reticular dermis and into the subcutaneous fat (Fig. 26–6). Extension of the atypical lymphocytes into follicular epithelium is a frequent finding [16]. Eosinophils are present in small amounts in most cases, but are not essential for making the diagnosis. The following entities must be con-

sidered in the differential diagnosis of this pattern of atypical lymphoid infiltrate:

- Arthropod bite reaction
- Follicular center cell lymphoma
- Jessner's lymphocytic infiltrate
- Lymphocytoma cutis
- Lymphomatoid papulosis
- Persistent nodular scabetic reaction

Special Studies. Immunophenotyping reveals the predominant dermal lymphocyte to be a T cell, with an admixture of CD4-positive and CD8-positive cells in cases that histologically and clinically simulate mycosis fungoides. The cases that are histologically more similar to B-cell lymphomas demonstrate a predominantly

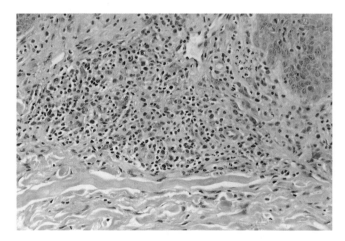

Fig. 26–4. Higher magnification demonstrates a mixed population of lymphocytes, some of which are large and atypical in anticonvulsant-induced pseudolymphoma.

B-cell infiltrate [16]. CD30-positive lymphocytes have been described in patients with a carbamazepine-associated lymphoid reaction [14]. Electron microscopic examination of the lymphocytes seen in the phenytoin-induced pseudolymphoma demonstrates marked nuclear hyperconvolution with cells showing a similarity to the Lutzner's cells seen in mycosis fungoides [15].

Pathogenesis. It has been proposed that a dysregulatory state, caused by depression of T-suppressor lymphocyte function, is the pathogenesis of these drug-induced lymphoid reactions [17, 18]. It has also been speculated that patients who have a deficiency in epoxide hydrolase are not able to rapidly degrade the offending agents. The increased levels of breakdown products stimulate an immune response [14].

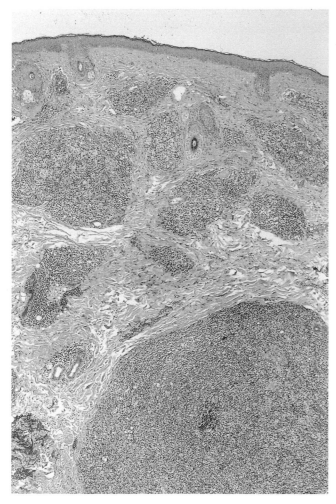

Fig. 26–5. Anticonvulsant-induced pseudolymphoma demonstrates a superficial and deep nodular infiltrate of lymphocytes extending into the deep reticular dermis.

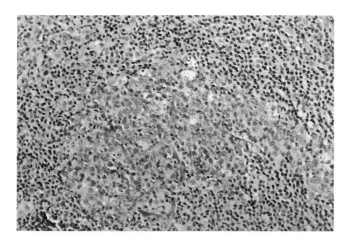

Fig. 26–6. A germinal center is present within the dense dermal infiltrate of lymphocytes in anticonvulsant-induced pseudolymphoma.

References

1. Beylot, C., Doutre, M. S., and Beylot-Barry, M., *Acute generalized exanthematous pustulosis.* Semin Cutan Med Surg, 1996. 15:244–249.
2. Roujeau, J. C., Bioulac-Sage, P., Bourseau, C., Guillaume, J. C., Bernard, P., Lok, C., Plantin, P., Claudy, A., et al., *Acute generalized exanthematous pustulosis. Analysis of 63 cases.* Arch Dermatol, 1991. 127:1333–1338.
3. Manders, S. M., and Heymann, W. R., *Acute generalized exanthematic pustulosis.* Cutis, 1994. 54:194–196.
4. Feio, A. B., Apetato, M., Costa, M. M., Sa, J., and Alcantara, J., *Acute generalized exanthematous pustulosis due to Coxsackie B4 virus.* Acta Med Port, 1997. 10:487–491.
5. Haro-Gabaldon, V., Sanchez-Sanchez-Vizcaino, J., Ruiz-Avila, P., Gutierrez-Fenandex, J., Linares, J., and Naranjo-Sintes, R., *Acute generalized exanthematous pustulosis with cytomegalovirus infection.* Int J Dermatol, 1996. 35:735–737.
6. Burrows, N. P., and Russell Jones, R., *Pustular drug eruptions: A histopathologic spectrum.* Histopathology, 1993. 22:569–573.
7. Kuchler, A., Hamm, H., Weidenthaler-Barth, B., Kampgen, E., and Brocker, E.-B., *Acute generalized exanthematous pustulosis following oral nystatin therapy: A report of three cases.* Br J Dermatol, 1997. 137:808–811.
8. Rosenthal, C. J., Noguera, C. A., Coppola, A., and Kapelner, S. N., *Pseudolymphoma with mycosis fungoides manifestations, hyperresponsiveness to diphenylhydantoin and lymphocyte disregulation.* Cancer, 1982. 49:2305–2314.
9. Sigal-Nahum, M., Petit, A., Gaulier, A., Torrent, J., Mourier, C., and Karmochkine, M., *A nodular cutaneous lymphoproliferative disorder during carbamazepine administration.* Br J Dermatol, 1992. 127:545–547.
10. Harris, D. W. S., Ostlere, L., Buckley, C., Whittaker, S., Sweny, P., and Rustin, M. H. A., *Phenytoin-induced*

pseudolymphoma. A report of a case and review of the literature. Br J Dermatol, 1992. 127:403–406.

11. D'Incan, M., Souteyrand, P., Bignon, Y. J., Fonck, Y., and Roger, H., *Hydantoin-induced cutaneous pseudolymphoma with clinical, pathologic, and immunologic aspects of Sezary syndrome.* Arch Dermatol, 1992. 128:1371–1374.

12. Kramlinger, K. G., Phillips, K. A., and Post, R. M., *Rash complication carbamazepine treatment.* J Clin Psychopharmacol, 1994. 14:408–413.

13. Schreiber, M. M., and McGregor, J. G., *Pseudolymphoma syndrome. A sensitivity to anticonvulsant drugs.* Arch Dermatol, 1968. 97:297–300.

14. Nathan, D. L., and Belsito, D. V., *Carbamazepine-induced pseudolymphoma with CD30 positive cells.* J Am Acad Dermatol, 1998. 38:806–809.

15. Wolf, R., Kahane, E., and Sandbank, M., *Mycosis fungoides-like lesions associated with phenytoin therapy.* Arch Dermatol, 1985. 121:1181–1182.

16. Crowson, A. N., and Magro, C. M., *Antidepressant therapy. A possible cause of atypical cutaneous lymphoid hyperplasia.* Arch Dermatol, 1995. 131:925–929.

17. Dosch, H.-M., Jason, J., and Gelfand, E. W., *Transient antibody deficiency and abnormal T-suppressor cells induced by phenytoin.* N Engl J Med, 1982. 306:406–409.

18. Bluming, A., Homer, S., and Khiroya, R., *Selective diphenylhydantoin-induced suppression of lymphocyte reactivity in vitro.* J Lab Clin Med, 1976. 88:417–422.

19. Watsky, K. L., *Acute generalized exanthematous pustulosis induced by metronidazole: The role of patch testing.* Arch Dermatol, 1999. 135:93–94.

20. Jan, V., Machet, L., Gironet, N., Martin, L., Machet, M. C., Lorette, G., and Vaillant, L., *Acute generalized exanthematous pustulosis induced by diltiazem: Value of patch testing.* Dermatology, 1998. 197:274–275.

21. Kuno, Y., and Tsuji, T., *Acute generalized exanthematous pustulosis upon ingestion of a progesterone preparation.* Acta Derm Venereol, 1998. 78:383.

22. Bosonnet, S., Dandurand, M., Moati, L., and Guillot, B., *Acute generalized exanthemic pustulosis after intake of clozapine (leponex). First case.* Ann Dermatol Venereol, 1997. 124:547–548.

23. Rosenberger, A., Tebbe, B., Treudler, R., and Orfanos, C. E., *Acute generalized exanthematous pustulosis, induced by nystatin.* Hautarzt, 1998. 49:492–495.

24. Condon, C. A., Downs, A. M., and Archer, C. B., *Terbinafine-induced acute generalized exanthematous pustulosis.* Br J Dermatol, 1998. 138:709–710.

25. Loche, F., Durieu, C., and Bazex, J., *Acute generalized exanthematous pustulosis induced by amoxapine.* Acta Derm Venereol, 1998. 78:224.

26. Leger, F., Machet, L., Jan, V., Machet, C., Lorette, G., and Vaillant, L., *Acute generalized exanthematous pustulosis associated with paracetamol.* Acta Derm Venereol, 1998. 78:222–223.

27. Machet, L., Jan, V., Machet, M. C., Lorette, G., and Vaillant, L., *Acute generalized exanthematous pustulosis induced by nifuroxazide.* Contact Dermatitis, 1997. 36:308–309.

28. Park, Y. M., Kim, J. W., and Kim, C. W., *Acute generalized exanthematous pustulosis induced by itraconazole.* J Am Acad Dermatol, 1997. 36:794–796.

29. Yamamato, T., and Minatohara, K., *Minocycline-induced acute generalized exanthematous pustulosis in a patient with generalized pustular psoriasis showing elevated level of sELAM-1.* Acta Derm Venereol, 1997. 77:168–169.

30. Assier-Bonnet, H., Saada, V., Bernier, M., Clerici, T., and Saiaig, P., *Acute generalized exanthematous pustulosis induced by hydroxychloroquine.* Dermatology, 1996. 193:70–71.

31. Ballmer-Weber, B. K., Widmer, M., and Burg, G., *Acetylsalicylic acid-induced generalized pustulosis.* Schweiz Med Wochenschr, 1993. 123:542–546.

32. Marce, S., Schaweverbeke, T., Bannwarth, B., Marty, L., and Dehais, J., *Generalized acute exanthematous pustulosis after ingestion of sulfasalazine.* Presse Med, 1993. 22:271.

33. Trueb, R. M., and Burg, G., *Acute generalized exanthematous pustulosis due to doxycycline.* Dermatology, 1993. 186:75–78.

34. Ogoshi, M., Yamada, Y., and Tani, M., *Acute generalized exanthematic pustulosis induced by cefaclor and acetazolamide.* Dermatology, 1992. 184:142–144.

35. Young, P. C., Turiansky, G. W., Bonner, M. W., and Benson, P. M., *Acute generalized exanthematous pustulosis inducecd by chromium picolinate.* J Am Acad Dermatol, 1999. 41:820–823.

36. Raymond, J. Z., and Goldman, H. M., *An unusual cutaneous reaction secondary to allopurinol.* Cutis, 1988. 41:323–326.

37. Brown, M. D., Ellis, C. N., Billings, J., Cooper, K. D., Baadsgaard, O., Headington, J. T., and Voorhees, J. J., *Rapid occurrence of nodular cutaneous T-cell infiltrates with cyclosporine therapy.* Arch Dermatol, 1988. 124:1097–1100.

38. Magro, C. M., and Crowson, A. N., *Drugs with antihistaminic properties as a cause of atypical cutaneous lymphoid hyperplasia.* J Am Acad Dermatol, 1995. 32:419–428.

39. Handfield-Jones, S. E., Jenkins, R. E., Whittaker, S. J., Besse, C. P., and McGibbon, D. H., *The anticonvulsant hypersensitivity syndorme.* Br J Dermatol, 1992. 129:175–177.

40. Kalimo, K., Rasanen, L., Aho, H., Maki, J., Pekka Mustikkamaki, U., and Rantala, I., *Persistent cutaneous pseudolymphoma after intradermal gold injection.* J Cutan Pathol, 1996. 23:328–334.

41. Gupta, A. K., Cooper, K. C., Ellis, C. N., Nickoloff, B. J., Hanson, C. A., Brown, M. D., and Voorhes, J. J., *Lymphocytic infiltrates of the skin in association with cyclosporine therapy.* J Am Acad Dermatol, 1990. 23:1137–1141.

42. Callot, V., Roujeau, J.-C., Bagot, M., Wechsler, J., Chosidow, O., Souteyrand, P., Morel, P., Dubertret, L., et al., *Drug-induced pseudolymphoma and hypersensitivity syndrome. Two different clinical entities.* Arch Dermatol, 1996. 132:1315–1321.

PART VI

Internal Malignant Neoplasms and Skin Diseases

CHAPTER 27

Cutaneous Neoplasms and Cysts Associated with Internal Malignancy

Muir-Torre Syndrome

Epidemiology. Muir-Torre syndrome is the constellation of multiple cutaneous neoplasms occurring in conjunction with low-grade visceral neoplasms [1]. The definition of the syndrome is the occurrence of at least one sebaceous neoplasm (excluding sebaceous hyperplasia and nevus sebaceus of Jadassohn) and one visceral cancer [1]. Either the cutaneous sebaceous neoplasm or the visceral malignancy may occur first. Although it is difficult to gauge the frequency of this relationship, in one retrospective study, 42% of patients diagnosed as having sebaceous adenoma, sebaceous carcinoma, or sebaceous epithelioma over a 60 year period had one or more primary visceral malignancies [2]. In another study, 61% of patients with Muir-Torre syndrome had a positive family history [3]. Muir-Torre syndrome is inherited in an autosomal dominant manner with a high degree of penetrance [3, 4]. There is a slight female predominance, and the syndrome becomes manifest primarily in middle-aged adults. Patients with Muir-Torre syndrome tend to have a relatively favorable prognosis after the appearance of the visceral malignancy.

Cutaneous Features. The cutaneous neoplasms that are associated with Muir-Torre syndrome include sebaceous tumors such as adenomas, epitheliomas, and carcinomas. Many patients will have only a solitary sebaceous neoplasm, but it is common to observe multiple such neoplasms in affected patients. These can number in the hundreds in rare patients.

Sebaceous adenoma is the most frequent cutaneous neoplasm associated with the Muir-Torre syndrome. These tumors are flesh-colored to yellow papules or nodules. In patients with Muir-Torre syndrome, sebaceous adenomas occur more frequently on the trunk than on the head and neck, whereas in patients with sporadic-appearing sebaceous neoplasms, most are concentrated on the head and neck [5]. The tumors are usually less than 1 cm in diameter, but can be greater than 5 cm in rare cases. Some sebaceous adenomas will have an obvious central keratotic pore, giving an appearance similar to that of keratoacanthoma.

Sebaceous epitheliomas are also commonly seen in patients with Muir-Torre syndrome. These tumors may also have a yellow color and have been reported to clinically resemble both basal cell carcinomas and keratoacanthomas. These tumors are most common on the head and neck and are usually less than 1 cm in diameter.

Sebaceous carcinomas occur in patients with Muir-Torre syndrome. Most of these tumors occur in association with the meibomian gland, but extraocular sebaceous carcinomas can also occur. These tumors occur in middle-aged to elderly patients and are more common in men [6]. In general, sebaceous carcinomas have a high rate of metastasis, but those occurring in patients with Muir-Torre syndrome appear to metastasize less frequently [3, 6].

Sebaceoma is a controversial term; some use it to designate a sebaceous epithelioma [1] and others to designate a distinct histologic entity [7]. In either case, it is important to note that this neoplasm is also a marker for Muir-Torre syndrome. These neoplasms present as yellow-orange papules or nodules, most commonly on the face or scalp [7].

Large studies of patients with sebaceous hyperplasia have found no evidence of increased incidence of gastrointestinal carcinomas. It thus seems unwise to consider sebaceous hyperplasia a component of the Muir-Torre syndrome [8]. Similarly, there is no evidence to support steatocystoma as part of the syndrome.

Keratoacanthomas can be seen as part of the syndrome. These can be single or multiple. In one series, 22% of patients with Muir-Torre syndrome had at least one keratoacanthoma [9]. Keratoacanthomas in the syndrome are clinically identical to sporadically occurring ones. They are rapidly growing, symmetric hyperkeratotic papules that have a central keratin-filled crater.

Associated Disorders. An average of two visceral malignant neoplasms is found in patients with Muir-Torre syndrome. These tend to be histologically low-grade neoplasms As many as 10% of patients manifest four to nine separate primary cancers. Colon carcinoma is the most common visceral malignancy associated with Muir-Torre syndrome and accounts for about half of all cancers in some studies [2]. Most of these neoplasms are in the proximal portion of the colon, and they tend to occur at a younger age than colon carcinomas in the general population. Colonic polyps occur in about one-fourth of all patients with the syndrome [1].

Genitourinary carcinomas account for 24% of all of the primary cancers associated with Muir-Torre syndrome. Other reported associated malignancies include breast carcinoma, Hodgkin's disease, non-Hodgkin's lymphoma, chronic lymphocytic leukemia, squamous cell carcinomas of the head and neck, chondrosarcomas, and parotid neoplasms [1]. A family history of carcinoma can be elicited in up to 70% of patients with the syndrome [3].

Rarely, benign neoplasms are reported in patients with Muir-Torre syndrome. These have included ovarian granulosa cell tumors, hepatic angiomas, schwannomas, and leiomyomas.

Histologic Features. Histologic features of the sebaceous neoplasms associated with Muir-Torre syndrome are identical to those of sporadically occurring neoplasms. Sebaceous adenomas have one or several lobules of sebaceous epithelium growing down from the

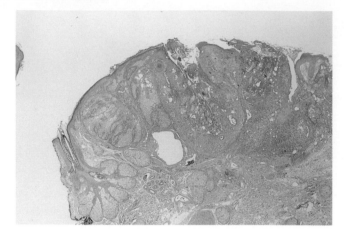

Fig. 27–1. Lobules of keratinocytes displaying sebaceous differentiation extend downward from the overlying epidermis in sebaceous adenoma.

overlying epidermis (Fig. 27–1). The lobules are composed of basaloid cells at the periphery that show gradual progression to mature sebocytes as they progress toward the center of the lobules (Fig. 27–2). The basaloid cells comprise less than 50% of the total area of the tumor lobules. Sebaceous adenomas have sharply circumscribed, smooth margins. Central cystic areas may be present, as can sebaceous ductules.

Sebaceous epitheliomas are architecturally similar to sebaceous adenomas. The primary difference is in the relative proportion of basaloid cells and mature sebocytes. In sebaceous epitheliomas, more than half of the mass in the tumor lobules consists of basaloid cells (Figs. 27–3 and 27–4). It remains unclear how this neoplasm differs from a basal cell carcinoma with sebaceous differentiation or a sebaceoma.

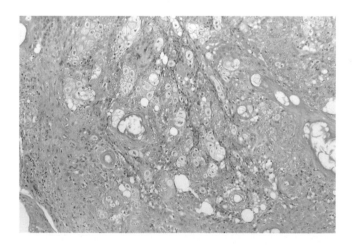

Fig. 27–2. Up to half of the cells, usually at the periphery of the lobules, remain basaloid, while the more centrally located cells demonstrate sebaceous differentiation in sebaceous adenoma.

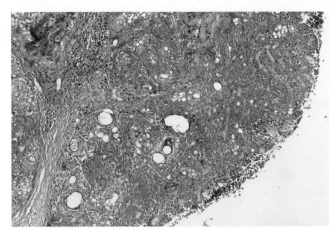

Fig. 27–3. Sebaceous epithelioma demonstrates a higher percentage of basaloid cells than mature sebocytes.

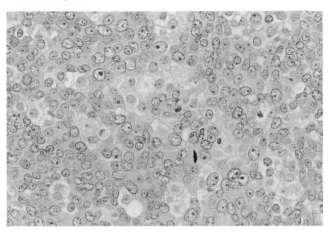

Fig. 27–5. Sebaceous carcinomas are characterized by little differentiation, nuclear pleomorphism, mitotic activity, and often an infiltrative growth pattern.

Sebaceoma is described as having aggregations of basaloid, undifferentiated cells admixed with mature-appearing sebocytes. The tumors may extend directly from the epidermis, but the connection is not always observed. Sebaceomas are sharply circumscribed and located in the upper portions of the dermis. The tumor nodules are surrounded by dense, eosinophilic collagen. Mitoses are rare, and cytologic atypia is not present [7].

Sebaceous carcinomas are histologically malignant neoplasms, characterized by atypical, hyperchromatic, pleomorphic cells, mitotic activity, and an infiltrative growth pattern. Sebaceous differentiation may be extensive or minimal and difficult to find (Fig. 27–5). Pagetoid extension of malignant sebocytes can be seen in sebaceous carcinomas arising on the eyelid, but is not ordinarily associated with these neoplasms when they arise in patients with Muir-Torre syndrome [1].

Keratoacanthomas associated with Muir-Torre syndrome are similar to sporadically occurring ones. In rare cases, sebaceous differentiation has been reported in these neoplasms associated with the syndrome [1]. The histologic features consist of a hyperkeratotic, symmetric cup-shaped proliferation of keratinocytes (Fig. 27–6). Symmetric buttressing of the adjacent epidermis is present. The neoplastic keratinocytes are large and have abundant pale staining, glassy cytoplasm (Fig. 27–7). Nuclear atypia may be present, and mitotic activity is often brisk. Neutrophilic abscesses are frequently identified in the center of the nests of atypical squamous cells. The atypical cells can invade the dermis as small angular nests. Elastophagocytosis by the neoplastic keratinocytes has been reported in keratoacanthomas. A brisk host immune response is present in the dermis beneath the keratinocytic proliferation. In

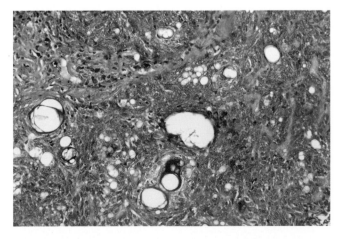

Fig. 27–4. The pattern of sebaceous differentiation is slightly less ordered in sebaceous epithelioma than in sebaceous adenoma.

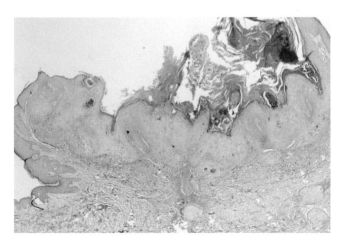

Fig. 27–6. A keratoacanthoma demonstrates a symmetric cup-like invagination extending downward from the surrounding epidermis.

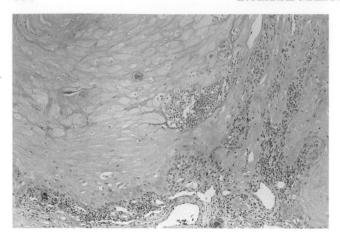

Fig. 27–7. Keratinocytes have abundant glassy cytoplasm in keratoacanthomas.

late, regressing tumors, the epidermis becomes flattened (Fig. 27–8). The immune response may be less intense, and scarring is present. It is difficult to distinguish a keratoacanthoma from a well-differentiated squamous cell carcinoma in many cases, and some authors believe keratoacanthomas to be a variant of well-differentiated squamous cell carcinoma [10]. The following entities must be considered in the histologic differential diagnosis of keratoacanthoma:

- Blastomycosis
- Halogenodermas
- Hyperplastic actinic keratosis
- Lupus vulgaris
- Pemphigus vegetans
- Pyoderma vegetante
- Squamous cell carcinoma
- Trichilemmoma
- Verruca vulgaris

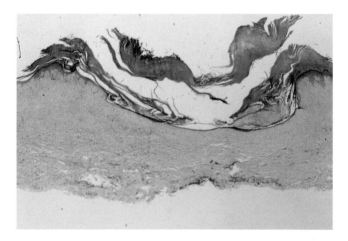

Fig. 27–8. Late, regressing keratoacanthomas demonstrate a flattened appearance and have a scar-like immune response in the dermis beneath them.

Special Studies. Special studies are not ordinarily required to make a diagnosis of a sebaceous neoplasm or keratoacanthoma in Muir-Torre syndrome; however, in some poorly differentiated sebaceous carcinomas, sebaceous differentiation may be difficult to identify. In these situations, immunolabeling may helpful. Sebocytes display epithelial membrane antigen very strongly, as opposed to surrounding keratinocytes, which do not express this antigen. Staining with cytokeratins may be helpful, but is not a specific finding. In some series, carcinoembryonic antigen has been shown to be expressed by sebaceous carcinomas.

Pathogenesis. Although the exact cause of Muir-Torre syndrome remains unknown, there has been some evidence linking the disease to a locus on chromosome 2p [11, 12]. Other investigators have suggested that microsatellite instabililty may be central to the development of neoplasms in patients with Muir-Torre syndrome [13].

Cowden's Syndrome (Multiple Hamartoma and Neoplasia Syndrome)

Epidemiology. Cowden's syndrome is defined as a constellation of mucocutaneous tumors associated with abnormalities of the breast, thyroid, and gastrointestinal tract [14]. The syndrome is inherited in an autosomal dominant manner. In some series, there is a female predominance [15]. A definitive diagnosis is based on a combination of major and minor criteria [16].

Cutaneous Features. Trichilemmomas are the most frequent cutaneous marker for Cowden's syndrome, occurring in more than 80% of affected patients [16]. Trichilemmomas are skin-colored papules that have a verrucous appearance. They are characteristically located on the face and may appear during childhood [17]. There is a predilection for facial orifices and for the extremities.

Punctate, hyperkeratotic papules may appear on the palms and soles in more than half of patients with Cowden's syndrome [18]. These papules may have a central depression, are skin colored, and are located primarily on the dorsa of the hands and feet, on the heels, and on the extensor surfaces of legs and forearms [18].

The oral mucosa may develop 1–3 mm papules or papillomas, which are so abundant as to give a "cobblestone" appearance [19]. Another, more recently described cutaneous tumor associated with Cowden's syndrome is the sclerotic fibroma. These are well-circumscribed dermal nodules that, when multiple, are a useful marker for Cowden's syndrome [20]. A wide range of less specific cutaneous tumors including lipomas, angiolipomas, hemangiomas, and fibroepithelial polyps have been described in patients with Cowden's syndrome [14].

Associated Disorders. Seventy-six percent of women with Cowden's syndrome have fibrocystic changes or fibroadenomas of the breast. Breast carcinoma is found in 25%–36% of women with the syndrome [18].

Up to two-thirds of patients with Cowden's syndrome suffer from thyroid disease. Goiters, thyroid adenomas, thyroglossal duct cysts, and follicular carcinomas have been reported in these patients [18].

Multiple benign polyps may be present throughout the gastrointestinal tract in patients with Cowden's syndrome [21]. These polyps can be in any location from the esophagus to the anus and have only a minimal risk for malignant degeneration. They are usually less than 5 mm. In one study, 60% of patients with the syndrome had gastrointestinal polyps [15].

Less frequent extracutaneous manifestations of Cowden's syndrome include ovarian cysts and leiomyomas, as well as cervical carcinomas, Gardner's duct cysts, transitional cell carcinomas of the renal pelvis, renal cell carcinomas, and urethral polyps [14]. Craniomegaly is present in up to 80% of patients with Cowden's syndrome, and about one-third have other skeletal anomalies [15], including high-arched palate. Kyphosis, bone cysts, and pectus excavatum have also been described [22]. A bird-like face is reported in some patients [23]. Eye abnormalities such as myopia and angioid streaks are reported in 13% of patients with Cowden's syndrome [18]. Prostate cancer [24] and osteosarcoma [25] have also been reported in association with Cowden's syndrome.

Rare cases of coexistent Cowden's syndrome and Lhermitte-Duclos disease, characterized by dysplastic cerebellar gangliocytomas, have been described [26]. Giant meningiomas have been seen in patients with this association [27]. In another family, coexistence with Bannayan-Riley-Ruvalcaba syndrome has been reported. It is believed that these syndromes are both caused by defects in the same chromosome [28].

Histologic Features. Trichilemmomas associated with Cowden's syndrome are histologically similar to sporadically occurring trichilemmomas. Histologic variants such as cylindric and lobulate trichilemmomas have been described in association with the syndrome [29], but these histologic differences are relatively minor. Trichilemmomas are basically lobular acanthomas that grow down from the epidermis, often surrounding a hair follicle (Fig. 27–9). Focal parakeratosis frequently overlies the tumor. The tumor lobules are composed of pale staining or clear keratinocytes that resemble the outer root sheath of the hair follicle. A thick, eosinophilic basement membrane is frequently seen surrounding the tumor lobules (Fig. 27–10). Occasional mitoses may be present. In some cases, the tumor lobules become separated by desmoplastic stroma, giving rise to a pseudoinvasive

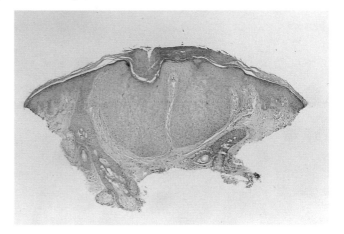

Fig. 27–9. Trichilemmomas grow down from the surface in a cup-shaped, symmetric pattern.

appearance. These neoplasms are termed *desmoplastic trichilemmomas.*

Acral keratoses have a nonspecific histologic appearance. Papillomatous growths demonstrate extensive hyperkeratosis and focal parakeratosis. Hypergranulosis may be present. There is no cytologic atypia to the keratinocytes. Unlike actinic or solar keratoses, increased dermal elastosis is not a feature of these growths. These tumors may resemble verrucae or acrokeratosis verruciformis histologically. Although some authors have suggested that these keratoses (as well as trichilemmomas) may be virally induced, ultrastructural examinations have failed to confirm that hypothesis [30].

Oral fibromas have a nonspecific histologic appearance. There is flattening of the mucosal surface and an increased amount of dense, eosinophilic collagen in the submucosa (Fig. 27–11). Fibroblasts may be

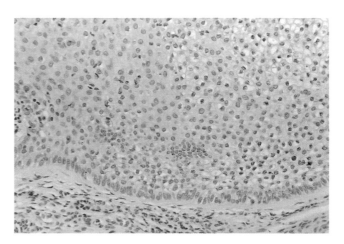

Fig. 27–10. The keratinocytes have pale-staining cytoplasm and demonstrate a characteristic peripheral palisading in trichilemmomas. Often, an eosinophilic band is seen at the periphery of the epithelial islands.

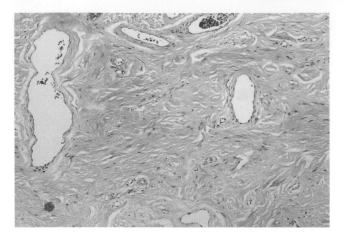

Fig. 27–11. Oral fibroma is characterized by dense submucosal fibrosis and ectatic blood vessels.

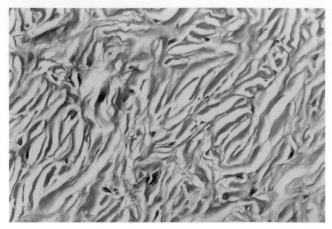

Fig. 27–13. Broad bands of collagen are present separated by clear spaces and relatively few cells in sclerotic fibroma.

slightly increased in number and demonstrate a stellate morphology.

Sclerotic fibromas are characterized by a dermal overgrowth of collagen underlying a flattened epider-

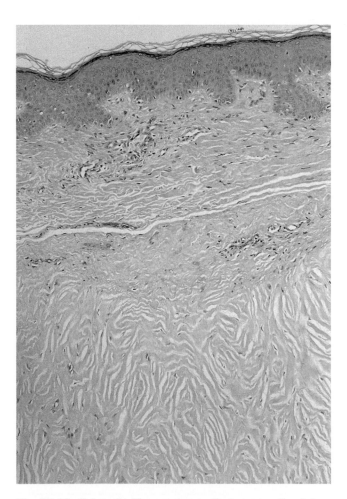

Fig. 27–12. Sclerotic fibroma is a well-circumscribed dermal nodule separated from the overlying epidermis.

mis. The dermis is paucicellular, and the affected collagen bundles are well-demarcated and separated from the epidermis by a grenz zone (Fig. 27–12). Interwoven fascicles of collagen are arranged in parallel bundles that are widely spaced and stain with increased eosinophilia [29] (Fig. 27–13). The following entities must be considered in the histologic differential diagnosis of sclerotic fibroma:

- Acquired digital fibrokeratoma
- Dermatofibroma
- Neurofibroma
- Scar

Special Studies. Special studies are not required to make a diagnosis of the cutaneous tumors associated with Cowden's syndrome.

Pathogenesis. The PTEN/MMAC1 gene has been identified as the gene responsible for Cowden's syndrome. Affected patients have demonstrated a wide range of mutations in the gene [31]. This gene is located on chromosome 10q22–23 [32]. Abnormalities in T-cell function have been reported in patients with Cowden's syndrome, but the significance of this finding is still unclear [33].

Gardner's Syndrome

Epidemiology. Gardner's syndrome is inherited in an autosomal dominant manner and is characterized by gastrointestinal, osseous, and cutaneous findings [34].

Cutaneous Features. The cutaneous features most commonly associated with Gardner's syndrome include follicular cysts, desmoid tumors, fibromas, and lipomas [35]. Follicular cysts are the most common cutaneous finding, occurring in virtually all patients with Gardner's syndrome. These are dermally located nodules that usually have no overlying surface change. They are usually asymptomatic and occur in any location on the body.

Associated Disorders. Adenomatous polyps of the colon are the major finding in patients with Gardner's syndrome. More than half of all affected patients will develop colon adenocarcinoma as a result of malignant degeneration of the adenomatous polyps [36]. Similar polyps may be found in the small intestine and stomach in almost one-half of these patients.

Congenital hypertrophic retinal pigmentation has been identified in patients with Gardner's syndrome and may be a specific marker [37]. Other associated disorders include osteomas, often within the mandible, and a wide range of dental anomalies [38].

Histologic Features. The histologic features of the follicular cysts are varied. Pilomatrical differentiation, partial or complete, has been described in these cysts [39]. In some patients, the cysts are histologically identical to sporadically occurring pilomatricomas, with basaloid cells, shadow cells, and calcification. In these cases, the cystic structures are present within the midreticular dermis. The histologic features of pilomatricoma are described fully in Chapter 9. Other authors have described these follicular cysts as evolving from follicular stem cells, showing a wide range of follicular differentiation extending from cysts with follicular infundibular or trichilemmal keratinization to those with well-develop hair matrix-like structures [40].

Special Studies. Special studies are not required to make histologic diagnoses of the various tumors associated with Gardner's syndrome.

Pathogenesis. The pathogenesis of Gardner's syndrome is currently unknown. An increased incidence of chromatid damage in fibroblasts from patients with Gardner's syndrome is, however, seen after exposure to ultraviolet light. Authors postulate a defect in DNA repair due to incomplete excision of DNA damage during the G2 phase of the cell cycle. This may play a role in the subsequent development of multiple neoplasms in these patients [41].

Birt-Hogg-Dube Syndrome

Epidemiology. Patients with Birt-Hogg-Dube syndrome present with hundreds of small, skin-colored papules on the face, neck, and upper torso. Cutaneous manifestations usually appear during the third or fourth decade. This rare syndrome has an autosomal dominant inheritance pattern [42].

Cutaneous Features. Innumerable nonspecific, small, skin-colored papules are present on the face, trunk, and upper torso of patients afflicted with BHD. Although some of the growths are simply acrochordons, it is difficult to distinguish these from the other associated follicular-based growths on clinical examination. Large and disfiguring lipomas have also been reported in this group of patients [43].

Associated Diseases. Renal oncocytomas and papillary renal cell carcinomas have been reported in patients with BHD. In one study, pulmonary cysts occurred in four patients from two separate families with BHD. Collagenomas were also present in these patients [43]. Multiple oral fibromas are present in some patients with BHD [43]. The syndrome has also been associated with intestinal polyposis [44].

Histologic Features. The histologic features of the three major cutaneous growths found in patients with BHD are identical to similar growths occurring spontaneously. Acrochordons, or fibroepithelial polyps, are exophytic polyps with a flattened epidermis and an overgrowth of dermal collagen. In most cases, cutaneous appendages are not present. Adipose tissue is occasionally seen in the lower portion of larger growths, and mucin accumulation may be observed in traumatized acrochordons. In these cases, dermal fibroblasts may have a stellate appearance.

Fibrofolliculomas consist of interanastamosing strands of benign, basaloid keratinocytes growing downward from the overlying epidermis. Follicular differentiation is present, and sebocytes may also be present. The strands of keratinocytes are surrounded by myxoid stroma that contains abundant hyaluronic acid [43] (Fig. 27–14). The following entities must be considered in the histologic differential diagnosis of a fibrofolliculoma:

- Basaloid follicular hamartoma
- Infundibulocystic basal cell carcinoma
- Trichoepithelioma
- Tumor of the follicular infundibulum

Trichodiscomas demonstrate a flattened epidermis with proliferation of spindle-shaped cells enmeshed in a myxoid papillary dermis. Increased amounts of acid mucopolysaccharides are present. At either lateral margin of the proliferation, there is often a hair follicle that has a distorted orientation (Figs. 27–15 and 27–16). The sharp circumscription and bordering hair follicles are helpful in distinguishing this entity from a neurofi-

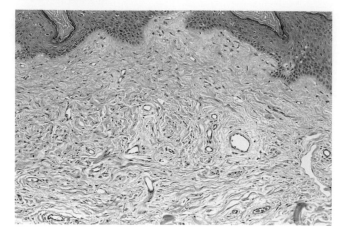

Fig. 27–16. Abundant mucin is present within the cellular papillary dermis in trichodiscoma

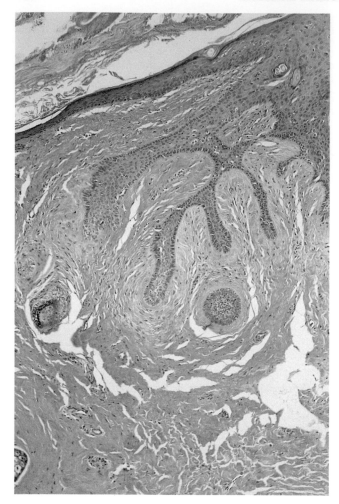

Fig. 27–14. Interanastamosing strands of basaloid keratinocytes with follicular differentiation extend down from the overlying epidermis in fibrofolliculoma.

broma. The following entities must be considered in the differential diagnosis of trichodiscoma:

- Myxoma
- Neurofibroma
- Neurothekeoma
- Pretibial myxedema
- Scleromyxedema

It has been postulated that fibrofolliculomas and trichodiscomas may represent a spectrum of the same lesion [43].

Special Studies. Special studies are not required to make a diagnosis of any of the cutaneous neoplasms identified in patients with BHD. A colloidal iron or Alcian blue stain performed at pH 2.5 may be helpful in identifying the increased amounts acid mucopolysaccharides in the superficial dermis.

Pathogenesis. It has been speculated that there is a BHD gene that behaves as a tumor suppressor gene that controls cell growth. Aberrations in the gene lead to multiple cutaneous and internal growths. The gene has not yet been localized [43].

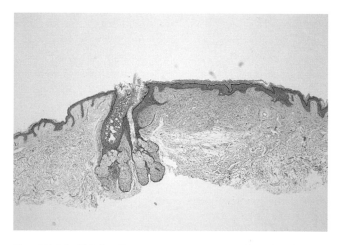

Fig. 27–15. Trichodiscoma appears as a sharply demarcated, dome-shaped papule with a flattened epidermis.

References

1. Schwartz, R. A., and Torre, D. P., *The Muir-Torre syndrome: a 25–year retrospect.* J Am Acad Dermatol, 1995. 33:90–104.
2. Finan, M. C., and Connoly, S. M., *Sebaceous gland tumors and systemic disease: A clinicopathologic analysis.* Medicine, 1984. 63:232–242.

3. Cohen, P. R., Kohn, S. R., and Kurzrock, R., *Association of sebaceous gland neoplasms and internal malignancy: The Muire-Torre syndrome*. Am J Med, 1991. 90:606–613.

4. Schwartz, R. A., Fliedger, D. N., and Saied, N. K., *The Torre syndrome with gastrointestinal polyposis*. Arch Dermatol, 1980. 116:312–314.

5. Rulon, D. B., and Helwig, E. B., *Multiple sebaceous neoplasms of the skin: An association with multiple visceral carcinomas, especially of the colon*. Am J Clin Pathol, 1973. 60:745–752.

6. Wick, M. R., Goellner, J. R., Wolfe, J. T. I., and Su, W. P. D., *Adnexal carcinomas of the skin. II. Extraocular sebaceous carcinomas*. Cancer, 1985. 56:1163–1172.

7. Troy, J. L., and Ackerman, A. B., *Sebaceoma: A distinctive benign neoplasm of adnexal epithelium differentiating toward sebaceous cells*. Am J Dermatopathol, 1984. 6:7–13.

8. Sciallis, G. F., and Winkelmann, R. K., *Multiple sebaceous adenomas and gastrointestinal carcinoma*. Arch Dermatol, 1974. 110:913–916.

9. Rao, N. A., Hidayat, A. A., McLean, I. W., and Zimmerman, L. E., *Sebaceous carcinomas of the ocular adnexa: A clinicaopathologic study of 104 cases with five-year follow-up data*. Hum Pathol, 1982. 13:113–122.

10. Hodak, E., Jones, R. E., and Ackerman, A. B., *Solitary keratoacanthoma is a squamous cell carcinoma: Three examples with metastases*. Am J Dermatopathol, 1993. 15:332–342.

11. Nystrom-Lahti, M., Parsons, R., Sistonen, P., Pylkkanen, L., Aaltonen, L. A., Leach, F. S., Hamilton, S. R., et al., *Mismatch repair genes on chromosomes 2p and 3p account for a major share of hereditary nonpolyposis colorectal cancer families evaluable by linkage*. Am J Hum Genet, 1994. 55:659–665.

12. Hall, N. R., Murday, V. A., Chapman, P., Williams, M. A., Burn, J., Finlay, P. J., and Bishop, D. T., *Genetic linkage in Muir-Torre syndrome to the same chromosomal region as cancer family syndrome (abstract)*. Eur J Cancer, 1994. 30:180–182.

13. Quinn, A. G., Healy, E., Rehman, I., Sikkink, S., and Rees, J. L., *Microsatellite instability in human nonmelanoma and melanoma skin cancer*. J Invest Dermatol, 1995. 104:309–312.

14. Mallory, S. B., *Cowden syndrome (multiple hamartoma syndrome)*. Dermatol Clin, 1995. 13:27–31.

15. Starink, T. M., Van der Veen, J. P., Arwert, F., de Waal, L. P., de Lange, G. G., Gille, J. J., and Eriksson, A. W., *The Cowden syndrome: A clinical and genetic study in 21 patients*. Clin Genet, 1986. 29:222–223.

16. Salem, O. S., and Steck, W. D., *Cowden's disease (multiple hamartoma and neoplasia syndrome)*. J Am Acad Dermatol, 1983. 8:686–696.

17. Takenoshita, Y., Kubo, S., Takeuchi, T., and Iida, M., *Oral and facial leisons in Cowden's disease: Report of two cases and a review of the literature*. J Oral Maxillofac Surg, 1993. 51:682–687.

18. Starink, T. M., *Cowden's disease: Analysis of fourteen new cases*. J Am Acad Dermatol, 1984. 11:1127–1141.

19. Wade, T. R., and Kopf, A. W., *Cowden's disease: A case report and review of the literature*. J Dermatol Surg Oncol, 1978. 4:459–464.

20. Metcalf, J. S., Maize, J. C., and LeBoit, P. E., *Circumscribed storiform collagenoma (sclerosing fibroma)*. Am J Dermatopathol, 1991. 13:122–129.

21. Chen, Y. M., Ott, D. J., Wu, W. C., and Gclfand, D. W., *Cowden's disease: A case report and literature review*. Gastrointest Radiol, 1987. 12:325–329.

22. Gentry, W. C., Reed, W. B., and Siegel, J. M., *Coden disease*. Birth Defects, 1975. 11:137–141.

23. Shapiro, S. D., Lambert, C., and Schwartz, R. A., *Cowden's disease. A marker for malignancy*. Int J Dermatol, 1988. 27:232–237.

24. Inagaki, T., and Ebisuno, S., *A case of Cowden's disease accompanied by prostatic cancer*. Br J Urol, 1996. 77:918–919.

25. Yen, B. C., Kahn, H., Schiller, A. L., Klien, M. J., Phelps, R. G., and Lebwohl, M. G., *Multiple hamartoma syndrome with osteosarcoma*. Arch Pathol Lab Med, 1993. 117:1252–1254.

26. Chapman, M. S., Perry, A. E., and Baughman, R. D., *Cowden's syndrome, Lhermitte-Duclos disease, and sclerotic fibroma*. Am J Dermatopathol, 1998. 20:413–416.

27. Lindboe, C. F., Helseth, E., and Myhr, G., *Lhermitte-Duclos disease and giant meningioma as manifestations of Cowden's disease*. Clin Neuropathol, 1995. 14:327–330.

28. Perriard, J., Saurat, J.-H., and Harms, M., *An overlap of Cowden's disease and Bannayan-Riley-Ruvalcaba syndrome in the same family*. J Am Acad Dermatol, 2000. 42:348–350.

29. Starink, T. M., Meijer, C. J. L. M., and Brownstein, M. H., *The cutaneous pathology of Cowden's disease: New findings*. J Cutan Pathol, 1985. 12:83–93.

30. Johnson, B. L., Kramer, E. M., and Lavker, R. M., *The keratotic tumors of Cowden's disease: An electron microscopic study*. J Cutan Pathol, 1987. 14:291–298.

31. Kohno, T., Takahashi, M., Fukutomi, T., Ushio, K., and Yokota, J., *Germline mutations of the PTEN/MMAC1 gene in Japanese patients with Cowden disease*. Jpn J Cancer Res, 1998. 89:471–474.

32. Eng, C., *Genetics of Cowden syndrome: Through the looking glass of oncology*. Int J Oncol, 1998. 12:701–710.

33. Halevy, S., Sandbank, M., Pick, A. I., and Feuerman, E. J., *Cowden's disease in three siblings: Electron-microscopic and immunologic studies*. Acta Derm Venereol, 1985. 65:126–131.

34. Poole, S., and Fenske, N. A., *Cutaneous markers of internal malignancy. I. Malignant involvement of the skin and the genodermatoses*. J Am Acad Dermatol, 1993. 28:1–13.

35. Schiffman, M. A., *Familial multiple polyposis associated with soft tissue and hard tissue tumors*. J Am Med Assoc, 1962. 179:514–522.

36. Sanchez, M. A., Zali, M. R., and Khalil, A. A., *Be aware of Gardner's syndrome*. Am J Gastroenterol, 1979. 71:68–73.

37. Traboulsi, E. I., Maumenee, I. H., and Krush, A. J., *Pigmented ocular fundus lesions in the inherited gastrointestinal polyposis syndromes and in hereditary nonpolyposis colorectal cancer.* Ophthalmology, 1988. 95:964–969.

38. Pujol, R. M., Casanova, J.M., Egido, R., Pujol, R., and de Moragas, J. M., *Multiple familial pilomatricomas: A cutaneous marker for Gardner syndrome?* Pediatr Dermatol, 1995. 12:331–335.

39. Cooper, P. H., and Fechner, R. E., *Pilomatricoma-like changes in the epidermal cysts of Gardner's syndrome.* J Am Acad Dermatol, 1983. 8:639–644.

40. Narisawa, Y., and Kohda, H., *Cutaneous cysts of Gardner's syndrome are similar to follicular stem cells.* J Cutan Pathol, 1995. 22:115–121.

41. Parshad, R., Sanford, K. K., and Jones, G. M., *Chromatid damage induced by fluorescent light during G2 phase in normal and Gardner syndrome fibroblasts. Interpretation in terms of deficient DNA repair.* Mutat Res, 1985. 151:57–63.

42. Birt, A. R., Hogg, G. R., and Dube, J., *Hereditary multiple fibrofolliculomas with trichodiscomas and acrochordons.* Arch Dermatol, 1977. 113:1674–1677.

43. Toro, J. R., Glenn, G., Duray, P., Darling, T., Weirich, G., Zbar, B., Linehan, M., et al., *Birt-Hogg-Dube syndrome. A novel marker of kidney disease.* Arch Dermatol, 1999. 135:1195–1202.

44. Rongioletti, F., Hazini, R., Gianotti, G., and Rebora, A., *Fibrofolliculomas, trichodiscomas and acrochordons (Birt-Hogg-Dube) associated with intestinal polyposis.* Clin Exp Dermatol, 1989. 14:72–74.

CHAPTER 28

Epidermal Proliferative Processes Associated with Internal Malignancy

Acanthosis Nigricans

Epidemiology. Acanthosis nigricans is a common cutaneous disorder. It usually occurs as an isolated condition, but can be seen in association with malignant neoplasms, obesity, or other conditions as described later. In one large study, acanthosis nigricans was found in 7.1% of unselected children. It was commonly associated with obesity in these children and was present in 66% of children weighing more than 200% of their ideal body weight. It was found in 13.3% of black children, 5.5% of Hispanic children, and <1% of white non-Hispanic children [1]. In adults, up to three-fourths of obese individuals will demonstrate acanthosis nigricans [2]. Acanthosis nigricans associated with malignant neoplasms is much less common and shows none of the same racial predilections [3].

Eight types of acanthosis nigricans have been described and are summarized briefly in Table 28–1. The variant known as malignant acanthosis nigricans is characterized by a rapid onset occurring in conjunction with an underlying neoplasm.

Cutaneous Features. Acanthosis nigricans appears as velvety, hyperpigmented patches and plaques present in intertriginous regions and/or over the knuckles. The posterior and lateral neck, axillae, and inguinal folds are the most commonly affected areas of the body. An-

tecubital and popliteal fossae, abdominal and breast folds, and the anogenital region are other common sites. In children, the back of the neck is the most frequently affected site [1]. The earliest changes are those of apparent hyperpigmentation. Over time, the skin becomes progressively thicker, probably due to hyperkeratosis, with increased skin markings. There is, however, no induration.

Acanthosis nigricans involving the palms and soles is seen much more commonly in patients with underlying malignant neoplasms than in acanthosis nigricans unassociated with neoplasia [4]. Mucosal acanthosis nigricans has been reported. It can appear as papillomatous thickening of the mucosal surfaces or as hyperpigmentation without significant thickening. Acanthosis nigricans can involve the lips, buccal mucosa, tongue, conjunctival surfaces and laryngeal mucosa. In addition, vaginal and anal mucosa can show similar changes. Mucosal involvement is more common in acanthosis nigricans associated with underlying malignant neoplasms [4].

Associated Disorders. Acanthosis nigricans is often associated with underlying endocrinopathies. Acanthosis nigricans was present in about one-fourth of children suffering from Cushing's disease [5]. Diabetes mellitus was found in about half of African-American adults with acanthosis nigricans, and the authors suggest that

Table 28–1. Subtypes of Acanthosis Nigricans

Subtype of Acanthosis Nigricans	Associations
Idiopathic	Rare; autosomal dominant
Obesity associated	Most common form
Syndromic	Many syndromes (see [3])
Malignant	Underlying neoplasms
Acral	Dorsum of hands and feet of dark-skinned people
Unilateral	Nevoid (hamartomous process)
Drug induced	Rare, associated with corticosteroids, estrogens, nicotinamide
Mixed type	Associated with more than one of the above associations

From references 3 and 68–71.

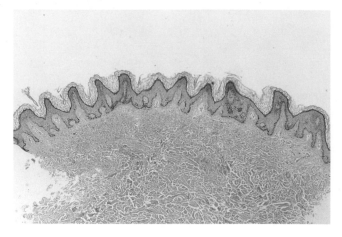

Fig. 28–1. Acanthosis nigricans is characterized by papillomatous epidermal hyperplasia.

acanthosis nigricans is a marker for hyperinsulinemia in these patients [6].

Malignant acanthosis nigricans is associated with underlying neoplasms that promote the cutaneous changes. In most cases, the associated neoplasm is an adenocarcinoma [7]. Acanthosis nigricans has also been associated with mycosis fungoides [8] and squamous cell carcinoma of the lung [9].

Acanthosis nigricans is reported in association with other unusual diseases, including Wilson's disease [10] and primary biliary cirrhosis [11]. It is also included as part of the Bannayan-Riley-Ruvalcaba syndrome, along with multiple lipomas and vascular malformations, lentigines of the penis and vulva, and verrucae [12], and as part of Costello's syndrome, with postnatal growth deficiency, coarse facies, redundant skin on the neck, dark skin, and multiple skin papillomas [13]. Acanthosis nigricans has been reported in conjunction with florid cutaneous papillomatosis and bronchogenic carcinoma [9].

Histologic Features. The histologic features of acanthosis nigricans are the same, regardless of the type as classified earlier. The skin has overlying hyperkeratosis, and the epidermis is papillomatous and occasionally mildly acanthotic (Fig. 28–1). Foci of epidermal atrophy can also be present. The dermal papillae are elongated, and upward projections of these papillae into the thinned overlying epidermis give rise to the papillomatous architecture [14]. Increased melanin is only occasionally present within basal keratinocytes and can be detected at higher levels within the epidermis (Fig. 28–2). There is no significant increase in numbers of melanocytes within lesional skin. It is generally believed that the apparent hyperpigmentation is more a function of increased thickness of the stratum corneum with retained melanin than due to a true increase in melanin

production. The dermis is unremarkable. The following entities must be considered in the histologic differential diagnosis of acanthosis nigricans:

- Confluent and reticulated papillomatosis of Gougerot and Carteaud
- Epidermal nevus
- Lichen simplex chronicus
- Seborrheic keratosis
- Tinea versicolor

Special Studies. Special studies are not required to make a diagnosis of acanthosis nigricans.

Pathogenesis. It is generally believed that acanthosis nigricans is caused by an increased level of some growth factor that is stimulating both keratinocytes and dermal fibroblasts [15]. Fasting plasma insulin levels cor-

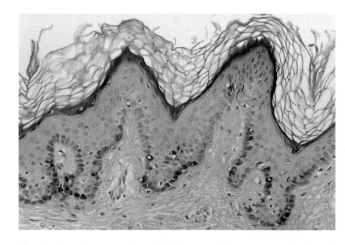

Fig. 28–2. Increased melanin may be present in basal keratinocytes in acanthosis nigricans, but no increase in melanocytes is detected.

relate with presence of acanthosis nigricans [1], and increased insulin levels are most often implicated in patients with acanthosis nigricans and no associated neoplasms. In patients with acanthosis nigricans associated with neoplasms, insulin-like tumor products are implicated in the pathogenesis of the cutaneous changes [16]. Transforming growth factor-α production was detected in a person with gastric adenocarcinoma and acanthosis nigricans, and the keratinocyte proliferation was attributed to this growth factor [17].

Bazex's Syndrome (Acrokeratosis Paraneoplastica)

Epidemiology. Bazex's syndrome is a rare paraneoplastic syndrome that is almost always associated with carcinomas of the upper aerodigestive tract. The mean age of onset is 61 years, and there is an overwhelming male predominance (perhaps in part related to the male predominance of bronchogenic carcinomas) [18].

Cutaneous Features. Bazex's syndrome is characterized by a papulosquamous eruption characterized by erythematous scaling patches and plaques on the ears, nose, hands, and feet [19]. This is accompanied by marked hyperkeratosis of the palms and soles [20]. Nail dystrophy occurs in conjunction with the skin changes and often persists after the cutaneous eruption has resolved [19]. Associated severe pain has been reported in one patient [21]. Less commonly, vesicles and bullae are present [19]. In some patients, the psoriasiform lesions extend to involve the arms and legs. The cutaneous eruption precedes the appearance of the malignancy by an average of 11 months in two-thirds of cases [18, 19]. In another 20% of patients, the onset of the cutaneous changes appeared simultaneously with the detection of the malignancy [18]. Cutaneous manifestations resolve with treatment of the underlying neoplasm [22]. Reappearance of skin lesions has been reported with tumor recurrence [18].

Associated Disorders. Bazex's syndrome is usually found in association with bronchogenic carcinomas. Other neoplasms, including Hodgkin's disease [22], cutaneous squamous cell carcinoma [20], metastatic neuroendocrine tumor [23], prostate carcinoma [24], and bladder carcinoma [25], have also been associated.

Co-occurrence of Bazex's syndrome and ichthyosis has been described [22]. In another patient, vitiligo and alopecia areata appeared at the same time as Bazex's syndrome, in conjunction with a cutaneous squamous cell carcinoma [20].

Histologic Features. The changes seen in the skin of patients with Bazex's syndrome are those of a chronic,

spongiotic dermatitis [26]. There is hyperkeratosis and focal parakeratosis overlying a spongiotic and acanthotic epidermis. Exocytosis of lymphocytes into the epidermis is present. Basal vacuolization is an inconstant finding. A mild superficial perivascular lymphocytic infiltrate is present within the dermis. The following entities must be considered in the histologic differential diagnosis of Bazex's syndrome:

- Contact dermatitis
- Dermatophytosis
- Dyshidrotic eczema
- Gianotti-Crosti syndrome
- Id reaction
- Nummular dermatitis

Special Studies. Special studies are not usually required to make a diagnosis of Bazex's syndrome. In one case, immunoglobulin deposition was reported along the dermal–epidermal junction of affected skin [27]. The significance of this finding is not known.

Pathogenesis. It has been suggested that transforming growth factor-α produced by tumor cells may play a role in the hyperproliferation of keratinocytes and acanthosis seen in Bazex's syndrome [22]. Others have suggested an immunologic mechanism for the pathogenesis of this syndrome [20].

Acquired Ichthyosis

Epidemiology. Acquired ichthyosis occurs after a range of inflammatory and neoplastic conditions, as discussed later.

Cutaneous Features. The cutaneous features of acquired ichthyosis are virtually identical to those of ichthyosis vulgaris except that the former develops later in life. Broad, rhomboid or square-shaped, white scales appear most commonly on the extensor surfaces of extremities and impart a resemblance to fish scales. Flexural surfaces are usually spared. The scalp is occasionally involved. The degree of scaling is quite variable and can be relatively minimal or very striking.

Associated Disorders. Acquired ichthyosis occurs in association with many types of neoplasms, including rhabdomyosarcoma [28], leiomyosarcoma [29], breast carcinoma [30], and carcinoma of the lung and cervix [31]. It is seen most commonly, however, in association with hematopoietic malignancies, including mycosis fungoides [32], non-Hodgkin's lymphoma [33], Hodgkin's disease [34], chronic myelogenous leukemia [35], polycythemia rubra vera [36], and lymphomatoid papulosis [37]. Acquired ichthyosis has also been reported to occur in patients with collagen vascular diseases, including lupus erythematosus [38, 39], eosinophilic fasciitis [40], and dermatomyositis [41].

Acquired ichthyosis also occurs in association with other systemic disease processes, including leprosy, hypothyroidism, chronic renal failure, nutritional deficiencies [34], hyperparathyroidism [42], diabetes mellitus [43], and sarcoidosis [44].

Acquired ichthyosis is seen about 7% of patients with acquired immunodeficiency syndrome [45] and has also been reported as many as 22% patients with concomitant human immunodeficiency virus type one and human T-lymphotropic virus type II infections [46]. Acquired ichthyosis has been reported in association with the use of clofazamine and nafoxidine [47] and with other cutaneous changes, including pityriasis rotunda [48] and Bazex's syndrome [49].

Histologic Features. Acquired ichthyosis is histologically indistinguishable from ichthyosis vulgaris. The stratum corneum is moderately hyperkeratotic, compacted, and orthokeratotic. The epidermis is either normal or slightly acanthotic. The granular layer is either markedly attenuated or completely absent (Fig. 28–3). Cutaneous appendages are decreased in size and number in many cases.

Special Studies. Special studies are not necessary to make a diagnosis of acquired ichthyosis; however, a complete patient history is necessary to distinguish it from ichthyosis vulgaris.

Pathogenesis. The exact pathogenesis of acquired ichthyosis is not known. Ichthyosis vulgaris, which is clinically and histologically identical to the acquired form of the disease, is known to be caused by a defect

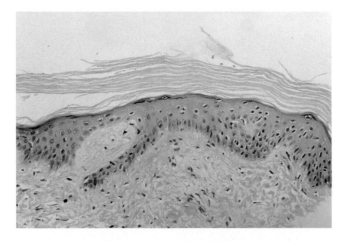

Fig. 28–3. The stratum corneum is thickened, with loss of the normal basket weave pattern, and the granular layer is markedly attenuated in acquired ichthyosis.

in profilaggrin. This causes a defect in the formation of keratohyaline granules [50]. It has not yet been established if a similar defect occurs in acquired ichthyosis and, if so, what triggers the loss or abnormal production of this protein. In one study, impaired lipogenesis was observed in a patient with acquired ichthyosis and Hodgkin's disease [51]. The significance of this finding remains unknown.

Leser-Trelat Syndrome

Epidemiology. Leser-Trelat is a controversial syndrome characterized by the rapid onset of multiple seborrheic keratoses in association with visceral malignant neoplasms [52]. Based on large epidemiologic studies, several groups have called into question the validity of this sign [53–55]. Others cite associations with acanthosis nigricans, a known paraneoplastic condition, as evidence in support of the existence of the syndrome [52]. There is a report in the literature of hereditary onset of multiple seborrheic keratoses in a cancer-prone family [56].

Cutaneous Features. The sign of Leser-Trelat is characterized by the rapid onset of multiple seborrheic keratoses. These neoplasms are similar in appearance to sporadically occurring seborrheic keratoses. They are mainly truncally distributed and follow skin lines. They appear as "stuck on," sharply demarcated exophytic tumors. They are covered by a thick, greasy scale. Some seborrheic keratoses are densely pigmented, while others have minimal pigment changes. Pruritus has been associated with the seborrheic keratoses associated with Leser-Trelat.

Associated Disorders. The sign of Leser-Trelat has been reported in association with many internal malignant neoplasms, including pancreatic carcinoma [57], lung carcinoma [9, 58], esophageal carcinoma [59], transitional cell carcinoma of the bladder [60], osteogenic sarcoma [61], breast carcinoma [62], and melanoma [63]. The Leser-Trelat sign has also been described in patients with Sézary syndrome [64]. In some of these patients, the seborrheic keratoses have resolved as the disease was treated and went into remission [65, 66]. It has also been reported with benign neoplasms, including Leydig's cell tumors [67]. The association appears to be most frequent with gastrointestinal tract neoplasms [57]. The sign of Leser-Trelat has been observed in conjunction with acanthosis nigricans and florid cutaneous papillomatosis, two other paraneoplastic processes [9, 58].

Histologic Features. The histologic features of seborrheic keratoses associated with the Leser-Trelat sign are identical to those of sporadically appearing seborrheic keratoses. There is hyperkeratosis overlying an acan-

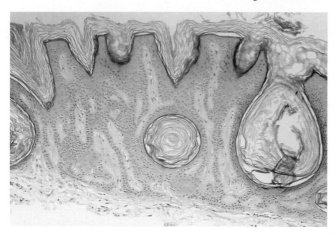

Fig. 28–4. Seborrheic keratoses demonstrate a proliferation of basaloid keratinocytes without cytologic atypia. Cystic structures are frequently present in these lesions.

thotic, and sometimes papillomatous, epidermis. The thickened epidermis is populated by basaloid keratinocytes that are not cytologically atypical. In some tumors, there is increased melanin within basal keratinocytes (Fig. 28–4). Mitoses are rare, and atypical forms are not present. Papillary dermal fibrosis may be present. The following entities must be considered in the histologic differential diagnosis of a seborrheic keratosis:

- Acanthosis nigricans
- Condyloma acuminatum
- Dermatofibroma, surface change
- Epidermal nevus
- Nevus sebaceus of Jadassohn
- Verruca vulgaris

Special Studies. Special studies are not required to make a diagnosis of seborrheic keratosis.

Pathogenesis. The pathogenesis of this controversial sign remains unknown. Those who believe in its existence postulate that the production of a human epidermal growth factor by some tumors may give rise to the development of multiple seborrheic keratoses [9, 58]. In one study, epidermal growth factor receptors and HER-2/neu oncoprotein were found in the proliferating epidermis, suggesting a possible role for growth factors in the pathogenesis of these lesions [56].

References

1. Stuart, C. A., Pate, C. J., and Peters, E. J., *Prevalence of acanthosis nigricans in an unselected population.* Am J Med, 1989. 87:269–272.

2. Hud, J. A. Jr., Cohen, J. B., Wagner, J. M., and Cruz, P. D. Jr., *Prevalence and significance of acanthosis nigricans in an adult obese population.* Arch Dermatol, 1992. 128:941–944.

3. Schwartz, R. A., *Acanthosis nigricans.* J Am Acad Dermatol, 1994. 31:1–19.

4. Curth, H. O., *Malignant acanthosis nigricans.* Arch Dermatol, 1970. 102:479–481.

5. Stratakis, C. A., Mastorakos, G., Mitsiades, N. S., Mitsiades, C. S., and Chrousos, G. P., *Skin manifestations of Cushing disease in children and adolescents before and after the resolution of hyercortisolemia.* Pediatr Dermtatol, 1998. 15:253–258.

6. Stuart, C. A., Gilkison, C. R., Keenan, B. S., and Nagamani, M., *Hyperinsulinemia and acanthosis nigricans in African Americans.* J Natl Med Assoc, 1997. 89:523–527.

7. Curth, H. O., Hilberg, A. W., and Machacek, G. F., *The site and histology of the cancer associated with malignant acanthosis nigricans.* Cancer, 1962. 15:364–382.

8. Schweitzer, W. J., Goldin, H. M., Bronson, D. M., and Brody, P. E., *Acanthosis nigricans associated with mycosis fungoides.* J Am Acad Dermatol, 1988. 19:951–953.

9. Gheeraert, P., Goens, J., Schwartz, R. A., Lambert, W. C., Schroeder, F., and Debusscher, L., *Florid cutaneous papillomatosis, malignant acanthosis nicricans, and pulmonary squamous cell carcinoma.* Int J Dermatol, 1991. 30:193–197.

10. Thaipisuttikul, Y., *Acanthosis nigricans associated with hepatolenticular degeneration.* J Dermatol, 1997. 24:395–400.

11. Pham, T. H., Kaushik, S., Lin, B. P., and Jones, D. B., *Case report: Acanthosis nigricans in association with primary biliary cirrhosis: Resolution after liver transplantation.* J Gastroenterol Hepatol, 1996. 11:1021–1023.

12. Fargnoli, M. C., Orlow, S. J., Semel-Concepcion, J., and Bolognia, J. L., *Clinicopathologic findings in Bannayan-Riley-Ruvalcaba syndrome.* Arch Dermatol, 1996. 132:1214–1218.

13. Philip, N., and Sigaudy, S., *Costello syndrome.* J Med Genet, 1998. 35:238–240.

14. Hall, J. M., Moreland, A., Cox, C. J., and Wade, T. R., *Oral acanthosis nigricans: Report of a case and comparison of oral and cutaneous pathology.* Am J Dermatopathol, 1988. 10:68–73.

15. Abeloff, M. D., *Paraneoplastic syndrome: A window on the biology of cancer.* N Engl J Med, 1987. 317:1598–1600.

16. Lerner, A. B., *On the cause of acanthosis nigricans.* N Engl J Med, 1969. 281:106–107.

17. Koyama, S., Ikeda, K., Sato, M., Shibahara, K., Yuhara, K., Fukutomi, H., Fukunaga, K., Kanazawa, N., et al., *Transforming growth factor alpha (TGF alpha)-producing gastric carcinoma with acanthosis nigricans: An endocrine effect of TGF alpha in the pathogenesis of cutaneous paraneoplastic syndrome and epithelial hyperplasia of the eosphagus.* J Gastroenterol, 1997. 32:71–77.

18. Bolognia, J. L., *Bazex syndrome: Acrokeratosis paraneoplastica.* Semin Dermatol, 1995. 14:84–89.

19. Bolognia, J. L., Brewer, Y. P., and Cooper, D. L., *Bazex syndrome (acrokeratosis paraneoplastica). An analytic review.* Medicine (Baltimore), 1991. 70:269–280.

20. Hara, M., Hunayama, M., Aiba, S., Suetake, T., Watanabe, M., Tanaka, M., and Tagami, H., *Acrokeratosis paraneoplastica (Bazex syndrome) associated with primary cutaneous squamous cell carcinoma of the lower leg, vitiligo and alopecia areata.* Br J Dermatol, 1995. 133:121–124.

21. O'Brien, T. J., *Basex syndrome (acrokeratosis paraneoplastica).* Austral J Dermatol, 1995. 36:91–93.

22. Lucker, G. P., and Steijlen, P. M., *Acrokeratosis paraneoplastica (Bazex syndrome) occurring with acquired ichthyosis in Hodgkin's disease.* Br J Dermatol, 1995. 133:322–325.

23. Halpern, S. M., O'Donnell, L. J., and Makunura, C. N., *Acrokeratosis paraneoplastica of Bazex in association with a metastatic neuroendocrine tumour.* J R Soc Med, 1995. 88:353P–354P.

24. Obasi, O. E., and Garg, S. K., *Bazex paraneoplastic acrokeratosis in prostate carcinoma.* Br J Dermatol, 1987. 117:647–651.

25. Arregui, M. A., Raton, J. A., Landa, N., Izu, R., Eizaquirre, X., and Diaz-Perez, J. L., *Bazex's syndrome (acrokeratosis paraneoplastica)—first case report of association with a bladder carcinoma.* Clin Exp Dermatol, 1993. 18:445–448.

26. Huges, B. R., and Cotterill, J. A., *The relationship of psoriasis to malignancy: A clinical report.* Clin Exp Dermatol, 1993. 18:41–44.

27. Pecora, A. L., Landsman, L., Imgrund, S. P., and Lambert, W. C., *Acrokeratosis paraneoplastica (Bazex's syndrome). Report of a case and review of the literature.* Arch Dermatol, 1983. 119:820–826.

28. Grattan, C. E., Williams, D. M., Raafat, F., and Manna, V., *Acquired ichthyosis in a child with rhabdomyosarcoma.* Pediatr Dermatol, 1988. 5:167–169.

29. Farrell, A. M., Ross, J. S., Thomas, J. M., Fisher, C., and Bunker, C. B., *Acquired ichthyosis, alopecia and loss of hair pigment associated with leiomyosarcoma.* J Eur Acad Dermatol Venereol, 1998. 10:159–163.

30. Polisky, R. B., and Bronson, D. M., *Acquired ichthyosis in a patient with adenocarcinoma of the breast.* Cutis, 1986. 38:359–360.

31. Flint, G. L., Flam, M., and Soter, N. A., *Acquired ichthyosis. A sign of nonlymphoproliferative malignant disorders.* Arch Dermatol, 1975. 111:1446–1447.

32. Kutting, B., Metze, D., Luger, T. A., and Bonsmann, G., *Mycosis fungoides presenting as an acquired ichthyosis.* J Am Acad Dermatol, 1996. 34:887–889.

33. Tamura, J., Shinohara, M., Matsushima, T., Sawamura, M., Murakami, H., and Kubota, K., *Acquired ichthyosis as a manifestation of abdominal recurrence of non-Hodgkin's lymphoma.* Am J Hematol, 1994. 45:191–192.

34. Schwartz, R. A., and Williams, M. L., *Acquired ichthyosis: A merker for internal disease.* Am Fam Physician, 1984. 29:181–184.

35. Dilek, I., Demirer, T., Ustun, C., Arat, M., Koc, H., Beksac, M., Erdi, H., Anadolu, R., et al., *Acquired ichthyosis associated with graft vs. host disease following allogeneic peripheral stem cell transplantation in a patient with chronic myelogenous leukemia.* Bone Marrow Transplant, 1998. 21:1159–1161.

36. Bergman, R., Friedman-Birnbaum, R., and Carter, A., *Acquired ichthyosis in a patient with polycythemia rubra vera.* Cutis, 1985. 36:157–158.

37. Yokote, R., Iwatsuki, K., Hashizume, H., and Takigawa, M., *Lymphomatoid papulosis associated with acquired ichthyosis.* J Am Acad Dermatol, 1994. 30:889–892.

38. Roger, D., Aldigier, J. C., Peyronnet, P., Bonnetblanc, J. M., and Leroux-Robert, C., *Acquired ichthyosis and pyoderma gangrenosum in a patient with systemic lupus erythematosus.* Clin Exp Dermatol, 1993. 18:268–270.

39. Labauge, P., Meunier, L., Combe, B., Barneon, G., Beauvais, L., Sany, J., and Meynadier, J., *Acquired ichthyosis and disseminated lupus erythematosus.* Ann Dermatol Venereol, 1992. 119:41–43.

40. de la Cruz-Alvarez, J., Allegue, F., and Oliver, J., *Acquired ichthyosis associated with eosinophilic fasciitis.* J Am Acad Dermatol, 1996. 34:1079–1080.

41. Roselino, A. M., Souza, C. S., Andrade, J. M., Tone, L. G., Soares, F. A., Llorach-Velludo, M. A., and Foss, N. T., *Dermatomyositis and acquired ichthyosis as paraneoplastic manifestations of ovarian tumor.* Int J Dermatol, 1997. 36:611–614.

42. London, R. D., and Lebwohl, M., *Acquired ichthyosis and hyperparathyroidism.* J Am Acad Dermatol, 1989. 21:801–802.

43. Yosopovitch, G., Hodak, E., Vardi, P., Shraga, I., Karp, M., Sprecher, E., and David, M., *The prevalence of cutaneous manifestations of IDDM patients and their association with diabetes risk factors and microvascular complications.* Diabetes Care, 1998. 21:506–509.

44. Banse-Kupin, L., and Pelachyk, J. M., *Ichthyosiform sarcoidosis. Report of two cases and review of the literature.* J Am Acad Dermatol, 1987. 17:616–620.

45. Sadick, N. S., McNutt, N. S., and Kaplan, M. H., *Papulosquamous dermatoses of AIDS.* J Am Acad Dermatol, 1990. 22:1270–1277.

46. Kaplan, M. H., Sadick, N. S., McNutt, N. S., Talmor, M., Coronesi, M., and Hall, W. W., *Acquired ichthyosis in concomitant HIV-1 and HTLV-II infection: A new association with intravenous drug abuse.* J Am Acad Dermatol, 1993. 29:701–708.

47. Aram, H., *Acquired ichthyosis and related conditions.* Int J Dermatol, 1984. 23:458–461.

48. Griffin, L. J., and Massa, M. C., *Acquired ichthyosis and pityriasis rotunda.* Clin Dermatol, 1993. 11:27–32.

49. Bazex, J., el Sayed, F., Sans, B., Marguery, M. C., and Samalens, G., *Basex paraneoplastic acrokeratosis associated with acquired ichthyosis, pigmentation disorders and pruritis: A late disclosure of laryngeal neoplasms.* Ann Dermatol Venereol, 1992. 119:483–485.

50. Sybert, V. P., Dale, B. A., and A., H. K., *Ichthyosis vulgaris: Identification of a defect in synthesis of filaggrin correlated with an absence of keratohyaline granules.* J Invest Dermatol, 1985. 84:191–194.

51. Cooper, M. F., Wilson, P. D., Hartop, P. J., and Shuster, S., *Acquired ichthyosis and impaired dermal lipoge-*

nesis in Hodgkin's disease. Br J Dermatol, 1980. 102: 689–693.

52. Schwartz, R. A., *Sign of Leser-Trelat.* J Am Acad Dermatol, 1996. 35:88–95.

53. Grob, J. J., Rava, M. C., Gouvernet, J., Fuentes, P., Piana, L., Gamerre, M., Sarlews, J. C., and Bonerandi, J. J., *The relation between seborrheic keratoses and malignant solid tumors. A case-controlled study.* Acta Derm Venereol, 1991. 71:166–169.

54. Lindelof, B., Sigurgeirsson, B., and Melander, S., *Seborrheic keratosis and cancer.* J Am Acad Dermatol, 1992. 26:947–950.

55. Rampen, H. J., and Schwengle, L. E., *The sign of Leser-Trelat: Does it exist?* J Am Acad Dermatol, 1989. 21:50–55.

56. Yamamoto, T., and Yokoyama, A., *Hereditary onset of multiple seborrheic keratoses: A variant of Leser Trelat sign.* J Dermatol, 1996. 23:191–195.

57. Ohashi, N., and Hidaka, N., *Pancreatic carcinoma associated with the Leser-Trelat sign.* Int J Pancreatol, 1997. 22:155–160.

58. Hattori, A., Umegae, Y., Kataki, S., and Nakahima, T., *Small cell carcinoma of the lung with the Leser-Trelat sign.* Arch Dermatol, 1982. 118:1017–1018.

59. Chiba, T., Shitomi, T., Nakano, O., Shimotono, H., Yamada, H., Fujimaki, E., Orii, S., Sato, K., et al., *The sign of Leser-Trelat associated with esophageal carcinoma.* Am J Gastroenterol, 1996. 91:802–804.

60. Yaniv, R., Servadio, Y., Feinstein, A., and Trau, H., *The sign of Leser-Trelat associated with transitional cell carcinoma of the urinary bladder—a case report and short review.* Clin Exp Dermatol, 1994. 19:142–145.

61. Barron, L. A., and Prendiville, J. S., *The sign of Leser-Trelat in a young woman with osteogenic sarcoma.* J Am Acad Dermatol, 1992. 26:344–347.

62. Friedman-Birnbaum, R., and Haim, S., *Seborrheic ker-* *atosis and papillomatosis: Markers of breast adenocarcinoma.* Cutis, 1983. 32:161–162.

63. Fanti, P. A., Metri, M., and Patrizi, A., *The sign of Leser-Trelat associated with malignant melanoma.* Cutis, 1989. 44:39–41.

64. Horiuchi, Y., Katsuoka, K., Tsukamoto, K., and Takezaki, S., *Leser-Trelat sign associated with Sézary syndrome.* Cutis, 1985. 36:409–410.

65. Cohen, J. H., Lessin, S. R., Vowels, B. R., Benoit, B., Witmer, W. K., and Rook, A. H., *The sign of Leser-Trelat in association with Sézary syndrome: Simultaneous disappearance of seborrheic keratoses and malignant T-cell clone during combined therapy with photopheresis and interferon alpha.* Arch Dermatol, 1993. 129:1213–1215.

66. Ikari, Y., Ohkura, M., Morita, M., Seki, K., Kubota, Y., and Mizoguchi, M., *Leser-Trelat sign associated with Sézary syndrome.* J Dermatol, 1995. 22:62–67.

67. Martin, R. W. 3rd, Rady, P., Arany, I., and Tyring, S. K., *Benign Leydig cell tumor of the testis associated with human papillomavirus type 33 presenting with the sign of Leser-Trelat.* J Urol, 1993. 150:1246–1250.

68. Curth, H. O., Macklin, M. T., and Aschner, B., *The genetic basis of acanthosis nigricans.* In *The Eleventh International Congress of Dermatology Stockholm 1957 Proceedings*, S. Hellerstom, K. Wikstrom, and A. M. Hellerstom, Eds. 1960, Kadan Ohlssons Boktryckeri, Lund, pp. 689–692.

69. Cormia, F. E., Curth, H. O., and Fellner, M., *Pseudoacanthossis nigricans and psoriasis.* Arch Dermatol, 1965. 91:678.

70. Krishnaram, A. S., *Unilateral nevoid acanthosis nigricans.* Int J Dermatol, 1991. 30:452–453.

71. Pavithran, K., *Oestrogen-induced acanthosis nigricans.* Ind J Dermatol Venereol Leprol, 1990. 56:460–461.

CHAPTER 29

Histiocytic Proliferations and Internal Malignancy

Necrobiotic Xanthogranuloma with Paraproteinemia

Epidemiology. Necrobiotic xanthogranuloma (NXG) is an uncommon disorder in which cutaneous disease is often associated with lymphoproliferative disorders. Paraproteinemia is present in more than 90% of patients [1]. In one study, the risk of associated overt multiple myeloma, amyloidosis, or macroglobulinemia was assessed at 9%–11% of patients with NXG [2]. Most commonly, the association is with multiple myeloma. The cutaneous manifestations may predate or appear concomitantly with the hematologic diseases. The average age of affected patients is about 54 years [3]. In one study, 13 of 22 patients affected with NXG and concomitant multiple myeloma survived for a mean duration of 9.5 years after the onset of cutaneous disease [1]. These patients eventually succumbed to their hematologic neoplasms.

Cutaneous Features. Necrobiotic xanthogranuloma presents as multiple, slowly growing, erythematous, yellowish plaques and subcutaneous nodules [1]. Overlying dyspigmentation is common. These are most commonly located periorbitally. Similar lesions can also occur on flexural surfaces and on the trunk, and not all patients demonstrate the periorbital findings [4]. Ulceration is a common finding in well-developed plaques [5]. In other cases, pruritic papules may be the presenting feature [2].

Associated Disorders. Necrobiotic xanthogranuloma has been shown occasionally to affect internal viscera. The following internal organs have been reported to be involved [3, 6–10]:

- Myocardium
- Pulmonary
- Spleen
- Ocular
- Liver
- Laryngeal mucosa
- Kidney

Myocardial involvement may be present in the majority of patients [6]. Ocular involvement may manifest as keratitis, sclerosis, episcleritis, or uveitis [7]. Nodular transformation of the liver has been reported at autopsy in several patients with NXG [8]. Involvement of the musculoskeletal system is a rare occurrence [3].

Monoclonal IgG paraproteinemia is present in up to two-thirds of patients [3]. Less commonly, IgA paraproteinemia has been described [9, 11]. Hyperlipidemia, hypocomplementemia, and cryoglobulinemia have also been reported in patients with NXG [5]. Affected patients may also demonstrate hepatosplenomegaly, leukopenia, and an elevated sedimentation rate [12].

Necrobiotic xanthogranuloma has been reported in a patient who was a carrier for human T-lymphotropic virus type I (HTLV-I) and who had a high titer of circulating anti-HTLV-1 antibodies [13]. Hodgkin's disease has also been associated with NXG [14]. Patients with chronic lymphocytic leukemia and NXG have also been reported [15].

Histologic Features. Histologic features of NXG include a dense dermal infiltrate of suppurative granulomas. Neutrophils and nuclear dust are present in the centers of large palisades of lipid-laden histiocytes. Multinucleated giant cells are abundant. Touton-type giant cells are present, along with more bizarre-appearing foreign-body giant cells [16]. Large areas of pale staining or homogeneous collagen are present within the centers of the histiocytic palisades (Fig. 29–1). Large cholesterol clefts are present in the reticular dermis in up to 80% of cases [15] (Fig. 29–2). These are usually seen within zones of degenerated dermis. Lymphoid nodules present in a perivascular distribution [15]. Plasma cells are usually present at the periphery of the lymphoid nodules. These lymphoid

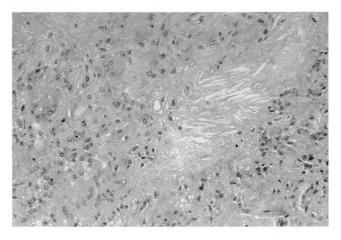

Fig. 29–2. Multinucleated giant cells and cholesterol clefts are commonly present in the dermis in necrobiotic xanthogranuloma.

nodules are found in more than half of all cases of NXG and are composed primarily of B lymphocytes [13] (Fig. 29–3).

Asteroid bodies are found within the cytoplasm of giant cells in up to one-third of cases [16]. The following entities must be considered in the histologic differential diagnosis of NXG:

- Infection—tuberculosis; deep fungus
- Necrobiosis lipoidica diabeticorum
- Rheumatoid nodule
- Xanthoma
- Xanthogranuloma

Special Studies. Immunophenotyping reveals the inflammatory process to be composed of non-X histio-

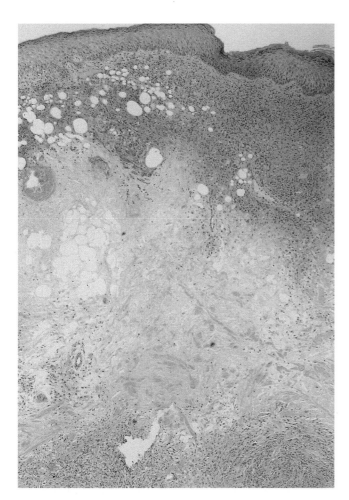

Fig. 29–1. A large area of zonal degeneration of collagen is present throughout the dermis in necrobiotic xanthogranuloma.

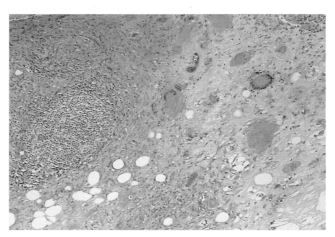

Fig. 29–3. Lymphoid nodules are present at the periphery of the degenerating collagen in many cases of necrobiotic xanthogranuloma.

cytes and T-helper lymphocytes [15]. These studies are not necessary for establishing the diagnosis.

Pathogenesis. The pathogenesis of NXG remains unknown at this time.

Multicentric Reticulohistiocytosis

Epidemiology. Multicentric reticulohistiocytosis (MR) is a rare disease that is characterized by cutaneous nodules and destructive arthritis [17]. Multicentric reticulohistiocytosis is more common in women and affects patients in the fourth and fifth decades. Occasional cases have been reported in children [18]. Underlying malignant neoplasm is reported in up to 30% of patients with MR [19]. Solitary reticulohistiocytomas also occur and are not associated with any systemic diseases.

Cutaneous Features. Multicentric reticulohistiocytosis presents as widespread papules and nodules that range in size from several millimeters to 2 cm. They are yellow-red or yellow-brown. Fingers, palms and backs of hands, face, and extremities are the most common sites of involvement. Oral and nasal mucosal surfaces are affected in about half of patients [20]. Cutaneous manifestations are the first signs of the disease in 90% of cases [21].

Associated Disorders. The most frequent process associated with the cutaneous changes of MR is destructive arthritis. The arthritis is diffuse and involves the hands in 80% of cases, the knees in 70%, and the wrists in 65%. After several years of progressive degeneration, the destructive arthritis may stabilize, but usually not until after the development of marked disability [22].

Malignant tumors are present in about 30% of patients. A wide range of malignancies have been associated, including malignant tumors of the breast [19], cervix [23], ovary [24], stomach, lung, colon, and pleura [21]. Malignant melanoma has also been reported in association with MR [25]. Myelodysplastic syndrome has been similarly associated [26].

Involvement of the eyes, muscles, and cardiovascular and pulmonary systems has been reported [20]. The thyroid is involved in rare cases of MR [27]. Several patients have been reported with coexisting MR and Sjögren's syndrome [28].

Histologic Features. The histologic features of MR consist of a dermal infiltrate of large histiocytes underlying an unremarkable or flattened epidermis (Fig. 29–4). The histiocytes have abundant "ground-glass" cytoplasm that has been described as "dusty rose"–colored and is strongly positive when stained with pe-

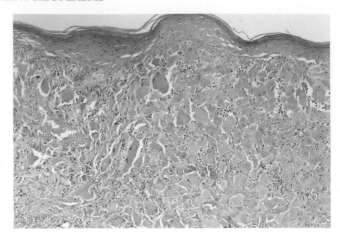

Fig. 29–4. A diffuse proliferation of histiocytes is present within the dermis in multicentric reticulohistiocytosis.

riodic acid–Schiff (Fig. 29–5). Multinucleated giant cells may be prominent. In early lesions, a dense lymphoid infiltrate may be present. Lymphocytic infiltrate is no longer extensive in older, well-developed lesions. The infiltrates are usually confined to the upper portions of the dermis. Collagen phagocytosis by the histiocytes is reported in patients with MR [29]. The earliest lesions may be indistinguishable from xanthomas, and the only clue may be correlation with the history of arthritis. The following entities must be considered in the histologic differential diagnosis of MR:

- Fibrous histiocytoma
- Granular cell tumor
- Juvenile xanthogranuloma
- Langerhans' cell histiocytosis
- Reticulohistiocytoma

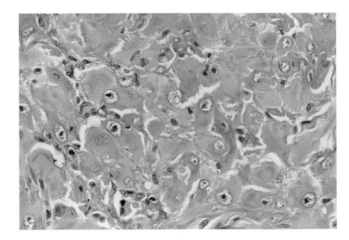

Fig. 29–5. Histiocytes in multicentric reticulohistiocytosis have a characteristic "ground-glass" appearance to the cytoplasm.

Solitary reticulohistiocytomas are histologically indistinguishable from the mulicentric ones, and clinical correlation is essential to make the correct diagnosis.

Special Studies. With electron microscopic studies, pleomorphic cytoplasmic inclusions have been found in about 40% of histiocytes studied in MR [30]. Ultrastructural examination is not ordinarily required to make a diagnosis of MR. In most cases, the histiocytes are S100 negative and express CD68.

Pathogenesis. It has been suggested that the infiltration of bones by histiocytes and multinucleated giant cells causes articular destruction by causing oversecretion of cytokines such as tumor necrosis factor-α, interleukin-1β, and interleukin-6 [31]. There is, however, no direct evidence of tumor infiltration of bone and cartilage lining joints.

Normolipemic Planar Xanthoma

Epidemiology. Normolipemic planar xanthomas occur in association with multiple myeloma and paraproteinemias in some patients who have no other lipid abnormalities. The incidence of this association is not well established.

Cutaneous Features. Planar xanthomas are yellow macules or soft papules that are usually less than 0.5 cm. Occasional xanthomas may be larger and form thin plaques. In some patients with paraproteinemias, extensive xanthomas have been described on the face, neck, trunk, and arms. These are yellow-orange colored [32].

Associated Disorders. Normolipemic planar xanthomas are most commonly associated with lymphoproliferative disorders. The most common association is with plasma cell dyscrasias, especially multiple myeloma [33]. In these patients, a circulating monoclonal gammopathy is frequently found. IgG-kappa is the most commonly reported gammopathy associated with this condition [34–36]. Mycosis fungoides has also been reported in association with normolipemic planar xanthomas [37], as has leukemia [38]. Association with hepatic disease has also been described [39]. Rare patients are reported who have normolipemic planar xanthomas and other inflammatory conditions, including erythrodermic atopic dermatitis [40] and relapsing polychondritis [41].

Histologic Features. Histologic sections reveal a perivascular infiltrate of neutrophils and lipid-containing histiocytes. Neutrophilic dust is present around the superficial vascular plexus. The histiocytes percolate out between collagen bundles of the dermis [41]. The epidermis is unremarkable or flattened (Figs. 29–6 and

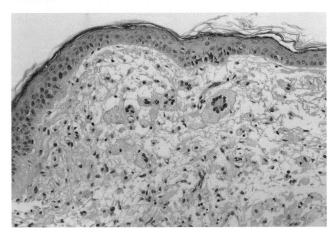

Fig. 29–6. Normolipemic planar xanthomas are characterized by abundant lipid-laden histiocytes within the papillary and reticular dermis.

29–7). The following entities must be considered in the histologic differential diagnosis of normolipemic planar xanthoma:

- Fibrous histiocytoma with lipidization
- Leprosy
- Tendinous xanthoma
- Tuberous xanthoma
- Xanthelasma
- Xanthogranuloma

Special Studies. Immunophenotyping studies reveal that the infiltrating histiocytes are CD1a-negative reactive histiocytes, similar to those seen in noninfectious granulomas [40].

Pathogenesis. Antilipoprotein activity due to a circulating monoclonal immunoglobulin has been reported

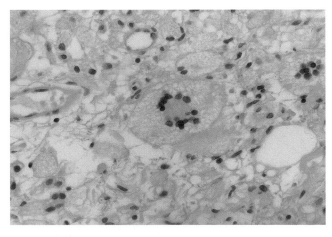

Fig. 29–7. Touton giant cells are present in normolipemic planar xanthomas.

in several patients with normolipemic planar xanthomas [35, 36]. This suggests the possibility of a causal relationship that needs to be further investigated [36]. Others have further suggested that the autoantibody activity of myeloma proteins against serum lipoproteins may result in normolipemic xanthomas [42].

References

1. Finan, M. C., and Winkelmann, R. K., *Necrobiotic xanthogranuloma with paraproteinemia. A review of 22 cases*. Medicine (Baltimore), 1986. 65:376–388.

2. Johnston, K. A., Grimwood, R. E., Meffert, J. J., and Deering, K. C., *Necrobiotic xanthogranuloma with paraproteinemia: An evolving presentation*. Cutis, 1997. 59:333–336.

3. Mehregan, D. A., and Winkelman, R. K., *Necrobiotic xanthogranuloma*. Arch Dermatol, 1992. 128:94–100.

4. McGregor, J. M., Miller, J., Smith, N. P., and Hay, R. J., *Necrobiotic xanthogranuloma without periorbital lesions*. J Am Acad Dermatol, 1993. 29:466–469.

5. Kossard, S., and Winkelmann, R. K., *Necrobiotic xanthogranuloma with paraproteinemia*. J Am Acad Dermatol, 1980. 3:257–270.

6. Umbert, I., and Winkelmann, R. K., *Necrobiotic xanthogranuloma with cardiac involvement*. Br J Dermatol, 1995. 133:438–443.

7. Hohenleutner, S., Hohenleutner, U., Stolz, W., and Landthaler, M., *Necrobiotic xanthogranuloma with eye involvement. Overview and case report*. Hautarzt, 1995. 46:330–334.

8. Novak, P. M., Robbins, T. O., and Winkelmann, R. K., *Necrobiotic xanthogranuloma with myocardial lesions and nodular transformation of the liver*. Hum Pathol, 1992. 23:195–196.

9. Fortson, J. S., and Schroeter, A. L., *Necrobiotic xanthogranuloma with IgA paraproteinemia and extracutaneous involvement*. Am J Dermatopathol, 1990. 12:579–584.

10. Winkelmann, R. K., Dahl, P. M., and Perniciaro, C., *Asteroid bodies and other cytoplasmic inclusions in necrobiotic xanthogranuloma with paraproteinemia*. J Am Acad Dermatol, 1998. 38:967–970.

11. Valentine, E. A., Friedman, H. D., Zamkoff, K. W., and Streeten, B. W., *Necrobiotic xanthogranuloma with IgA multiple myeloma: A case report and literature review*. Am J Hematol, 1990. 35:283–285.

12. Robertson, D. M., and Winkelmann, R. K., *Ophthalmic features of necrobiotic xanthogranuloma with paraproteinemia*. Am J Ophthalmol, 1984. 97:173–183.

13. Nishimura, M., Takano-Nishimura, Y., Yano, I., Hayashi, N., and Toshitani, S., *Necrobiotic xanthogranuloma in a human T-lymphotropic virus type 1 carrier*. J Am Acad Dermatol, 1992. 27:886–889.

14. Reeder, C. B., Connolly, S. M., and Winkelmann, R. K., *The evolution of Hodgkin's disease and necrobiotic xanthogranuloma syndrome*. Mayo Clin Proc, 1991. 66:1222–1224.

15. Scupham, R. K., and Fretzin, D. F., *Necrobiotic xanthogranuloma with paraproteinemia*. Arch Pathol Lab Med, 1989. 113:1389–1391.

16. Finan, M. C., and Winkelmann, R. K., *Histopathology of necrobiotic xanthogranuloma with paraproteinemia*. J Cutan Pathol, 1987. 14:92–99.

17. Barrow, M. V., and Holubar, K., *Multicentric reticulohistiocytosis: A review of 33 patients*. Medicine (Baltimore), 1969. 48:287–305.

18. Candell Chalom, E., Elenitsas, R., Rosenstein, E. D., and Kramer, N., *A case of multicentric reticulohistiocytosis in a 6-year-old child*. J Rheumatol, 1998. 25:794–797.

19. Valencia, I. C., Colsky, A., and Berman, B., *Multicentric reticulohistiocytosis associated with recurrent breast carcinoma*. J Am Acad Dermatol, 1998. 39:864–866.

20. Chevrant-Breton, J., *La reitculohistiocytose multicentrique: Revue de la litterature recente (depuis 1969)*. Ann Dermatol Venereol, 1977. 104:830–840.

21. Nunnick, J. C., Krusinski, P. A., and Yates, J. W., *Multicentric reticulohistiocytosis and cancer: A case report and review of the literature*. Med Pediatr Oncol, 1985. 13:273–279.

22. Gianotti, F., and Caputo, R., *Histiocytic syndromes: A review*. J Am Acad Dermatol, 1985. 13:383–404.

23. Ridgway, H. A., and Rhodes, E. L., *Multicentric reticulohistiocytosis with carcinoma-in-situ of the cervix*. Br J Dermatol, 1979. 101(Suppl 17):61–62.

24. Hall-Smith, P., *Multicentric reticulohistiocytosis with ovarian carcinoma*. Proc R Soc Med, 1976. 69:380–381.

25. Gibson, G., Cassidy, M., O'Connell, P., and Murphy, G. M., *Multicentric reticulohistiocytosis associated with recurrence of malignant melanoma*. J Am Acad Dermatol, 1995. 32:134–136.

26. Bauer, A., Garbe, C., Detmar, M., Kreuser, E. D., and Gollnick, H., *Multicentric reticulohistiocytosis and myelodysplastic syndrome*. Hautarzt, 1994. 45:91–96.

27. Finelli, L. G., Tenner, L. K., Ratz, J. L., and Long, B. D., *A case of multicentric reticulohistiocytosis with thyroid involvement*. J Am Acad Dermatol, 1986. 15:1097–1100.

28. Shiokawa, S., Shingu, M., Nishimura, M., Yasuda, M., Yamamoto, M., Tawara, T., Wada, T., and Nobunaga, M., *Multicentric reticulohistiocytosis associated with subclinical Sjögren's syndrome*. Clin Rheumatol, 1991. 10:201–205.

29. Caputo, R., Alessi, E., and Berti, E., *Collagen phagocytosis in multicentric reticulohistiocytosis*. J Invest Dermatol, 1981. 76:342–346.

30. Caputo, R., Crosti, C., and Cainelli, T., *A unique cytoplasmic structure in papular histiocytoma*. J Invest Dermatol, 1977. 68:98–104.

31. Nakamura, H., Yoshino, S., Shiga, H., Tanaka, H., and Katsumata, S., *A case of spontaneous femoral neck fracture associated with multicentric reticulohistiocytosis: Oversecretion of interleukin-1β, interleukin-6, and tumor necrosis factor [al by affected synovial cells*. Arthritis Rheum, 1997. 40:2266–2270.

32. Feiwel, M., *Xanthomatosis in cryoglobulinemia and other paraproteinemias with report of a case.* Br J Dermatol, 1968. 80:719–729.

33. Possick, P., *Plasma cell dyscrasia (monoclonal gammopathy) associated with diffuse normolipemic plane xanthomatosis; basal-cell epitheliomatosis.* Arch Dermatol, 1969. 100:252–254.

34. Rotteleur, G., Gaveau, D., Guieu, M., Dejobert, Y., Krivosic, I., and Thomas, P., *Normolipemic diffuse xanthomatosis disclosing IgG kappa myeloma.* Ann Dermatol Venereol, 1988. 115:175–178.

35. Piccinno, R., Menni, S., Cavicchini, S., and Gianotti, R., *Normolipemic plane xanthomas and IgG-κ multiple myeloma. Description of a clinical case.* G Ital Dermatol Venereol, 1990. 125:449–451.

36. Modiano, P., Gillet-Terver, M. N., Reichert, S., Francois-Griffaton, A., Beaumont, J. L., Weber, M., and Schmutz, J. L., *Normolipemic plane xanthoma, monoclonal gammopathy, anti-lipoprotein activity, hypocomplementemia.* Ann Dermatol Venereol, 1995. 122:507–508.

37. McCadden, M. E., Glick, A. D., and King, L. E. Jr., *Mycosis fungoides associated with dystrophic xanthomatosis.* Arch Dermatol, 1987. 123:91–94.

38. Winkelmann, R. K., *Normolipemic xanthoma planum and its associated syndromes.* Hautarzt, 1983. 34:159–163.

39. Rudolph, R. L., *Diffuse "essential" normolipemic xanthomatosis.* Int J Dermatol, 1975. 14:651–656.

40. Goerdt, S., Kretzchmar, L., Bonsmann, G., Luger, T., and Kolde, G., *Normolipemic papular xanthomatosis in erythrodermic atopic dermatitis.* J Am Acad Dermatol, 1995. 32:326–333.

41. Yoshimura, T., Aiba, S., Tadaki, T., and Tagami, H., *Generalized normolipemic plane xanthomatosis associated with relapsing polychondritis.* Acta Derm Venereol, 1994. 74:221–223.

42. Doutre, M. S., Conri, C., Beylot, C., Fleury, B., Chapoulard, H., and Biolac, P., *Normolipemic plane xanthomas and IgGk myeloma with anti-lipoprotein activity. A propos of a case. Review of the literature.* Dermatologica, 1985. 170:157–164.

CHAPTER 30

Miscellaneous Cutaneous Lesions

Paraneoplastic Pemphigus

Epidemiology. Paraneoplastic pemphigus is a rare blistering disease that occurs most commonly with malignant hematologic diseases and less commonly with tumors of solid organs. The cutaneous eruption often parallels the course of the neoplasm and is almost invariably rapidly fatal; however, rare long-term survivors have been reported [1].

Cutaneous Features. The eruptions in patients with paraneoplastic pemphigus have a polymorphous appearance. In some patients, the disease resembles erythema multiforme, with targetoid macules that have necrotic centers. Other patients develop flaccid blisters that spread easily (positive Nikolski's sign) and greatly resemble pemphigus vulgaris [2]. Rare patients have been reported with tense bullae resembling bullous pemphigoid [3]. Scaling and erythema may be present [4]. A papulosquamous eruption is rarely the presenting feature, and vesicles are also reported in some cases. Some cases have a lichenoid appearance. Pruritus is a common complaint. The trunk, extremities, palms, and soles are often involved [5].

Mucosal surfaces are always involved in this process [5]. Conjunctiva [6] and oral and genital mucosa are most frequently involved, and tracheal mucosa [7] and pulmonary bronchial mucosa [2, 8] are rarely affected. The mucosal ulcerations are typically quite painful, and the oral manifestations are often the most severe within the disease spectrum.

Associated Diseases. Paraneoplastic pemphigus is seen most commonly in patients with leukemia [7] (especially chronic lymphocytic leukemia), Hodgkin's disease [9], and non-Hodgkin's lymphoma [10]. Paraneoplastic pemphigus has been reported in rare patients with Castleman's disease [8] and thymoma [4]. It has also been reported, although less frequently, in association with many solid tumors, including adenocarcinoma of the colon [11], pancreatic carcinoma [12], and bronchogenic squamous cell carcinoma [13]. Radiotherapy has been implicated in inducing paraneoplastic pemphigus in one case [14].

Histologic Features. The histologic features of paraneoplastic pemphigus are similar but not identical to those seen in pemphigus vulgaris. Suprabasilar acantholysis resulting in blister formation is seen in virtually all cases (Fig. 30–1). In addition, dyskeratosis is seen in about half of cases. Basal vacuolization is also frequently present [15]. Spongiosis is often present. An interface dermatitis with exocytosis of lymphocytes into the epidermis is seen in most cases [4] (Fig. 30–2). The combination of inflammatory interface changes and suprabasal bulla formation via acantholysis are highly suggestive of the diagnosis. The following entities must be considered in the differential diagnosis of paraneoplastic pemphigus:

- Erythema multiforme
- Lichen planus
- Pemphigus vulgaris

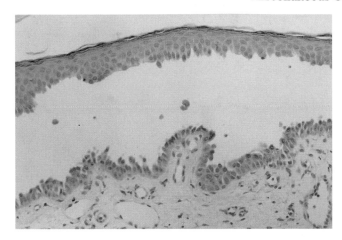

Fig. 30–1. An acantholytic suprabasilar blister resembling pemphigus vulgaris is present in most cases of paraneoplastic pemphigus.

Special Studies. Direct immunofluorescence examination performed on perilesional skin demonstrates intercellular staining with IgG and C3 in most cases. Additional staining along the basement membrane zone is also present in a minority of cases [4]. Similar immunostaining is detected on affected mucosal surfaces [3]. Rarely, IgA deposition may be seen in a similar distribution.

Western blotting demonstrates the circulating autoantibodies to be directed against a number of different proteins, including those with molecular weights of 250 (desmoplakin I), 230 (bullous pemphigoid antigen), 210 (desmoplakin II) and 190 kD (not yet further characterized) [2] and periplakin in patients with paraneoplastic pemphigus [16]. Indirect immunofluorescence performed on rat bladder epithelium has been shown to be positive in 75%–90% of patients with paraneoplastic pemphigus and to be 83% specific for

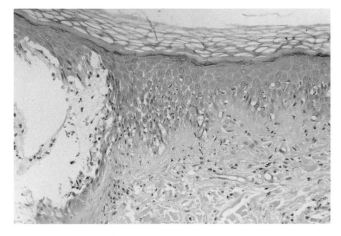

Fig. 30–2. Interface dermatitis with basal vacuolization is present in more than half of cases of paraneoplastic pemphigus.

this entity [17, 18]. Similar positive staining is also detected when monkey esophagus is used as the substrate.

Pathogenesis. Autoantibodies directed against a complex of desmosomal proteins, including desmoplakin, periplakin, envoplakin [19], plectin [20], and the bullous pemphigoid antigen, destroy affected desmosomes, resulting in acantholysis and blister formation of epithelia. The mechanism by which neoplasia induces the autoimmune reaction has not yet been elucidated [21].

Erythema Gyratum Repens

Epidemiology. Erythema gyratum repens (EGR) is a rare cutaneous eruption that is almost always an indicator of underlying internal malignancy [22]. Two studies have suggested that the incidence of associated underlying malignancy is 80%–85% in patients with EGR [23, 24]. Reports of EGR unassociated with systemic disease appear in the literature [25].

Cutaneous Features. Erythema gyratum repens is a slowly expanding eruption that is characterized by a "wood grain" appearance. The trunk and proximal extremities are most commonly affected, and the face is usually spared. A slight scale is present overlying parallel curving bands of erythema alternating with less erythematous skin in an arcuate pattern. The pattern migrates at up to 1 cm per day. Pruritus is common.

Associated Disorders. Erythema gyratum repens is associated with internal malignancy in most cases. The most frequent association is with bronchogenic carcinoma [26]. It has also been associated with esophageal carcinoma [27], Hodgkin's disease [28], and adrenal cell carcinoma [29]. Erythema gyratum repens has also been associated with pulmonary tuberculosis [30] and hypereosinophilic syndrome [31].

Histologic Features. The histologic features of EGR are not specific. There is parakeratosis overlying foci of mild spongiosis. A lymphohistiocytic infiltrate is present around the vessels of the superficial vascular plexus, occasionally extending down to the deeper dermal blood vessels. The infiltrate varies from sparse to moderately intense [32]. Eosinophils are present in small numbers in most cases. The following entities must be considered in the histologic differential diagnosis of EGR:

- Arthropod bite reaction
- Dermal hypersensitivity reaction
- Drug eruption
- Erythema annulare centrifugum
- Erythema migrans
- Pityriasis rosea
- Small plaque parapsoriasis

Special Studies. Direct immunofluorescence demonstrated granular deposits of immunoglobulins along the basement membrane zone of affected skin in some patients with EGR. Circulating antibasement membrane zone antibodies were detected by indirect immunofluorescence [33]. It is not known how often these findings are seen in cases of EGR or what the significance of these observations is in terms of pathogenesis.

Pathogenesis. The pathogenesis of EGR is not known. Epidermal growth factor and other cytokines have been implicated in the pathogenesis [33].

Superficial (Migratory) Thrombophlebitis

Epidemiology. Superficial migratory thrombophlebitis occurs in patients with a variety of hypercoagulable conditions. In one series, 12% of patients with thrombophlebitis were found to harbor an occult malignancy [34]. The association of spontaneously occurring venous thrombosis and internal malignancy is termed *Trousseau's syndrome* [35]. Superficial venous thrombosis of the breast has been termed *Mondor's disease.* In most cases, this is secondary to trauma or previous surgery [36].

Cutaneous Features. Superficial thrombophlebitis is most common on the lower extremities, although other superficial veins are occasionally affected. The overlying skin is erythematous and tender. A firm, linear cord is palpable beneath the surface of the skin. In some cases, superficial ulceration may occur in older lesions.

Associated Disorders. Superficial thrombophlebitis is associated with both primary and secondary hypercoagulable states [37, 38]. Primary states include deficiencies of antithrombin III, heparin cofactor 2, protein C [39], protein S, factor XII [40], and dysfibrinogenemia [38]. In addition, patients with a lupus anticoagulant [41] or anticardiolipin antibodies [39] are also predisposed toward developing superficial thrombophlebitis.

Secondary hypercoagulable states associated with superficial thrombophlebitis include malignancies, pregnancy, use of oral contraceptives, Beçhet's disease, and Buerger's disease [42]. Pancreatic carcinoma is the most frequently associated malignancy, with superficial thrombophlebitis observed in about 7% of these patients [43]. Superficial thrombophlebitis has, however, been associated with many other types of cancer, including cholangiocarcinoma [44], ovarian carcinoma [45], and cancers of the prostate, breast, lungs, uterus, and brain [34]. In one large series, the incidence of venous thrombosis in a population of cancer patients was assessed at 0.4% [46].

Histologic Features. Histologic sections of superficial thrombophlebitis reveal skin with an unremarkable epidermis and superficial dermis. At the interface between the deep reticular dermis and the subcutaneous fat, an inflammatory infiltrate is present surrounding and infiltrating affected vessels. In some cases, the vessels have more of an oblong shape than a completely circular one, as is characteristic of veins with less vascular wall support than arteries (Fig. 30–3). This becomes important in distinguishing superficial thrombophlebitis from polyarteritis nodosa, which involves similar-caliber vessels located in similar anatomic locations within the skin. The nature of the inflammatory infiltrate in superficial thrombophlebitis depends on the age of the lesion sampled. Early lesions will demonstrate almost entirely neutrophils, whereas older lesions have more of a mixed infiltrate with abundant lymphocytes, histiocytes, and multinucleated giant cells admixed with neutrophils. The vessel lumen is ordinarily completely occluded with thrombus. The inflammatory infiltrate frequently extends slightly into the surrounding deep dermis and subcutaneous fat, giving rise to a panniculitis. Multiple levels through the tissue block may be necessary to isolate the affected vessel or vessels. The following entities must be considered in the histologic differential diagnosis of superficial thrombophlebitis:

- Erythema induratum
- Erythema nodosum
- Infectious etiology
- Nodular vasculitis
- Polyarteritis nodosa—classic
- Polyarteritis nodosa—cutaneous

Special Studies. In some cases, a Verhoeff-van Gieson stain is helpful in evaluating the affected vessels for the presence of an internal elastic lamina (Fig. 30–4). If present, this is strong evidence in favor of arterial involvement and a diagnosis of polyarteritis nodosa. If no elas-

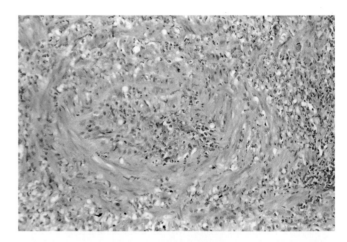

Fig. 30–3. Superficial thrombophlebitis is characterized by a marked transmural neutrophilic infiltrate involving veins located in the subcutaneous fat.

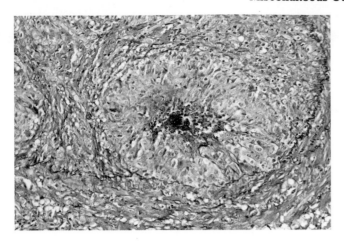

Fig. 30–4. A Verhoeff-van Gieson stain is helpful in determining that the affected vessel is a vein as characterized by no internal elastic lamina.

tic lamina is identified, either the affected vessel is a vein or extensive damage has occurred secondary to the inflammatory infiltrate.

Pathogenesis. It has been suggested that the expression of tissue factor by malignant cells predisposes patients affected with Trousseau's syndrome to thrombophlebitis [35]. Tissue factor is a cell surface glycoprotein that is responsible for initiating the extrinsic pathway of the coagulation cascade. It has been shown that in these patients the tumors do express tissue factor on the cell surfaces [47].

Paraneoplastic Vasculitis

Epidemiology. Approximately 5%–8% of patients with malignancies develop vasculitis [48, 49]. About two-thirds of cases occur with hematologic malignancies and the others with solid tumors [48]. Paraneoplastic vasculitis occurs equally in men and women. The vasculitis may occur before or concurrent with the onset of the malignancies. In a few cases, evidence of systemic paraneoplastic vasculitis is present in the absence of cutaneous changes [50].

Cutaneous Features. Paraneoplastic vasculitis can have one of several cutaneous morphologies, including the appearance of a leukocytoclastic vasculitis, polyarteritis nodosa [51], Henoch-Schönlein purpura (leukocytoclastic vasculitis) [52], or urticarial vasculitis [53]. Leukocytoclastic vasculitis is the most common pattern seen in this condition. Leukocytoclastic vasculitis and polyarteritis nodosa are described in Chapter 4 and Henoch-Schönlein purpura in Chapter 8.

Associated Disorders. Paraneoplastic vasculitis is most commonly seen with hematologic malignancies [48]. The

association has been reported with non-Hodgkin's lymphomas, angioimmunoblastic lymphadenopathy, chronic lymphocytic leukemia [54], and myelodysplastic syndromes [52]. Among solid tumors, the association is most frequent with lung cancer [48], cancers of the gastrointestinal tract [51], and renal carcinomas [55].

Histologic Features. The histologic features of paraneoplastic vasculitis vary depending on the type of vasculitis. Microscopic descriptions of leukocytoclastic vasculitis and polyarteritis nodosa are provided in Chapter 4 and Henoch-Schönlein purpura in Chapter 8.

A pattern of lymphocytic vasculitis has also been described in patients with lymphoproliferative disorders and paraneoplastic vasculitis [54]. In these cases, lymphocytes infiltrate the walls of vessels within the superficial vascular plexus. These were found to be reactive T lymphocytes. Extravasation of erythrocytes was occasionally seen [52]. The existence of a true lymphocytic vasculitis has been questioned and remains a controversial entity.

Special Studies. Antineutrophil cytoplasmic antibodies have been detected in a patient with paraneoplastic vasculitis [56]. The frequency of this observation is not known. Direct immunofluorescence may be helpful in detecting immune complex deposits within the affected vessel walls.

Pathogenesis. Although the pathogenesis of paraneoplastic vasculitis remains unknown, it seems likely that immune complexes associated with the underlying malignancies play some role in the development of the vasculitis. It has also been suggested that chemotactic factors or deficient phagocytic cells may play some role [57].

Sweet's Syndrome (Acute Febrile Neutrophilic Dermatosis)

Epidemiology. Sweet's syndrome is an uncommon dermatosis that has an estimated incidence of 2.7 cases per 10^6 people [58]. The female to male ratio is approximately 2.5:1 [59]. The mean age of onset is 52.6 years, with most cases reported in patients aged 30 to 60 years [59]. There are two peaks of incidence, one at about age 35 years and the other at age 60 years [59]. Sweet's syndrome rarely affects children [60]. In one series, the cutaneous eruption preceded the onset of an underlying condition in 61% of patients [61].

Cutaneous Features. Sweet's syndrome presents as the abrupt onset of multiple, tender or painful erythematous papules that are most common on the face, trunk, and extremities. These papules enlarge to form edematous plaques or nodules. The plaques are sharply demarcated, range in size from 1 to 20 cm, and frequently cause a burning sensation. Pseudovesiculation and pustules may be present. A palmoplantar pustulosis appearance has been reported [62]. An erythema multiforme-like appearance has been described in some patients. Mucosal involvement has been reported in a few patients [58], and genital lesions are rare [63]. Pathergy (see Chapter 5) has been reported in about 8% of patients with Sweet's syndrome [64].

Associated Disorders. Sweet's syndrome is not associated with other underlying disease processes in about 76% of cases. Approximately 11% of cases are associated with underlying neoplasia, 16% with other inflammatory processes, and 2% of cases are associated with pregnancy [64]. Table 30–1 summarizes the systemic diseases that have been associated with Sweet's syndrome.

Acute myelogenous leukemia accounts for approximately 42% of patients with Sweet's syndrome and an underlying malignancy [65]. In patients with Sweet's syndrome and solid tumors, 37% of the tumors were from the genitourinary system, 23% from the breast, and 17% from the gastrointestinal tract [61, 66]. In this subset of patients with Sweet's syndrome, there is no female predominance [67].

In rare cases, drugs have been implicated in the development of Sweet's syndrome. Furosemide [68] and minocycline [69] have been reported to cause the syndrome.

From 48% [58] to 83% [70] of patients with Sweet's syndrome are intermittently febrile. Arthralgias or arthritis are present in about half of patients [58]. Conjunctivitis, uveitis, and episcleritis have also been reported in about one-third of patients [64]. Neutrophilia is present in up to 60% of patients [61]. Headaches, nausea, vomiting, and malaise are also commonly observed [71].

Internal organ involvement with a neutrophilic inflammatory infiltrate has been described in patients with Sweet's syndrome. Segmental acute aortitis and myositis have been reported [72]. Acute pneumonitis is reported in rare patients [59]. Heart involvement has been described in a single patient [59]. Renal involvement leading to acute renal failure occurs in rare patients [73].

Histologic Features. The histologic features of Sweet's syndrome consist of a diffuse, moderately dense inflammatory infiltrate of neutrophils throughout the papillary and superficial reticular dermis (Fig. 30–5 A). In a few cases, the neutrophilic infiltrate extends into the deeper portions of the dermis and into the subcutaneous fat [61]. In most cases, papillary dermal edema is pronounced, leading to subepidermal blister formation in some cases (Fig. 30–5 B). The epidermis is usu-

Table 30–1. Systemic Diseases Associated with Sweet's Syndrome
Hematologic malignancies
Acute myelogenous leukemia
Chronic myelogenous leukemia
Multiple myeloma
Hairy cell leukemia
Polycythemia vera
Hodgkin's disease
Non-Hodgkin's lymphoma
Nonhematologic malignancies
Breast carcinoma
Melanoma
Lung carcinoma
Renal cell carcinoma
Transitional cell carcinoma of the bladder
Gastric adenocarcinoma
Prostate carcinoma
Colonic adenocarcinoma
Follicular carcinoma of the thyroid
Ovarian carcinoma
Inflammatory conditions
Infectious processes
Salmonella
Tuberculosis
Cytomegalovirus
Leprosy
Human immunodeficiency virus
Yersinia
Toxoplasmosis
Autoimmune diseases
Lupus erythematosus
Rheumatoid arthritis
Thyroiditis
Sjögren's syndrome
Mixed connective tissue disease
Inflammatory bowel disease
Behçet's disease
Other
Pregnancy
Sarcoidosis
Complement deficiency

From references 61, 64, 65, 67, and 71.

ally unaffected, but slight spongiosis is occasionally seen. In addition, intraepidermal pustules may be present. Karyorrhectic debris is common within the dermis. Endothelial swelling may be present, but true vasculitis is not identified [67]. A deeper, perivascular lymphocytic inflammatory infiltrate is often present. It has been reported that a lymphocytic infiltrate characterizes the earliest changes seen in Sweet's syndrome and that the classic neutrophilic infiltrate occurs in later, well-developed lesions [74]. In late lesions, histiocytes predominate and neutrophils are less pronounced [64]. Eosinophils are also present in most cases. The following entities must be considered in the histologic differential diagnosis of Sweet's syndrome:

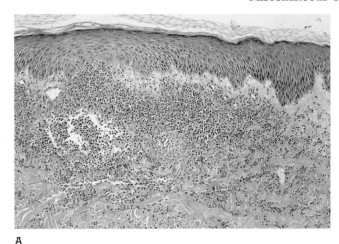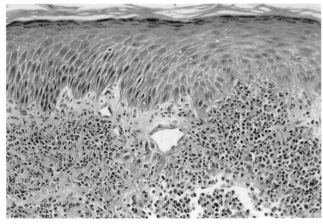

A   B

Fig. 30–5. *A,* Sweet's syndrome or acute febrile neutrophilic dermatosis demonstrates sheets of neutrophils in the papillary and superficial reticular dermis, along with papillary dermal edema. *B,* The vessels are predominantly spared, despite the abundance of neutrophils and karyorrhectic debris.

- Bowel-associated dermatitis/arthritis syndrome
- Cellulitis
- Leukocytoclastic vasculitis
- Metastatic Crohn's disease
- Palisaded and neutrophilic dermatosis of rheumatoid arthritis
- Pyoderma gangrenosum

Special Studies. Direct immunofluorescence studies may be helpful in distinguishing Sweet's syndrome from leukocytoclastic vasculitis. Immune complexes are not detected in vessel walls in Sweet's syndrome, but are commonly seen in active lesions of leukocytoclastic vasculitis. Circulating antibodies directed against neutrophil cytoplasmic antigens are present in many patients with Sweet's disease and may be helpful in making the diagnosis [75].

Pathogenesis. It has been suggested that Sweet's syndrome represents an abnormal immunologic response toward unknown antigens [59]. Interleukin-1, a neutrophil activator, might play a role in this process [76]. The process is thought to be mediated by helper T-cell type I cytokines [77]. A similar pathogenesis may be responsible for the cutaneous eruption seen after administration of granulocyte-macrophage colony-stimulating factor that demonstrates many of the same histologic changes [78].

Pityriasis Rotunda

Epidemiology. Pityriasis rotunda is a rare dermatosis that has been described most commonly in Japanese, black South African, and black West Indian patients [79]. This form of the disease represents the sporadic form that

has been associated with underlying systemic diseases. There also appears to be a familial form of the disease [80], which has been described in Sardinia, Italy [81], and which does not appear to be associated with underlying systemic disease. Although exceedingly rare, pityriasis rotunda has been reported in white patients [82].

Men and women are equally affected, and the disease is most prevalent in young adults. The cutaneous eruption lasts from months to years and may worsen in the winter months [83].

Cutaneous Features. Pityriasis rotunda is characterized by multiple round or oval, sharply defined patches with overlying scale. The patches are usually either hypochromic or hyperchromic and are asymptomatic. The trunk and proximal extremities are the usual site for this cutaneous eruption. One or multiple patches may be present and range in size from less than 1 to 25–30 cm in diameter. White patients tend to have fewer lesions than black or Asian patients with pityriasis rotunda [84].

Associated Disorders. Pityriasis rotunda has been described in association with internal malignancies. The association is strongest in patients with hepatocellular carcinoma. Approximately 16% of patients with hepatocellular carcinoma in South Africa demonstrated pityriasis rotunda [85]. In the same study population, about 5% of patients with tuberculosis also demonstrated the cutaneous changes [85]. Pityriasis rotunda has also been reported in association with multiple myeloma [80], leukemia [86], and carcinoma of the prostate [87], stomach [88], and esophagus [86]. Pityriasis rotunda has been reported in patients with uterine leiomyomas and ovarian cysts [86].

Histologic Features. The histologic features of pityriasis rotunda have not been well described. In some patients, the changes have resembled ichthyosis vulgaris. The stratum corneum is characterized by increased orthokeratotic keratin. The granular layer is slightly diminished to absent, and the epidermis is slightly acanthotic. No inflammation is present [79]. Ultrastructural studies revealed lipid vacuoles in the corneocytes, and focal diminution in the size of keratohyaline granules was seen, as was increased intercellular cementing substance [84].

Special Studies. Special studies are not required to make a diagnosis of pityriasis rotunda.

Pathogenesis. Several investigators have suggested that pityriasis rotunda represents a variant of ichthyosis [80] with a similar defect in keratinization. Some authors consider it to be a variant of ichthyosis vulgaris [79]. Others suggest that it represents a localized form of acquired ichthyosis [89] or a variant of some other type of congenital ichthyosis [84].

References

1. Perniciaro, C., Kuechle, M., Colon-Otero, K. G., Raymond, M. G., Spear, K. L., and Pittelkow, M. R., *Paraneoplastic pemphigus: A case of prolonged survival.* Mayo Clin Proc, 1994. 69:851–855.

2. Segard-Drouard, M., Lefebvre, L., Catteau, B., Pannequin, C., Delaporte, E., Janin, A., and Thomas, P., *Paraneoplastic pemphigus with tracheobronchial involvement.* Ann Dermatol Venereol, 1997. 124(615–618).

3. Fullerton, S. H., Woodley, D. T., Smoller, B. R., and Anhalt, G. J., *Paraneoplastic pemphigus with autoantibody deposition in bronchial epithelium after autologous bone marrow transplantation.* JAMA, 1992. 267:1500–1502.

4. Mehregan, D. R., Oursler, J. R., Leiferman, K. M., Muller, S. A., Anhalt, G. J., and Peters, M. S., *Paraneoplastic pemphigus: A subset of patients with pemphigus and neoplasia.* J Cutan Pathol, 1993. 20:203–210.

5. Mutasim, D. F., Pelc, N. J., and Anhalt, G. J., *Paraneoplastic pemphigus, pemphigus vulgaris, and pemphigus foliaceus.* Clin Dermatol, 1993. 11:113–117.

6. Meyers, S. J., Varley, G. A., Meisler, D. M., Camisa, C., and Wander, A. H., *Conjunctival involvement in paraneoplastic pemphigus.* Am J Ophthalmol, 1992. 114:621–624.

7. Osmanski, J. P. 2nd, Fraire, A. E., and Schaefer, O. P., *Necrotizing tracheobronchitis with progressive airflow obstruction associated with paraneoplastic pemphigus.* Chest, 1997. 112:1704–1707.

8. Kim, S. C., Chang, S. N., Lee, I. J., Park, S. D., Jeong, E. T., Lee, C. W., Ahn, C. M., et al., *Localized mucosal*

9. Dega, H., Laporte, J. L., Joly, P., Gabarre, J., andre, C., Delpech, A., Frances, C., et al., *Paraneoplastic pemphigus associated with Hodgkin's disease.* Br J Dermatol, 1998. 138:196–198.

10. Schlesinger, T., McCarron, K., Camisa, C., and Anhalt, G. J., *Paraneoplastic pemphigus occurring in a patient with B-cell non-Hodgkin's lymphoma.* Cutis, 1998. 1998:61.

11. Chamberland, M., *Paraneoplastic pemphigus and adenocarcinoma of the colon.* Union Med Can, 1993. 122:201–203.

12. Matz, H., Milner, Y., Frusic-Zlotkin, M., and Brenner, S., *Paraneoplastic pemphigus associated with pancreatic carcinoma.* Acta Derm Venereol, 1997. 77:289–291.

13. Lam, S., Stone, M. S., Goeken, J. A., Massicotte, S. J., Smith, A. C., Folberg, R., and Krachmer, J. H., *Paraneoplastic pemphigus, cicatricial conjunctivitis, and acanthosis nigricans with patchy dermatoglyphy in a patient with bronchogenic squamous cell carcinoma.* Ophthalmology, 1992. 99:108–113.

14. Lee, M. S., Kossard, S., Ho, K. K., Barneston, R. S., and Ravich, R. B., *Paraneoplastic pemphigus triggered by radiotherapy.* Austral J Dermatol, 1995. 36:206–210.

15. Horn, T. D., and Anhalt, G.J., *Histologic features of paraneoplastic pemphigus.* Arch Dermatol, 1992. 128:1091–1095.

16. Mahoney, M. G., Aho, S., Uitto, J., and Stanley, J. R., *The members of the plakin family of proteins recognized by paraneopalstic pemphigus antibodies include periplakin.* J Invest Dermatol, 1998. 111:308–313.

17. Helou, J., Albritton, J., and Anhalt, G. J., *Accuracy of indirect immunofluorescence testing in the diagnosis of paraneoplastic pemphigus.* J Am Acad Dermatol, 1995. 32:441–447.

18. Liu, A. Y., Valenzuela, R., Helm, T. N., Camisa, C., Melton, A. L., and Bergfeld, W. F., *Indirect immunofluorescence on rat bladder transitional epithelium: A test with high specificity for paraneoplastic pemphgus.* J Am Acad Dermatol, 1993. 28:696–699.

19. Kiyokawa, C., Ruhrberg, C., Nie, Z., Karashima, T., Mori, O., Nishikawa, T., Green, K. J., et al., *Envoplakin and periplakin are components of the paraneoplastic pemphigus antigen complex.* J Invest Dermatol, 1998. 111:1236–1238.

20. Proby, C., Fujii, Y., Owaribe, K., Nishikawa, T., and Amagai, M., *Human antibodies against HD1/plectin in paraneoplastic pemphigus.* J Invest Dermatol, 1999. 112:153–156.

21. Anhalt, G. J., *Paraneoplastic pemphigus.* Adv Dermatol, 1997. 12:77–96.

22. White, J. W. Jr., *Gyrate erythema.* Dermatol Clin, 1985. 3:129–139.

23. Kawakami, T., and Saito, R., *Erythema gyratum repens unassociated with underlying malignancy.* J Dermatol, 1995. 22:587–589.

24. Boyd, A. S., Neldner, K. H., and Menter, A., *Erythema*

gyratum repens: A paraneoplastic eruption. J Am Acad Dermatol, 1992. 26:757–762.

25. Langlois, J. C., Shaw, J. M., and Odland, G. F., *Erythema gyratum repens unassociated with internal malignancy.* J Am Acad Dermatol, 1985. 12:911–913.

26. Rojo Sanchez, S., Suarez Fernandez, R., de Eusebio Murillo, E., Lopez Bran, E., Sanchez de Paz, F., and Robledo Aguilar, A., *Erythema gyratum repens: Another case of a rare disorder but no new insight into pathogenesis.* Dermatology, 1996. 193:336–337.

27. Barriere, H., Litoux, P., Bureau, B., Preel, J. L., and Thebaud, Y., *Gammel's erythema gyratum repens and aqcuired ichthyosis associated with eosphageal carcinoma.* Ann Dermatol Venereol, 1978. 105:319–321.

28. Yobra Sotillo, I., Garcia Bravo, B., and Camacho Martinez, G., *Erythema gyratum repens of Gammel and Hodgkin's disease.* Med Cutan Ibero Lat Am, 1983. 11:281–286.

29. Kwatra, A., McDonald, R. E., and Corriere, Jr., J. N., *Erythema gyratum repens in association with renal cell caricnoma.* J Urol, 1998. 159:2077.

30. Barber, P. V., Doyle, L., Vickers, D. M., and Hubbard, H., *Erythema gyratum repens with pulmonary tuberculosis.* Br J Dermatol, 1978. 98:465–468.

31. Morita, A., Sakakibara, N., and Tsuji, T., *Erythema gyratum repens associated with hypereosinophilic syndrome.* J Dermatol, 1994. 21:612–614.

32. Bressler, G. S., and Jones, Jr., R. E., *Erythema annulare centrifugum.* J Am Acad Dermatol, 1981. 4:597–602.

33. Caux, F., Lebbe, C., Thomine, E., Benyahia, B., Flageul, B., Joly, P., Rybojad, M., et al., *Erythema gyratum repens. A case studied with immunoflurescence, immunoelectron microscopy and immunohistochemistry.* Br J Dermatol, 1994. 131:102–107.

34. Monreal, M., Fernandez-Llamazares, J., Perandreu, J., Urrutia, A., Sahuquillo, J. C., and Contel, E., *Occult cancer in patients with venous thromboembolism: Which patients, which cancers.* Thromb Haemost, 1997. 78:1316–1318.

35. Callander, N., and Rapaport, S. I., *Trousseau's syndrome.* West J Med, 1993. 158:364–371.

36. Pugh, C. M., and DeWitty, R. L., *Mondor's disease.* J Natl Med Assoc, 1996. 88:359–363.

37. Samlaska, C. P., and James, W. D., *Superficial thrombophlebitis. II. Secondary hypercoagulable states.* J Am Acad Dermatol, 1990. 23:1–18.

38. Samlaska, C. P., and James, W. D., *Superficial thrombophlebitis. I. Primary hypercoaguable states.* J Am Acad Dermatol, 1990. 22:975–989.

39. Fiehn, C., Pezzuto, A., and Hunstein, W., *Superficial migratory thrombophlebitis in a patient with reversible protein C deficiency and anticardiolipin antibodies.* Ann Rheum Dis, 1994. 53:843–844.

40. Samlaska, C. P., James, W. D., and Simel, D. L., *Superficial migratory thrombophlebitis and factor XII deficiency.* J Am Acad Dermatol, 1990. 22:939–943.

41. Blum, F., Gilkeson, G., Greenberg, C., and Murray, J., *Superficial migratory thrombophlebitis and the lupus anticoagulant.* Int J Dermatol, 1990. 29:190–192.

42. Olin, J. W., Young, J. R., Graor, R. A., Ruschhaupt, W. F., and Bartholomew, J. R., *The changing clinical spectrum of thromboangiitis obliterans (Buerger's disease).* Circulation, 1990. 82(5 Suppl):IV3–8.

43. Pinzon, R., Drewinko, B., Trujillo, J. M., Guinee, V., and Giacco, G., *Pancreatic carcinoma and Trousseau's syndrome: Experience at a large cancer center.* J Clin Oncol, 1986. 4:509–514.

44. Martins, E. B., Fleming, K. A., Garrido, M. C., Hine, K. R., and Chapman, R. W., *Superficial thrombo-phlebitis, dysplasia, and cholangiocarcinoma in primary sclerosing cholangitis.* Gastroenterology, 1994. 107:537–542.

45. Evans, T. R., Mansi, J. L., and Bevan, D. H., *Trousseau's syndrome in association with ovarian carcinoma.* Cancer, 1996. 77:2544–2549.

46. Giauffret, F., Pottier, P., Pistorius, M. A., and Planchon, B., *Venous thrombosis of the legs and cancer. Evaluation of risk factors of venous thrombosis in the medical environment.* J Mal Vasc, 1997. 22:234–238.

47. Rao, L. V., *Tissue factor as a tumor procoagulant.* Cancer Metastasis Rev, 1992. 11:249–266.

48. Hayem, G., Gomez, M. J., Grossin, M., Meyer, O., and Kahn, M. F., *Systemic vasculitis and epithelioma. A report of three cases with a literature review.* Rev Rhum Eng Ed, 1997. 64:816–824.

49. Sanchez, N. P., Van Hale, H. M., and Su, W. P. D., *Clinical and histopathologic spectrum of necrotizing vasculitis.* Arch Dermatol, 1985. 121:220–224.

50. Sanchez-Guerrero, J., Gutierre-Urena, S., Vidaller, A., Reyes, E., Iglesias, A., and Alarcon-Segovia, D., *Vasculitis as a paraneoplastic syndrome. Report of 11 cases and review of the literature.* J Rheumatol, 1990. 17:1458–1462.

51. Poveda, F., Gonzalez-Garcia, J., Picazo, M. L., Giminez, A., Camacho, J., Barvado, F. J., and Vazques-Rodriguez, J. J., *Systemic polyarteritis nodosa as the initial manifestation of a gastric adenocarcinoma.* J Intern Med, 1994. 236:679–683.

52. Blanco, R., Gonzalez-Gay, M. A., Ibanez, D., Lopez-Viana, A., Ferran, C., Regueira, A., and Gonzalez-Vela, C., *Henoch-Schönlein purpura as clinical presentation of a myelodysplastic syndrome.* Clin Rheumatol, 1997. 16:626–628.

53. Lewis, J. E., *Urticarial vasculitis occurring in association with visceral malignancy.* Acta Derm Venereol, 1990. 70:345–347.

54. Pavlidis, N. A., Klouvas, G., Tsokos, M., Bai, M., and Moutsopoulos, H. M., *Cutaneous lymphocytic vasculopathy in lymphoproliferative disorders—a paraneoplastic lymphocytic vasculitis of the skin.* Leuk Lymphoma, 1995. 16:477–482.

55. Hoag, G. N., *Renal cell carcinoma and vasculitis: Report of two cases.* J Surg Oncol, 1987. 35:35–38.

56. Navarro, J. F., Quereda, C., Rivera, M., Navarro, F. J., and Ortuno, J., *Anti-neutrophil cytoplasmic antibody-associated paraneoplastic vasculitis.* Postgrad Med J, 1994. 70:373–375.

57. Beylot, J., Malou, M., Doutre, M. S., Beylot, C., Broustet, A., Reiffers, J., Lacost, D., et al., *Leukocytoclastic vasculitis and malignant hematologic diseases (12 cases).* Rev Med Interne, 1989. 10:509–514.

58. Kemmett, D., and Hunter, J. A. A., *Sweet's syndrome: A clinicopathologic review of 29 cases.* J Am Acad Dermatol, 1990. 23:503–607.

59. Sitjas, D., Puig, L., Cuatrecasas, M., and De Moragas, J. M., *Acute febrile neutrophilic dermatosis (Sweet's syndrome).* Int J Dermatol, 1993. 32:261–268.

60. Collins, P., Rogers, S., Keenan, P., and McCabe, M., *Acute febrile neutrophilic dermatosis in childhood (Sweet's syndrome).* Br J Dermatol, 1991. 124:203–206.

61. Cohen, P. R., Holder, W. R., Tucker, S. B., Kono, S., and Kurzock, R., *Sweet syndrome in patients with solid tumors.* Cancer, 1993. 72:2723–2731.

62. Sommer, S., Wilkinson, S. M., Merchant, W. J., and Goulden, V., *Sweet's syndrome presenting as palmoplantar pustulosis.* J Am Acad Dermatol, 2000. 42:332–334.

63. Lindskov, R., *Acute febrile neutrophilic dermatatosis with genital involvement.* Acta Derm Venereol (Stockh), 1984. 64:559–561.

64. von den Driesch, P., *Sweet's syndrome (acute febrile neutrophilic dermatosis).* J Am Acad Dermatol, 1994. 31:535–556.

65. Cohen, P. R., Talpaz, M., and Kurzock, R., *Malignancy-associated Sweet's syndrome: Review of the world literature.* J Clin Oncol, 1988. 6:1887–1897.

66. Inomata, N., Sasaki, T., and Nakajima, H., *Sweet's syndrome with gastric cancer.* J Am Acad Dermatol, 1999. 41:1033–1034.

67. Cohen, P. R., and Kurzock, R., *Sweet's syndrome and cancer.* Clin Dermatol, 1993. 11:149–157.

68. Cobb, M. W., *Furosemide-induced eruption simulating Sweet's syndrome.* J Am Acad Dermatol, 1989. 21:339–343.

69. Mensinng, H., and Kowalszick, L., *Acute febrile neutrophilic dermatosis (Sweet's syndrome) caused by minocycline.* Dermatologica, 1991. 182:43–46.

70. Gunawardena, D. A., Gunawardena, K. A., Ratnayaka, M. R. S., and Vasanthanathan, N. S., *The clinical spectrum of Sweet's syndrome (acute febrile neutrophilic dermatosis): Report of eighteen casese.* Br J Dermatol, 1975. 92:363–373.

71. Chan, H.-L., Lee, Y.-S., and Kuo, T.-T., *Sweet's syndrome: Clinicopathologic study of eleven cases.* Int J Dermatol, 1994. 33:425–432.

72. Attias, D., Laor, R., Zuckerman, E., Naschitz, J. E., Luria, M., Misselvitch, I., and Boss, J. H., *Acute neutrophilic myositis in Sweet's syndrome: Late phase transformation into fibrosing myositis and panniculitis.* Human Pathol, 1995. 26:688–690.

73. Frayha, R., Matta, M., and Kurban, A., *Sweet's syndrome simulating systemic lupus erythematosus.* Dermatologica, 1972. 144:321–324.

74. Jordaan, H. F., *Acute febrile neutrophilic dermatosis: A histolopathological study of 37 patients and a review of the literature.* Am J Dermatopathol, 1989. 11:99–111.

75. Kemmett, D., Harrison, D. J., and Hunter, J. A. A., *Antibodies to neutrophil cytoplasmic antigens: A serologic marker for Sweet's syndrome.* J Am Acad Dermatol, 1991. 24:967–969.

76. Going, J. J., *Is the pathogenesis of Sweet's syndrome mediated by interleukin-1?* Br J Dermatol, 1987. 116:282–286.

77. Giasuddin, A. S. M., El-Orfi, A. H. A. M., Ziu, M., and El-Barnawi, N. Y., *Sweet's syndrome: Is the pathogenesis mediated by helper T cell type I cytokines.* J Am Acad Dermatol, 1998. 39:943–943.

78. Horn, T. D., Burke, P. J., Karp, J. E., and Hood, A. F., *Intravenous administration of recombinant granulocyte-macrophage colony-stimulating factor causes a cutaneous eruption.* Arch Dermatol, 1991. 127:49–52.

79. Pinto, G. M., Tapadinhas, C., Moura, C., and Alfonso, A., *Pityriasis rotunda.* Cutis, 1996. 58:406–408.

80. Lodi, A., Betti, R., Chiarelli, G., Carducci, M., and Crosti, C., *Familial pityriasis rotunda.* Int J Dermatol, 1990. 29:483–485.

81. Aste, N., Pau, M., Aste, N., and Biggio, P., *Pityriasis rotunda: A survey of 42 cases observed in Sardinia, Italy.* Dermatology, 1997. 194:32–35.

82. el-Hefnawi, H., and Rasheed, A., *Pityriasis rotunda.* Arch Dermatol, 1966. 93:84–86.

83. Kahanna, M., Levy, A., Ronnen, M., Schewach-Millet, M., and Stempler, D., *Pityriasis rotunda in a white patient. Report of the second case and review of the literature.* J Am Acad Dermatol, 1986. 15:362–265.

84. Grimault, R., Gelmetti, C., Brusasco, A., Tadini, G., and Caputo, R., *Pityriasis rotunda: Report of a familial occurrence and review of the literature.* J Am Acad Dermatol, 1994. 31:866–871.

85. Berkowitz, I., Hokinson, H. J., Kew, M. C., and DiBisceglie, A. M., *Pityriasis rotunda as a cutaneous marker of hepatocellular carcinoma: A comparison with its prevalence in other diseases.* Br J Dermatol, 1989. 120:545–549.

86. Leibowitz, M. R., Weiss, R., and Smith, E. H., *Pityriasis rotunda: A cutaneous sign of malignant diseases in two patients.* Arch Dermatol, 1983. 119:607–609.

87. Rubin, M. G., and Mathes, B., *Pityriasis rotunda: Two cases in black Americans.* J Am Acad Dermatol, 1986. 14:74–78.

88. Ito, M., and Tanaka, T., *Pseudo-ichthyose acquise en taches circulaires: "Pityriasis circinata Toyama."* Ann Dermatol Syph, 1960. 87:26–37.

89. Combemale, P., L'Henaff, N., and Guennoc, B., *Pityriasis rotunda.* Ann Dermatol Venereol, 1993. 120:287–288.

CHAPTER
31

The Skin and Metastatic Diseases

Epidemiology. The skin is a frequent site of tumor metastasis and may be the initial presenting sign of an internal malignant neoplasm. An estimated 9% of patients with cancer have cutaneous metastases at time of autopsy [1]. The exact incidences are difficult to ascertain, as each group of investigators studying this problem includes and excludes different types of tumors when compiling statistics. Skin metastases are the first sign of metastatic spread in 7.6% of patients [2, 3]. In one large series, the skin was estimated to be the twelfth most common metastatic site for all tumors [4].

Malignant tumors from virtually all organs can metastasize to the skin. In general, the relative frequencies of cutaneous involvement parallel the frequencies of primary malignant tumors. Table 31–1 lists the distributions of primary tumors giving rise to cutaneous metastases in a large series from 1972. Almost 75% of all cutaneous metastases in women arise from breast carcinomas [5]. Colon carcinoma, another common neoplasm, often gives rise to cutaneous metastases. Hypernephromas (renal cell carcinomas) can be the initial presenting sign or can appear many years after initial diagnosis [6]. Gastric, esophageal, and ovarian carcinomas give rise to cutaneous metastases less frequently. Uterine carcinoma is a relatively uncommon source for cutaneous metastatic disease [6, 7]. In children, neuroblastomas and leukemias are the most frequent tumors to metastasize to the skin [8]. The incidence of primary malignancies has changed in the years

since these data were accumulated, and the relative incidences of cutaneous metastases reflect these changes.

Although there is obvious variation related to the type of primary neoplasm involved, in general, cutaneous metastasis is associated with a poor prognosis [9]. In one series, mean survival ranged from 1 to 34 months, depending on the tumor type [3].

Cutaneous Features. The clinical features of cutaneous metastases are, in some cases, dependent on the site of origin of the primary tumor. Metastases from internal malignant neoplasms can display manifold appearances. The most common presentation is that of one to several firm, dermal nodules, occasionally located within or near a surgical scar at the site of excision of the primary tumor. These metastatic tumors are often nondescript and usually painless.

Breast carcinoma is by far the most frequent neoplasm to demonstrate cutaneous metastases. Several patterns of cutaneous involvement have been described, and each of these has a slightly different cutaneous appearance. Inflammatory breast carcinoma demonstrates an erythematous and edematous patch or plaque, usually on the skin of the breast, and resembles erysipelas [10]. Less commonly, other types of metastatic cancer, including those originating from the gastrointestinal tract, salivary glands, lungs, and genitourinary system, can have a similar clinical appearance [5]. Metastatic breast cancer can also cause a morphea-like induration of the skin with scattered ery-

Table 31–1. Frequency (%) of Primary Site Accounting for Cutaneous Metastasis

Organ	Men	Women
Breast	2	69
Esophagus	3	
Kidney	6	
Large intestine	19	9
Liver	1	
Lung	24	4
Melanoma	13	5
Ovary		4
Pancreas	2	2
Prostate	1	
Salivary glands	2	
Sarcoma	3	2
Squamous cell carcinoma (head and neck)	12	1
Stomach	6	
Thyroid	1	
Urinary bladder	2	1
Uterine cervix		2

From reference 6.

thematous nodules (en cuirasse) [5]. A lymphangioma circumscriptum-like appearance with multiple violaceous papulovesicles has been termed *telangiectatic metastatic breast carcinoma* [11]. Alopecia neoplastica is an uncommon presentation usually associated with metastatic breast carcinoma that is characterized by circular plaques of alopecia that appear much like alopecia areata [6]. Other neoplasms can present with a similar clinical picture. Densely pigmented metastatic tumors usually represent melanoma [12].

Renal cell carcinoma most frequently metastasizes to the scalp and presents as a highly vascular erythematous nodule that resembles a pyogenic granuloma [13]. Lesions can be solitary or multiple.

Tumors originating in the gastrointestinal tract often display metastatic disease in the skin of the perineum or abdomen. These cutaneous tumors can be inflammatory and solitary or multiple and appear more like chronic fistulas or hidradenitis suppurativa [5].

Other rare patterns of metastatic spread to the skin display cutaneous features that appear to be unrelated to the type of primary neoplasm. In one series, a zosteriform pattern was detected in two patients with metastatic carcinoma. In one patient, the primary tumor was a breast carcinoma, and in the other the primary tumor was an undifferentiated carcinoma that came from an unknown site [14]. In children, neuroblastoma and leukemia often present with cutaneous involvement characterized by multiple, disseminated blue-gray nodules [8].

Cutaneous metastases are typically patterned. Most cutaneous metastases arise in sites relatively close to the site of the primary tumor [15]. For instance, lung cancer metastatic to the skin is found most frequently on the chest [9] and gastrointestinal carcinomas and genitourinary carcinomas on the skin of the abdomen. In one large study, scalp metastases were most commonly from tumors of the lung and kidney in men and from the breast in women [6]. Metastases on the face often derived from squamous cell carcinomas of the head and neck. Abdominal skin was the most frequent site of metastasis in both men and women. Primary tumors were most commonly from the colon, lung, stomach, and ovary [6].

Umbilical metastases derive from several types of primary internal neoplasms. This peculiar presentation of metastatic disease has been termed a "Sister Mary Joseph nodule" (named for its describer, a nun at the Mayo Clinic) and is associated with primary gastrointestinal and genitourinary tract carcinomas [16].

Systemic lymphomas of all types can secondarily involve the skin. Many of these lymphomas have primary cutaneous counterparts that are discussed in Chapter 10. A discussion of other systemic lymphomas that may secondarily involve the skin is beyond the scope of this volume, and the reader is referred to textbooks of hematopathology.

Associated Disorders. Metastatic neoplasms are seen most commonly in patients with known underlying cancer; however, cutaneous metastasis can be the first indication of systemic disease. There are no additional specific diseases especially associated metastatic disease.

Histologic Features. The histologic appearance of a cutaneous metastasis depends on the type of primary neoplasm that is infiltrating the skin. The most common histologic pattern of a metastatic carcinoma is that of a dermal nodule, usually located in the deeper reticular dermis (Fig. 31–1). Strands or cords of tumor cells may emanate from the central nodule in a "starburst" pattern (Fig. 31–2). Cutaneous appendages are often destroyed by the infiltrating tumor mass. The epidermis is often flattened, but rarely involved or infiltrated. Metastatic tumors will often ulcerate. The specific architectural and cytologic features of the dermal tumor mass are directly related to the type of primary neoplasm that has spread to involve the skin.

Breast carcinoma metastatic to the skin can be found limited mainly or in part to lymphatic spaces or diffusely throughout the dermis. The pattern of metastatic tumor filling and occluding the lymphatic

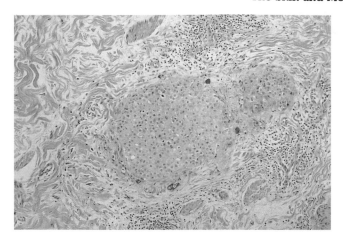

Fig. 31–1. Dermal nodule of metastatic ductal carcinoma of the breast metastasized to the skin.

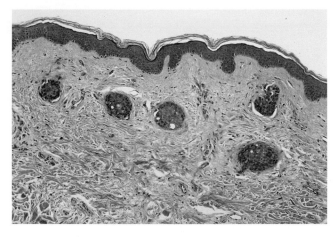

Fig. 31–3. Nests of metastatic breast carcinoma are present in lymphatic spaces throughout the dermis in inflammatory carcinoma.

spaces is associated with the clinical appearance of "inflammatory carcinoma" (Fig. 31–3). Although usually associated with metastatic breast carcinoma, this pattern has been described in colon carcinoma [17]. Glandular differentiation may be present, and in other cases cords of malignant cells course throughout the dermis. Evidence of glandular differentiation supports an adenocarcinoma that can arise from many different primary sites (Fig. 31–4). Evidence of keratinization supports a primary squamous cell carcinoma giving rise to a different list of potential sites of tumor origins. Immunopathology has proved to be very helpful in further isolating the organ of origin of metastatic tumors with unrecognized primary tumors (Table 31–1).

Metastatic renal cell carcinoma demonstrates a dense dermal infiltrate of clear cells growing in a glandular pattern. There is marked vascularity within the surrounding dermis. The tumor cells are large, with oval nuclei and extensive clear cytoplasm (Fig. 31–5). There is some histologic resemblance to sebaceous carcinoma [13].

In rare cases, epidermotropism of neoplastic cells into the epidermis and invading follicular epithelium is seen in metastatic disease. This has been reported with colon carcinoma [18], breast carcinoma [19], prostatic carcinoma [20], and laryngeal carcinoma [21]. It has also been described in melanoma that has metastasized to the skin [22].

Special Studies. Immunopathology can be especially helpful in determining the origin of the primary neoplasm is many cases. Relatively organ-specific antigens exist that can be helpful in distinguishing between

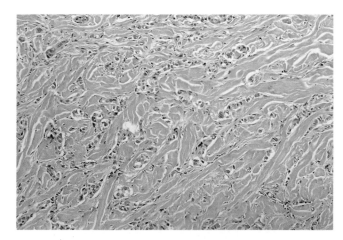

Fig. 31–2. Individual cells of metastatic lobular carcinoma percolate through dermal collagen bundles.

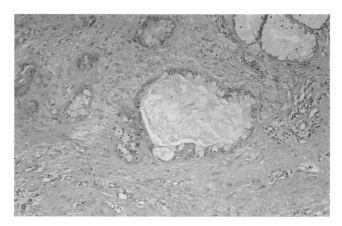

Fig. 31–4. Glandular differentiation and prominent goblet cells may be present in colon carcinoma that has metastasized to the skin.

Table 31–2. Antibodies Useful in Determining Site of Origin of Primary Neoplasm

Antibody	*Primary Neoplasms Recognized*
Carcinoembyronic antigen (CEA)	Gastrointestinal, breast, lung adenocarcinoma
Common leukocyte antigen	Lymphoma, leukemia
Cytokeratin	Squamous cell carcinomas of multiple sites
Cytokeratin 20	Merkel cell carcinomas
Epithelial membrane antigen (EMA)	Most carcinomas
Estrogen receptors	Ovarian, endometrial, breast carcinomas
Gross cystic fluid protein-15	Breast
HMB-45	Melanocytic neoplasms
MART-1	Melanocytic neoplasms
Neuron-specific enolase	Neuroendocrine neoplasms, neural tumors
Progesterone receptors	Breast, ovary, endometrium
Prostate acid phosphatase	Prostate
Prostate-specific antigen	Prostate
S100	Melanocytic, neural neoplasms; less commonly chondroid, lipomatous tumors
Smooth muscle actin	Smooth muscle
Thyroid-stimulating hormone	Thyroid
Vimentin	Mesenchymal tumors, renal cell carcinoma, melanoma

neoplasms that have similar histologic appearances. Table 31–2 lists antibodies that are useful in attempting to determine the site of origin from a cutaneous metastasis from an unknown primary site. As with any immunostaining methods, it is important to keep in mind that cross-reactivity can be extensive and that the results of a staining profile must be interpreted in conjunction with the clinical situation and the routine histologic appearance of the neoplasm. It is important to construct a panel of antibodies that will provide a checkerboard pattern of staining results designed to maximize the sensitivity and specificity for each type of primary neoplasm in the list of differential diagnostic possibilities.

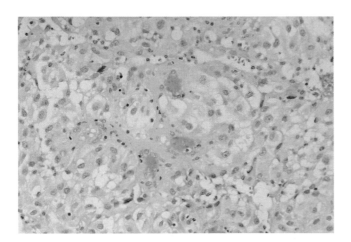

Fig. 31–5. Metastatic renal cell carcinoma is characterized by large cells with abundant clear cytoplasm and marked vascularity.

Pathogenesis. The skin can be secondarily involved by malignant tumors by direct extension from the primary tumor or by either distant or localized metastases. Distant metastases can occur via lymphatic spread, as is suggested in cases of inflammatory carcinoma of the breast [5], or via hematogenous channels, as has been suggested for cases of alopecia neoplastica [23].

References

1. Spencer, P. S., and Helma, T. N., *Skin metastases in cancer patients.* Cutis, 1987. 39:119–121.
2. Lookingbill, D. P., Spangler, N., and Sexton, F. M., *Skin involvement as the presenting sign of internal carcinoma.* J Am Acad Dermatol, 1990. 22:19–26.
3. Lookingbill, D. P., Spangler, N., and Helm, K. F., *Cutaneous metastases in patients with metastatic carcinoma: A retrospective study of 4020 patients.* J Am Acad Dermatol, 1993. 29:228–236.
4. Enticknap, J. B., *An analysis of 1000 cases of cancer with special reference to metastases.* Guys Hosp Rep, 1952. 101:273–279.
5. Schwartz, R. A., *Cutaneous metastatic disease.* J Am Acad Dermatol, 1995. 33:161–182.
6. Brownstein, M. H., and Helwig, E. B., *Metastatic tumors of the skin.* Cancer, 1972. 29:1298–1307.
7. Brady, L. W., O'Neill, E. A., and Farber, S. H., *Unusual sites of metastases.* Semin Oncol, 1977. 4:59–64.
8. Maher-Wiese, V. L., Wenner, N. P., and Grant-Kels, J. M., *Metastatic cutaneous lesions in children and adolescents with a case report of metastatic neuroblastoma.* J Am Acad Dermatol, 1992. 26:620–628.

9. Reingold, I. M., *Cutaneous metastases from internal carcinoma.* Cancer, 1966. 19:162–168.

10. Chevallier, B., Asselain, B., Kunlin, A., Veyret, C., Bastit, P., and Graic, Y., *Inflammatory breast cancer: Determination of prognostic factors by univariate and multivariate analysis.* Cancer, 1987. 60:897–902.

11. Van Vonno, N. C., *A case of caricnoma telangiectaticum.* Br J Derm Syphilol, 1933. 45:423–424.

12. Poiares-Baptista, A., and Abreu de Vasconcelos, A., *Cutaneous pigmented metastasis from breast carcinoma simulating malignant melanoma.* Int J Dermatol, 1988. 27:124–125.

13. Menter, A., Boyd, A. S., and McCaffree, D. M., *Recurrent renal cell carcinoma presenting as askin nodules: Two case reports and review of the literature.* Cutis, 1989. 44:305–308.

14. Manteaux, A., Cohen, P. R., and Rapini, R. P., *Zosteriform and epidermotropic metastasis.* J Dermatol Surg Oncol, 1992. 18:97–100.

15. Beerman, H., *Some aspects of cutaneous malignancy.* Am J Med Sci, 1957. 233:456–472.

16. Steck, W. D., and Helwig, E. B., *Tumors of the umbilicus.* Cancer, 1965. 18:907–915.

17. Kauffman, C. L., and Sina, B., *Metastatic inflammatory carcinoma of the rectum: Tumor spread by three routes.* Am J Dermatopathol, 1997. 19:528–532.

18. Oku, T., Nakayama, F., and Takigawa, M., *A peculiar form of epidermotropism in cutaneous metastatic carcinoma.* J Dermatol, 1990. 17:59–61.

19. Requena, L., Sanchez Yus, E., Nunez, C., White, C. R. Jr., and Sangueza, O. P., *Epidermotropically metastatic breast carcinoma. Rare histopathologic variants mimicking melanoma and Paget's disease.* Am J Dermatopathol, 1996. 18:385–395.

20. Segal, R., Penneys, N. S., and Nahass, G., *Metastatic prostatic carcinoma histologically mimicking malignant melanoma.* J Cutan Pathol, 1994. 21:280–282.

21. Aguilar, A., Schoendorff, C., Lopez Redondo, M. J., Ambrojo, P., Requena, L., and Sanchez Yus, E., *Epidermotropic metastases from internal carcinomas.* Am J Dermatopathol, 1991. 13:452–458.

22. Abernethy, J. L., Soyer, H. P., Kerl, H., Jorizzo, J. L., and White, W. L., *Epidermotropic metastatic malignant melanoma simulating melanoma in situ. A report of 10 examples from two patients.* Am J Surg Pathol, 1994. 18:1140–1149.

23. Cohen, I., Levy, E., and Schrieber, H., *Alopecia neoplastica due to breast carcinoma.* Arch Dermatol, 1961. 84:490–492.

PART VII

Pediatric Diseases with Prominent Cutaneous Features

CHAPTER
32

Congenital Disorders

Down's Syndrome

Epidemiology. Down's syndrome is due to trisomy 21. It has a prevalence rate of 9.6/10,000 live births [1] and is the most common chromosomal syndrome in humans. The occurrence of Down's syndrome is strongly related to maternal age.

Cutaneous Features. There are protean cutaneous manifestations in patients with Down's syndrome. Palmoplantar hyperkeratosis is present in about 41% of patients with Down's syndrome. Seborrheic dermatitis was present in 31% of patients and xerosis in about 10% of patients in one series [2].

Elastosis perforans serpiginosa is more frequent in patients with Down's syndrome than in other patients [3, 4]. This presents as hyperkeratotic papules arranged in a serpiginous pattern and can be localized or generalized. The neck and upper extremities are the most commonly affected sites. Elastosis perforans serpiginosa is also associated with many other conditions, such as

- Acrogeria
- Chronic renal failure
- Down's syndrome
- Ehler's-Danlos syndrome
- Marfan's syndrome
- Osteogenesis imperfecta
- Penicillamine therapy
- Pseduoxanthoma elasticum
- Scleroderma

Syringomas are present in many patients with Down's syndrome and are more common in affected women [5]. Syringomas have a predilection for the periorbital regions of the face and appear as firm 1–2 mm papules with no surface changes. Less commonly, miliary calcinosis of the extremities has been reported in patients with Down's syndrome [6, 7]. Rare associations include multiple collagenomas [6, 8] and Cowden's disease [9]. Norwegian scabies is more frequent in patients with Down's syndrome [10, 11]. This form of the disease is characterized by the presence of widespread pruritic, hyperkeratotic, and crusted plaques. Organisms are easily found in skin scrapings. Alopecia areata was present in 9% of patients with Down's syndrome in one study and vitiligo in 2% of these patients [5]. Other manifestations include cutis marmorata, geographic tongue, and fissured tongue [2]. Widespread pustular eruptions have also been described in patients with Down's syndrome and may represent folliculitis [12] or leukemoid reactions [13].

Associated Disorders. Congenital leukemia and leukemoid reactions are strongly associated with Down's syndrome [13]. As many as 10% of infants with Down's syndrome develop a form of megakaryoblastic leukemia, many of which spontaneously disappear within a few months [14, 15]. These patients are at higher risk for developing subsequent, fatal leukemias [14]. Congenital leukemia may be acute myelogenous leukemia [13], myelomonocytic leukemia [16], acute megakaryoblastic leukemia [17], acute lymphocytic leukemia [18], or chronic myelogenous leukemia. Many genetic abnormalities have been reported as present within the leukemic cell lines [17, 19].

Congenital heart disease is present in many patients with Down's syndrome. About 35% of patients with heart defects had ventricular septal defects, 8% had isolated secundum atrial septal defects, 7% had isolated persistent patent ductus arteriosus, and 4% had tetralogy of Fallot [1].

Renal disease is also frequently associated with patients with Down's syndrome and usually occurs after the first decade of life. These diseases include focal segmental glomerulosclerosis, acute glomerulonephritis, minimal change disease, and membranous nephropathy [20]. Renal hypoplasia is also frequently seen, along with glomerular microcysts and dilated renal tubules. Obstructive uropathy has also been reported [21].

Pulmonary development is occasionally abnormal in patients with Down's syndrome. Reduced branching of the airways has been reported [22]. Liver disease is uncommon in patients with Down's syndrome, but hepatic fibrosis has been reported in a small series [23].

In addition to childhood leukemias, a number of other neoplasms has been reported to occur with increased frequency in patients with Down's syndrome. Lymphomas, extragonadal germ cell tumors, especially intracranial [24], and, to a lesser degree, retinoblastomas, and pancreatic and bone tumors are seen more often than expected in this population. Men and boys with Down's syndrome have a higher risk for developing these neoplasms [25]. There is a still not fully understood association between Down's syndrome and Alzheimer's disease [26, 27].

Histologic Features. Congenital leukemia and leukemoid reactions may be histologically indistinguishable [13]. There is a dense, diffuse infiltrate of immature myeloid cells that completely inundates the dermis and all cutaneous appendages. There is marked cellular pleomorphism. Mitotic activity is brisk, and extensive karyorrhectic debris may be present.

Syringomas associated with Down's syndrome are histologically indistinguishable from sporadically occurring ones. The epidermis is normal to slightly flattened. Within the papillary dermis and extending into the very superficial portion of the reticular dermis, there is a well-circumscribed proliferation of small nests of bland-appearing keratinocytes demonstrating ductular differentiation (Fig. 32–1). The ductules are lined by two rows of cells, and a central cuticle is present in many cases. Tadpole-like or comma-like structures are formed by the keratinocytes. The epithelial structures are enmeshed in dense fibrous stroma that ordinarily stains much more eosinophilic than the surrounding dermal collagen (Fig. 32–2). Cytologic atypia is not present, and mitotic activity is unusual. The following entities must be considered in the histologic differential diagnosis of syringoma:

- Basal cell carcinoma, morpheaform type
- Microcystic adnexal carcinoma
- Trichoepithelioma, desmoplastic

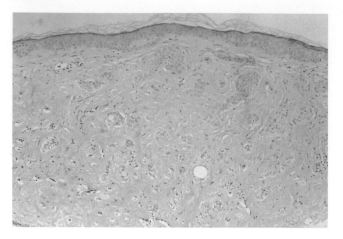

Fig. 32–1. Syringoma is characterized by a well-circumscribed dermal nodule of nests and cords of cells enmeshed in a dense fibrous stroma.

Elastosis perforans serpiginosa is a transepidermal elimination disorder that may occur sporadically, as well as in association with Down's syndrome. A similar histologic process has been associated with penicillamine use. The epidermis is progressively acanthotic, leading up to an area of central disruption (Fig. 32–3). Wavy, refractile, eosinophilic fibers extend from the underlying dermis up into and through channels within the epidermis. There is often a dense collection of debris and similar fibers in the stratum corneum overlying the transepidermal channels. Within the dermis, there are increased numbers of fragmented elastic tissue fibers, many of which have a deep eosinophilic hue (Fig. 32–4). More basophilic debris is also present at the site of epidermal elimination in many cases. A moderate inflammatory infiltrate is often present localized to the region of degenerating elastic tissue fibers. Multinucleated giant cells are often seen (Fig. 32–5). In patients with elastosis perforans serpiginosa, the elastic

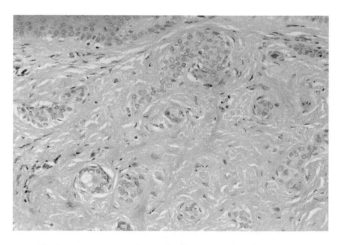

Fig. 32–2. Ductular and "tadpole-like" structures are present within the papillary dermis in syringoma.

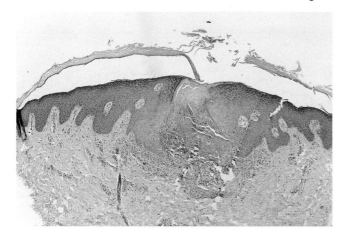

Fig. 32–3. A central channel demonstrating transepidermal elimination is present in elastosis perforans serpiginosa.

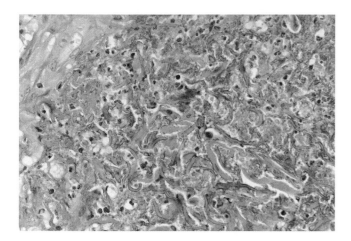

Fig. 32–4. Degenerating elastic tissue fibers, often with an eosinophilic hue, are present within and beneath the channel in elastosis perforans serpiginosa.

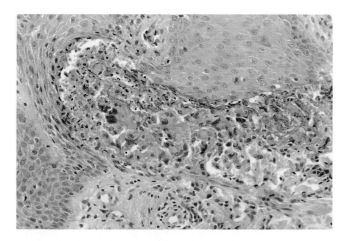

Fig. 32–5. Clusters of multinucleated giant cells are often present beneath the area of degenerating elastic tissue fibers in elastosis perforans serpiginosa.

tissue fibers have a knobby appearance. The following entities must be considered in the histologic differential diagnosis of elastosis perforans serpiginosa:

- Excoriation
- Kyrle's disease
- Perforating calcific elastosis
- Perforating folliculitis
- Reactive perforating collagenosis

Special Studies. Special studies are not required to make a diagnosis of any of the entities described above. A Verhoeff-van Gieson stain is, however, sometimes helpful in demonstrating the perforating elastic tissue fibers in elastosis perforans serpiginosa. In addition, increased numbers of coarse elastic tissue fibers are seen throughout the papillary dermis.

Pathogenesis. The pathogenesis of Down's syndrome is not known. In most cases, there is no explanation for the cutaneous findings associated with the syndrome. In rare cases, abnormal vitamin A levels have been implicated in the pathogenesis of elastosis perforans serpiginosa occurring in patients with Down's syndrome [4].

Rothmund-Thomson Syndrome

Epidemiology. Rothmund-Thomson syndrome (RTS), also known as *poikiloderma congenitale*, is a rare, autosomal recessive condition characterized by poikiloderma, photosensitivity, skeletal anomalies, and increased risk for developing cancer [28]. A gene assigned to chromosome 8 may be the cause of RTS [29]. Approximately 200 published cases are present in the literature. There is a 4:1 female predominance [30].

Cutaneous Features. Patients with RTS are often diagnosed based on the cutaneous manifestations. Patients have a characteristic poikiloderma and photosensitivity. The poikilodermatous changes are most prominent on sun-exposed areas of the face and upper extremities [31]. Poikiloderma consists of reticulated areas of hyperpigmentation and hypopigmentation and telangiectasia. Telangiectasias are also present in well-developed lesions. The changes develop in infancy. The earliest findings include erythematous and edematous plaques that may develop blisters. The trunk and flexural surfaces are generally spared.

Verrucous, hyperkeratotic plaques appear on the hands in about one-third of patients with RTS [32, 33]. The hyperkeratosis is typically present on the palmar and plantar surfaces. There is some suggestion that these verrucous lesions may be predisposed to malignant transformation [34].

Sparse hair density involving eyebrows and eyelashes, including alopecia, is present in up to 80% of patients and onychodystrophy in up to one-third of patients [35]. Anhidrosis is encountered less frequently [31]. Calcinosis universalis has been described in rare patients [36].

Associated Disorders. Rothmund-Thomson syndrome involves many organ systems. Patients are characteristically short statured and have small hands and feet and bony defects [35]. These include frontal bossing, saddle nose, and prognathism [28]. Other anomalies may include complete agenesis of the tibia and radius [37]. Dentition is abnormal in about 40% of patients. Mental retardation is infrequent [38].

Patients with RTS are at a slightly increased risk for developing mesenchymal neoplasms. Osteogenic sarcoma is seen with a low increase in frequency [39, 40]. Non-Hodgkin's lymphoma has also been reported in patients with RTS [40], as have fibrosarcoma and parathyroid adenoma [28].

Glaucoma is frequently encountered in patients with RTS, as are juvenile cataracts [41]. Other ocular anomalies include exophthalmos, corneal atrophy, and retinal coloboma [28]. Hypogonadism is often present [35].

Rare complications include esophageal stenosis [35], and increased infections may be present due to altered immunologic function [31]. Rare patients have been reported with associated myopathies [32]. Rare gastrointestinal anomalies, including annular pancreas and duodenal stenosis, have also been described in patients with RTS [33].

Histologic Features. Early cutaneous lesions of RTS are characterized by papillary dermal edema. Vasodilation is prominent, and there is a moderate infiltrate of lymphocytes and histiocytes surrounding vessels of the superficial vascular plexus. As the lesions age, the epidermis becomes progressively atrophic, with overlying hyperkeratosis. The basal layer is hyperpigmented. Dermal appendages are lost, elastic tissue fibers in the superficial dermis are fragmented, and pigment incontinence is prominent. The following entities must be considered in the histologic differential diagnosis of RTS:

- Bloom's syndrome
- Dermatomyositis
- Erythema dyschromicum perstans
- Graft-versus-host disease
- Lupus erythematousus
- Poikiloderma atrophican vasculare

Keratinocyte atypia may be present at an early age [42]. This may be related to the slight increase in squamous cell carcinomas and basal cell carcinomas that are reported to occur at young ages in patients with RTS [28].

Special Studies. Special tissue studies are not helpful in establishing a tissue diagnosis of RTS.

Pathogenesis. Defective DNA-repair mechanisms have been found in patients with RTS and are thought to be the cause of the increased rate of malignant tumors acquired by these patients [38, 43–45]. Abnormalities in numbers and distribution of Langerhans' cells have been reported in a patient with RTS, and it has been postulated that this may indicate a functional impairment predisposing such individuals to the infection and increased development of cutaneous malignant tumors [46]. Most patients with RTS, however, have normal immune function [28]. Others have suggested a defect in connective tissue metabolism in patients with RTS [28].

Bloom's Syndrome

Epidemiology. Bloom's syndrome is an autosomal recessive disorder that manifests early as growth retardation, often in conjunction with increased sun sensitivity, multiple neoplasms, and infections [47].

Cutaneous Features. Extreme photosensitivity is the most prominent cutaneous feature in patients with Bloom's syndrome. In some cases the cutaneous manifestations are strongly reminiscent of lupus erythematosus [48]. Erythematous and edematous, scaly plaques are present in photodistributed areas, most commonly on the cheeks. In later cases, the skin has widespread areas of hyperpigmentation and hypopigmentation.

Associated Disorders. Patients with Bloom's syndrome demonstrate growth retardation, malar hypoplasia, and multiple malignant neoplasms [49]. Mental retardation is unusual [50]. Leukemias occur in about 5% of patients with Bloom's syndrome, and Hodgkin's disease is reported somewhat less commonly in these patients [50, 51]. Retinoblastomas [49], Wilms' tumors [52], skin carcinomas, and lung carcinomas are reported in patients with Bloom's syndrome [53].

Patients with Bloom's syndrome are also predisposed toward developing multiple infections, leading to chronic lung disease. This includes pulmonary fibrosis and bronchiectasis. The incidence of diabetes mellitus is increased in patients with Bloom's syndrome [47]. Conjunctival telangiectasias may be present in patients with Bloom's syndrome [54].

Histologic Features. The histologic changes of the lupus-like skin eruption have been well documented. There is a marked interface dermatitis, with extensive basal vacuolization and pigment incontinence. Within

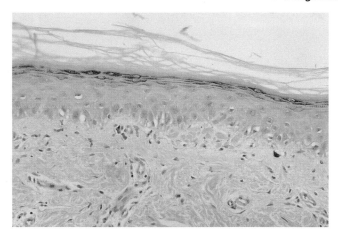

Fig. 32–6. Bloom's syndrome is characterized by an atrophic epidermis, interface dermatitis with dying keratinocytes, and a superficial perivascular lymphocytic inflammatory infiltrate.

the dermis, there is a superficial perivascular lymphocytic infiltrate surrounding dilated capillaries [48] (Fig. 32–6). The following entities must be considered in the histologic differential diagnosis of Bloom' syndrome:

- Dermatomyositis
- Erythema dyschromicum perstans
- Graft-versus-host disease
- Lupus erythematosus
- Poikiloderma atrophicans
- Rothmund-Thomson syndrome

Special Studies. Despite Bloom's syndrome's histologic similarities to lupus erythematosus, direct immunofluorescence examination fails to demonstrate deposits of immunoglobulins along the basement membrane in patients with Bloom's syndrome [48].

Pathogenesis. Bloom's syndrome is caused by chromosomal instability [47]. Chromosomal aberrations and sister chromatid exchanges are frequent in these patients [50, 53].

Ataxia-Telangiectasia

Epidemiology. Ataxia-telangiectasia (AT) is an autosomal recessive disorder. It is slightly more common in male patients [55]. Onset of symptoms is during early childhood. Approximately 1% of the general population are heterozygous carriers for the gene [56]. Instability of chromosomes 7 and 14 is present in almost all cases [57]. Deletions on chromosomes 4 and 6 have also been reported [58]. The observed clinical anomalies have been linked to an ATA gene located on chromosome 11q22–23 [59]. Consanguinity is found in

some series [55]. Early mortality is frequent in these patients and is most often due to pulmonary infections or to cancer [55].

Cutaneous Features. The most frequent cutaneous manifestation of AT is diffuse telangiectasias. The telangiectasias are not always in a photodistribution [60]. This is often the presenting feature of the disease. Ocular telangiectasias are also common and may be the presenting feature in some patients. The skin may demonstrate other signs of premature aging, including actinic keratoses and actinic lentigines [56, 61].

Another less common cutaneous presentation is that of noninfectious granulomas [58, 62, 63]. These may present as atrophic, scarred, violaceous plaques or nodules and are mainly on the limbs [58].

Café-au-lait macules are present in many patients with AT [60, 64]. Other rare associations include acanthosis nigricans, vitiligo, impetigo, hirsutism, lipoatrophy, gray hair, and progeroid changes [60]. Necrobiosis lipoidica has been reported in a patient with AT [65]. Sarcoidosis has also been associated in rare cases [66]. Diffuse hyperpigmentation may be present in some affected patients [67].

Associated Disorders. Patients with AT suffer from progressive neurologic disabilities such as cerebellar ataxia [56, 57]. Diffuse cerebellar atrophy is present in advanced cases.

Growth retardation is present in most patients with AT [55]. Defects in cellular and humoral immunity lead to increased incidence of cancer and infection [56]. Bronchopulmonary infections are common, affecting up to two-thirds of patients with AT [55, 57]. Most patients have low circulating lymphocyte counts and low serum IgG and IgA levels. IgM levels may be increased [55].

Histologic Features. The telangiectasias present in patients with AT are histologically identical to other, sporadically appearing telangiectasias. Ectatic, thin-walled vessels are present within the papillary dermis. The endothelial cells appear flattened. Increased elastotic material may be present around the dilated vessels (Fig. 32–7).

The histologic changes of the granulomatous lesions demonstrate sarcoidal granulomas. There is no degeneration of collagen within the center of these palisading granulomas [58]. The histologic changes seen in café-au-lait macules are identical to those seen in the café-au-lait macules associated with neurofibromatosis (Chapter 9).

Special Studies. Special stains are necessary to exclude infectious processes such as fungi and mycobacteria in

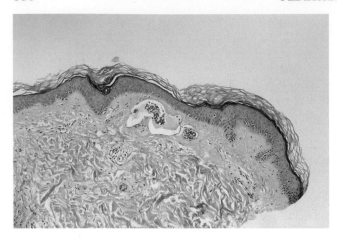

Fig. 32–7. Telangiectatic vessels from a patient with ataxia-telangiectasia are seen within the superficial vascular plexus.

the granulomatous lesions found in the skin of patients with AT.

Pathogenesis. Fibroblasts from patients with AT are far more radiosensitive than normal controls, necessitating far more DNA repair after exposure to irradiation [68]. This chromosomal fragility may play a role in the predisposition that these patients have to develop malignant neoplasms [69]. It has been postulated that the noninfectious granulomas present in the skin of some patients with AT may represent an attempt to localize antigens in the setting of a dysfunctional immune system [63].

Progeria

Epidemiology. There are many progeroid syndromes. The best described one is also known as the Hutchinson-Gilford progeria syndrome. It is a very rare, autosomally inherited condition characterized by premature aging. Both dominant and recessive transmissions have been proposed, and as has sporadic mutation [70, 71]. Most affected patients die by the age of 10–15 years, largely due to cardiovascular disease.

Cutaneous Features. Cutaneous changes occur early in life in patients with progeria. The earliest include irregular pigmentary changes at any location. Occipital alopecia occurs within the first 3–4 years of life. Scleroderma-like atrophy is present later in the disease [72]. Other patients are reported to have loose skin with wrinkling [73].

Other changes include the absence of ear lobes, coarse hairs, delayed and abnormal tooth development, and dystrophic nails [74]. Scar-like plaques are present in patients with progeria [75, 76].

Associated Disorders. Patients with progeria are of normal intelligence and have normal emotional development. Patients with progeria have attenuation of the terminal phalanges, resorption of the distal ends of their clavicles, and diffuse osteopenia [74]. There may be stiffness in the joints.

The cardiovascular system is also affected in patients with progeria [70]. Atherosclerosis of large arteries is common. Cardiac hypertrophy is also present [72].

Histologic Features. The histologic features of the scar-like lesions in progeria include an atrophic epidermis, often with basal cell degeneration. The dermis is thickened, with markedly increased amounts of reticular dermal collagen [75]. Elastotic degeneration of the skin has also been reported [77].

Special Studies. Patients with progeria have increased urinary excretion of hyaluronic acid [70]. There are no special skin biopsy studies necessary to help with the diagnosis.

Pathogenesis. It is believed that abnormalities in the metabolism of hyaluronic acid may be the underlying pathogenesis of progeria [70]. This leads to an increased accumulation of collagen [76].

Albinism

Epidemiology. Oculocutaneous albinism (OCA) and primary ocular albinism are a complex series of genetic anomalies associated with a range of diseases. They are characterized by hypopigmentation or depigmentation of the skin, eyes, and hair. Tyrosinase-negative OCA is classified as type IA. Type II OCA is tyrosinase positive. Oculocutaneous albinism has an incidence of 1 in 17,000 within the United States, and more than 1% of the population is heterozygous for the gene that causes albinism [78]. Most cases are inherited in an autosomal recessive manner [79]. Primary ocular albinism is an X-linked trait [80]. At least six genetic mutations have been described in patients with different subtypes of albinism [81]. Albinism is a part of several syndromes, including Hermansky-Pudlak syndrome, Chediak-Higashi syndrome [82], and Griscelli-Prunieras syndrome [79].

Cutaneous Features. Patients with albinism have a partial or total lack of melanin pigment throughout their skin, depending on the type of albinism. In all cases, melanocytes are present within the epidermis, essentially in normal numbers, but fail to produce normal amounts of melanin.

In one study, 82% of patients with type I OCA demonstrated pigmented lesions [83]. Dendritic hyperpigmented macules are present in 43% of these patients and occur on sun-exposed skin [83]. Melanocytic nevi, including dysplastic nevi, have been described in patients with albinism [84, 85].

Associated Disorders. The most common extracutaneous manifestations of albinism are defects in visual acuity, which range from 20/40 to 20/400. Foveal hypoplasia and defects in the optic nerves are also common findings in patients with albinism [86]. Photophobia, nystagmus, and strabismus are frequent findings.

The incidences of squamous cell carcinoma, basal cell carcinoma, and actinic keratosis are markedly increased in patients with albinism [87]. Interestingly, although rare cases of malignant melanoma are reported in these patients, the incidence does not appear to be markedly elevated [87, 88]. In an African population, 23.4% of albinos developed skin cancer, most commonly of the squamous cell type [89]. This is a common cause of death in these patients.

Oculocutaneous albinism is part of the Hermansky-Pudlak syndrome, in conjunction with platelet dysfunction and ceroid deposition [82]. Progressive pulmonary fibrosis, leading to restrictive lung disease, occurs in these patients [90]. Patients also have decreased levels of von Willebrand's factor [91]. Ceroid pigment accumulates in monocytes and lymphocytes, possibly due to lysosomal dysfunction [92].

Histologic Features. The histologic changes in albinism are restricted largely to the melanocytes. They have been shown to have short dendritic processes and markedly decreased numbers of melanosomes [91]. Melanosomes are limited mainly to stage I or II in the skin and retinal pigment epithelium [91, 93]. Stage I melanosomes contain no melanin, and stage II melanosomes contain only minimal melanin.

Histologic findings in the ephilides present in patients with albinism include flattened rete ridges. There is no increase in the number of melanocytes, but there is a focal increase in melanin pigment within basal keratinocytes [83].

Melanocytic nevi have been described in patients with albinism and are histologically quite similar to melanocytic nevi occurring in patients without the disease. In one study, an increased number of giant melanocytes was found in nevi from patients with albinism [84]. Features of congenital nevus were found in 8.8% of nevi in the same series. Despite the fact that the nevi were for the most part on sun-protected skin, there was marked solar elastosis present in the surrounding dermis.

Special Studies. Special studies are not necessary on histologic sections to make a diagnosis of albinism.

Dopa stains for melanin can be helpful in demonstrating the absence of melanin production, but are rarely necessary. S100 stains demonstrate normal distribution and number of melanocytes. Ultrastructural examination demonstrates melanocytes with short dendritic processes and decreased numbers of fully developed melanosomes.

Pathogenesis. Type I OCA is caused by a deficiency in the catalytic activity of tyrosinase, important in a least three steps within the melanin biosynthetic pathway. Type II OCA is due to abnormalities in polypeptide P that may be involved in the transport of tyrosine within melanosomes [94].

McCune-Albright Syndrome

Epidemiology. McCune-Albright syndrome (MAS) is a rare, autosomal dominant disorder. Large, irregularly shaped café-au-lait macules, precocious puberty, and fibrous dysplasia characterize the syndrome. It has been suggested that the survival of a lethal gene in a mosaic condition is responsible for MAS [95].

Cutaneous Features. The most common cutaneous manifestation of MAS is the presence of multiple café-au-lait macules. In some patients, these hyperpigmented macules appear to follow Blaschko's lines [95]. They have been described as being quite large, with irregular outlines resembling the "coast of Maine" in some patients.

Another frequent finding is that of cutaneous osteomas, which appear as cutaneous nodules that can be present in any part of the body [96]. Less common cutaneous anomalies reported in these patients include patchy or diffuse alopecia [97, 98], pili torti, dermal cysts, preauricular appendix (accessory tragus), and verrucous epidermal nevi [97, 99, 100].

Associated Disorders. McKune-Albright syndrome displays protean manifestations involving many organ systems. Some patients are very short, with marked obesity and stocky extremities, and have cataracts, hearing deficits, and dental anomalies [101].

Multiple endocrinopathies have been reported in patients with MAS. Sexual precocity is the most commonly encountered anomaly. Other patients demonstrate multinodular goiters, hyperthyroidism, hyperparathyroidism, hypophosphatemic hyperphosphaturic rickets, Cushing's syndrome, pituitary adenomas, and acromegaly [102–104]. Polyostotic fibrous dysplasia of bone has been described in these patients [102]. Facial fibrous dysplasia can result in visual loss [105].

Histologic Features. The histologic changes seen in café-au-lait macules are indistinguishable from those described in association with neurofibromatosis (see Chapter 9). The histologic features of the diffuse alopecia include fibrous overgrowth replacing follicular epithelium [98].

Special Studies. Special studies are not necessary to make a diagnosis of MAS.

Pathogenesis. McKune-Albright syndrome is caused by the postzygotic mutation in gene encoding alpha S (GNAS1), which causes enhanced function of the G alpha S protein [106].

Waardenburg's Syndrome

Epidemiology. Waardenburg's syndrome (WS) is inherited in an autosomal dominant manner. Four subtypes of the syndrome have been described. Estimates of the overall incidence range from 1:20,000 to 1:40,000 [107]. Waardenburg's syndrome type I is characterized by sensoneurial hearing loss, pigment abnormalities in the hair, skin, and eyes, and dystopia canthorum. A mutation in the PAX3 gene, located on chromosome 2q, has been identified as the cause of these anomalies [108, 109]. Waardenburg's syndrome type III has a similar genetic defect and differs from type I WS by the presence of upper extremity anomalies [110]. Waardenburg's syndrome type II is caused by a mutation in the microphthalmia-associated transcription factor (MITF) [111]. Waardenburg's syndrome type IV is associated with Hirschprung's disease and is caused by mutations in the genes for endothelin-3 or its receptors [110].

Cutaneous Features. Depigmentation of the skin is seen in 17%–58% of patients with WS, with a white forelock being the most common presentation [107]. Spontaneous repigmentation of leukodermic patches has been reported in rare patients with the syndrome [107].

Associated Disorders. Congenital deafness occurs in 9%–38% of patients with WS type I [107]. Hearing loss occurs in up to 77% of patients with type II WS [109]. Heterochromic or hypochromic irides are present in about 20% of patients with type I disease and in 47% of patients with WS type II [109]. Type I WS is characterized by dystopia canthorum, but this finding is not seen in type II WS. Congenital cataracts may also be present [112]. Dystopia canthorum is present in virtually all patients. A broad nasal root is seen in 78% of affected patients [107]. Other findings include hypoplastic alae, smooth philtrum, bushy eyebrows with synophrys, and premature graying of hair [113]. Multicystic dysplastic kidneys have been reported in a patient with WS [114].

Histologic Features. Melanocytes are decreased in number in the leukodermic skin, as well as in the affected irides.

Special Studies. Electron microscopic examination of leukodermic skin demonstrates a marked decrease in the number of melanocytes. Melanosome size is also markedly reduced [112]. At the edge of the hypopigmented skin, melanocytes appear decreased in number and degenerating. Normal skin demonstrates similar changes [115].

Pathogenesis. Waardenburg's syndrome is believed to be due to a defect in neural crest migration and melanin synthesis [112]. In WS type II, it is known that the defective gene transactivates the gene for tyrosinase. Failure of this gene results in faulty melanocyte differentiation [111]. The cause for the abnormal migration and function of melanocytes in types I and II WS is not understood, but it is believed that the affected PAX3 gene in some way interacts with the transcription factor responsible for the type II WS [111].

Xeroderma Pigmentosa

Epidemiology. Xeroderma pigmentosum (XP) is a rare autosomal disease caused by defects in DNA repair capabilities. The overall incidence in the United States is estimated to be approximately 1 per 1 million [116]. There is an equal male to female incidence of the disease [117, 118]. In some series consanguinity of parents is present in a high percentage of cases [118, 119]. Multiple defects in the DNA repair process have been found responsible for the syndrome known as XP. These have been classified into complementation groups A–I [118]. The incidences of the different groups vary geographically. The most common subtypes seen in the United States are A (29.4% of cases), C (27.3% of cases), variant (24.1% of cases), and D (15% of cases) [118]. The different subtypes of XP display marked differences in the severity of the clinical features, as well as cellular and genetic features [120].

There is a 90% probability of surviving to age 13 years, 80% to age 28 years, and 70% to age 40 years for patients with XP [118]. Thus, the mortality rate is greatly increased. Approximately one-third of deaths can be attributed to the development of cancer and another 11% to infectious processes [118].

Cutaneous Features. Cutaneous manifestations are among the earliest detectable changes in patients with XP. Pigmentary changes occur within months of birth and are followed rapidly by the development of cutaneous atrophy, solar-induced keratoses, and carcinomas. Freckles are present on the face of all affected patients and appear within 6–9 months of birth [119]. Less than 5% of patients will have no symptoms until after 14 years of age [118]. Other early changes include hypopigmented macules with or without atrophy, dryness of the skin, and telangiectasias. Later developments include actinic keratoses, keratoacanthomas, and pyogenic granulomas [119].

By 10 years of age, up to 79% of affected patients will develop their first cutaneous carcinoma [118, 121]. The neoplasms develop most frequently in sun-exposed areas of the skin. These are most commonly squamous cell carcinomas, but basal cell carcinomas also occur with greatly increased frequency. In other studies, the incidence of cutaneous carcinoma is somewhat lower, but is found in at least half of all patients with XP [118]. The incidence of basal cell carcinoma or squamous cell carcinoma is 4800 times greater in patients with XP than in the general U.S. population [122]. Melanomas have been reported in approximately 5% of patients with XP, about a 2000-fold increase over that of the U.S. population [118, 122]. Melanomas occurring on patients with XP have more of a sun-exposed distribution than that seen in the population at large. All of the types of malignant tumors appearing on the skin of patients with XP are known to metastasize. Oral changes include the development of actinic cheilitis, squamous cell carcinoma and basal cell carcinoma of the lips, erosions and gingivostomatitis, and squamous cell carcinoma of the tongue [119].

Associated Disorders. Eye changes caused by sun-exposure are found in up to 95% of patients with XP [118]. These changes include photophobia in approximately 20% of cases [118], hyperpigmentation and telangiectasias of the eyelids and conjunctivae, atrophy and ectropion of eyelids, and corneal scarring [119]. Squamous and basal cell carcinomas of the eyelids are also encountered frequently.

Neurologic abnormalities have been described in a minority of patients [118]. These include low intelligence, abnormal motor activity, deterioration of neurologic status, decreased hearing, abnormal speech, and microencephaly [118]. These changes are especially prominent in the DeSanctis-Caccione variant, associated with XP, dwarfism, and immature sexual development [123].

Patients with XP rarely develop internal malignant neoplasms, including follicular carcinoma of the thyroid, astrocytoma and medulloblastoma, pancreatic and gastric adenocarcinoma, bronchogenic carcinoma, and leukemia [118, 119]. It is not known if these occur with increased frequencies in these patients.

Other associations include anemia, growth retardation, and hypothyroidism [119]. Rare patients with XP have been reported with systemic lupus erythematosus, sarcoidosis, hepatitis, and hyperlipoproteinemia [118].

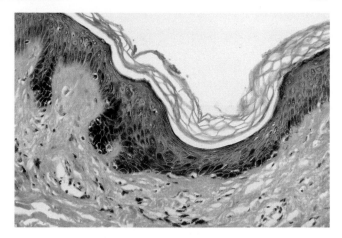

Fig. 32–8. Increased numbers of melanocytes and increased basal keratinocyte melanin are present in patients with xeroderma pigmentosum.

Histologic Features. There are no specific histologic changes associated with XP. Extensive solar elastosis is present in skin taken from sun-exposed areas, even in biopsy specimens from very young children. Other ultraviolet light-induced changes are also present, including increased numbers and altered distribution of melanocytes, irregular clumping of pigment, and epidermal atrophy (Fig. 32–8). The neoplasms associated with XP are histologically indistinguishable from similar-appearing neoplasms occurring in patients who do not have XP (Fig. 32–9).

Special Studies. DNA repair studies are helpful in making a diagnosis of XP. In vitro complementation studies are required to fully delineate the type of disease any individual with XP has [124]. There are no

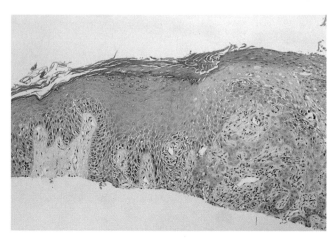

Fig. 32–9. A cutaneous squamous cell carcinoma arising within a patient with xeroderma pigmentosum has the same histologic characteristics as squamous cell carcinomas not associated with this disease.

special studies that can be performed on histologic sections to aid in the diagnosis.

Pathogenesis. Cellular hypersensitivity to ultraviolet-induced DNA damage results in the development of cutaneous neoplasms [118]. Deficiencies in various gene products involved in repair and excision of nucleotides result in increased genetic aberrations [125]. Defects may take place at the time of excision or postreplication [126]. It has also been postulated that defects in natural killer cell activity may contribute to the increased incidence of these tumors [127].

Cockayne's Syndrome

Epidemiology. Cockayne's syndrome is an autosomal recessive disorder. It is a disease caused by defects in DNA repair, but it is not associated with the development of cancer. Consanguinity is reported in the families of many affected patients [128]. The mean age of death is approximately 12 years [129]. Rare patients have milder disease and survive into adulthood [130].

Cutaneous Features. Irregular pigmentation of the skin is present in patients with Cockayne's syndrome. Intense freckling is found commonly. Extreme photosensitivity is seen in up to 85% of patients [128]. Facial erythema is a common finding in children. Telangiectasias are described in many patients with Cockayne's syndrome. Inability to perspire has been reported in patients with Cockayne's syndrome [131].

Associated Disorders. Cockayne's syndrome is characterized by motor, growth, and mental retardations, which usually become apparent during the second year of life [132]. Patients develop progeroid features in approximately 85% of cases [128]. Intracranial calcification and hypogonadism are also encountered in these patients. Dental caries are frequent. Hypertension, hepatic dysfunction, and osteoporosis are also reported in patients with Cockayne's syndrome [131].

Neurologic abnormalities are the most frequent and most severe complications in patients with Cockayne's syndrome [129]. These include sensorineural hearing loss, retinal pigment degeneration, and cataracts in almost 90% of patients [128]. Development of cataracts before the age of 3 years predicts severe disease and early death [129]. Gait disturbances are present in approximately 84% of patients [128]. Cerebral atrophy is seen in most affected patients [128].

Renal failure due to focal segmental glomerulosclerosis and adrenocortical failure have been reported in association with Cockayne's syndrome [133]. Other histologic abnormalities within the kidneys have also been reported [134]. Cockayne's syndrome has been re-

ported to occur simultaneously with xeroderma pigmentosum in rare patients [135].

Histologic Features. The histologic changes seen in the telangiectasias and pigment irregularities are not specific and resemble those seen in sporadically occurring lesions. Eccrine glands are small for age in patients with Cockayne's syndrome [132].

Special Studies. Special stains on histologic studies are not helpful in making the diagnosis of Cockayne's syndrome. Nerve conduction studies and cytogenetic tests are useful.

Pathogenesis. Extreme photosensitivity of fibroblasts has been demonstrated in patients with Cockayne's syndrome; however, these patients demonstrate near-normal levels of ultraviolet light–induced unscheduled DNA synthesis [130]. Cockayne's syndrome cells are deficient in transcription coupled DNA repair [136]. The defect appears to be limited to the repair of cyclobutane dimers [137]. There is reduced recovery of RNA synthesis [138].

Dyskeratosis Congenita

Epidemiology. Dyskeratosis congenita is a rare inherited disorder. Most cases are inherited in an X-linked manner and thus are seen in boys [139]. Several forms of autosomal dominant inheritance may, however, be seen with this disease, as well [140]. In these cases, girls can also be affected. Autosomal recessive cases have also been reported [141, 142]. Cutaneous signs are often the first manifestation of the disease and usually appear by age 10 years.

Cutaneous Features. Reticulated hyperpigmentation of the skin is the usual presenting sign and occurs by the end of the first decade of life. In most cases, these changes are limited to the neck, chest, and proximal extremities. In one patient, accentuation along Blashko's lines was reported [142]. In some cases, a poikilodermatous appearance is seen. Fingernails are routinely dystrophic. Thickened, white plaques are present on the buccal mucosa. Atrophic lingual papillae are also seen in some patients. Rarely, palmoplantar hyerkeratosis and/or scarring alopecia may be present.

Associated Disorders. Bone marrow failure is an expected complication in patients with dyskeratosis congenita. Aplastic anemia is the most commonly observed hematologic disturbance seen in these patients, occurring in greater than 90% of patients with dyskeratosis congenita [143]. Pancytopenia, as well as humoral and cellular immunologic disturbances, are reported [144].

Increased risk of infection by organisms such as *Pneumocystis carinii* is characteristic of dyskeratosis congenita.

Predisposition to malignancies has also been described in these patients. Signet ring carcinoma of the rectum in a young adult has been reported [145]. Squamous cell carcinomas of the tongue, cervix, and esophagus are also reported with increased frequencies [146–148]. Hodgkin's disease has been associated with dyskeratosis congenita [149].

Imparied cellular immunity is seen in patients with dyskeratosis congenita. This defect is the likely cause of increased susceptibility to infections and development of malignancies [150].

Less common associations include microcephaly, mental retardation, and cerebellar hypoplasia [140]. Dyskeratosis congenita has been associated with X-linked ocular albinism, juvenile-onset diabetes mellitus, and elevated levels of fetal hemoglobin [151]. Congenital meatal atresia with resultant urinary tract obstruction has also been reported in a patient with dyskeratosis congenita [147].

Gastrointestinal complications such as abdominal pain, vomiting, dysphagia, and hematochezia occur in some patients with dyskeratosis congenita [146]. Usual interstitial pneumonia may also occur in these patients [152, 153].

Histologic Features. Histologic changes in well-developed cases of dyskeratosis congenita demonstrate epidermal atrophy with diminution of the rete ridges. There is overlying hyperkeratosis. In some cases, small clefts may be seen at the dermal–epidermal junction [154]. The dermis is characterized by telangiectatic blood vessels and an infiltrate of melanin-laden macrophages.

Special Studies. Electron microscopy reveals vacuoles within basal keratinocytes and decreased keratin tonofilaments within the same cells [154].

Pathogenesis. The dyskeratosis congenita gene has been localized to Xq28 in several affected families [139]. A mutation in the gene encoding for dyskerin has been implicated in the pathogenesis of the X-linked form of the disease [155], although others dispute this observation [156]. This results in chromosomal instability due to lower levels of telomerase activity.

Proteus Syndrome

Epidemiology. Proteus syndrome is composed of a constellation of skeletal anomalies, hamartomas, and multiple mesodermal malformations, including hemihypertrophy with overgrowth of long bones and an-

giomatous proliferations [157]. The syndrome is named after the Greek god Proteus and means *polymorphous*. Most reported cases have been sporadic, although there have been isolated reports of mother–daughter and father–son transmission [158]. It is believed that the syndrome is due to the action of a dominant lethal gene that survives by mosaicism [159, 160]. A somatic mutation has been postulated [161].

Cutaneous Features. Verrucous epidermal nevi are present in most patients with Proteus syndrome. These are usually unilateral and may be extensive. "Cerebriform," or deeply rugated, masses have also been described on the palmar and plantar surfaces [157]. Linear areas of hyperpigmentation and depigmentation have been described in some patients with Proteus syndrome [162]. Focal dermal hypoplasia can also occur [163]. These areas appear atrophic, with prominence of the dermal vasculature.

Associated Disorders. Hemihypertrophy resulting in regional gigantism, macrodactyly, exocytoses, especially of the skull, and scoliosis are found in most patients with Proteus syndrome [157]. Overgrowth of the long bones is often present. Subcutaneous masses occur in more than half of these patients. These tumors have been shown to be lipomas, hamartomas, and angiomatous proliferations [157]. It has been demonstrated that most of the vascular proliferations are composed of lymphatic vessels [164, 165]. Port-wine stain vascular hamartomas and angiokeratomas have also been reported [166]. Diffuse, panlobar cystic emphysematous pulmonary disease occurs in rare cases [167].

Less commonly, ambiguous genitalia have been reported in patients with Proteus syndrome [168]. Nephrogenic diabetes insipidus has been reported [169] as has cardiomyopathy [170]. A unique pattern of muscular dysgenesis has also been described [171]. Rarely, central nervous system abnormalities, including hemimegalencephaly, subependymal calcified nodules, occipital dysmyelination, compression of the corpus callosum, and periventricular cysts may be seen, as can peripheral neuropathies [172–174]. Rare other tumors, including cystic teratoma and ovarian cystadenomas, have been reported in patients with Proteus syndrome [175, 176].

Histologic Features. The thickened, cerebriform proliferations present on the soles and palms demonstrate elongation of the cytoplasm of basal keratinocytes and marked hyperkeratosis [162]. They are not specific changes and can be seen in many hyperkeratotic conditions.

Epidermal nevi seen in Proteus syndrome are similar to those seen in other syndromes or those occurring sporadically (see Chapter 11). The linear lesions with altered pigmentation are characterized by acanthosis and hyperkeratotic orthokeratin.

The lymphangiomas seen in patients with Proteus syndrome are not histologically distinguishable from lymphangiomas occurring sporadically. Thin-walled, markedly ectatic vessels are lined by flattened endothelial cells. These vessels may be present at any layer of the dermis or subcutaneous fat. Although occasional traumatized lesions may demonstrate blood and fibrin within the vascular spaces, in most cases the spaces are empty or filled with eosinophilic, proteinaceous material.

Special Studies. Ultrastructural examination of the linear lesions reveals extensive vacuolization in the region of keratinocytes and melanocytes with large aggregates of melanosomes in the intercellular spaces. There is slight degeneration of melanocytes [177].

Pathogenesis. The pathogenesis of Proteus syndrome remains unknown.

Basal Cell Nevus Syndrome (Gorlin's Syndrome)

Epidemiology. Basal cell nevus syndrome (BCNS) is an autosomal dominant syndrome that predisposes patients to the development of basal cell carcinomas, ovarian fibromas, medulloblastomas, and other neoplasms and hamartomas [178]. The chromosomal defect has been localized to a deletion on chromosome 9q22.3–q31 [179]. The inherited condition demonstrates complete penetrance and variable expressivity [180].

Cutaneous Features. Basal cell carcinomas are present in up to 80% of white patients and 38% of black patients with BCNS [179]. The mean age of onset of the first basal cell carcinoma is approximately 23 years of age, and patients have been reported with over 1000 such lesions [179].

In addition to multiple basal cell carcinomas, BCNS is associated with epidermal cysts and palmar and plantar pits. Palmar and plantar pits are present in 87% of patients with BCNS [179].

Associated Disorders. Basal cell nevus syndrome is associated with many types of neoplasms. The following is a partial list of these neoplasms [182–186]:

- Cardiac fibroma
- Fibrosarcoma
- Leiomyosarcoma
- Meningioma
- Medulloblastoma
- Ovarian fibrothecoma
- Ovarian fibroma
- Ovarian fibrosarcoma
- Rhabdomyosarcoma
- Rhabdomyoma

Skeletal anomalies are frequent in patients with BCNS. These include cleft lip and palate [187]. Spina bifida occulta is present in up to 45% of these patients and anomalies of the ribs in approximately 50% [188]. Jaw cysts are present in approximately 75% of patients with BCNS and present before the age of 20 years in more than 80% of patients [179]. These cysts tend to recur [181]. Other skeletal deformities include macrocephaly in 50% of patients, hypertelorism in 42% of patients, frontal bossing in approximately one-fourth of patients, and a pectus deformity in 13% [179]. Exotrophia and delayed dental development are also reported [189, 190].

Calcifications in the dural folds or falx cerebri are also found in most patients with BCNS [187]. Neural hamartomas and heterotopias are also present in some patients and may give rise to symptoms such as epilepsy [190]. A bridged sella turcica is found in 68% of patients [179].

Histologic Features. Basal cell carcinomas from patients with BCNS are histologically quite similar to those occurring sporadically. Specifically, nests of basaloid cells are present in the dermis, usually growing down from the overlying epidermis. The nests are surrounded by a palisade of basaloid cells with high nuclear/cytoplasmic ratios. There are abundant mitoses, and necrosis is present in the centers of some of the larger epithelial islands. Tumor stroma is often hypercellular and myxoid and is often retracted away from the epithelial islands, leaving a cleft. A nodular or solid growth pattern is seen in approximately 80% of neoplasms arising on the head and neck and 50% of those arising from other body sites [192]. Multiple cystic structures containing keratin, similar to those seen in trichoepithelioma, are present in many of the basal cell carcinomas arising in this population [192].

Odontogenic keratin-filled cysts of the jaw display an epithelial-lined cyst comprised of two to five layers of squamous cells and is frequently ulcerated [193]. The cyst cavity is filled with orthokeratotic keratin, and there is a brisk inflammatory infiltrate [194]. Cysts from patients with BCNS tend to have more epithelial proliferation and a higher mitotic rate than those from control patients [195].

Palmar and plantar pits demonstrate trichoblastic formation with multiple proliferations of basaloid cells with peripheral palisading. Cleft formation is not present and is helpful in distinguishing these benign follicular neoplasms from basal cell carcinomas.

Special Studies. Special studies are not helpful in making a diagnosis of BCNS on histologic sections; however, karyotyping and genetic analyses may be used to make a definitive diagnosis of this syndrome.

Pathogenesis. Blue cell nevus syndrome has been shown to be related to mutations in the tumor suppressor gene PATCHED. Animal studies have demonstrated that mutations in PATCHED lead to developmental anomalies and hamartomas, as well as multiple neoplasms, some of which resemble basal cell carcinomas [196].

The frequency of basal cell carcinoma within individuals with BCNS appears to be related to exposure to ultraviolet light and skin color [197], although this relationship is not found in all studies [198]. A high rate of sister chromatid exchange has been demonstrated in response to ultraviolet and x-ray irradiation in patients with BCNS [199].

Lipoid Proteinosis
(Hyalinosis Cutis et Mucosae)

Epidemiology. Lipoid proteinosis, also known as hyalinosis cutis et mucosae and Urbach-Wiethe disease, is a rare, autosomal recessive disease.

Cutaneous Features. Patients with lipoid proteinosis develop papules and nodules that may be hyperkeratotic or verrucous, usually on the head and extremities [200]. The oral mucosal surfaces including the labia, buccal surfaces, tongue, and frenulum are thickened and nodular. Gingival hyperplasia is also present [201]. Late cutaneous lesions heal with varicella-like scars and hyperpigmentation [202]. In some patients, multiple small papules are seen along the eyelids with a "string of pearls" appearance.

Associated Disorders. Lipoid proteinosis can involve the central nervous system, lungs, lymph nodes, gastrointestinal tract, and striated muscles [200, 203]. Infantile hoarseness due to deposits of material in the larynx is the most common presentation [204]. Deposits of similar material may be found in each of these organs and lead to symptoms such as lymphadenopathy, dysphagia, muscle weakness, respiratory difficulties, and neuropsychiatric disorders. Small bowel involvement has led to acute gastrointestinal bleeding [205].

Histologic Features. Large amounts of amorphous, eosinophilic material are present within the stroma of affected tissues [206]. This material is most prevalent surrounding the eccrine apparatus and the dermal blood vessels, but can also be seen expanding the papillary dermis (Figs. 32–10 and 32–11).

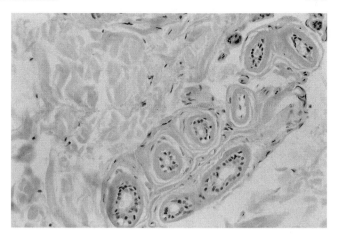

Fig. 32–10. Lipoid proteinosis is characterized by dense deposits of amorphous eosinophilic material surrounding eccrine ducts.

Special Studies. Periodic acid–Schiff stains demonstrate the amorphous material within the dermis to be strongly positive and are helpful in making the diagnosis. Ultrastructural studies demonstrate an accumulation of lipid-containing material within lysosomes of eccrine sweat glands and in dermal histiocytes [206]. Immunologic studies have demonstrated increased amounts of type IV collagen surrounding the dermal appendages and blood vessels and along the dermal–epidermal junction [207].

Pathogenesis. It has been suggested that lipoid proteinosis may be caused by two separate defects—impaired collagen production and a metabolic defect leading to the accumulation of intracellular lipids [206, 208]. The exact nature of the material has not yet been fully elucidated. Studies have demonstrated decreased

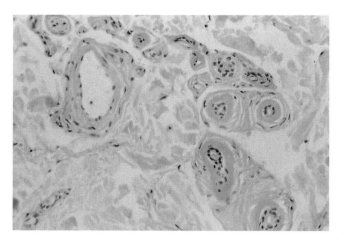

Fig. 32–11. Deposits similar to those in Figure 32–10 are present within vessel walls in a patient with lipoid proteinosis.

amounts of type I collagen and elevated levels of types III and IV collagen in the dermis of affected individuals [202, 208].

Epidermolysis Bullosa

Epidemiology. Epidermolysis bullosa is an inherited, trauma-induced blistering disorder that is traditionally divided into three categories based on the level of blister formation. The categories include epidermolysis bullosa simplex (EBS), with the most superficial blisters located in the basal layer of the epidermis; junctional epidermolysis bullosa (JEB), with blisters at the level of the hemidesmosomes; and dystrophic epidermolysis bullosa (DEB), with blisters in the superficial papillary dermis. Within each category of epidermolysis bullosa there are many well-described variants [209, 210].

Most subtypes of EBS are inherited in an autosomal dominant manner, although an autosomal recessive inheritance pattern is described for some subtypes. This is the most common variant of epidermolysis bullosa and usually presents at birth or shortly thereafter.

Junctional epidermolysis bullosa is most commonly inherited in an autosomal recessive pattern. The extent of the disease varies from mild to rapidly lethal at birth.

Dystrophic epidermolysis bullosa can be inherited in an autosomal dominant or recessive manner. Patients with recessive disease are much more severely affected and have markedly shortened life expectancies. Many of these patients now live into their fourth decades, with extensive medical support and death frequently due to infection or development of cutaneous squamous cell carcinomas. Those with dominantly inherited disease tend to have relatively mild cutaneous manifestations and normal life expectancies.

Cutaneous Features. Epidermolysis bullosa simplex manifests as trauma-induced blisters, predominantly on the hands and feet, occurring at or shortly after birth. The disease is usually minimally disabling and tends to improve with age. Milia and scarring are uncommon sequelae, as is mottled postinflammatory pigmentation. By adulthood, blisters formation is generally only a minimal concern for patients.

Patients with JEB present with generalized blister formation at the time of birth. Nails are absent or marked dystrophic. Lesions heal with scarring in many cases. In some cases, blisters are so extensive that they put the patient at greatly increased risk for complications such as infection, thermal dysregulation, and fluid retention problems.

Patients with the recessive form of DEB have a severe, generalized blistering eruption at the time of birth.

Table 32-1. Disorders Associated with Epidermolysis Bullosa
Epidermolysis bullosa simplex
Anodontia/hypodontia
Muscular dystrophy (rare)
Oral erosions
Anemia
Growth retardation
Esophageal webs (rare)
Myasthenia gravis (rare)
Keratitis
Junctional epidermolysis bullosa
Oral erosions
Esophageal and anal involvement (rare)
Laryngeal blisters
Corneal erosions
Enamel hypoplasia and "dysplatic" teeth
Pyloric atresia
Dystrophic epidermolysis bullosa
Erosions of gastrointestinal tract
Erosions of genitourinary tract
Keratitis
Cutaneous squamous cell carcinoma
Growth retardation

From reference 209.

Blisters heal with scarring and milia formation, leading to flexion contractures.

Associated Disorders. Table 32–1 lists some of the major associated disorders occurring in patients with each of the major subtypes of epidermolysis bullosa. Epidermolysis bullosa simplex is only rarely associated with other disorders. The rare autosomal dominant variant has been associated with muscular dystrophy [211]. These patients may also demonstrate decaying teeth, urethral strictures, respiratory complications, and esophageal webs [211].

Rare patients with JEB have associated pyloric atresia [212]. This group of patients often have associated genitourinary involvement that may contribute to their shortened life expectancy. Most patients with JEB, however, have disease limited almost exclusively to mucocutaneous surfaces.

Histologic Features. Routine histology has limited utility in establishing a diagnosis of epidermolysis bullosa. All subtypes are characterized by noninflammatory "subepidermal" blisters (Fig. 32–12). Despite the fact that the split occurs within the basal layer keratinocytes in EBS, there is so little of the cell present on the floor of the blister that it is usually not possible to detect this on routine sections. Scarring and milia may be observed in cases of DEB (and rarely in the other subtypes), but this is not a reliable distinguishing characteristic. Special studies are required to make a more precise diagnosis.

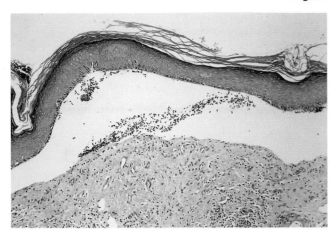

Fig. 32–12. Epidermolysis bullosa is characterized by a noninflammatory subepidermal blister.

The following entities must be considered in the histologic differential diagnosis of epidermolysis bullosa:

- Bullosis diabeticorum
- Bullous pemphigoid (cell poor)
- Friction blister
- Lichen sclerosis et atrophicus
- Porphyria cutanea tarda

Special Studies. Transmission electron microscopy remains a useful diagnostic tool for assessing the specific subtype of epidermolysis bullosa. Defects in basal keratinocytes and loss of hemidesmosomes or anchoring fibrils are helpful in making a diagnosis of EBS, JEB, or DEB, respectively. In some laboratories, however, electron microscopy has been largely superceded by immunologic techniques that enable direct observation of structural proteins within the basement membrane zone [209]. A less complicated method of immunomapping, using antibodies directed against type IV collagen (present within the lamina lucida), is also helpful in determining the level of the blister within the basement membrane zone [209].

Pathogenesis. The blister in EBS forms within the basal keratinocytes, immediately superficial to the hemidesmosomes. Defects in keratins 5 or 14 have been demonstrated in most afffected families [213]. In an autosomal recessive variant, a defect in the plectin gene has been demonstrated [211]. These patients often have coexistent muscular dystrophy.

Junctional epidermolysis bullosa is caused by a defect in hemidesmosomal proteins. This results in a split within the lamina lucida region of the basement membrane zone. In some cases, there is an absence of laminin-5 (nicein/kalinin) [214]. In others, GB3 and DEJ-1 proteins have been shown to be absent

[215]. $\alpha6\beta4$-Integrin is abnormal in some patients with JEB [216].

Dystrophic epidermolysis bullosa is caused by a defect in collagen type VII [214]. This protein makes up the anchoring fibrils located high in the papillary dermis and is essential for attachment of the dermis to the epidermis.

Congenital Nevus (Giant)

Epidemiology. Congenital melanocytic nevi are apparent in approximately 1% of newborns [217]. Congenital melanocytic nevi are generally categorized by size into small, intermediate, and large or giant. Small congenital melanocytic nevi are not associated with any systemic diseases and are not further discussed in this chapter. Similarly, the risk for malignant transformation in intermediate-sized congenital nevi is controversial and judged to be low [218]. Intermediate-sized neoplasms are also not associated with any other systemic processes and are not further addressed. Giant congenital melanocytic are much less common. The actual incidence is difficult to assess, however, with a reported range of approximately 1 in every 1160 newborns to 1 in 20,000 newborns in the United States [219, 220]. These very large nevi have been associated with increased risk for melanoma and with other, less common entities [220]. These nevi are discussed.

Cutaneous Features. Giant congenital melanocytic nevi can occur in any body site; however, most of the giant ones are present on the trunk [221]. They are often macular at birth, becoming more papular, nodular, and verrucous with age. A uniform tan or brown color is present throughout the nevus. Small foci of darker pigmentation may be present in areas with pigment incontinence. The nevus is sharply marginated. In some cases, increased numbers of densely pigmented terminal hairs may emanate from the surface of the nevus.

Associated Disorders. Malignant melanoma occurs with increased incidence in patients with giant congenital melanocytic nevi. The incidence of melanoma in these lesions ranges from 6.3% up to 15%, depending on the studies cited [222, 223]. The relative risk for developing melanoma has been assessed as high as 17-fold more than that in the normal population. When patients with giant congenital melanocytic nevi develop melanomas, the prognosis is generally quite poor [224]. Although less than 1% of melanomas occur before puberty, approximately one-third of melanomas arising in these patients do so within large congenital nevi [221]. In patients with large congenital nevi who develop melanomas, one-fourth occur within the first 2 years of life and 66% by the age of 5 years [221].

Giant congenital nevi have also been associated with other neural crest–derived neoplasms, including malignant schwannoma [225]. Rare rhabdomyosarcomas and liposarcomas have also been described within these lesions [226].

Giant congenital melanocytic nevi are associated with leptomeningeal melanosis and with subsequent neurologic abnormalities, including seizures [219]. Transplacental extension of giant congenital melanocytic nevi into the fetal side of the placenta has been reported in a small series of patients [227]. Atrophy of the lower and upper limbs has been reported in patients with giant melanocytic nevi on the extremities [228].

Histologic Features. The histologic features of giant congenital nevi are variable, depending on the age of the patient at the time of the biopsy. In younger patients, the intraepidermal proliferation of melanocytes is often quite pronounced, while in older patients only slightly increased numbers of melanocytes may be present within the epidermis (Fig. 32–13). Melanocytes are aggregated into nests in the upper portion of the dermis and disperse as single cells in the lower portions. Melanocytes are dispersed throughout the dermis. The melanocytes present in the superficial dermis often have ample cytoplasm, vesicular nuclei, and inconspicuous nucleoli. The cytoplasm diminishes with progressive descent into the dermis, the nuclei become more hyperchromatic, and nucleoli are no longer visible (Fig. 32–14). This process of "maturation" is similar to that seen in acquired melanocytic nevi.

Slight degrees of cytologic atypia may be observed in the intraepidermal and superficial dermal components of the nevus [229]. Dermal melanocytes are pres-

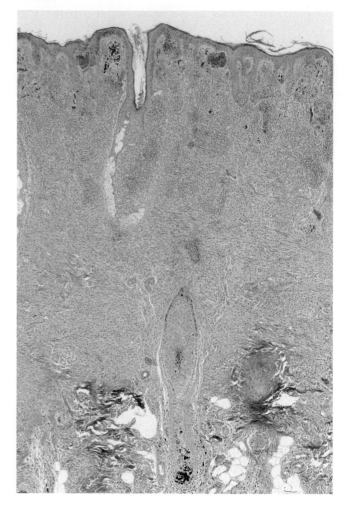

Fig. 32–14. Dermal melanocytes demonstrate maturation, with cells becoming smaller and darker with progressive descent into the dermis.

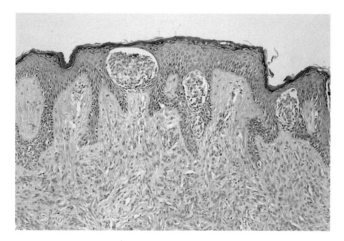

Fig. 32–13. Congenital melanocytic nevi in young patients are characterized by nests of melanocytes as well as single melanocytes along the dermal–epidermal junction.

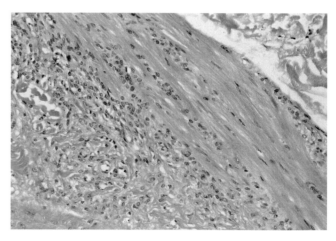

Fig. 32–15. Dermal melanocytes are present within the arrector pili muscles in some congenital melanocytic nevi.

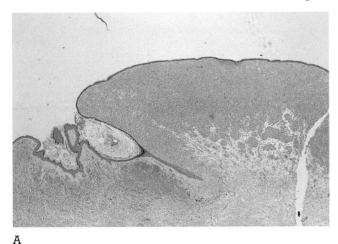
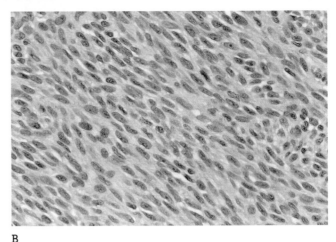

A   B

Fig. 32–16. *A,* An expansile nodule of dermal melanocytes is present within this congenital melanocytic nevus. *B,* Melanocytes within it demonstrate cytologic features distinct from melanocytes within the remainder of the melanocytic nevus.

ent within the adventitial dermis surrounding cutaneous appendages and may extend into the follicular epithelium. They are also found within arrector pili muscles in many cases (Fig. 32–15). The collection of dermal nevus cells extends into the lower half of the reticular dermis in virtually all giant congenital nevi and extends into the subcutaneous fat in 75% of these cases [229].

Melanomas can arise from the intraepidermal component of the congenital nevus, analogous to melanomas that arise from acquired melanocytic nevi. Alternatively, melanomas arising de novo from within the dermis have also been described within giant congenital nevi [219, 230]. In these cases, "expansile nodules" of clonal-appearing melanocytes are present within the dermis and appear cytologically different from the surrounding benign nevus cells (Fig. 32–16). Increased mitotic activity, lack of maturation, and nuclear atypia are present within the malignant cells. It is often difficult to distinguish these malignant clones of cells from benign "expansile clones" that have also been described in giant congenital melanocytic nevi. The benign clones can also display cytologic atypia, scattered mitoses, and occasionally necrosis. They tend to blend in with the surrounding nests of melanocytes. The cells within the benign clones are less pleomorphic and have less chromatin clumping than those seen within the malignant counterparts [231]. Especially when occurring in the neonatal population, dermal nodules within giant congenital nevi tend to be biologically benign [232]. Heterologous elements, including cartilage, have been described within giant congenital nevi [226].

Special Studies. Special studies are not helpful in making a diagnosis of a giant congenital melanocytic nevus.

Pathogenesis. The pathogenesis of giant congenital melanocytic nevi is not understood. They are believed to be hamartomatous proliferations.

References

1. Freeman, S. B., Taft, L. F., Dooley, K. J., Allran, K., Sherman, S. L., Hassold, T. J., Khoury, M. J., et al., *Population-based study of congenital heart defects in Down syndrome.* Am J Med Genet, 1998. 80:213–217.
2. Ercis, M., Balci, S., and Atakan, N., *Dermatological manifestations of 71 Down syndrome children admitted to a clinical genetics unit.* Clin Genet, 1996. 50:317–320.
3. O'Donnell, B., Kelly, P., Dervan, P., and Powell, F. C., *Generalized elastosis perforans serpiginosa in Down's syndrome.* Clin Exp Dermatol, 1992. 17:31–33.
4. Jan, V., Saugier, J., Arbeille, B., Maurage, C., Callens, A., and Lorette, G., *Elastosis perforans serpiginosa with vitamin A deficiency in a child with trisomy 21.* Ann Dermatol Venereol, 1996. 123:188–190.
5. Carter, D. M., and Jegasothy, B. V., *Alopecia areata and Down syndrome.* Arch Dermatol, 1976. 112:1397–1399.
6. Sais, G., Jucgla, A., Moreno, A., and Peyri, J., *Milia-like idiopathic calcinosis cutis and multiple connective tissue nevi in a patient with Down syndrome.* J Am Acad Dermatol, 1995. 32:129–130.
7. Delaporte, E., Gosselin, P., Catteau, B., Nuyts, J. P., Piette, F., and Bergoend, H., *Perforating milia-like id-*

iopathic calcinosis of the extremities in Down syndrome. Ann Dermatol Venereol, 1997. 124:159–161.

8. Smith, J. B., Hogan, D. J., Glass, L. F., and Fenske, N. A., *Multiple collagenomas in a patient with Down syndrome.* J Am Acad Dermatol, 1995. 33:835–837.

9. de la Torre, C., and Cruces, M. J., *Cowden's disease and Down syndrome. An exceptional association.* J Am Acad Dermatol, 1991. 25:909–911.

10. Chouvet, B., Ortonne, J. P., Perrot, H., and Thivolet, J., *Norweigian scabies: Etiological grounds.* Ann Dermatol Venereol, 1979. 106:569–574.

11. Espy, P. D., and Jolly, Jr., H. W., *Norweigian scabies: Occurrence in a patient undergoing immunosuppression.* Arch Dermatol, 1976. 112:193–196.

12. Kavanagh, G. M., Leeming, J. P., Marshman, G. M., Reynolds, N. J., and Burton, J. L., *Folliculitis in Down's syndrome.* 1993. 129:696–699.

13. Lerner, L. H., Wiss, K., Gellis, S., and Barnhill, R., *An unusual pustular eruption in an infant with Down syndrome and a congenital leukemoid reaction.* J Am Acad Dermatol, 1996. 35:330–333.

14. Zipursky, A., Brown, E., Christensen, H., Sutherland, R., and Doyle, J., *Leukemia and/or myeloproliferative syndrome in neonates with Down syndrome.* Semin Perinatol, 1997. 21:97–101.

15. Zipursky, A., Poon, A., and Doyle, J., *Leukemia in Down syndrome: A review.* Pediatr Hematol Oncol, 1992. 9:139–149.

16. Crombet, O., and Svarch, E., *Down syndrome and juvenile myelomonocytic leukemia.* Pediatr Hematol Oncol, 1999. 16:181–182.

17. Ma, S. K., Ha, S. Y., Wan, T. S., and Chan, L. C., *t(5;7)(q34;q21) in acute megakaryoblastic leukemia associated with Down syndrome.* Cancer Genet Cytogenet, 1997. 96:177.

18. Kalwinsky, D. K., Raimondi, S. C., Bunin, N. J., Fairclough, D., Pui, C. H., Relling, M. V., Ribeiro, R., et al., *Clinical and biological characteristics of acute lymphocytic leukemia in children with Down syndrome.* Am J Med Genet Suppl, 1990. 7:267–271.

19. Seghezzi, L., Dellacecchia, C., Maserati, E., Minelli, A., Carra, A., Locatelli, F., Argusti, A., et al., *Ph-positive CML in blastic phase with monosomy 7 in a Down syndrome patient. Monitoring by interphase cytogenetics and demonstration of maternal allelic loss.* Cancer Genet Cytogenet, 1997. 99:77–80.

20. Lo, A., Brown, H. G., Fivush, B. A., Neu, A. M., and Racusen, L. C., *Renal disease in Down syndrome: Autopsy study with emphasis on glomerular lesions.* Am J Kidney Dis, 1998. 31:329–335.

21. Ariel, I., Wells, T. R., Landing, B. H., and Singer, D. B., *The urinary system in Down syndrome: A study of 124 autopsy cases.* Pediatr Pathol, 1991. 11:879–888.

22. Schloo, B. L., Vawter, G. F., and Reid, L. M., *Down syndrome: Patterns of disturbed lung growth.* Hum Pathol, 1991. 22:919–923.

23. Inoue, T., Kobayashi, Y., and Kusuda, S., *Unusual hepatic fibrosis in three cases of Down syndrome.* Rinsho Byori, 1996. 44:590–594.

24. Chik, K., Li, C., Shing, M. M., Leung, T., and Yuen, P. M., *Intracranial germ cell tumors in children with and without Down syndrome.* J Pediatr Hematol Oncol, 1999. 21:149–151.

25. Satge, D., Sommelet, D., Geneix, A., Nishi, M., Malet, P., and Vekemans, M., *A tumor profile in Down syndrome.* Am J Med Genet, 1998. 78:207–216.

26. Schweber, M. S., *Alzheimer's disease and Down syndrome.* Prog Clin Biol Res, 1989. 317:247–267.

27. Heston, L. L., *Alzheimer's dementia and Down's syndrome: Genetic evidence suggesting an association.* Ann NY Acad Sci, 1982. 396:29–37.

28. Vennos, E. M., Collins, M., and James, W. D., *Rothmund-Thomson syndrome: Review of the world literature.* J Am Acad Dermatol, 1992. 27:750–762.

29. Miozzo, M., Castorina, P., Riva, P., Dalpra, L., Fuhrman Conti, A. M., Volpi, L., Hoe, T. S., et al., *Chromosomal instability in fibroblasts and mesenchymal tumors from 2 sibs with Rothmund-Thomson syndrome.* Int J Cancer, 1998. 77:504–510.

30. Moss, C., *Rothmund-Thomson syndrome: A report of two patients and a review of the literature.* Br J Dermatol, 1990. 122:821–829.

31. Snels, D. G., Bavinck, J. N., Muller, H., and Vermeer, B. J., *A female patient with the Rothmund-Thomson syndrome associated with anhidrosis and severe infections of the respiratory tract.* Dermatology, 1998. 196:260–263.

32. Blaheta, H. J., Dummer, W., Machetanz, G., and Drosner, M., *Congenital poikiloderma of the verrucous type in Thomson syndrome with associated myopathy.* Hautarzt, 1994. 45:499–503.

33. Blaustein, H. S., Stevens, A. W., Stevens, P. D., and Grossman, M. E., *Rothmund-Thomson syndrome associated with annular pancreas and duodenal stenosis: A case report.* Pediatr Dermatol, 1993. 10:159–163.

34. Rodermund, O. E., and Hausmann, D., *Verrucous type of Thomson's syndrome. A contribution to the congenital poikilodermas.* Hautarzt, 1977. 28:308–313.

35. Guler, O., Aydin, M., Ugras, S., Kisli, E., and Metin, A., *Rothmund-Thomson syndrome associated with eosphageal stenosis: Report of a case.* Surg Today, 1998. 28:839–842.

36. Aydemir, E. H., Onsun, N., Ozan, S., and Hatemi, H. H., *Rothmund-Thomson syndrome with calcinosis universalis.* Int J Dermatol, 1988. 27:591–592.

37. Febrer Bosch, M. I., Martinez Aparicio, A., Clemente Garcia, J., and Aliaga Boniche, A., *Thomson-type congenital poikiloderma with major bone dysplasias.* Ann Dermatol Venereol, 1984. 111:429–433.

38. Kerr, B., Ashcroft, G. S., Scott, D., Horan, M. A., Ferguson, M. W., and Donnai, D., *Rothmund-Thomson syndrome: Two case reports show heterogeneous cutaneous abnormalities, an association with genetically programmed aging changes, and increased chromosomal radiosensitivity.* J Med Genet, 1996. 33:928–934.

39. Baro, P. R., Bastart, F. M., Batrina, J. R., Mateo, J. M., and Vidal, M. T., *Case 529: osteosarcoma of calcaneus with Rothmund-Thompson syndrome (RTS).* Skeletal Radiol, 1989. 18:136–139.

40. Spurney, C., Gorlick, R., Meyers, P. A., Healey, J. H., and Huvos, A. G., *Multicentric osteosarcoma, Roth-*

mund-Thomson syndrome, and secondary nasopharyngeal non-Hodgkin's lymphoma: A case report and review of the literature. J Pediatr Hematol Oncol, 1998. 20:494–497.

41. Nathanson, M., Dandine, M., Gaudelus, J., Mousset, S., Lasry, D., and Perelman, R., Rothmund-Thompson syndrome with glaucoma. Endocrine study. Semin Hop, 1983. 59:3379–3384.

42. Shuttleworth, D., and Marks, R., Epidermal dysplasia and skeletal deformity in congenital poikiloderma (Rothmund-Thomson syndrome). 1987. 117:377–384.

43. el-Koury, J. M., Haddad, S. N., and Atallah, N. G., Osteosarcomatosis with Rothmund-Thomson syndrome. Br J Radiol, 1997. 70:215–218.

44. Vennos, E. M., and James, W. D., Rothmund-Thomson syndrome. Dermatol Clin, 1995. 13:143–150.

45. Shinya, A., Nishigori, C., Moriwaki, S., Takebe, H., Kubota, M., Ogino, A., and Imamura, S., A case of Rothmund-Thomson syndrome with reduced DNA repair capacity. Arch Dermatol, 1993. 129:332–336.

46. Sillevis Smitt, J. H., Gons, M. H., Oorthuys, J. W., Krieg, S. R., and Bos, J. D., The poikiloderma of Rothmund-Thomson syndrome: Changes in Langerhans cell morphology and distribution. Dermatologica, 1989. 179:187–190.

47. German, J., Bloom's syndrome. Dermatol Clin, 1995. 13:7–18.

48. Grob, M., Wyss, M., Spycher, M. A., Dommann, S., Schinzel, A., Burg, G., and Trueb, R. M., Histopathologic and ultrastructural study of lupus-like skin lesions in a patient with Bloom syndrome. J Cutan Pathol, 1998. 25:275–278.

49. Gibbons, B., Scott, D., Hungerford, J. L., Cheung, K. L., Harrison, C., Attard-Montalto, S., Evans, M., et al., Retinoblastoma in association with the chromosome breakage syndromes Fanconi's anaemia and Bloom's syndrome: Clinical and cytogenetic studies. Clin Genet, 1995. 47:311–317.

50. Werner-Favre, C., Wyss, M., Cabrol, C., Felix, F., Guenin, R., Laufer, D., and Engel, E., Cytogenetic study in a mentally retarded child with Bloom syndrome and acute lymphoblastic leukemia. Am J Med Genet, 1984. 18:215–221.

51. Passarge, E., Bloom's syndrome: The German experience. Ann Genet, 1991. 34:179–197.

52. Berger, C., Frappaz, D., Leroux, D., Blez, F., Vercherat, M., Bouffet, E., Jalbert, P., et al., Wilms tumor and Bloom syndrome. Arch Pediatr, 1996. 3:802–805.

53. Takemiya, M., Shiraishi, S., Teramoto, T., and Miki, Y., Bloom's syndrome with porokeratosis of Mibelli and multiple cancers of the skin, lung and colon. Clin Genet, 1987. 31:35–44.

54. Sahn, E. E., Jussey, 3rd, R. H., and Chrismann, L. M., A case of Bloom syndrome with conjunctival telangiectasia. Pediatr Dermatol, 1997. 14:120–124.

55. Ersoy, F., Berkel, A. I., Sanal, O., and Oktay, H., Twenty-year follow-up of 160 patients with ataxia-telangiectasia. Turk J Pediatr, 1991. 33:205–215.

56. Hansen, L. K., Wulff, K., and Seersholm, N. J., Ataxia telangiectasia. Ugeskr Laeger, 1995. 157:2134–2138.

57. Farina, L., Uggetti, C., Ottolini, A., Martelli, A., Bergamaschi, R., Sibilla, L., Zappoli, F., et al., Ataxia-telangiectasia: MR and CT findings. J Comput Assist Tomogr, 1994. 18:724–727.

58. Joshi, R. K., al Asiri, R. H., Haleem, A., Abanmi, A., and Patel, C. K., Cutaneous granuloma with ataxia telangiectasia—a case report and review of the literature. Clin Exp Dermatol, 1993. 18:458–461.

59. Gatti, R., Ataxia-telangiectasia (group A): Localization of ATA gene to chromosome 11q22–23 and pathogenetic implications. Allergol Immunopathol (Madr), 1991. 19:42–46.

60. Cohen, L. E., Tanner, D. J., Schaefer, H. G., and Levis, W. R., Common and uncommon cutaneous findings in patients with ataxia-telangiectasia. J Am Acad Dermatol, 1984. 10:431–438.

61. Korting, G. W., and Bork, K., Overall progeroid aspect of the Louis-Bar syndrome: Pigmentary and keratotic phenomena. Hautarzt, 1979. 30:273–275.

62. Drolet, B. A., Brolet, B., Zvulunov, A., Jacobsen, R., Troy, J., and Esterly, N. B., Cutaneous granulomas as a presenting sign in ataxia-telangiectasia. Dermatology, 1997. 194:273–275.

63. Paller, A. S., Massey, R. B., Curtis, M. A., Pelachyk, J. M., Dombrowski, H. C., Leickly, F. E., and Swift, M., Cutaneous granulomatous lesions in patients with ataxia-telangiectasia. J Pediatr, 1991. 119:917–922.

64. Ortonne, J. P., Claudy, A. L., and Freycon, F., Café au lait spots in ataxia-telangiectasia (A. T.). Histochemical and ultrastructural study in one case. Arch Dermatol Res, 1980. 268:91–99.

65. Gotz, A., Eckert, F., and Landthaler, M., Ataxia-telangiectasia (Louis-Bar's syndrome) associated with ulcerating necrobiosis lipoidica. J Am Acad Dermatol, 1994. 31:124–126.

66. Fleck, R. M., Myers, L. K., Wasserman, R. L., Tigelaar, R. E., and Freeman, R. G., Ataxia-telangiectasia associated with sarcoidosis. Pediatr Dermatol, 1986. 3:339–343.

67. Tsukahara, M., Masuda, M., Ohshiro, K., Kobayashi, K., Kajii, T., Ejima, Y., and Sasaki, M. S., Ataxia telangiectasia with generalized skin pigmentation and early death. Eur J Pediatr, 1986. 145:121–124.

68. Blocher, S., Sigut, D., and Hannan, M. A., Fibroblasts from ataxia telangiectasia (AT) and AT heterozygotes show an enhanced level of residual DNA double-strand breaks after low dose-rate gamma-irradiation as assayed by pulse field gel electrophoresis. Int J Radiat Biol, 1991. 60:791–802.

69. Becker, Y., Cancer in ataxia-telangiectasia patients: Analysis of factors leading to radiation—induced and spontaneous tumors. Anticancer Res, 1986. 6:1021–1032.

70. Badame, A. J., Progeria. Arch Dermatol, 1989. 125:540–544.

71. Monu, J. U., Benka-Coker, L. B., and Fatunde, Y., Hutchinson-Gilford progeria syndrome in siblings. Report of three new cases. Skeletal Radiol, 1990. 19:585–590.

72. Shozawa, T., Sageshima, M., and Okada, E., Progeria

with cardiac hypertrophy and review of 12 autopsy cases in the literature. Acta Pathol Jpn, 1984. 34:797–811.

73. Clark, M. A., and Weiss, A. S., *Elevated levels of glycoprotein gp200 in progeria fibroblasts.* Mol Cell Biochem, 1993. 120:51–60.

74. Gillar, P. J., Kaye, C. I., and McCourt, J. W., *Progressive early dermatologic changes in Hutchinson-Gilford progeria syndrome.* Pediatr Dermatol, 1991. 8:199–206.

75. Wollina, U., Reuter, A., Schaarschmidt, H., Muller, E., Maak, B., and Schmidt, U., *Hutchinson-Gilford syndrome.* Hautarzt, 1992. 43:453–457.

76. Jimbow, K., Kobayashi, H., Ishii, M., Oyanagi, A., and Ooshima, A., *Scar and keloid-like lesions in progeria. An electron-microscopic and immunohistochemical study.* Arch Dermatol, 1988. 124:1261–1266.

77. Ishii, T., *Progeria: Autopsy report of one case, with a review of pathologic findings reported in the literature.* J Am Geriatri Soc, 1976. 24:193–202.

78. King, R. A., and Summers, C. G., *Albinism.* Dermatol Clin, 1988. 6:217–228.

79. Lacour, J. P., and Ortonne, J. P., *Oculocutaneous albinism.* Ann Pediatr (Paris), 1992. 39:409–418.

80. Hoeft, W. W., *Albinism—a clinician's low vision perspective.* J Am Optom Assoc, 1991. 62:69–72.

81. Oetting, W. S., and King, R. A., *Molecular basis of albinism: Mutations and polymorphisms of pigmentation genes associated with albinism.* Hum Mutat, 1999. 13:99–115.

82. Toro, J., Turner, M., and Gahl, W. A., *Dermatologic manifestations of Heermansky-Pudlak syndrome in patients with and without a 16–base pair duplication in the HPS1 gene.* Arch Dermatol, 1999. 135:774–780.

83. Bothwell, J. E., *Pigmented skin lesions in tyrosinase-positive oculocutaneous albinos: A study in black South Africans.* Int J Dermatol, 1997. 36:831–836.

84. Perez, M. I., and Sanchez, J. L., *Histopathologic evaluation of melanocytic nevi oculocutaneous albinism.* Am J Dermatopathol, 1985. 7(suppl):23–28.

85. Pehamberger, H., Honigsmann, H., and Wolff, K., *Dysplastic nevus syndrome with multiple primary amelanotic melanomas in oculocutaneous albinism.* J Am Acad Dermatol, 1984. 11:731–735.

86. Oetting, W. S., Summers, C. G., and King, R. A., *Albinism and the associated ocular defects.* Metab Pediatr Syst Ophthalmol, 1994. 17:5–9.

87. Ihn, H., Nakamura, K., Abe, M., Furue, M., Takehara, K., Nakagawa, H., and Ishibashi, Y., *Amelanotic metastatic melanoma in a patient with oculocutaneous albinism.* J Am Acad Dermatol, 1993. 28:895–900.

88. Levine, E. A., Ronan, S. G., Shirali, S. S., and Das gupta, T. K., *Malignant melanoma in a child with oculocutaneous albinism.* J Surg Oncol, 1992. 51:138–142.

89. Kromberg, J. G., Castle, D., Zwane, E. M., and Jenkins, T., *Albinism and skin cancer in Southern Africa.* Clin Genet, 1989. 36:43–52.

90. Parker, M. S., Rosado Shipley, W., de Christenson, M. L., Slutzker, A. D., Carroll, F. E., Worrell, J. A., and White, J. G., *The Hermansky-Pudlak syndrome.* Ann Diagn Pathol, 1997. 1:99–103.

91. Husain, S., Marsh, E., Saenz-Santamaria, M. C., and McNutt, N. S., *Hermansky-Pudlak syndrome: Report of a case with histologic, immunohistochemical and ultrastructural findings.* J Cutan Pathol, 1998. 25:380–385.

92. Sakuma, T., Monma, N., Satodate, R., Satoh, T., Takeda, R., and Kuriya, S., *Ceroid pigment deposition in circulating blood monocytes and T lymphocytes in Hermansky-Pudlak syndrome: An ultrastructural study.* Pathol Int, 1995. 45:866–870.

93. Akeo, K., Shirai, S., Okisaka, S., Shimizu, H., Miyata, H., Kikuchi, A., Nishikawa, T., et al., *Histology of fetal eyes with oculocutaneous albinism.* Arch Ophthalmol, 1996. 114:613–616.

94. Spritz, R. A., *Molecular genetics of oculocutaneous albinism.* Hum Mol Genet, 1994. 3:1469–1475.

95. Rieger, E., Kofler, R., Borkenstein, M., Schwingshandl, J., Soyer, H. P., and Kerl, H., *Melanotic macules following Blaschko's lines in McCune-Albright syndrome.* Br J Dermatol, 1994. 130:215–220.

96. Lorette, G., Valat, J. P., Gatti, P., Fetissoff, F., Arbeille, B., Boistard, C., and Moraine, C., *Albright's hereditary osteodystrophy with multiple cutaneous osteomas.* Ann Dermatol Venereol, 1984. 111:1073–1079.

97. Pierini, A. M., Ortonne, J. P., and Floret, D., *Cutaneous manifestations of McCune-Albright syndrome: Report of a case.* Ann Dermatol Venereol, 1981. 108:969–976.

98. Schwartz, R. A., Spicer, M. S., Leevy, C. B., Ticker, J. B., and Lambert, W. C., *Cutaneous fibrous dysplasia: An incomplete form of the McCune-Albright syndrome.* Dermatology, 1996. 192:258–261.

99. Yu, A. C., Ng, V., Dicks-Mireaux, C., and Grant, D. B., *Epidermal naevus syndrome associated with polyostotic fibrous dysplasia and central precocious puberty.* Eur J Pediatr, 1995. 154:102–104.

100. Rustin, M. H., Bunker, C. B., Gilkes, J. J., Robinson, T. W., and Dowd, P. M., *Polyostotic fibrous dysplasia associated with extensive linear epidermal nevi.* Clin Exp Dermatol, 1989. 14:371–375.

101. Canillot, S., Chouvet, B., Besancon, C., and Perrot, H., *Cutaneous osteoma and Albright's hereditary osteodystrophy.* Ann Dermatol Venereol, 1994. 121:408–413.

102. Mauras, N., and Blizzard, R. M., *The McCune-Albright syndrome.* Acta Endocrinol Supple (Copenh), 1986. 279:207–217.

103. Abs, R., Beckers, A., Van de Vyver, F. L., De Schepper, A., Stevenaert, A., and Hennen, G., *Acromegaly, multinodular goiter and silent polyostotic fibrous dysplasia. A variant of the McCune-Albright syndrome.* J Endocrinol Invest, 1990. 13:671–675.

104. Brogan, P., Khadilkar, V. V., and Stanhope, R., *Occult T3 toxicosis in McCune-Albright syndrome.* Horm Res, 1998. 50:105–106.

105. Bocca, G., de Vries, J., Cruysberg, J. R., Boers, G. H., and Monnens, L. A., *Optic neuropathy in McCune-Albright syndrome: An indication for aggressive treatment.* Acta Pediatr, 1998. 87:599–600.

106. Ringel, M. D., Schwindinger, W. F., and Levine, M. A., *Clinical implications of genetic defects in G proteins. The molecular basis of McCune-Albright syndrome and*

Albright hereditary osteodystrophy. Medicine (Baltimore), 1996. 75:171–184.

107. Chang, T., Hashimoto, K., and Bawle, E. V., *Spontaneous contraction of leukodermic patches in Waardenburg syndrome.* J Dermatol, 1993. 20:707–711.

108. DeStefano, A. L., Cupples, L. A., Arnos, K. S., Asher, Jr., J. H., Baldwin, C. T., Blanton, S., Carey, M. L., et al., *Correlation between Waardenburg syndrome phenotype and genotype in a population of individuals with identified PAX3 mutations.* Hum Genet, 1998. 102: 499–506.

109. Liu, X. Z., Newton, V. E., and Read, A. P., *Waardenburg syndrome type II: Phenotypic findings and diagnostic criteria.* Am J Med Genet, 1995. 55:95–100.

110. Read, A. P., and Newton, V. E., *Waardenburg syndrome.* J Med Genet, 1997. 34:656–665.

111. Watanabe, A., Takeda, K., Ploplis, B., and Tachibana, M., *Epistatic relationship between Waardenburg syndrome genes MITF and PAX3.* Nat Genet, 1998. 18:283–286.

112. Mullaney, P. B., Parsons, M. A., Westherhead, R. G., and Karcioglu, Z. A., *Clinical and morphological features of Waardenburg syndrome type II.* Eye, 1998. 12:353–357.

113. da-Silva, E. O., *Waardenburg I syndrome: A clinical and genetic study of two large Brazilian kindreds, and literature review.* Am J Med Genet, 1991. 40:65–74.

114. Jankauskiene, A., Dodat, H., Deiber, M., Rosenberg, D., and Cochat, P., *Multicystic dysplastic kidney associated with Waardenburg syndrome type I.* Pediatr Nephrol, 1997. 11:744–745.

115. Perrot, H., Ortonne, J. P., and Thivolet, J., *Ultrastructural study of leukodermic skin in Waardenburg-Klein syndrome.* Acta Derm Venereol, 1977. 57:195–200.

116. Kraemer, K. H., and Slor, H., *Xeroderma pigmentosum.* Clin Dermatol, 1985. 3:33–69.

117. Butterworth, T., and Ladda, R. L., *Light-Sensitive Genodermatoses: Clinical Genodermatoses*, vol. 2. 1981, Praeger, New York, pp. 1–4.

118. Kraemer, K. H., Lee, M. M., and Scotto, J., *Xeroderma pigmentosum: Cutaneous, ocular and neurologic abnormalities in 830 published cases.* Arch Dermatol, 1987. 123:241–250.

119. Khatri, M. L., Shafi, M., and Mashina, A., *Xerodermal pigmentosum. A clinical study of 24 Libyan cases.* J Am Acad Dermatol, 1992. 26:75–78.

120. Stary, A., and Sarasin, A., *Xeroderma pigmentosum.* Presse Med, 1997. 20:1992–1997.

121. Jung, E. G., *Xeroderma pigmentosum—review.* Int J Dermatol, 1986. 25:629–633.

122. Kraemer, K. H., Lee, M. M., and Scotto, J., *DNA repair protects against cutaneous and internal neoplasia: Evidence from xeroderma pigmentosum.* Carcinogenesis, 1984. 5:511–524.

123. Reed, W. B., Sugarman, G. I., and Mathis, R. A., *DeSanctis-Caccione syndrome.* Arch Dermatol, 1977. 113:1561–1563.

124. Kaufmann, W. K., *In vitro complementation of xeroderma pigmentosum.* Mutagenesis, 1988. 3:373–380.

125. Copeland, N. E., Hanke, C. W., and Michalak, J. A.,

The molecular basis of xeroderma pigmentosum. Dermatol Surg, 1997. 23:447–455.

126. Pawsey, S. A., Magnus, I. A., Ramsay, C. A., Benson, P. F., and Giannelli, F., *Clinical, genetic and DNA repair studies on a consecutive series of patients with xeroderma pigmentosum.* Q J Med, 1979. 48:179–210.

127. Norris, P. G., Limb, G. A., Hamblin, A. S., and Hawk, J. L. M., *Impairment of natural-killer-cell activity in xeroderma pigmentosum.* N Engl J Med, 1988. 319:1668–1669.

128. Ozdirim, E., Topcu, M., Ozon, A., and Cila, A., *Cockayne syndrome: Review of 25 cases.* Pediatr Neurol, 1996. 15:312–316.

129. Nance, M. A., and Berry, S. A., *Cockayne syndrome: Review of 140 cases.* Am J Med Genet, 1992. 42:68–84.

130. Miyauchi, H., Horio, T., Akaeda, T., Asada, Y., Chang, H. R., Ishizaki, K., and Ikenaga, M., *Cockayne syndrome in two adult siblings.* J Am Acad Dermatol, 1994. 30:329–335.

131. O' Brien, F. C., and Ginsberg, B., *Cockayne syndrome: A case report.* AANA J, 1994. 62:346–348.

132. Landing, B. H., Sugarman, G., and Dixon, L. G., *Eccrine sweat gland anatomy in Cockayne syndrome: A possible diagnostic aid.* Pediatr Pathol, 1983. 1:349–353.

133. Reiss, U., Hofweber, K., Herterich, R., Waldherr, R., Bohnert, E., Jung, E., and Scharer, K., *Nephrotic syndrome, hypertension, and adrenal failure in atypical Cockayne syndrome.* Pedatir Nephrol, 1996. 10:602–605.

134. Hirooka, M., Hirota, M., and Kamada, M., *Renal lesions in Cockayne syndrome.* Pediatr Nephrol, 1988. 2:239–243.

135. Scott, R. J., Itin, P., Kleijer, W. J., Kolb, K., Arlett, C., and Muller, H., *Xeroderma pigmentosum-Cockayne syndrome complex in two patients: Absence of skin tumors despite severe deficiency of DNA excision repair.* J Am Acad Dermatol, 1993. 29:883–889.

136. Bohr, V. A., Dianov, G., Balajee, A., May, A., and Orren, D. K., *DNA repair and transcription in human premature aging disorders.* J Invest Dermatol Symp Proc, 1998. 3:11–13.

137. Kraemer, K. H., Levy, D. D., Parris, C. N., Gozukara, E. M., Moriwaki, S., Adelberg, S., and Seidman, M. M., *Xeroderma pigmentosum and related disorders: Examining the linkage between defective DNA repair and cancer.* J Invest Dermatol, 1994. 103(Suppl 5):96S–101S.

138. Miyauchi-Hashimoto, H., Akaeda, T., Maihara, T., Ikenaga, M., and Horio, T., *Cockayne syndrome without typical clinical manifestations including neurologic abnormalities.* J Am Acad Dermatol, 1998. 39:565–570.

139. Arngrimsson, R., Dokal, I., Luzzatto, L., and Connor, J. M., *Dyskeratosis congenita: Three additional families show linkage ot a locus in Xq28.* J Med Genet, 1993. 30:618–619.

140. Pai, G. S., Morgan, S., and Whetsell, C., *Etiology heterogeneity in dyskeratosis congenita.* Am J Med Genet, 1989. 32:63–66.

141. Elliott, A. M., Graham, G. E., Bernstein, M., Mazer,

B., and Teebi, A. S., *Dyskeratosis congenita: An auto-somal recessive variant*. Am J Med Genet, 1999. 83: 178–182.

142. Baselga, E., Drolet, B. A., van Tuinen, P., Esterly, N. B., and Happle, R., *Dyskeratosis congenita with linear areas of severe cutaneous involvement*. Am J Med Genet, 1998. 75:492–496.

143. Knight, S. W., Heiss, N. S., Vulliamy, T. J., Aalfs, C. M., McMahon, C., Richmond, P., Jones, A., et al., *Unexplained aplastic anaemia, immunodeficiency, and cerebellar hypoplasia (Hoyeraal-Hreidarsson syndrome) due to mutations in the dyskeratosis congenita gene, DKC1*. Br J Haematol, 1999. 107:335–339.

144. Solder, B., Weiss, M., Jager, A., and Belohradsky, B. H., *Dyskeratosis congenita: Multisystemic disorder with special consideration of immunologic aspects. A review of the literature*. Clin Pediatr (Phila), 1998. 37:521–530.

145. Kawaguchi, K., Sakamaki, H., Onozawa, Y., and Koike, M., *Dyskeratosis congenita (Zinsser-Cole-Engman syndrome). An autopsy case presenting with rectal carcinoma, non-cirrhotic portal hypertension and Pneumocystis carinii pneumonia*. Virchows Arch A Pathol Anat Histopathol, 1990. 417:247–253.

146. Anil, S., Beena, V. T., Raji, M. A., Remani, P., Ankathil, R., and Vijayakumar, T., *Oral squamous cell carcinoma in a case of dyskeratosis congenita*. Ann Dent, 1994. 53:15–18.

147. Olsen, T. G., Peck, G. L., and Lovegrove, R. H., *Acute urinary tract obstruction in dyskeratosis congenita*. J Am Acad Dermatol, 1981. 4:556–560.

148. Hyodo, M., Sadamoto, A., Hinohira, Y., and Yumoto, E., *Tongue cancer as a complication of dyskeratosis congenita in a woman*. Am J Otolaryngol, 1999. 20: 405–407.

149. Baykal, C., Buyukbabani, N., and Kavak, A., *Dyskeratosis congenita associated with Hodgkin's disease*. Eur J Dermatol, 1998. 8:385–287.

150. Lee, B. W., Yap, H. K., Quah, T. C., Chong, A., and Seah, C. C., *T cell immunodeficiency in dyskeratosis congenita*. Arch Dis Child, 1992. 67:524–526.

151. Reichel, M., Grix, A. C., and Isseroff, R. R., *Dyskeratosis congenita associated with elevated fetal hemoglobin, X-linked ocular albinism, and juvenile-onset diabetes mellitus*. Pediatr Dermatol, 1992. 9:103–106.

152. Imokawa, S., Sato, A., Toyoshima, M., Yoshitomi, A., Tamura, R., Suda, T., Suganuma, H., et al., *Dyskeratosis congenita showing usual interstitial pneumonia*. Intern Med, 1994. 33:226–230.

153. Vanbiervliet, P., Blockmans, D., and Bobbaers, H., *Dyskeratosis congenita and associated interstitial lung disease: A case report*. Acta Clin Belg, 1998. 53:198–202.

154. Kagoura, M., and Morohashi, M., *Dyskeratosis congenita: A light microscopic and ultrastructural study*. Eur J Dermatol, 1998. 8:307–309.

155. Mitchell, J. R., Wood, E., and Collins, K., *A telomerase component is defective in the human disease dyskeratosis congenita*. Nature, 1999. 402:551–555.

156. Heiss, N. S., Girod, A., Salowsky, R., Wiemann, S., Pep-perkok, R., and Poutska, A., *Dyskerin localizes to the nucleolus and its mislocalization is unlikely to play a role in the pathogenesis of dyskeratosis congenita*. Hum Mol Genet, 1999. 8:2515–2524.

157. Samlaska, C. P., Levin, S. W., James, W. D., Benson, P. M., Walker, J. C., and Perlik, P. C., *Proteus syndrome*. Arch Dermatol, 1989. 125:1109–1114.

158. Goodship, J., Redfearn, A., Milligan, D., Gardner-Medwin, D., and Burn, J., *Transmission of Proteus syndrome from father to son?* J Med Genet, 1991. 28: 781–785.

159. Lacombe, D., Taieb, A., Vergnes, P., Sarlangue, J., Chateil, J. F., Bucco, P., Nelson, J. R., et al., *Proteus syndrome in 7 patients: Clinical and genetic considerations*. Genet Couns, 1991. 2:93–101.

160. Happle, R., *How many epidermal nevus syndromes exist? A clinicogenetic classification*. J Am Acad Dermatol, 1991. 25:550–556.

161. Schwartz, C. E., Brown, A. M., Der Kaloustian, V. M., McGill, J. J., and Saul, R. A., *DNA fingerprinting: The utilization of minisatellite probes to detect a somatic mutation in the Proteus syndrome*. EXS, 1991. 58:95–105.

162. Viljoen, D. L., Saxe, N., and Temple-Camp, C., *Cutaneous manifestations of the Proteus syndrome*. Pediatr Dermatol, 1988. 5:14–21.

163. Happle, R., Steijlen, P. M., Theile, U., Karitzky, D., Tinschert, S., Albrecht-Nebe, H., and Kuster, W., *Patchy dermal hypoplasia as a characteristic feature of Proteus syndrome*. Arch Dermatol, 1997. 133:77–80.

164. Vaughn, R. Y., Selinger, A. D., Howell, C. G., Parrish, R. A., and Edgerton, M. T., *Proteus syndrome: Diagnosis and surgical management*. J Pediatr Surg, 1993. 28:5–10.

165. Vaughn, R. Y., Lesher, Jr., J. L., Chandler, F. W., O'Quinn, J. L., Hobbs, J. L., Howell, C. G., and Edgerton, M. T., *Histogenesis of vascular tumors in the Proteus syndrome*. South Med J, 1994. 87:228–232.

166. Plotz, S. G., Abeck, D., Plotz, W., and Ring, J., *Proteus syndrome with widespread portwine stain nevus*. Br J Dermatol, 1998. 139:1060–1063.

167. Newman, B., Urbach, A. H., Orenstein, D., and Dickman, P. S., *Proteus syndrome: Emphasis on the pulmonary manifestations*. Pediatr Radiol, 1994. 24:189–193.

168. Frydman, M., Kauschansky, A., and Vrsano, I., *Ambiguous genitalia in the Proteus syndrome*. Am J Med Genet, 1990. 36:511–512.

169. Hotamisligil, G. S., and Ertogan, F., *The Proteus syndrome: Association with nephrogenic diabetes insipidus*. Clin Genet, 1990. 38:139–144.

170. Shaw, C., Bourke, J., and Dixon, J., *Proteus syndrome with cardiomyopathy and a myocardial mass*. Am J Med Genet, 1993. 46:145–148.

171. Sarnat, H. B., Diadori, P., and Trevenen, C. L., *Myopathy of the Proteus syndrome: Hypothesis of muscular dysgenesis*. Neuromusc Disord, 1993. 3:293–301.

172. Dietrich, R. B., Glidden, D. E., Roth, G. M., Martin, R. A., and Demo, D. S., *The Proteus syndrome: CNS manifestations*. AJNR Am J Neuroradiol, 1998. 19: 987–990.

173. Choi, M. L., Wey, P. D., and Borah, G. L., *Pediatric peripheral neuropathy in Proteus syndrome*. Ann Plast Surg, 1998. 40:528–532.

174. del Rosario Barona-Mazuera, M., Hidalgo-Galvan, L. R., de la Luz Orozco-Covarrubias, M., Duran-McKinster, C., Tamayo-Sanchez, L., and Ruiz-Maldanado, R., *Proteus syndrome: New findings in seven patients*. Pediatr Dermatol, 1997. 14:1–5.

175. Zachariou, Z., Krug, M., Benz, G., and Daum, R., *Proteus syndrome associated with a sacrococcygeal teratoma: A rare combination*. Eur J Pediatr Surg, 1996. 6:259–251.

176. Gordon, P. L., Wilroy, R. S., Lasater, O. E., and Cohen, Jr., M. M., *Neoplasms in Proteus syndrome*. Am J Med Genet, 1995. 22:74–78.

177. Nazzaro, V., Cambiaghi, S., Montagnani, A., Brusasco, A., Cerri, A., and Caputo, R., *Proteus syndrome. Ultrastructural study of linear verrucous and depigmented nevi*. J Am Acad Dermatol, 1991. 25:377–383.

178. Bale, A. E., Gailani, M. R., and Leffell, D. J., *Nevoid basal cell carcinoma syndrome*. J Invest Dermatol, 1994. 103(5 Suppl):126S–130S.

179. Kimonis, V. E., Goldstein, A. M., Pastakia, B., Yang, M. L., Kase, R., DiGiovanna, J. J., Bale, A. E., et al., *Clinical manifestations in 105 persons with nevoid basal cell carcinoma syndrome*. Am J Med Genet, 1997. 69:299–308.

180. Lo Muzio, L., Nocini, P. F., Savoia, A., Consolo, U., Procaccini, M., Zelante, L., Pannone, G., et al., *Nevoid basal cell carcinoma syndrome. Clinical findings in 37 Italian affected individuals*. Clin Genet, 1999. 55:34–40.

181. Gorlin, R. J., *Nevoid basal-cell carcinoma syndrome*. Medicine (Baltimore), 1987. 66:98–113.

182. Fox, R., Eckford, S., Hirschowitz, L., Browning, J., and Lindop, G., *Refractory gestational hypertension due to a renin-secreting ovarian fibrothecoma associated with Gorlin's syndrome*. Br J Ostet Gynaecol, 1994. 101:1015–1017.

183. Hardisson, D., Jiminez-Heffernan, J. A., Nistal, M., Picazo, M. L., Tovar, J. A., and Contreras, F., *Neural variant of fetal rhabdomyoma and naevoid basal cell caricnoma syndrome*. Histopathology, 1996. 29:247–252.

184. Garcia-Prats, M. D., Lopez-Carreira, M., Mayordomo, J. I., Ballestin, C., Rivera, F., Daz-Puente, M. T., Munoz, M., et al., *Leiomyosarcoma of the soft tissues in a patient with nevoid basal-cell carcinoma syndrome*. Tumori, 1994. 80:401–404.

185. Coffin, C. M., *Congenital cardiac fibroma associated with Gorlin syndrome*. Pediatr Pathol, 1992. 12:255–262.

186. Johnson, A. D., Hebert, A. A., and Esterly, N. B., *Nevoid basal cell carcinoma syndrome: Bilateral ovarian fibromas in a 3 ¹/₂ year-old girl*. J Am Acad Dermatol, 1986. 14:371–374.

187. Gorlin, R. J., *Nevoid basal cell carcinoma syndrome*. Dermatol Clin, 1995. 13:113–125.

188. Ratcliffe, J. F., Shanley, S., and Chenevix-Trench, G., *The prevalence of cervical and thoracic congenital skeletal abnormalities in basal cell naevus syndrome: a review of cervical and chest radiographs in 80 patients with BCNS*. Br J Radiol, 1995. 68:596–599.

189. Hall, J., Johnston, K. A., McPhillips, M. J., Barnes, S. D., and Elston, D. M., *Nevoid basal cell carcinoma syndrome in a black child*. J Am Acad Dermatol, 1998. 38:363–365.

190. Rosenblum, S. II., *Delayed dental development in a patient with Gorlin syndrome: Case report*. Pediatr Dent, 1998. 20:355–358.

191. Hogan, R. E., Tress, B., Gonzales, M. F., King, J. O., and Cook, M. J., *Epilepsy in the nevoid basal cell carcinoma syndrome (Gorlin syndrome): Report of a case due to focal neuronal heterotopia*. Neurology, 1996. 46:574–576.

192. Lindeberg, H., and Jepsen, F. L., *The nevoid basal cell carcinoma syndrome. Histopathology of the basal cell tumors*. J Cutan Pathol, 1983. 10:68–72.

193. Barr, R. J., Headley, J. L., Jensen, J. L., and Howell, J. B., *Cutaneous keratocysts of nevoid basal cell carcinoma syndrome*. J Am Acad Dermatol, 1986. 14:572–576.

194. Janse van Rensburg, L., Nortje, C. J., and Thompson, I., *Correlating imaging and histopathology of an odontogenic keratocyst in the nevoid basal cell carcinoma syndrome*. Dentomaxillofac Radiol, 1997. 26:195–199.

195. Woolgar, J. A., Rippin, J. W., and Browne, R. M., *A comparative histological study of odontogenic keratocysts in basal cell naevus syndrome and control patients*. J Oral Pathol, 1987. 16:75–80.

196. Oro, A. E., Higgins, K. M., Hu, Z., Bonifas, J. M., Epstein, Jr., E. H., and Scott, M. P., *Basal cell carcinomas in mice overexpressing sonic hedgehog*. Science, 1997. 276:817–821.

197. Shanley, S., Ratcliffe, J., Hockey, A., Haan, E., Oley, C., Ravine, D., Martin, N., et al., *Nevoid basal cell carcinoma syndrome: Review of 118 affected individuals*. Am J Med Genet, 1994. 50:282–290.

198. Goldstein, A. M., Bale, S. J., Peck, G. L., and DiGiovanna, J. J., *Sun exposure and basal cell carcinomas in the nevoid basal cell carcinoma syndrome*. J Am Acad Dermatol, 1993. 29:34–41.

199. Frentz, G., Munch-Petersen, B., Wulf, H. C., Niebuhr, E., and da Canha Bang, F., *The nevoid basal cell carcinoma syndrome: Sensitivity to ultraviolet and x-ray irradiation*. J Am Acad Dermatol, 1987. 17:637–643.

200. Rizzo, R., Ruggieri, M., Micali, G., Tine, A., Sanfilippo, S., and Pavone, L., *Lipoid proteinosis: A case report*. Pediatr Dermatol, 1997. 14:22–25.

201. Bazopoulou-Kyrkanidoe, E., Tosios, K. I., Zabelis, G., Charalampopoulou, S., and Papanicolaou, S. I., *Hyalinosis cutis et mucosae: Gingival involvement*. J Oral Pathol Med, 1998. 27:233–237.

202. Muda, A. O., Paradisi, M., Angelo, C., Mostaccioli, S., Atzori, F., Puddu, P., and Faraggiana, T., *Lipoid proteinosis: Clinical, histologic, and ultrastructural investigations*. Cutis, 1995. 56:220–224.

203. Ozbeck, S. S., Akyar, S., and Turgay, M., *Case report: Computed tomography findings in lipoid proteinosis: Report of two cases*. Br J Radiol, 1994. 67:207–209.

204. Chaudhary, S. J., and Dayal, P. K., *Hyalinosis cutis et*

mucosae. Review with a case report. Oral Surg Oral Med Oral Pathol Oral Radiol Endod, 1995. 80:168–171.

205. Caccamo, D., Jaen, A., Telenta, M., Varela, E., and Tiscornia, O., *Lipoid proteinosis of the small bowel.* Arch Pathol Lab Med, 1994. 118:572–574.

206. Navarro, C., Fachal, C., Rodriguez, C., Padro, L., and Dominguez, C., *Lipoid proteinosis. A biochemical and ultrastructural investigation of two new cases.* Br J Dermatol, 1999. 141:326–331.

207. Hausser, I., Biltz, S., Rauterberg, E., Frosch, P. J., and Anton-Lamprecht, I., *Hyalinosis cutis et mucosae (Urbach-Wiethe disease)—ultrastructural and immunologic characteristics.* Hautarzt, 1991. 42:28–33.

208. Harper, J. I., Duance, V. C., Sims, T. J., and Light, N. D., *Lipoid proteinosis: An inherited disorder of collagen metabolism?* Br J Dermatol, 1985. 113:145–151.

209. Fine, J.-D., Bauer, E. A., Briggman, R. A., Carter, D. M., Eady, R. A. J., Esterly, N. B., Holbrook, K. A., et al., *Revised clinical and laboratory criteria for subtypes of inherited epidermolysis bullosa.* J Am Acad Dermatol, 1991. 24:119–135.

210. Bergman, R., *Immunohistopathologic diagnosis of epidermolysis bullosa.* Am J Dermatopathol, 1999. 21:185–192.

211. Shimizy, H., Takizawa, Y., Pulkkinen, L., Murata, S., Kawai, M., Hachisuka, H., Udono, M., et al., *Epidermolysis bullosa simplex associated with muscular dystrophy: Phenotype–genotype correlations and review of the literature.* J Am Acad Dermatol, 1999. 41:950–956.

212. Valari, M. D., Phillips, R. J., Lake, B. D., and Harper, J. I., *Junctional epidermolysis bullosa and pyloric atresia: A distinct entity. Clinical and pathological studies in five patients.* Br J Dermatol, 1995. 133:732–736.

213. Kitajima, Y., Jokura, Y., and Yaoita, H., *Epidermolysis bullosa simplex, Dowling-Meara type. A report of two cases with different types of tonofilament clumping.* Br J Dermatol, 1993. 128:79–85.

214. Uitto, J., Pulkkinen, L., and Christiano, A. M., *Molecular basis of the sydtrophic and junctional forms of epidermolysis bullosa: Mutations in the type VII collagen and kalinin (laminin 5) genes.* J Invest Dermatol, 1994. 103:39S–46S.

215. Meneguzzi, G., Marinkvich, M. P., Aberdam, D., Burgeson, R. E., and Ortonne, J. P., *Abnormal expression of kalinin in the Herlitz's JEB epithelial basement membrane.* Exp Dermatol, 1992. 1:221–229.

216. Gil, S. G., Brown, T. A., Ryan, M. C., and Carter, W. G., *Junctional epidermolysis bullosa: Defects in expression of epiligrin/nicein/kalinin and integrin β4 that inhibit hemidesmosome formation.* J Invest Dermatol, 1994. 103(Suppl 5):31S–38S.

217. Walton, R. G., Jacobs, A. H., and Cox, A. J., *Pigmented lesions in newborn infants.* Br J Dermatol, 1976. 95:389–396.

218. Sahin, S., Levin, L., Kopf, A. W., Rao, B. K., Triola, M., Koenig, K., Huang, C., et al., *Risk of melanoma in*

medium-sized congenital melanocytic nevi: A follow-up study. J Am Acad Dermatol, 1998. 39:428–433.

219. Egan, C. L., Oliveria, S. A., Elenitsas, R., Hanson, J., and Halpern, A. C., *Cutaneous melanoma risk and phenotypic changes in large congenital nevi: A follow-up study of 46 patients.* J Am Acad Dermatol, 1998. 39:923–932.

220. Roth, M. E., and Grant-Kels, J. M., *Important melanocytic lesions in childhood and adolescence.* Pediatr Dermatol, 1991. 38:791–809.

221. Trozak, D. J., Rowland, W. D., and Hu, F., *Metastatic malignant melanoma in prepubertal children.* Pediatrics, 1975. 55:191–204.

222. Kaplan, E. W., *The risk of malignancy in large congenital nevi.* Plast Reconstr Surg, 1974. 530:421–428.

223. Rhodes, A. R., *Pigmented birthmarks and precursor melanocyte lesions of cutaneous melanoma identifiable in childhood.* Pediatr Clin North Am, 1983. 30:435–463.

224. Rhodes, A. R., Weinstock, M. A., and Fitzpatrick, T. B., *Risk factors for cutaneous melanoma. A practical method of recognizing predisposed individuals.* JAMA, 1987. 258:3146–3154.

225. Roth, M. J., Medeiros, J., Kapur, S., Wexler, L. H., Mims, S., Horowitz, M. E., and Tsokos, M., *Malignant schwannoma with melanocytic and neuroepithelial differentiation in an infant with congenital giant melanocytic nevus: A complex neurocristopathy.* Hum Pathol, 1993. 24:1371–1375.

226. Hendrickson, M. R., and Ross, J. C., *Neoplasms arising in congenital giant nevi.* Am J Surg Pathol, 1981. 5:109–135.

227. Jauniaux, E., de Meeeus, M. C., Verellen, G., Lachapelle, J. M., and Hustin, J., *Giant congenital melanocytic nevus with placental involvement: Long-term follow-up of a case and review of the literature.* Pediatr Pathol, 1993. 13:717–721.

228. Itin, P. H., and Lautenschlager, S., *Lower and upper extremity atrophy associated with a giant congenital melanocytic nevus.* Pediatr Dermatol, 1998. 15:287–289.

229. Barnhill, R. L., and Fleischli, M., *Histologic features of congenital melanocytic nevi in infants 1 year of age or younger.* J Am Acad Dermatol, 1995. 33:780–785.

230. Padilla, R. S., McConnell, T. S., Gribble, J. T., and Smoot, C., *Malignant melanoma arising in a giant congenital melanocytic nevus. A case report with cytogenetic and histopathologic analyses.* Cancer, 1988. 62:2589–2594.

231. Fleischi, M., and Barnhill, R. L., *Histologic features of congenital melanocytic nevi less than a year of age (abstract).* J Cutan Pathol, 1993. 20:541.

232. Barnhill, R. L., and Busam, K. J., *Congenital melanocytic neoplasms, congenital and childhood melanoma.* In *Pathology of Melanocytic Nevi and Malignant Melanoma.* 1995, Butterworth-Heinemann, Boston, p. 79.

INDEX

Note: Page numbers followed by "f" indicate figures; numbers followed by "t" indicate tables.